FIRST AID FOR THE®
Internal Medicine Boards

Third Edition

TAO LE, MD, MHS
Assistant Clinical Professor of Medicine and Pediatrics
Chief, Section of Allergy and Immunology
Department of Medicine
University of Louisville
Louisville, Kentucky

PETER V. CHIN-HONG, MD, MAS
Associate Professor of Medicine
Director, Transplant and Immunocompromised Host Infectious Diseases Program
University of California, San Francisco
San Francisco, California

THOMAS E. BAUDENDISTEL, MD, FACP
Program Director, Internal Medicine Residency
Kaiser Permanente, Oakland
Deputy Editor, *Journal of Hospital Medicine*

CINDY J. LAI, MD
Associate Professor of Medicine
Site Director, Medicine Clerkships
University of California, San Francisco
San Francisco, California

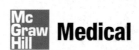 **Medical**

New York   Chicago   San Francisco   Lisbon   London   Madrid   Mexico City
Milan   New Delhi   San Juan   Seoul   Singapore   Sydney   Toronto

First Aid for the® Internal Medicine Boards, Third Edition

Copyright © 2011, 2008 by Tao Le. All rights reserved. Printed in China. Except as permitted under the United States Copyright Act of 1976, no part of this publication may be reproduced or distributed in any form or by any means, or stored in a data base or retrieval system, without the prior written permission of the publisher.

First Aid for the® is a registered trademark of The McGraw-Hill Companies, Inc.

1 2 3 4 5 6 7 8 9 0   CTP/CTP   15 14 13 12 11

ISBN 978-0-07-171301-6
MHID 0-07-171301-8
ISSN 1556-5386

NOTICE

Medicine is an ever-changing science. As new research and clinical experience broaden our knowledge, changes in treatment and drug therapy are required. The authors and the publisher of this work have checked with sources believed to be reliable in their efforts to provide information that is complete and generally in accord with the standards accepted at the time of publication. However, in view of the possibility of human error or changes in medical sciences, neither the authors nor the publisher nor any other party who has been involved in the preparation or publication of this work warrants that the information contained herein is in every respect accurate or complete, and they disclaim all responsibility for any errors or omissions or for the results obtained from use of the information contained in this work. Readers are encouraged to confirm the information contained herein with other sources. For example and in particular, readers are advised to check the product information sheet included in the package of each drug they plan to administer to be certain that the information contained in this work is accurate and that changes have not been made in the recommended dose or in the contraindications for administration. This recommendation is of particular importance in connection with new or infrequently used drugs.

This book was set in Electra LH by Rainbow Graphics.
The editors were Catherine A. Johnson and Brian Kearns.
The production supervisor was Phil Galea.
Project management was provided by Rainbow Graphics.
The designer was Alan Barnett.
China Translation & Printing Services, Ltd., was printer and binder.

McGraw-Hill books are available at special quantity discounts to use as premiums and sales promotions, or for use in corporate training programs. To contact a representative please e-mail us at bulksales@mcgraw-hill.com.

To the contributors to this and future editions, who took time to share their knowledge, insight, and humor for the benefit of residents and clinicians.

and

To our families, friends, and loved ones, who endured and assisted in the task of assembling this guide.

Contents

CHAPTER 1. Allergy and Immunology 1
Anuj Gaggar, MD, PhD
Marc Riedl, MD, MS

CHAPTER 2. Ambulatory Medicine 25
Christina A. Lee, MD
Nadine Dubowitz, MD

CHAPTER 3. Cardiovascular Disease 87
Anuj Gaggar, MD, PhD
Sanjiv Shah, MD

CHAPTER 4. Critical Care 147
Christina A. Lee, MD
Christian A. Merlo, MD, MPH

CHAPTER 5. Dermatology 157
Miten Vasa, MD
Siegrid S. Yu, MD

CHAPTER 6. Endocrinology 199
Christina A. Lee, MD
Diana M. Antoniucci, MD, MAS
Karen Earle, MD
Melissa Weinberg, MD

CHAPTER 7. Gastroenterology and Hepatology . . 245
Anuj Gaggar, MD, PhD
Ma Somsouk, MD, MAS
Scott W. Biggins, MD, MAS

CHAPTER 8. Geriatrics 311
Christina A. Lee, MD
Stephanie Rennke, MD

CHAPTER 9. Hematology 337
Miten Vasa, MD
Thomas Chen, MD, PhD

CHAPTER 10. Hospital Medicine 381
Miten Vasa, MD
Ellis A. Johnson, MD, MPH
Robert L. Trowbridge, MD

CHAPTER 11. Infectious Diseases 415
Anuj Gaggar, MD, PhD
José M. Eguía, MD, MPH

CHAPTER 12. Nephrology 477
Christina A. Lee, MD
Alan C. Pao, MD

CHAPTER 13. Neurology 507
Miten Vasa, MD
Joey English, MD, PhD
S. Andrew Josephson, MD

CHAPTER 14. Oncology 551
Miten Vasa, MD
Jonathan E. Rosenberg, MD

CHAPTER 15. Psychiatry 595
Anuj Gaggar, MD, PhD
Amin N. Azzam, MD, MA

CHAPTER 16. Pulmonary Medicine 617
Christina A. Lee, MD
Christian A. Merlo, MD, MPH

CHAPTER 17. Rheumatology 649
Miten Vasa, MD
Jonathan Graf, MD

CHAPTER 18. Women's Health 703
Christina A. Lee, MD
Linda Shiue, MD

AUTHORS

Anuj Gaggar, MD, PhD
Fellow, Division of Infectious Diseases
Department of Medicine
University of California, San Francisco

K. Pallav Kolli, MD
Imaging Editor
Resident, Department of Radiology and Biomedical Imaging
University of California, San Francisco

Christina A. Lee, MD
Chief Resident, Moffitt-Long Hospital
Department of Medicine
University of California, San Francisco

Miten Vasa, MD
Chief Resident
Department of Medicine
Kaiser Permanente, Oakland

SENIOR REVIEWERS

Diana M. Antoniucci, MD, MAS
Assistant Clinical Professor
Department of Medicine
University of California, San Francisco

Amin N. Azzam, MD, MA
Associate Professor
Department of Psychiatry
University of California, San Francisco

Scott W. Biggins, MD, MAS
Assistant Professor, Division of Gastroenterology
Department of Medicine
University of Colorado, Denver

Thomas Chen, MD, PhD
Physician
Southbay Oncology/Hematology

Nadine Dubowitz, MD
Instructor, Division of Geriatric Medicine and Gerontology
Department of Medicine
Emory University School of Medicine

Karen Earle, MD
Chief, Division of Endocrinology
California Pacific Medical Center

José M. Eguía, MD, MPH
Director of Infectious Disease
St. Mary's Medical Center, San Francisco

José M. Eguía, MD, MPH
Director of Infectious Disease
St. Mary's Medical Center, San Francisco

Jonathan Graf, MD
Assistant Professor, Division of Rheumatology
Department of Medicine
University of California, San Francisco

Ellis A. Johnson, MD, MPH
Resident, Department of Internal Medicine
Maine Medical Center

S. Andrew Josephson, MD
Assistant Professor, Department of Neurology
Director, Neurohospitalist Program
University of California, San Francisco

Christian A. Merlo, MD, MPH
Assistant Professor
Department of Medicine and Epidemiology
Johns Hopkins University

Alan C. Pao, MD
Assistant Professor, Division of Nephrology
Department of Medicine
Stanford University

Stephanie Rennke, MD
Assistant Clinical Professor, Division of Hospital Medicine
Department of Medicine
University of California, San Francisco

Marc Riedl, MD, MS
Assistant Professor, Division of Clinical Immunology and Allergy
Department of Medicine
University of California, Los Angeles

Sanjiv Shah, MD
Assistant Professor, Division of Cardiology
Department of Medicine
Northwestern University

Linda Shiue, MD
Physician, Palo Alto Medical Clinic
Assistant Clinical Professor
Department of Medicine
University of California, San Francisco

Ma Somsouk, MD, MAS
Assistant Professor
Department of Medicine
University of California, San Francisco

Robert L. Trowbridge, MD
Director, Undergraduate Medical Education
Department of Medicine
Maine Medical Center

Melissa Weinberg, MD
Assistant Clinical Professor
Department of Medicine
University of California, San Francisco

Siegrid S. Yu, MD
Assistant Professor
Department of Dermatology
University of California, San Francisco

Preface

With this revised and expanded edition of *First Aid for the Internal Medicine Boards*, we hope to provide residents and clinicians with the most useful and up-to-date preparation guide for the American Board of Internal Medicine (ABIM) certification and recertification exams. This edition represents an outstanding effort by a talented group of authors and includes the following:

- A new, full-color design for easier studying
- Updated summaries of thousands of board-testable topics
- Hundreds of revised high-yield tables, diagrams, and illustrations
- New vignette questions with answers throughout the text to help test your knowledge
- Mnemonics throughout, making learning memorable and fun

We invite you to share your thoughts and ideas to help us improve *First Aid for the Internal Medicine Boards*. See How to Contribute, p. xiii.

Tao Le
Louisville

Peter Chin-Hong
San Francisco

Tom Baudendistel
Oakland

Cindy Lai
San Francisco

Acknowledgments

This has been a collaborative project from the start. We gratefully acknowledge the thoughtful comments, corrections, and advice of the residents, international medical graduates, and faculty who have supported the authors in the development of *First Aid for the Internal Medicine Boards*.

Thanks to Joey English, MD, PhD, and Jonathan Rosenberg, MD, for their help with this edition. For support and encouragement throughout the process, we are grateful to Thao Pham, Linda Shiue, Lisa Kinoshita, Kerry Cho, Louise Petersen, and Selina Franklin.

Thanks to our publisher, McGraw-Hill, for the valuable assistance of their staff. For enthusiasm, support, and commitment to this challenging project, thanks to our editor, Catherine Johnson. For outstanding editorial support, we thank Andrea Fellows. A special thanks to Rainbow Graphics, especially David Hommel, Tina Castle, and Susan Cooper, for remarkable editorial and production work.

Tao Le
Louisville

Peter Chin-Hong
San Francisco

Tom Baudendistel
Oakland

Cindy Lai
San Francisco

Acknowledgements

How to Contribute

To continue to produce a high-yield review source for the ABIM exam, you are invited to submit any suggestions or corrections. We also offer **paid internships** in medical education and publishing ranging from three months to one year (see below for details). Please send us your suggestions for

- Study and test-taking strategies for the ABIM
- New facts, mnemonics, diagrams, and illustrations
- Low-yield topics to remove

For each entry incorporated into the next edition, you will receive a **$10 gift certificate**, as well as personal acknowledgment in the next edition. Diagrams, tables, partial entries, updates, corrections, and study hints are also appreciated, and significant contributions will be compensated at the discretion of the authors. Also let us know about material in this edition that you feel is low yield and should be deleted.

The preferred way to submit entries, suggestions, or corrections is via our blog at **www.firstaidteam.com** or e-mail at **firstaidteam@yahoo.com**. Please include your name, address, institutional affiliation, phone number, and e-mail address (if different from the address of origin).

NOTE TO CONTRIBUTORS

All entries become property of the authors and are subject to editing and reviewing. Please verify all data and spellings carefully. In the event that similar or duplicate entries are received, only the first entry received will be used. Include a reference to a standard textbook to facilitate verification of the fact. Please follow the style, punctuation, and format of this edition if possible.

INTERNSHIP OPPORTUNITIES

The author team is pleased to offer part-time and full-time paid internships in medical education and publishing to motivated physicians. Internships may range from three months (eg, a summer) up to a full year. Participants will have an opportunity to author, edit, and earn academic credit on a wide variety of projects, including the popular *First Aid* series. Writing/editing experience, familiarity with Microsoft Word, and Internet access are desired. For more information, e-mail a résumé or a short description of your experience along with a cover letter to **firstaidteam@yahoo.com**.

Introduction:
Guide to the ABIM Exam

KEY FACT

The majority of your patients will be aware of your certification status.

Introduction

For house officers, the American Board of Internal Medicine (ABIM) certification exam represents the culmination of three years of diligence and hard work. For practicing physicians, it is part of the maintenance-of-certification (MOC) process. However, the certification and recertification process represents far more than just another set of exams in a series of costly tests. To your patients, it means that you have attained the level of clinical knowledge and competency that is necessary to the provision of good clinical care. In fact, according to a poll conducted for the ABIM, about 72% of adult patients are aware of their physicians' board-certification status.

In this chapter, we will talk more about the ABIM exam and will provide you with proven approaches toward conquering that exam. For a detailed description of the ABIM exam, visit **www.abim.org**.

ABIM—The Basics

HOW DO I REGISTER TO TAKE THE EXAM?

KEY FACT

Register early to avoid an extra $400 late fee.

You can register for the ABIM exam online by going to "Physician Login" at www.abim.org and following the instructions given there. The registration fee for the exam is currently $1345. If you miss the application deadline, a $400 nonrefundable late fee is tacked on. There is also an international test-center fee of $500. Check the ABIM Web site for information on the latest registration deadlines, fees, and policies.

WHAT IF I NEED TO CANCEL THE EXAM OR CHANGE TEST CENTERS?

ABIM currently provides partial refunds if a written cancellation is received before certain deadlines. You can also change your test center by providing a written request for a specific deadline. Check the ABIM Web site for the latest information on its refund and cancellation policy as well as its procedures.

HOW IS THE ABIM EXAM STRUCTURED?

As of August 2010, the ABIM exam is a one-day computer-based test (CBT). The exam is divided into four two-hour sections with 60 questions in each section, yielding a total of 240 questions. Images (blood smears, radiographs, ECGs, patient photos) are embedded in certain questions. During the time allotted for each block, examinees can answer test questions in any order as well as review responses and change answers. However, examinees **cannot go back and change answers from previous blocks.** The CBT format allows you to make your own notes on each question using a pop-up box, and it also permits you to click a box to designate which questions you might wish to review before the end of the session (time permitting).

Please check the ABIM Web site to check for Web demos, updates, and details about the CBT format as well as to identify testing centers near you.

WHAT TYPES OF QUESTIONS ARE ASKED?

All questions on the ABIM exam are **single-best-answer** types only. You will be presented with a scenario and a question followed by 4–6 options. Virtually all questions on the exam are vignette based. A substantial amount of extraneous information may be given, or a clinical scenario may be followed by a question that you might be able to answer without actually reading the case. Some questions require interpretation of photomicrographs, radiology studies, photographs of physical findings, and the like. It is your job to determine which information is superfluous and which is pertinent to the case at hand.

Question content is based on a content "blueprint" developed by ABIM (see Table 1). This blueprint may change from year to year, so check the ABIM Web site for the latest information. About **75%** of the **primary content** focuses on traditional subspecialties such as cardiology and gastroenterology. The remaining **25%** pertains to certain outpatient or related specialties and to subspecialties such as allergy/immunology, dermatology, and psychiatry. There are also **cross-content** questions that may integrate information from multiple primary content areas.

KEY FACT

Virtually all questions are case based.

TABLE 1. ABIM Certification Blueprint

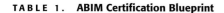

PRIMARY CONTENT AREAS	RELATIVE PROPORTIONS
Cardiovascular disease	14%
Pulmonary disease	10%
Gastroenterology	9%
Infectious disease	9%
Endocrinology/metabolism	8%
Rheumatology/orthopedics	8%
Oncology	7%
Hematology	6%
Nephrology/urology	6%
Neurology	4%
Psychiatry	4%
Allergy/immunology	3%
Dermatology	3%
Obstetrics/gynecology	2%
Ophthalmology	2%
Otolaryngology	2%
Miscellaneous	3%
Total	100%

(continues)

TABLE 1. **ABIM Certification Blueprint** *(continued)*

CROSS-CONTENT AREAS	RELATIVE PROPORTIONS
Critical care medicine	10%
Geriatric medicine	10%
Prevention	6%
Women's health	6%
Clinical epidemiology	3%
Ethics	3%
Nutrition	3%
Palliative/end-of-life care	3%
Adolescent medicine	2%
Occupational medicine	2%
Patient safety	2%
Substance abuse	2%

Source: www.abim.org, 2010.

HOW ARE THE SCORES REPORTED?

Passing scores are established before the administration of the ABIM exam, so your status will not be influenced by the relative performance of others taking the test with you. The scoring and reporting of test results may take up to **three months.** Once your score has been determined, however, your pass/fail status will become available to you on the ABIM Web site one day after your results have been mailed out. Note that you need to register in order to access this feature.

Your score report will give you a "pass/fail" decision; the overall number of questions you answered correctly with a corresponding percentile; and the number of questions you answered correctly with a corresponding percentile for the primary and cross-content subject areas noted in the blueprint. Each year, between **20 and 40 questions** on the exam do not count toward your final score. Again, these may be "experimental" questions or questions that are subsequently disqualified. Historically, between **85% and 94%** of first-time examinees pass on their first attempt (see Table 2). About 90% of examinees who are recertifying pass on their first attempt, and some 97% are ultimately successful with multiple attempts. There is no limit on the number of times you can retake the exam if you fail.

TABLE 2. Performance of First-Time Test Takers

Year	Number Taking	Percentage Passed
2009	7226	88%
2008	7194	91%
2007	7097	94%
2006	7007	91%
2005	7051	92%

Source: www.abim.org, 2010.

THE MAINTENANCE-OF-CERTIFICATION (MOC) EXAM

Physicians who have previously passed the ABIM exam are required to recertify every 10 years. The MOC exam is given twice per year, typically in April and October. It is a one-day exam that consists of three modules lasting two hours each. Each module has 60 questions for a total of 180 questions. Examinees are given two minutes per question. The MOC exam is currently administered as a CBT at a Pearson VUE testing site. Performance on the MOC exam is similar to that of the certification exam. Since 1996, 88% of MOC test takers have passed on their first attempt, and 96% have ultimately passed (see Table 3).

TEST PREPARATION ADVICE

The good news about the ABIM exam is that it tends to focus on the diagnosis and management of diseases and on conditions that you have likely seen as a resident and should expect to see as an internal medicine specialist. Assuming that you have performed well as a resident, *First Aid* and a good source of practice questions may be all that you need to pass. However, you might consider using *First Aid* as a **guide** along with multiple supplementary resources, such as a standard textbook, journal review articles, MKSAP, or a concise electronic text such as *UpToDate*, as part of your studies. Original research articles are low yield, and very new research (ie, research done less than 1–2 years before the exam) will not be tested. In addition, a number of high-quality board review courses are offered throughout the country. Such review courses are costly but can be of benefit to those who need some focus and discipline.

 KEY FACT

Check the ABIM Web site for the latest passing requirements.

 KEY FACT

Use a combination of *First Aid*, textbooks, journal reviews, and practice questions.

 KEY FACT

The ABIM exam tends to focus on the horses, not the zebras.

TABLE 3. MOC Exam Performance

Year	Percent Passed
2009	90%
2008	92%
2007	83%
2006	79%
2005	84%

Ideally, you should begin your preparation early in your **last year of residency,** especially if you are starting a demanding job or fellowship right after residency. Cramming in the period between the end of residency and the exam is **not advisable.**

As you study, concentrate on the **nuances of management,** especially for difficult or complicated cases. For **common diseases,** learn both common and **uncommon presentations;** for **uncommon diseases,** focus on **classic presentations** and manifestations. Draw on the experiences of your residency training to anchor some of your learning. When you take the exam, you will realize that you've seen most of the clinical scenarios in your three years of wards, clinics, morning report, case conferences, or grand rounds.

OTHER HIGH-YIELD AREAS

Focus on topic areas that are typically not emphasized during residency training but are board favorites. These include the following:

- Topics in outpatient specialties (eg, allergy, dermatology, ENT, ophthalmology)
- Formulas that are needed for quick recall (eg, alveolar gas, anion gap, creatinine clearance)
- Basic biostatistics (eg, sensitivity, specificity, positive predictive value, negative predictive value)
- Adverse effects of drugs

TEST-TAKING ADVICE

By this point in your life, you have probably gained more test-taking expertise than you care to admit. Nevertheless, here are a few tips to keep in mind when taking the exam:

- For long vignette questions, read the question stem and scan the options; **then** go back and read the case. You may get your answer without having to read through the whole case.
- There's no penalty for guessing, so you should **never** leave a question blank.
- Good pacing is key. You need to leave adequate time to get to all the questions. Even though you are allotted an average of two minutes per question, you should aim for a pace of 90–100 seconds per question. If you don't know the answer within a short period, make an educated guess and move on.
- It's okay to **second-guess** yourself. Research shows that our "second hunches" tend to be better than our first guesses.
- Don't panic when you confront "impossible" questions. These may be **experimental questions** that won't count toward your score. So again, take your best guess and move on.
- Note the age and race of the patient in each clinical scenario. When ethnicity is given, it is often relevant. Know these well, especially for more common diagnoses.
- Remember that questions often describe clinical findings rather than naming eponyms (eg, they cite "tender, erythematous bumps in the pads of the finger" instead of "Osler's nodes").
- Manage your break time. On exam day, it's important to return to the test area at least 10–15 minutes before your break ends to make sure the testing center official has time to check in all test takers.

KEY FACT

Never leave a question blank! Remember that there is no penalty for guessing.

Testing and Licensing Agencies

American Board of Internal Medicine
510 Walnut Street, Suite 1700
Philadelphia, PA 19106-3699
215-446-3500 or 800-441-2246
Fax: 215-446-3633
www.abim.org

Educational Commission for Foreign Medical Graduates (ECFMG)
3624 Market Street
Philadelphia, PA 19104-2685
215-386-5900
Fax: 215-386-9196
www.ecfmg.org

Federation of State Medical Boards (FSMB)
400 Fuller Wiser Road, Suite 300
Euless, TX 76039
817-868-4000
Fax: 817-868-4099
www.fsmb.org

NOTES

CHAPTER 1

Allergy and Immunology

Anuj Gaggar, MD, PhD
Marc Riedl, MD, MS

Diagnostic Testing in Allergy

ALLERGY SKIN TESTING

- A confirmatory test for the presence of **allergen-specific IgE antibody**.
  - **Prick-puncture skin testing:** Adequate for most purposes. A drop of allergen extract is placed on the skin surface, and epidermal puncture is performed with a specialized needle.
  - **Intradermal skin testing:** Used for venom and penicillin testing; allergen is injected intracutaneously.
- All skin testing should use ⊕ (histamine) and ⊖ (saline) controls.
- Skin-testing **wheal-and-flare reactions** are measured 15–20 minutes after placement.

LABORATORY ALLERGY TESTING

- Radioallergosorbent serologic testing (**RAST**) is performed to confirm the presence of **allergen-specific IgE antibody**.
  - Results are comparable to skin testing for pollen- and food-specific IgE.
  - Recommended when the subject has anaphylactic sensitivity to the antigen; useful when skin testing is either not available or not possible because of skin conditions or interfering medications (eg, antihistamine use).
- RAST testing alone is generally **not** adequate for **venom or drug allergy** testing.

DELAYED-TYPE HYPERSENSITIVITY SKIN TESTING

- An effective screening test for functional **cell-mediated immunity**.
- Involves **intradermal injection of 0.1 mL of purified antigen.** The standard panel includes *Candida*, **mumps, tetanus toxoid,** and **PPD.**
- The injection site is examined for **induration 48 hours** after injection.
- Approximately 95% of normal subjects will respond to one of the above-mentioned antigens.
- The absence of a response suggests deficient cell-mediated immunity or anergy.

ALLERGEN PATCH TESTING

- The appropriate diagnostic test for **allergic contact dermatitis.**
- Suspected substances are applied to the skin with adhesive test strips for 48 hours.
- The skin site is examined 48 and 72 hours after application for evidence of erythema, edema, and vesiculation (reproduction of contact dermatitis).

Diagnostic Testing in Immunology

COMPLEMENT DEFICIENCY TESTING

- The **complement pathway** consists of the **classic** (immune complex mediated), **alternative** (induced by microbial surfaces), and **mannose-binding lectin** (induced by microbial surfaces) **pathways.**

- **CH50** is a **screening** test for the **classic complement pathway.**
    - All nine elements of **C1–C9** are required to produce a normal CH50.
    - A normal CH50 does not exclude the possibility of low C3 or C4.
- **Deficiencies that lead to disease** include the following:
    - **CH50:** Any C1–C9.
    - **C1-INH:** Hereditary angioedema.
    - **C2, C3, C4:** Recurrent sinopulmonary infections (encapsulated bacteria such as *Streptococcus pneumoniae, Haemophilus influenzae,* and *Neisseria meningitidis*).
    - **C1, C2, C4:** SLE.
    - **C1, C3, C4:** Pyogenic bacterial infections.
    - **C5–C9:** *Neisseria* infections.

HUMORAL (B-CELL) AND CELLULAR (T-CELL) DEFICIENCY TESTING

Testing for B- and T-cell deficiency is as follows:

- **CD19:** For **B-cell** immunity.
- **IgG, IgM, IgA, IgD, IgE:** For antibody.
- **CD3, CD4, CD8:** For **T-cell** immunity.
- **CD16, CD56:** For **natural killer cell** immunity.

Gell and Coombs Classification of Immunologic Reactions

The traditional framework that is used to describe immune-mediated reactions. It is not inclusive of all complex immune processes.

MNEMONIC

Gell-Coombs classification system—

ACID

Anaphylactic: type I
Cytotoxic: type II
Immune complex: type III
Delayed hypersensitivity: type IV

TYPE I: IMMEDIATE REACTIONS (IgE MEDIATED)

- Specific antigen exposure causes **cross-linking of IgE on mast cell/basophil surfaces,** leading to the release of histamine, leukotrienes, prostaglandins, and **tryptase.**
- Mediator release leads to symptoms of **urticaria, rhinitis, wheezing, diarrhea, vomiting, hypotension,** and **anaphylaxis,** usually within **minutes** of antigen exposure.
- **Late-phase** type I reactions may cause **recurrent symptoms 4–8 hours** after exposure.

TYPE II: CYTOTOXIC REACTIONS

- Mediated by **antibodies,** primarily IgG and IgM, **directed at cell surface or tissue antigens.** Antigens may be native, foreign, or haptens (small foreign particles attached to larger native molecules).
- Antibodies **destroy cells** by **opsonization** (coating for phagocytosis), **complement-mediated lysis,** or **antibody-dependent cellular cytotoxicity.**
- Clinical examples include penicillin-induced autoimmune **hemolytic anemia** and certain forms of **autoimmune thyroiditis.**

TYPE III: IMMUNE COMPLEX REACTIONS

- Exposure to antigen in genetically predisposed individuals causes **antigen-antibody complex** formation.

- Antigen-antibody complexes **activate complement and neutrophil** infiltration, leading to tissue inflammation that most commonly affects the **skin, kidneys, joints,** and **lymphoreticular system.**
- Clinically presents with symptoms of "serum sickness" **10–14 days after exposure;** most frequently caused by β-lactam **antibiotics** or nonhuman antiserum (antithymocyte globulin, antivenoms).

TYPE IV: DELAYED HYPERSENSITIVITY REACTIONS (T-CELL MEDIATED)

- Exposure to antigen causes direct activation of **sensitized T cells,** usually CD4+ cells.
- T-cell activation causes tissue **inflammation 48–96 hours after exposure.**
- The most common clinical reaction is allergic contact dermatitis such as that resulting from **poison ivy.**

Asthma

A 19-year-old man with a history of asthma presents with persistent wheezing and coughing. He describes daily and nightly symptoms that occur twice per week. He currently takes an inhaled corticosteroid twice daily and albuterol as needed. What would be the next appropriate change in his medications?

↑ his corticosteroid dose to a medium-dose agent and add a long-acting β₂-agonist (salmeterol). The patient is describing moderate persistent symptoms and would thus benefit from the above interventions. Although one might also consider adding leukotriene modifiers, such agents should not be used in place of long-acting β₂-agonists or inhaled corticosteroids.

A **chronic inflammatory disorder** of the airway resulting in **airway hyperresponsiveness, airflow limitation,** and **respiratory symptoms.** Often begins in childhood, but may have adult onset. **Atopy** is a strong identifiable **risk factor** for the development of asthma. Subtypes include exercise-induced, occupational, aspirin-sensitive, and cough-variant asthma.

SYMPTOMS

- Symptoms include **dyspnea** (at rest or with exertion), **cough, wheezing,** mucus hypersecretion, chest tightness, and nocturnal awakenings with respiratory symptoms.
- Symptoms may have identifiable **triggers** (eg, exercise, exposure to cat dander, NSAIDs, cold exposure).

EXAM

- **Acute exacerbations: Expiratory wheezing;** a prolonged expiratory phase; ↑ respiratory rate.
- **Severe exacerbations: Pulsus paradoxus,** cyanosis, lethargy, use of accessory muscles of respiration, silent chest (absence of wheezing due to lack of air movement).
- **Chronic asthma without exacerbation:** Presents with minimal to no wheezing. Signs of allergic rhinosinusitis (boggy nasal mucosa, posterior

oropharynx cobblestoning, suborbital edema) are commonly found. **Exam may be normal** between exacerbations.

DIFFERENTIAL

- **Upper airway obstruction:** Foreign body, tracheal compression, tracheal stenosis, vocal cord dysfunction.
- **Other lung disease:** Emphysema, chronic bronchitis, CF, allergic bronchopulmonary aspergillosis, Churg-Strauss syndrome, chronic eosinophilic pneumonia, obstructive sleep apnea, restrictive lung disease, pulmonary embolism.
- **Cardiovascular disease:** CHF, ischemic heart disease.
- **Respiratory infection:** Bacterial or viral pneumonia, bronchiectasis, sinusitis.

DIAGNOSIS

Diagnosed by the history and objective evidence of **obstructive lung disease.**

- **PFTs:** Show a ↓ **FEV_1/FVC ratio** with **reversible obstruction** (> 12% ↑ in FEV_1 after bronchodilator use) and **normal diffusing capacity.**
- **Methacholine challenge:** Useful if baseline lung function is normal but clinical symptoms are suggestive of asthma. A ⊕ methacholine challenge test is not diagnostic of asthma, but a ⊖ test indicates that asthma is unlikely (**high sensitivity, lower specificity**).

> **KEY FACT**
>
> The role of a methacholine challenge is to exclude the diagnosis of asthma. A ⊕ challenge can be 2° to numerous etiologies and thus may not be definitive.

TREATMENT

Acute exacerbations are treated as follows:

- **Initial treatment: Inhaled rapid-acting β₂-agonists** (albuterol), one dose q 20 min × 1 hour; O_2 to keep saturation > 90%.
  - **Good response:** With a peak expiratory flow (PEF) > 80% of predicted or personal best after albuterol, continue albuterol q 3–4 h and institute appropriate chronic therapy (see below).
  - **Incomplete response:** With a PEF 60–80% of predicted or personal best, consider systemic corticosteroids; continue inhaled albuterol q 60 min × 1–3 hours if continued improvement is seen.
  - **Poor response or severe episode:** With a PEF < 60% of predicted or personal best, give systemic corticosteroids and consider systemic epinephrine (preferably IM), IV theophylline, and/or IV magnesium.
- **Follow-up:**
  - **Good response:** Patients with improved symptoms, a PEF > 70%, and an O_2 saturation > 90% for 60 minutes after the last treatment may be discharged home with appropriate outpatient therapy and follow-up. Oral corticosteroids are appropriate in most cases.
  - **Incomplete response:** Patients with **incomplete responses** after the initial two hours of treatment (persistent moderate symptoms, PEF < 70%, O_2 saturation < 90%) should be admitted for **inpatient therapy** and monitoring with inhaled albuterol, O_2, and **systemic corticosteroids.**
  - **Poor response:** Patients with a **poor response** to initial therapy (severe symptoms, lethargy, confusion, PEF < 30%, Po_2 < 60, Pco_2 > 45) should be admitted to the **ICU** for treatment with **inhaled albuterol, O_2, IV corticosteroids,** and **possible intubation** and mechanical ventilation.

Chronic asthma therapy (see Table 1.1) is based on asthma severity. The treatment regimen should be **reviewed every 1–6 months,** with changes made

> **KEY FACT**
>
> Asthma symptoms that occur more than twice weekly generally indicate the need for inhaled corticosteroid therapy.

> **KEY FACT**
>
> Long-acting β₂-agonists have been associated with asthma-related deaths. Never use these agents as monotherapy in severe asthma.

> **KEY FACT**
>
> Consider the addition of anti-IgE (omalizumab) for the treatment of severe persistent asthma.

TABLE 1.1.   Guidelines for the Treatment of Chronic Asthma

Asthma Classification	Symptoms[a]	Pulmonary Function	Recommended Treatment
Mild intermittent	≤ 2 days/week, ≤ 2 nights/month.	PEF ≥ 80%	Bronchodilator 2–4 puffs q 4 h as needed. No daily medications necessary.
Mild persistent	> 2 days/week but < 1 time/day or > 2 nights/month.	PEF ≥ 80%	Add low-dose inhaled corticosteroids. Leukotriene modifiers, theophylline, and cromolyn may also be added.
Moderate persistent	Daily symptoms or > 1 night/week.	PEF 60–80%	↑ to medium-dose inhaled corticosteroids and add a long-acting inhaled β_2-agonist. Leukotriene modifiers or theophylline may also be added.
Severe persistent	Continuous symptoms.	PEF < 60%	↑ to high-dose inhaled corticosteroids plus long-acting inhaled β_2-agonists. Daily oral corticosteroids may be added if necessary (60 mg QD).

[a]Dyspnea (at rest or with exertion), cough, wheezing, mucus hypersecretion, chest tightness, and nocturnal awakenings with respiratory symptoms.

KEY FACT

Think of reactive airway dysfunction syndrome (RADS) in a patient with symptoms of asthma following a single, large exposure to an irritant such as chlorine or mustard gas (biological warfare). Treat like asthma.

depending on symptom severity and clinical course. Additional treatment considerations for both acute and chronic asthma include the following:

- Recognize the exacerbating effects of **environmental factors** such as allergens, air pollution, smoking, and weather (cold and humidity).
- Use potentially **exacerbating medications** (ASA, NSAIDs, β-blockers) **with caution.**
- Always consider **medication compliance and technique** as possible complicating factors in poorly controlled asthma.
- Treatment of **coexisting conditions** (eg, **rhinitis, sinusitis, GERD**) may improve asthma.

COMPLICATIONS

- Hypoxemia, respiratory failure, pneumothorax or pneumomediastinum.
- Frequent hospitalizations and previous intubation are warning signs of potentially fatal asthma.
- A subset of patients with chronic asthma develop **airway remodeling** that leads to accelerated, irreversible loss of lung function.

Allergic Rhinitis

 A 35-year-old woman presents to your office with persistent symptoms of allergic rhinitis. She has previously tried antihistamines, pseudoephedrine, and nasal corticosteroids with only modest benefit. She returns for further evaluation. What is the best course of therapy for this patient?

Diagnostic allergy testing or immunotherapy. Empiric therapy is often an effective means of controlling allergy symptoms, and antihistamines, pseudoephedrine, and nasal steroids have generally shown the most benefit for such symptoms. Evaluation by allergy testing can help in planning allergen avoidance or determine the need for immunotherapy.

The **most common cause** of chronic rhinitis. Allergic factors are present in 75% of rhinitis cases. May be **seasonal or perennial;** incidence is greatest in adolescence and ↓ with advancing age. Usually persistent, with occasional spontaneous remission.

SYMPTOMS

- Sneezing, nasal itching, rhinorrhea, nasal congestion, sore throat, throat clearing, itching of the throat and palate.
- Sleep disturbance; association with obstructive sleep apnea.
- Concomitant conjunctivitis with ocular itching, lacrimation, and puffiness.

EXAM

Patients present with swollen nasal turbinates with pale or bluish mucosa, clear nasal discharge, clear to white secretions along the posterior wall of the oropharynx, infraorbital darkening, conjunctival erythema, and lacrimation.

DIFFERENTIAL

- **Nonallergic rhinitis:** Vasomotor or gustatory rhinitis.
- **Rhinitis medicamentosa:** Overuse of vasoconstricting nasal sprays, leading to rebound nasal congestion and associated symptoms.
- **Hormonal rhinitis:** Associated with pregnancy, use of OCPs, and hypothyroidism.
- **Drug-induced rhinitis:** Common causes include β-blockers, α-blockers, and cocaine.
- **Atrophic rhinitis:** Develops in elderly patients with atrophy of the nasal mucosa.
- **Infectious rhinosinusitis:** Acute viral syndromes lasting 7–10 days; bacterial sinusitis.
- **Nasal obstruction due to a structural abnormality:** Septal deviation, nasal polyposis, nasal tumor, foreign body.

DIAGNOSIS

Based on the history and ⊕ **skin testing** to common aeroallergens (eg, grass/tree/weed pollen, house dust mites, cockroaches, dog and cat dander, mold).

TREATMENT

- **Intranasal corticosteroids:** The most effective medication for allergic and nonallergic rhinitis. Have no significant systemic side effects; most beneficial when used regularly.
- **Allergen avoidance measures:** Most effective for house dust mites (involves the use of allergen-impermeable bed and pillow casings and washing of bedding in hot water). Indoor pollen exposure can be ↓ by keeping windows closed and using air conditioners.
- **Antihistamines:** ↓ sneezing, rhinorrhea, and pruritus. Less effective for nasal congestion; best if used regularly. Not effective for nonallergic rhinitis. Nonsedating antihistamines are preferable.
- **Oral decongestants:** Effectively ↓ nasal congestion in allergic and nonallergic rhinitis. May cause insomnia and exacerbate hypertension or arrhythmia.
- **Allergen immunotherapy:** Indicated as an alternative or adjunct to medications. The only effective therapy that has been demonstrated to modify the long-term course of the disease.

COMPLICATIONS

Chronic sinusitis and otitis; exacerbation of asthma.

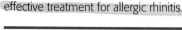

KEY FACT

Intranasal corticosteroids are the most effective treatment for allergic rhinitis.

Hypersensitivity Pneumonitis

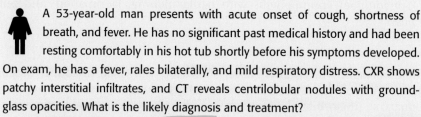

A 53-year-old man presents with acute onset of cough, shortness of breath, and fever. He has no significant past medical history and had been resting comfortably in his hot tub shortly before his symptoms developed. On exam, he has a fever, rales bilaterally, and mild respiratory distress. CXR shows patchy interstitial infiltrates, and CT reveals centrilobular nodules with ground-glass opacities. What is the likely diagnosis and treatment?
"Hot tub lung" due to hypersensitivity to *Mycobacterium avium* complex (MAC). Treatment involves avoidance of further antigen exposure and empiric steroids with a taper.

A complex immune-mediated lung disease resulting from repeated inhalational exposure to a wide variety of **organic dusts** (see Table 1.2). Presents in acute, subacute, and chronic forms.

SYMPTOMS

- **Acute:** Nonproductive cough, shortness of breath, fever, diaphoresis, myalgias occurring 6–12 hours after intense antigen exposure.
- **Chronic:** Insidious onset of dyspnea, productive cough, fatigue, anorexia, weight loss.

EXAM

- **Acute:** Patients appear ill with fever, respiratory distress, and dry rales (wheezing is **not** a prominent symptom). Exam may be normal in asymptomatic patients between episodes of acute hypersensitivity pneumonitis.
- **Chronic:** Dry rales, ↓ breath sounds, digital clubbing.

TABLE 1.2.   Selected Causes of Hypersensitivity Pneumonitis

DISEASE	ANTIGEN	SOURCE
Farmer's lung	*Micropolyspora faeni, Thermoactinomyces vulgaris.*	Moldy hay.
"Humidifier lung"	Thermophilic actinomycetes.	Contaminated humidifiers, heating systems, or air conditioners.
Bird fancier's lung ("pigeon breeder's disease")	Avian proteins.	Bird serum and excreta.
Bagassosis	*Thermoactinomyces facchari* and *T vulgaris.*	Moldy sugar-cane fiber (bagasse).
Sequoiosis	*Graphium, Aureobasidium,* and other fungi.	Moldy redwood sawdust.
Maple bark stripper's disease	*Cryptostroma (Coniosporium) corticale.*	Rotting maple tree logs or bark.
Mushroom picker's disease	Same as farmer's lung.	Moldy compost.
Suberosis	*Penicillium frequentans.*	Moldy cork dust.
Detergent worker's lung	*Bacillus subtilis* enzyme.	Enzyme additives.

(Reproduced with permission from McPhee SJ et al. *Current Medical Diagnosis & Treatment 2010.* New York: McGraw-Hill, 2010, Table 9-20.)

DIFFERENTIAL

- Acute:
    - **Pneumonia:** Bacterial, viral, or atypical.
    - **Toxic fume bronchiolitis:** Sulfur dioxide, ammonia, chlorine.
    - **Organic dust toxic syndrome:** Inhalation of dusts contaminated with bacteria and fungi.
- **Subacute or chronic:** Chronic bronchitis, idiopathic pulmonary fibrosis, chronic eosinophilic pneumonia, collagen vascular disease, sarcoidosis, 1° pulmonary histiocytosis, alveolar proteinosis.

DIAGNOSIS

- **PFTs:**
    - **Acute: Restrictive pattern** with ↓ FVC and FEV_1. ↓ DL_{CO} is common.
    - **Chronic:** Combined obstructive and restrictive pattern.
- Imaging:
    - **Acute:** CXR shows transient patchy, peripheral, bilateral interstitial infiltrates. CT typically shows ground-glass opacifications and diffuse consolidation.
    - **Subacute:** CXR shows nodular, patchy infiltrates; CT reveals centrilobular nodules with areas of ground-glass opacity and air trapping.
    - **Chronic:** CXR shows fibrotic changes with honeycombing and areas of emphysema; CT shows honeycombing, fibrosis, traction bronchiectasis, ground-glass opacities, and small nodules.
- Labs:
    - **Acute:** ↑ WBC count; ↑ ESR.
    - **Acute or chronic: High titers of precipitating IgG** against the offending antigen (indicates exposure, not necessarily disease). Double-gel immunodiffusion is preferred, as ELISA may be too sensitive.

- **Bronchoalveolar lavage:** Lymphocytosis with a predominance of CD8+ T cells.
- **Lung biopsy:** Interstitial and alveolar **noncaseating granulomas;** "foamy" macrophages; predominance of lymphocytes.
- **Inhalational challenge:** Not required or recommended for diagnosis; helpful when data are lacking or diagnosis is unclear. Performed only with careful medical monitoring.

TREATMENT

- Avoidance of the offending antigen.
- Oral corticosteroids at a dosage of 40–80 mg QD with tapering after clinical improvement has been achieved.

COMPLICATIONS

- Irreversible loss of lung function.
- Death is uncommon but has been reported.

Allergic Bronchopulmonary Aspergillosis (ABPA)

An immunologic reaction to antigens of *Aspergillus* present in the bronchial tree.

SYMPTOMS

Asthma (may be cough variant or exercise induced); expectoration of golden brown mucous plugs; fever with acute flare.

EXAM

Wheezing, rales, or bronchial breath sounds; digital clubbing and cyanosis (late-stage disease).

DIFFERENTIAL

Asthma without ABPA, pneumonia (bacterial, viral, fungal, acid-fast bacilli), Churg-Strauss syndrome, eosinophilic pneumonias, CF.

DIAGNOSIS

- **Essential criteria** for ABPA-S (seropositive ABPA) are as follows:
  - The presence of **asthma.**
  - ⊕ immediate **skin tests to *Aspergillus.***
  - ↑ total serum **IgE** (> 1000 ng/mL).
  - ↑ serum ***Aspergillus*-specific IgE and/or IgG.**
- Other features include the following:
  - The above plus central bronchiectasis = ABPA-CB (ABPA with central bronchiectasis).
  - Precipitating antibodies to *Aspergillus.*
  - Peripheral blood eosinophilia (> 1000/mm³).
  - CXR showing infiltrates (transient or fixed).
  - A sputum culture that is ⊕ for *Aspergillus* or that contains *Aspergillus* hyphae.

TREATMENT

- **Prednisone;** itraconazole may be used as an adjunctive medication.
- Chronic inhaled corticosteroids to control asthma.

COMPLICATIONS

Corticosteroid-dependent asthma, irreversible loss of pulmonary function, chronic bronchitis, pulmonary fibrosis, death due to respiratory failure or cor pulmonale.

Allergic Fungal Sinusitis

An immunologic reaction to fungal aeroallergens *(Aspergillus, Bipolaris, Curvularia, Alternaria, Fusarium)* that causes chronic, refractory sinus disease.

SYMPTOMS

Sinus congestion and obstruction that are refractory to antibiotics; thick mucoid **secretions** (**"peanut butter"** appearance); nasal polyposis; proptosis; asthma.

EXAM

Presents with thickening of the sinus mucosa, allergic mucin on rhinoscopy, and nasal polyps.

DIFFERENTIAL

- **Chronic rhinosinusitis:** Bacterial, allergic (nonfungal).
- **Invasive fungal disease:** Seen in immunocompromised patients (HIV, diabetes).
- **Other:** Nasal polyposis without allergic fungal sinusitis; mycetoma (fungus ball).

DIAGNOSIS

- **Diagnostic criteria** include the following:
  - Chronic sinusitis for > 6 months.
  - **Allergic mucin** containing many eosinophils and fungal hyphae.
  - **Sinus CT** showing opacification of the sinus (often unilateral) with **hyperattenuated,** expansile material.
  - Absence of invasive fungal disease.
- **Other supportive findings** include peripheral blood eosinophilia and immediate skin tests ⊕ to fungus.

TREATMENT

- **Surgical** removal of allergic mucin.
- **Prednisone** 0.5–1.0 mg/kg for weeks with slow tapering.
- Intranasal corticosteroids; nasal irrigation.

COMPLICATIONS

Bony erosions from expansion of allergic mucin; surgical complications; high recurrence rate despite therapy.

Urticaria and Angioedema

 An 18-year-old man presents to the ER with recurrent abdominal pain. He has had several similar episodes over the past several years, with each episode resolving slowly over time and associated with swelling of his arms bilaterally. His episode today is worse, and he again has arm swelling bilaterally. Which tests would be useful in determining the cause of his recurrent symptoms?

C1 inhibitor (C1-INH) assay and C1q level. This patient has symptoms consistent with recurrent angioedema, which can be acquired or hereditary. Treatment involves replacement of inhibitor, often via C1-INH concentrate or FFP. Angioedema often presents with abdominal pain, as gut edema is common.

Localized edema in the skin or mucous membranes. Individual wheals (hives) typically last < 24 hours. May be acute (< 6 weeks of symptoms) or chronic (> 6 weeks).

SYMPTOMS

- Presents with pruritic hives and painful soft tissue swelling on the lips, oral mucosa, periorbital area, hands, and feet (see Figure 1.1).
- **Individual skin lesions** resolve in < 24 hours without residual scarring. Angioedema may take longer to fully resolve.

EXAM

- Erythematous, blanching skin wheals; soft tissue swelling as described above. No scarring or pigmentary changes can be seen at previously affected sites.
- Exam may be normal between symptomatic flares.

> **KEY FACT**
>
> Think of hereditary angioedema in a patient presenting with recurrent episodes of angioedema **without** pruritus or urticaria. Check a C1-INH assay, which will be low.

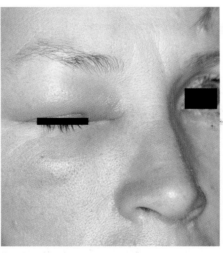 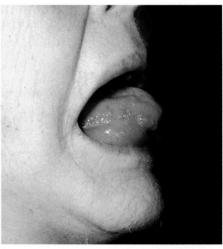

A   B

FIGURE 1.1. **Angioedema.** (A) Angioedema leading to closure of the right eye. (B) Sublingual angioedema. (Reproduced with permission from Wolff K, Johnson RA. *Fitzpatrick's Color Atlas & Synopsis of Clinical Dermatology*, 6th ed. New York: McGraw-Hill, 2009, Fig. 22-7B.)

DIFFERENTIAL

- **IgE-mediated allergic reaction:** Food, medication, insect stings.
- **Non-IgE reactions:** ASA, narcotics, radiocontrast media.
- **Physical urticaria:** Pressure, vibratory, solar, cholinergic, local heat and cold.
- **Autoimmunity:** Vasculitis, associated thyroiditis.
- **Infections:** Mononucleosis, viral hepatitis, fungal and parasitic disease.
- **Idiopathic:** Accounts for most cases of chronic urticaria.
- **Isolated angioedema:** Consider hereditary angioedema or acquired angioedema (associated with vasculitis and neoplasms).
- **Other:** Dermatographism; cutaneous mastocytosis.

DIAGNOSIS

- The clinical history suggests diagnostic testing.
- Provocative testing for physical urticarias.
- Labs include ESR, ANA, skin biopsy (if necessary to exclude vasculitis), and antithyroid antibodies if autoimmunity is suspected.
- Order a CBC, a viral hepatitis panel, and a stool O&P if the history is suggestive of infection.
- In the setting of angioedema alone, obtain a C1-INH assay to exclude hereditary angioedema; determine the C1q level to exclude acquired angioedema.

TREATMENT

- Avoid inciting exposure or treat the underlying condition if it is identified.
- **Antihistamines:** Regular use of nonsedating H_1 antagonists is preferred. Sedating H_1 antagonists may also be used QHS; H_2 antagonists may be helpful adjunctive medication.
- **Other:**
  - Ephedrine (OTC) is helpful for acute flares.
  - Leukotriene modifiers are beneficial in some cases.
  - Oral corticosteroids for severe, refractory cases.
  - Epinephrine for life-threatening laryngeal edema.
  - Danazol, stanozolol, or C1-INH concentrate for chronic treatment of hereditary angioedema.

COMPLICATIONS

Laryngeal edema.

Atopic Dermatitis (Eczema)

A chronic inflammatory skin disease that is often associated with a personal or family **history of atopy.** Usually begins in childhood.

SYMPTOMS

- Characterized by intense **pruritus** and an erythematous papular rash typically occurring in the flexural areas of the elbows, knees, ankles, and neck (see Figure 1.2). Pruritus precedes the rash (**"an itch that rashes"**).
- Chronic atopic dermatitis manifests as thickened nonerythematous plaques of skin (lichenification).

KEY FACT

Most cases of chronic urticaria are idiopathic. Extensive laboratory evaluation in the absence of systemic symptoms or unusual features is generally not beneficial.

KEY FACT

A patient with angioedema and well-controlled hypertension? Think ACEIs.

KEY FACT

When used regularly at adequate doses, antihistamines successfully treat most cases of urticaria.

KEY FACT

In contrast to angioedema associated with anaphylaxis, hereditary angioedema does not respond to epinephrine. Treat with FFP or C1-INH concentrate.

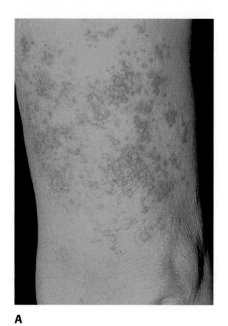
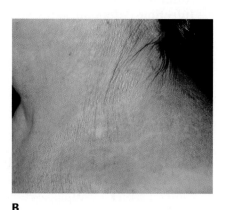

A   **B**

FIGURE 1.2.   Atopic dermatitis. (A) Erythematous papules of subacute atopic dermatitis on the extensor surface of the upper arm. (B) Lichenification of the skin of the shoulder and neck in chronic atopic dermatitis. (Reproduced with permission from Wolff K et al. *Fitzpatrick's Dermatology in General Medicine*, 7th ed. New York: McGraw-Hill, 2008, Figs. 14-4 and 14-2.)

EXAM

Presents with an erythematous papular rash in **flexural areas** as well as with excoriations, serous exudate, lichenification (if chronic), and other findings of atopic disease (boggy nasal mucosa, conjunctival erythema, expiratory wheezing).

DIFFERENTIAL

- **Other dermatitis:** Seborrheic, irritant, contact, psoriasis.
- **Neoplasia:** Cutaneous T-cell lymphoma.
- **Infectious:** Scabies, candidiasis, tinea versicolor.
- **Hyper-IgE syndrome:** Usually diagnosed in childhood.

DIAGNOSIS

- Diagnosis is readily made through the history and physical.
- Consider skin biopsy to rule out cutaneous T-cell lymphoma in new-onset eczema in an adult.

TREATMENT

- **Skin hydration:** Lotions, emollients.
- **Topical corticosteroids.**
- **Antihistamines** to reduce pruritus.
- Avoid skin irritants (eg, abrasive clothing, temperature extremes, harsh soaps).
- Avoid allergic triggers if identified (food, aeroallergens; more common in children).
- Treat bacterial, fungal, and viral **superinfection** as necessary.
- Topical **tacrolimus/pimecrolimus** and oral corticosteroids for severe disease.

COMPLICATIONS

- **Chronic skin changes:** Scarring, hyperpigmentation.
- **Cutaneous infection:** Bacterial (primarily *S aureus*), viral (primarily HSV); risk of eczema vaccinatum with smallpox vaccine.

Allergic Contact Dermatitis

A lymphocyte-mediated delayed hypersensitivity reaction causing a skin rash on an antigen-exposed area.

SYMPTOMS

- Characterized by a **pruritic** rash that typically appears 5–21 days after the initial exposure or 12–96 hours after reexposure in sensitized individuals.
- The typical pattern is **erythema** leading to **papules** and then **vesicles**. The rash precedes pruritus and appears in the distribution of antigen exposure (see Figure 1.3).

EXAM

- **Acute stage:** Skin erythema, papules, vesicles.
- **Subacute or chronic stage:** Crusting, scaling, lichenification, and thickening of the skin.

DIFFERENTIAL

Atopic dermatitis, seborrheic dermatitis, irritant dermatitis (antigen-nonspecific irritation, usually due to chemicals or detergents), psoriasis.

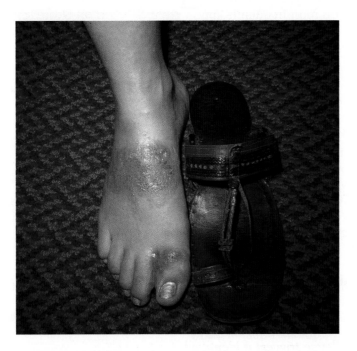

FIGURE 1.3.   Contact dermatitis. Erythematous papules, vesicles, and serous weeping localized to areas of contact with the offending agent are characteristic. (Reproduced with permission from Hurwitz RM. *Pathology of the Skin: Atlas of Clinical-Pathological Correlation.* Stamford, CT: Appleton & Lange, 1991: 3.)

DIAGNOSIS

- **Location of the rash:** Suggests the cause—eg, feet (shoes), neck/ears (jewelry), face (cosmetics/hair products).
- **Allergy patch testing:** See above.

TREATMENT

Antigen avoidance, topical corticosteroids, antihistamines for pruritus; oral prednisone in severe or extensive cases.

COMPLICATIONS

2° infection from scratching affected skin.

Anaphylaxis

A systemic type I (IgE-mediated) hypersensitivity reaction that is often life threatening. Requires **previous exposure** (known or unknown) for sensitization. Risk factors include parenteral antigen exposure and repeated interrupted antigen exposure. Common causes are **foods** (especially peanuts and shellfish), **drugs** (especially penicillin), **latex, stinging insects,** and **blood products.**

SYMPTOMS

- Symptoms include skin erythema, pruritus, urticaria, angioedema, laryngeal edema, wheezing, chest tightness, cramping abdominal pain, nausea, vomiting, diarrhea, diaphoresis, dizziness, a sense of "impending doom," hypotension, syncope, and shock.
- Symptoms most frequently appear **seconds to minutes after exposure** but may be delayed several hours for ingested agents.

EXAM

Urticaria, angioedema, flushing, wheezing, stridor, diaphoresis, hypotension, tachycardia.

DIFFERENTIAL

- **Other types of shock:** Cardiogenic, endotoxic, hemorrhagic.
- **Cardiovascular disease:** Arrhythmia, MI.
- **Scombroid:** Histamine poisoning from spoiled fish.
- **Anaphylactoid reaction:** Nonspecific mast cell activation (**not** IgE).
- **Other:** Carcinoid syndrome, pheochromocytoma, severe cold urticaria, vasovagal reaction, systemic mastocytosis, panic attack.

DIAGNOSIS

- ↑ **serum tryptase** drawn 30 minutes to three hours after onset can help confirm the diagnosis.
- Presence of **allergen-specific IgE antibody** by skin or RAST testing (best performed one month after event).

TREATMENT

- **Epinephrine** 1:1000 0.3 mL IM. Repeat every 15 minutes as needed.
- **Maintain airway:** O$_2$; inhaled bronchodilators; intubation if necessary.
- Rapid IV fluids if the patient is hypotensive.
- **Diphenhydramine:** Give 50 mg IV/IM/PO.

KEY FACT

The treatment of anaphylaxis consists of the prompt administration of epinephrine. Mortality is strongly associated with delays in epinephrine administration.

- **Corticosteroids** (prednisone 60 mg or equivalent) IV/IM/PO: Reduce late-phase recurrence of symptoms 4–8 hours later.
- Vasopressor medications in the presence of persistent hypotension.
- IV epinephrine 1:10,000 0.3 mL should be given only in terminal patients.
- Consider **glucagon and/or atropine for patients on β-blockers** whose symptoms are refractory to therapy.
- Monitor patients for 8–12 hours after the reaction.
- Ensure that patients have access to injectable epinephrine and antihistamines on discharge.

COMPLICATIONS

Respiratory obstruction, cardiovascular collapse, death.

MNEMONIC

The ABCs of anaphylaxis treatment:

Airway
Breathing
Circulation
Drugs
Exposure
Note: Epinephrine should be administered as soon as anaphylaxis is suspected.

Anaphylactoid Reactions

Clinically indistinguishable from anaphylactic reactions, but caused by non-specific mast cell activation (**not IgE mediated**). May occur with initial exposure to medication. Common causes include radiocontrast media, vancomycin, amphotericin, opiates, and general anesthetics (induction agents and muscle relaxants).

DIAGNOSIS

- ↑ **serum tryptase** drawn 30 minutes to three hours after onset helps confirm mast cell release.
- **Absence of allergen-specific IgE** antibody to suspected antigens by skin or RAST testing (best performed one month after the event).

TREATMENT

- The same as that for anaphylaxis.
    - **Vancomycin:** Slow infusion rate.
    - **Radiocontrast media:** Use low-osmolality forms.
- Anaphylactoid reactions are **generally preventable with pretreatment** through use of corticosteroids and antihistamines. Pretreatment is recommended for patients with a history of reactions to radiocontrast media.

Food Allergy

True (IgE-mediated) food allergy in adults is most commonly caused by **peanuts, crustaceans, tree nuts,** and **fish.** Sensitivities to these foods tend to be lifelong. Multiple food allergies are rare in adults. Anaphylactic signs and symptoms occur **minutes to two hours after ingestion.**

DIFFERENTIAL

- Nonallergic food intolerance (lactase deficiency, celiac disease, symptoms due to vasoactive amines).
- Food poisoning, including scombroid.
- Anaphylaxis due to other causes.
- Eosinophilic gastroenteritis.

DIAGNOSIS

- Anaphylaxis may be confirmed with ↑ **serum tryptase** if the test is conducted 30 minutes to three hours after the reaction.
- ⊕ **allergy skin or RAST tests** to food antigen.
- Conduct a double-blind placebo-controlled food challenge if the diagnosis is unclear.

TREATMENT

- Treat anaphylaxis in an acute setting (see above).
- Eliminate implicated foods from the diet.
- Ensure patient access to injectable epinephrine.

Stinging Insect Allergy

Allergic reactions occur to three major stinging insect families: **vespids** (yellow jackets, hornets, wasps), **apids** (honeybees and bumblebees), and **fire ants.** Reactions are classified as **local** (symptoms at the sting site) or **systemic** (anaphylactic).

SYMPTOMS/EXAM

- **Local reaction:** Swelling and erythema; pain at the sting site lasting several hours.
- **Large local reaction:** Extensive swelling and erythema at the sting site lasting up to one week; nausea and malaise.
- **Systemic reaction:** Anaphylactic symptoms occurring within 15 minutes of sting.

DIFFERENTIAL

- **Toxic venom reaction:** Results from large venom burden delivery by **multiple simultaneous stings.** The pharmacologic properties of venom may cause hypotension and shock.
- Anaphylaxis due to other causes.

DIAGNOSIS

- Systemic reactions may be confirmed by an ↑ **serum tryptase** if drawn 30 minutes to three hours after the reaction.
- Any systemic reaction should be confirmed with **venom-specific IgE by allergy skin or RAST testing** given the risk of recurrence with repeat stings. Testing should be performed several weeks after the reaction in view of mast cell depletion.

TREATMENT

- **Large local:** Antihistamines; analgesics; a short prednisone course for severe or disabling local reactions.
- **Systemic:** Treatment is the same as that for anaphylaxis (see above).
- **Venom immunotherapy:** Recommended for patients with a history of systemic reaction and ⊕ venom-specific IgE tests. Immunotherapy is 98% effective in preventing systemic allergic reactions on resting.
- Insect avoidance.
- Ensure patient access to antihistamines and injectable epinephrine.

KEY FACT

Any adult who reacts systemically to an insect sting, regardless of reaction severity, should be evaluated for venom immunotherapy.

KEY FACT

People who have an anaphylactic reaction to insect stings should be educated about their venom sensitivity and provided with self-administered injectable epinephrine (EpiPen).

Drug Allergy

A 32-year-old man with HIV is diagnosed with neurosyphilis. He states that he is allergic to penicillin and had difficulty breathing when he received penicillin as a child. He is admitted for treatment and has a skin test that confirms a reaction to penicillin. What is the appropriate treatment course for this patient?

Desensitization. Inasmuch as penicillin is the treatment of choice for neurosyphilis and he has confirmed IgE-mediated allergy to penicillin, the next step would be systematic desensitization. The patient would likely be admitted to the ICU, given serially ↑ doses of penicillin, and monitored closely.

Only a small portion of adverse drug reactions are drug hypersensitivity reactions (immune mediated), of which a small subset represents true drug allergy (IgE mediated).

SYMPTOMS

Immunologic drug reactions may present with a wide range of symptoms. Common symptoms include urticaria, angioedema, morbilliform rash, blistering mucocutaneous lesions, cough, dyspnea, wheezing, anaphylaxis, arthralgias, fever, and lymphadenopathy.

EXAM

- **Dermatologic findings:** Urticaria, angioedema, morbilliform rash, purpura, petechiae, exfoliative dermatitis, bullous skin lesions.
- **Other:** Wheezing, lymphadenopathy, jaundice, fever.

DIFFERENTIAL

- **Nonimmunologic adverse drug reaction:** Dose-related toxicity, pharmacologic side effects, drug-drug interactions.
- **Pseudoallergic reaction:** Direct mast cell release (opiates, vancomycin, radiocontrast media).
- Nondrug causes of presenting symptoms.

DIAGNOSIS

- Diagnosed on the basis of clinical judgment using the following **general criteria:**
  - The patient's symptoms are consistent with an immunologic drug reaction.
  - The patient was administered a drug known to cause the symptoms.
  - The temporal sequence of drug administration and the appearance of symptoms is consistent with a drug reaction.
  - Other causes of the symptoms have effectively been excluded.
- When available, **diagnostic testing** supportive of an immunologic mechanism to explain the drug reaction (see Table 1.3).
- The drug challenge procedure is the definitive diagnostic test but should be performed only by an experienced clinician if an absolute indication exists for the drug.

KEY FACT

The vast majority of adverse drug reactions are due to predictable drug effects and do not represent true drug allergy.

KEY FACT

Diagnostic drug allergy skin testing is standardized and predictive only for penicillin.

TABLE 1.3. **Diagnostic Testing and Therapy for Drug Hypersensitivity**

Immunologic Reaction	Clinical Manifestations	Laboratory Tests	Therapeutic Considerations
Type I	Anaphylaxis, angioedema, urticaria, bronchospasm.	Skin testing, RAST testing, serum tryptase.	Discontinue drug; epinephrine, antihistamines, systemic corticosteroids, bronchodilators; inpatient monitoring if severe.
Type II	Hemolytic anemia, thrombocytopenia, neutropenia.	Direct/indirect Coombs' test.	Discontinue drug; consider systemic corticosteroids; transfusion in severe cases.
Type III	Serum sickness, vasculitis, glomerulonephritis.	Immune complexes, ESR, complement studies, ANA/ANCA, C-reactive protein, tissue biopsy for immunofluorescence studies.	Discontinue drug; NSAIDs, antihistamines; systemic corticosteroids or plasmapheresis if severe.
Type IV	Allergic contact dermatitis; maculopapular drug rash.[a]	Patch testing; lymphocyte proliferation assay.[b]	Discontinue drug; topical corticosteroids, antihistamines; systemic corticosteroids if severe.

[a]Suspected type IV reaction; mechanism not fully elucidated.

[b]Investigational test.

TREATMENT

- **Discontinuation of the drug:**
    - In most instances, symptoms promptly resolve if the diagnosis is correct.
    - If the drug is absolutely indicated, refer the patient for **graded challenge/desensitization.**
- **Symptomatic treatment for specific symptoms:** Antihistamines, topical corticosteroids, bronchodilators; oral corticosteroids in severe cases.
- **Patient education:** Educate patients with regard to the risk of future reaction, drug avoidance, and cross-reactive medications.

COMPLICATIONS

- **Fatal drug hypersensitivity:** Anaphylaxis, toxic epidermal necrolysis.
- **"Multiple drug allergy syndrome":** Lack of patient/physician understanding of adverse drug reactions can lead to multiple medication avoidance and restrictive, ineffective medical therapy.

Mastocytosis

A disease characterized by **excessive numbers of mast cells** in the skin, internal organs, and bone marrow. Caused by a somatic **kit gene mutation.** Has variable severity ranging from the isolated cutaneous form to indolent systemic disease to aggressive lymphoma-like disease or mast cell leukemia.

SYMPTOMS

Pruritus, flushing, urticaria, diarrhea, nausea, vomiting, abdominal pain, headache, hypotension, anaphylaxis.

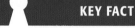

KEY FACT

Mastocytosis should be suspected when an **urticarial rash** is accompanied by abdominal (eg, diarrhea), lymphatic (eg, splenomegaly), or anaphylactic signs and symptoms.

EXAM

Presents with **urticaria pigmentosa** (a pigmented macular skin rash that urticates with stroking) as well as with lymphadenopathy, hepatomegaly, and splenomegaly.

DIFFERENTIAL

- **Anaphylaxis:** Drugs, foods, venoms, exercise induced, idiopathic.
- **Flushing syndromes:** Scombroid, carcinoid, VIPoma, pheochromocytoma.
- **Shock:** Cardiogenic, hemorrhagic, endotoxic.
- **Angioedema:** Hereditary or acquired.
- **Other:** Panic attack.

DIAGNOSIS

Diagnosed by the presence of one major plus one minor or three minor criteria.

- **Major criteria:** Characteristic multifocal dense **infiltrates of mast cells on bone marrow** biopsy.
- **Minor criteria:**
  - Spindle-shaped morphology of mast cells on **tissue biopsy.**
  - Detection of the **c-kit mutation.**
  - **Flow cytometry** of bone marrow mast cells coexpressing CD117, CD2, and CD25.
  - **Serum tryptase** levels of > 20 ng/mL.

TREATMENT

- H_1 and H_2 antagonists.
- Epinephrine for episodes of anaphylaxis.
- Topical steroids for skin lesions; oral corticosteroids for advanced disease.
- Hematopoietic stem cell transplantation or chemotherapy for patients with aggressive disease or associated hematologic disorders.

1° Immunodeficiency in Adults

A 32-year-old man presents to his primary care physician for cough and fever and is noted on CXR to have a right middle lobe pneumonia. This is the fourth time in the past 18 months that he has presented with pneumonia requiring antibiotics, and he has also had several sinus infections that have necessitated treatment over this time. Laboratory evaluation shows normal IgG levels, including all subclasses, and an undetectable IgA level. What is the appropriate treatment for this patient?

Vaccination and antibiotics as needed. The patient has selective IgA deficiency. There is no role for IVIG in this patient in light of its unclear benefit and potential adverse reactions. The patient should be monitored for potential complications such as lymphoproliferative diseases and celiac disease. Patients with evidence of celiac disease by history will have ⊖ serologies (which are IgA antibodies) and will require endoscopy for diagnosis.

Adult 1° immunodeficiencies (non-HIV) generally present in the second or third decade of life with **recurrent respiratory infections** due to antibody deficiency (hypogammaglobulinemia). Conditions include **common variable immunodeficiency (CVID)**, **selective IgA deficiency** (most common, with an incidence of 1:500), IgG subclass deficiency, and selective antibody deficiency with normal immunoglobulins (SADNI).

SYMPTOMS

- Presents with frequent **respiratory tract infections** (sinusitis, otitis, pneumonia); a need for IV or prolonged oral antibiotic courses to clear infections; and **chronic GI symptoms** such as diarrhea, cramping abdominal pain, and malabsorption.
- IgG subclass deficiency and selective IgA deficiency are often asymptomatic.

EXAM

Nasal congestion and discharge; respiratory wheezing or rales; digital clubbing 2° to chronic lung disease; lymphadenopathy; splenomegaly.

DIFFERENTIAL

- Hypogammaglobulinemia due to loss (GI, renal).
- Hypogammaglobulinemia due to medications (immunosuppressants, anticonvulsants).
- HIV, CF, allergic respiratory disease.

DIAGNOSIS

- A **history** of recurrent infection.
- **Antibody deficiency by laboratory testing:** Order quantitative immunoglobulins initially (IgG, IgA, IgM), after which IgG subclasses may be obtained.
    - **CVID: Low IgG** (< 500 mg/dL), usually with low IgA and/or IgM.
    - **Selective IgA deficiency: Absence of IgA** (< 7 mg/dL) **with normal IgG** and IgM (the most common 1° immunodeficiency).
    - **IgG subclass deficiency:** Low levels of one or more IgG subclasses (IgG1, IgG2, IgG3, IgG4). Clinical significance is unclear.
    - **SADNI:** Normal immunoglobulin levels with failure to produce protective antibody levels against specific immunizations (most commonly pneumococcus; rarely tetanus).
- Exclude other causes of hypogammaglobulinemia (antibody loss due to protein-losing enteropathy or nephropathy, medication, lymphopenia).

TREATMENT

- **CVID:**
    - **IVIG** 400–500 mg/kg monthly.
    - Aggressive treatment of infection.
    - Monitor lung function; pulmonary hygiene for bronchiectasis.
- **Selective IgA deficiency:**
    - **Antibiotic therapy and/or prophylaxis** as necessary.
    - **IVIG is contraindicated** owing to possible anti-IgA IgE antibody.
    - Patients should receive only **washed blood products** in view of the **risk of anaphylaxis** with exposure to IgA.

KEY FACT

Suspect IgA deficiency in a patient with an anaphylactic reaction that occurs seconds to minutes after a blood transfusion. Treat by immediately administering epinephrine and discontinuing the transfusion.

- **IgG subclass deficiency and SADNI:**
    - Antibiotic therapy as needed.
    - IVIG is reserved for rare patients with significant infection despite preventive antibiotics.

COMPLICATIONS

- **CVID:** Variable T-cell deficiency, **GI malignancy** (gastric cancer, small bowel lymphoma), **bronchiectasis, lymphoproliferative** disease, noncaseating granulomas of internal organs, **autoimmune disease.**
- **Selective IgA deficiency: Celiac disease, lymphoproliferative** disease, GI **malignancy** (gastric cancer, small bowel lymphoma), **autoimmune** disease.

NOTES

CHAPTER 2

Ambulatory Medicine

Christina A. Lee, MD
Nadine Dubowitz, MD

Screening for Common Diseases

HYPERLIPIDEMIA

> A 55-year-old man with hypertension presents for his annual checkup. On exam, his BP is 130/85 mm Hg, and routine labs show a total cholesterol level of 280 mg/dL, an LDL of 200 mg/dL, an HDL of 40 mg/dL, and a triglyceride level of 200 mg/dL with normal LFTs. What is your first-line treatment, and how will you counsel this patient?
>
> Counsel the patient on lifestyle modifications, including diet, exercise, and smoking cessation (if applicable). This patient has two cardiac risk factors, hypertension and age (male > 45), and his LDL goal should be < 130 mg/dL. Begin by initiating low-dose statin therapy. Counsel the patient about uncommon but possible side effects of statins, including muscle aches, myositis, and liver enzyme elevation. Repeat LFTs in eight weeks and with any new concerns such as muscle cramps.

Hyperlipidemia is a risk factor for CAD, stroke, and peripheral vascular disease. Major risk factors for CAD are as follows:

- Age (men > 45, women > 55), cigarette smoking, hypertension, a family history of premature CAD (in a first-degree male relative < 55 years of age or female relative < 65 years of age), HDL < 40 mg/dL (HDL > 60 mg/dL is protective).
- Risk factor equivalents to CAD include DM and symptomatic noncoronary atherosclerotic disease (eg, carotid artery disease, peripheral arterial disease, abdominal aortic aneurysm).

DIAGNOSIS

- Obtain a fasting total cholesterol, LDL, HDL, and triglycerides (TG).
- The United States Preventive Services Task Force (USPSTF) recommends screening all men ≥ 35 years of age and all women ≥ 45 years of age. Begin screening at age 20 if any major cardiovascular risk factors are present.
- The National Cholesterol Education Program Adult Treatment Panel III (ATP III) recommends that adults ≥ 20 years of age be screened at least once every five years.
- The optimal age at which to stop screening is unknown. There is insufficient evidence to support the screening of patients > 65 years of age unless multiple cardiovascular risk factors are present.

TREATMENT

- Therapeutic lifestyle changes (TLC) are indicated for all patients with an LDL above the goal LDL level. Such changes include a low-saturated-fat, low-cholesterol, high-fiber diet; plant stanols/sterols (eg, vegetable oil, nuts, legumes, whole grains, vegetables, fruits, and supplements); and ↑ physical activity.
- Cholesterol-lowering medications are appropriate for patients who are at high or moderately high risk for CAD or for those who have not reached their LDL goal after three months of TLC. **Statins** are considered first-line therapy by virtue of their improved clinical cardiovascular outcomes.

KEY FACT

Combining statins and fibrates ↑ the risk of myositis and rhabdomyolysis. Muscle toxicity may occur in 1–5% of patients treated with both a statin and gemfibrozil.

KEY FACT

The goal of therapy is to reduce LDL by 30–40%, which reduces CAD risk by 30–40%. For patients at high cardiovascular risk, the goal is < 100 mg/dL.

KEY FACT

Myalgias occur in a minority of patients who take statins, but myositis with ↑ CK and rhabdomyolysis with renal failure are rare. Treat by stopping the statin and providing supportive care.

TABLE 2.1. **Drugs Used for the Treatment of Hyperlipidemia**

Drug Class	Examples/ Comments	LDL	HDL	TG	Applications	Adverse Effects
HMG-CoA reductase inhibitors	Statins (eg, atorvastatin, simvastatin, pravastatin).	↓↓	↑	↓	**First-line** medication for lowering the risk of cardiovascular events in most patients requiring lipid-lowering medication. Primarily lower LDL.	Elevated LFTs, myositis. **Myositis is more common when fibrates, and possibly niacin, are used with a statin.** Monitor LFTs and CK.
Niacin (nicotinic acid)	B vitamin; ↓ lipoprotein (a).	↓	↑↑	↓↓	Raise HDL; lower TG and LDL **(near-ideal effects on lipid profile).**	**Flushing** limits use (affects > 50% of patients; ↓ with ASA). Can exacerbate gout and PUD; can cause elevated liver enzymes and blood glucose.
Fibrates	Gemfibrozil, fenofibrate.	↓	↑	↓↓	Hypertriglyceridemia.	Gallstones, hepatitis, myositis (especially when used with statins).
Bile acid–binding resins	Cholestyramine.	↓↓	↑	↑	Used to treat elevated LDL only. The only lipid-lowering medication that is **safe in pregnancy.**	GI upset (bloating/gas, constipation); impaired absorption of fat-soluble vitamins and some medications; worsening of high TG.
Ezetimibe	Inhibitor of intestinal cholesterol transporter.	↓	↑	↓	Used to treat elevated LDL. Often **used with a statin** when LDL goal is not reached with a statin alone, although clinical benefits are unclear.	Elevated LFTs when used in combination with statins.

- Table 2.1 identifies the effects of and indications for the major classes of cholesterol-lowering agents. Table 2.2 identifies risk categories that determine LDL cholesterol goals.

DIABETES MELLITUS (DM)

- The American Diabetes Association (ADA) recommends that DM screening be conducted every three years for those ≥ 45 years of age. However, the USPSTF states that evidence is insufficient to recommend for or against DM screening except in patients with hypertension or hyperlipidemia.
- The ADA's diagnostic criteria include any of the following:
    - A hemoglobin A_{1c} (HbA_{1c}) ≥ 6.5%. **This is a new recommendation by the ADA.**
    - A **fasting blood glucose level ≥ 126 mg/dL.**
    - **Symptoms of DM** (polyuria, polydipsia, weight loss) and a random blood glucose level ≥ 200 mg/dL.
    - A two-hour blood glucose level ≥ 200 mg/dL during an oral glucose **tolerance test.**
- "Impaired fasting glucose" is defined as a fasting blood glucose level of 110–126 mg/dL.

KEY FACT

Although niacin is a "jack of all trades" medication, its negative impact on skin flushing, gout, PUD, diabetes, and liver disease can limit its use. Taking ASA 30 minutes before taking niacin can ↓ flushing.

TABLE 2.2. **LDL Goals and Treatment Thresholds**[a]

Risk Category	Definition	LDL Goal	Initiate TLC[b]	Consider Drug Therapy
High risk	CAD or CAD risk equivalents (10-year risk > 20%).	< 100 mg/dL (optional goal < 70 mg/dL)	≥ 100 mg/dL	≥ 130 mg/dL (100–129 mg/dL: drug optional).
Moderate risk	Two or more risk factors (10-year risk < 20%).	< 130 mg/dL	≥ 130 mg/dL	≥ 130 mg/dL if 10-year risk is 10–20%. ≥ 160 mg/dL if 10-year risk is < 10%.
Lower risk	0–1 risk factor.	< 160 mg/dL	≥ 160 mg/dL	≥ 190 mg/dL (160–189 mg/dL: LDL-lowering drug optional).

[a]Derived from recommendations from the ATP III, 2004.

[b]TLC measures include a low-fat, low-cholesterol, high-fiber diet; weight control; and exercise.

- An HbA_{1c} of 5.7–6.4% is associated with an ↑ risk of developing DM. The HbA_{1c} treatment goal is < 7%.

ABDOMINAL AORTIC ANEURYSM (AAA)

- The USPSTF recommends one-time AAA screening for men 65–75 years of age who have ever smoked. The preferred modality is ultrasound (see Figure 2.1).
- Surgical repair of AAAs ≥ 5.5 cm ↓ AAA-specific mortality in this population.

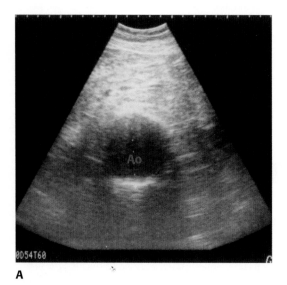

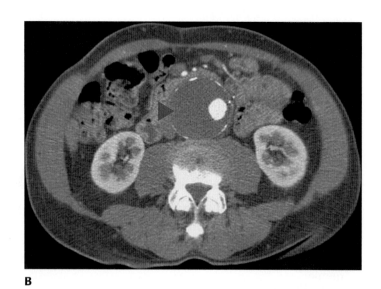

A   **B**

FIGURE 2.1. **Abdominal aortic aneurysm.** (A) Bedside ultrasound image of a 6.5-cm abdominal aortic aneurysm (Ao = aorta). (B) Transaxial image from a contrast-enhanced CT showing a 5.5-cm aneurysm with extensive mural thrombus (arrowhead). (Image A reproduced with permission from Tintinalli JE et al. *Tintinalli's Emergency Medicine: A Comprehensive Study Guide,* 6th ed. New York: McGraw-Hill, 2004, Fig. 58-2. Image B reproduced with permission from Doherty GM. *Current Diagnosis & Treatment: Surgery,* 13th ed. New York: McGraw-Hill, 2010, Fig. 34-16.)

Cancer Screening

Refer to Table 2.3 for an overview of USPSTF cancer screening guidelines.

BREAST CANCER

The most common cancer in all major ethnic groups. Caucasians have the highest rates of breast cancer, followed by African Americans, but the highest mortality rates are found among African Americans. The strongest risk factors are age (> 40 years) and gender (female). Other risk factors include the following:

- A personal history of invasive or in situ breast cancer (associated with an ↑ risk of invasive breast cancer in the contralateral breast).
- A family history, particularly of premenopausal breast cancer, in one or more first-degree relatives.
- ⊕ mutations of BRCA1 or BRCA2.
- Current or prior use of HRT (> 5 years).
- Early menarche (< 12 years); later menopause (> 55 years); later pregnancy (age at first birth > 30 years). ↑ estrogen exposure leads to a higher risk of breast cancer.
- A previous breast biopsy with proliferative changes (eg, complex fibroadenoma, moderate hyperplasia), especially with cytologic atypia, on breast biopsy.
- Heavy alcohol use.
- Obesity (for postmenopausal breast cancer).
- OCP use is probably not a risk factor in average-risk women but may be in those with a ⊕ family history.

SCREENING

Screening recommendations based on USPSTF guidelines are as follows:

- **Mammography: Biennial (not annual) screening** is recommended for women 50–74 years of age. The decision to screen women < 50 years of age should be individualized and should incorporate the patient's values regarding relative benefits and harms, as the mortality benefit is small and the risk of false ⊕s high. There is insufficient evidence to assess screening in women ≥ 75 years of age.
  - The sensitivity of mammography is approximately 90% and is higher in older than in younger women.
  - There is insufficient evidence to recommend digital mammography or MRI over film mammography.
- **Breast self-examination (BSE):** Not shown to have benefit. Recommend against teaching BSE.
- **Clinical breast examination (CBE):** There is insufficient evidence to recommend for or against CBE.
- **Genetic counseling** and consideration of BRCA1/BRCA2 mutation testing are recommended for those with the following risk factors:
  - A family history of breast cancer in two or more first-degree relatives (at least one premenopausal) or three or more first- or second-degree relatives.
  - Breast and ovarian cancer in the same patient or in any first- and second-degree relatives in the patient's family.

KEY FACT

Breast cancer screening in women 40–49 years of age remains a controversial issue, and physicians and patients should engage in shared decision making. Previously, the USPSTF recommended that screening start at age 40.

KEY FACT

Lifestyle modifications to ↓ breast cancer risk:
- ↓ the duration of HRT use.
- Have first child at an earlier age.
- Avoid adult weight gain.
- ↓ alcohol intake.

KEY FACT

Testing for BRCA1 and BRCA2 mutations should not be performed without prior genetic counseling. It should be considered only for women with family histories highly suggestive of a genetic susceptibility to breast and/or ovarian cancer.

TABLE 2.3. USPSTF Cancer Screening Guidelines

	BREAST	COLON	CERVIX	PROSTATE
Target population	All women.	All women and men.	All women who have ever had sex and who have a cervix.	All men.
Strength of recommendation[a]	B	A	A	I
Age to start	Age 50. Screening between 40 and 49 years of age is controversial and should be an individual decision made by patients and their physicians.	Age 50.	Within three years of onset of sexual activity or age 21, whichever comes first.	The men most likely to benefit are those $\geq$ 50 years of age. Men with risk factors should consider starting at age 40–45.
Age to stop	Age 74, although women $\geq$ 75 years of age may still benefit if they do not have significant comorbid disease.	Age 75. Consider screening patients between 76 and 85 years of age if there are no significant comorbid conditions. Screening is not recommended in patients > 85 years of age.	Age 65 if a woman has had regular screening with normal results and is not otherwise at high risk.	Screening is not recommended for men $\geq$ 75 years of age.
Screening modality	Mammography.	Fecal occult blood testing (FOBT) annually, flexible sigmoidoscopy every 5 years, or colonoscopy every 10 years. Each has different risks and advantages; there is no clear best test. There is insufficient evidence for CT colonography and fecal DNA testing.	Pap smear. There is insufficient evidence to recommend for or against newer modalities, including HPV testing.	PSA +/– DRE (PSA is more sensitive).
Frequency of screening	Every two years.	**FOBT:** Annual. **Flexible sigmoidoscopy:** Every 5 years. **Colonoscopy:** Every 10 years.	At least every three years.	If screening has benefit, every year.

[a]Strength of USPSTF recommendations: A—strongly recommended. B—recommended. C—no recommendation for or against. D—against recommendation. I—insufficient evidence.

- A family history of male breast cancer or of women with bilateral breast cancer.
- Ashkenazi Jewish heritage plus a first-degree relative (or two second-degree relatives) with breast or ovarian cancer.

PREVENTION

- Women with mutations of BRCA1 or BRCA2 should undergo intensive surveillance and may consider prophylactic mastectomy and/or oophorectomy.
- Tamoxifen and raloxifene are selective estrogen receptor modulators (SERMs) that may ↓ the risk of invasive breast cancer in **high-risk** patients > 35 years of age. Adverse effects include an ↑ risk of thromboembolism (tamoxifen > raloxifene) and uterine cancer.

CERVICAL CANCER

Caused by high-risk types of human papillomavirus (HPV-16 and -18). HPV is an STD, and **risk factors** include multiple sexual partners, early onset of intercourse, other STDs, smoking, low socioeconomic status, and HIV/immunosuppression.

SCREENING

USPSTF guidelines for Pap screening are as follows:

- Screen sexually active women at least every three years starting at age 21 or within three years of the onset of sexual activity, whichever comes first. Those with known risk factors or a history of abnormal Pap smears should be screened annually.
- Stop screening at age 65 in women who have had adequate prior screening with normal results and who are otherwise at low risk. Older women who have not had a recent Pap test should be screened.
- There is no need to screen those who had a total hysterectomy that was done for benign reasons.
- HPV serotype testing for high-risk strains on Pap smear is FDA approved as an adjunct to Pap smears in women ≥ 30 years of age. The USPSTF states that more evidence is needed to evaluate the utility of HPV plus Pap testing as a 1° testing strategy.
- Abnormalities on Pap smear are followed up with diagnostic colposcopy and biopsy.

PREVENTION

- Safer sexual practices (barrier contraceptives, fewer sexual partners) may help prevent cervical cancer.
- A vaccine against HPV strains 6, 11, 16, and 18 has been developed and is recommended for all women and girls aged 9–26 (see the discussion of immunizations below). Pap smear screening remains the same in vaccinated and unvaccinated patients.

COLORECTAL CANCER

A 45-year-old Caucasian man presents for a routine checkup. He is healthy and takes no medications. His father was diagnosed with colon cancer at 52 years of age. He wants to know if he should undergo colon cancer screening.

With a family history of colon cancer before age 50, this patient should begin colon cancer screening 10 years prior to his father's colon cancer diagnosis. Thus, he should have started screening at age 42. He can select from any cancer screening modality, but given his strong family history, colonoscopy would generally be preferred.

KEY FACT

In high-risk patients, consider tamoxifen and raloxifene (SERMs) to ↓ the risk of invasive breast cancer.

KEY FACT

Screening for colorectal, breast, and cervical cancer has been proven to reduce mortality. Screening for prostate cancer has not been shown to lower mortality.

- There is no one "best" screening modality for colorectal cancer ("any screening is better than no screening"). Options include annual FOBT, flexible sigmoidoscopy every 5 years, or colonoscopy every 10 years.
- Screening should begin at age 50. High-risk patients should begin colonoscopy screening at age 40, or 10 years before the youngest affected relative was diagnosed.
- Risks for colon cancer include a personal or strong family history of colorectal cancer or adenomatous polyps, and a family history of hereditary colon cancer syndromes (familial adenomatous polyposis, hereditary non-polyposis colon cancer).
- There is insufficient evidence to recommend newer screening technologies such as CT colonography ("virtual colonoscopy") or fecal DNA.

PROSTATE CANCER

- Screening with serum PSA testing and DRE are controversial because of their **lack of proven effectiveness in improving health outcomes or mortality.** The USPSTF states that there is insufficient evidence to recommend for or against PSA and/or DRE.
- Most groups recommend that physicians **discuss both the potential advantages of PSA screening (early detection of possibly harmful cancers) and its disadvantages** (false-⊕ and false-⊖ results, overdiagnosis of highly indolent cancers, more biopsies, anxiety, morbidity associated with prostate cancer treatment).
- Consider screening men if they are ≥ 50 years of age and are expected to live at least 10 years. Begin at a younger age (40–45 years) if patients are at ↑ risk (eg, African American men, those with a first-degree relative with prostate cancer, those with the BRCA1 or BRCA2 mutation).

OTHER CANCERS

The USPSTF makes no recommendations for routine screening of lung, ovarian, or other cancers.

Immunizations

 A 26-year-old woman in her first trimester of pregnancy asks about routine vaccinations. She is already immune to measles, mumps, and rubella (MMR) but is not immune to varicella. Which vaccinations should she receive?
Do not give live attenuated vaccines, including varicella and MMR, during pregnancy. This patient should receive inactivated influenza vaccine if her pregnancy will extend during the fall and winter seasons. If indicated, tetanus, diphtheria, and acellular pertussis (Td and Tdap) can also be given during pregnancy.

Table 2.4 describes the indications for and uses of common vaccines.

TABLE 2.4. **Adult Immunization Recommendations**

Vaccine	Indications	Schedule	Special Considerations
Td/Tdap	All adults.	Td booster every 10 years. 1° series of three doses for adults with an uncertain history of 1° vaccination. A single dose of Tdap should be given once, in place of Td, to adults < 65 years of age.	Give Tdap as soon as two years after the last Td for adults in close contact with infants < 12 months of age (eg, immediately postpartum) as well as to all health care workers.
HPV	Women and girls 9–26 years of age regardless of any prior history of HPV infection, genital warts, or cervical dysplasia.	Three doses at 0, 2, and 6 months. Vaccinate at 11 or 12 years of age with catch-up vaccination between 13 and 26 years.	Ideally, should be administered before the onset of sexual activity. Not recommended during pregnancy.
Herpes zoster (shingles)	Adults > 60 years of age, whether or not they have had a prior episode of VZV.	One dose.	Contraindicated in severely immunocompromised patients (eg, those with advanced HIV, with a hematologic malignancy, or on high-dose chronic steroids).
MMR	Adults born after 1957 without documentation of prior vaccination. Particular targets for vaccination include college students, health care workers, international travelers, and women of childbearing age.	One or two doses. A second dose is recommended for those at risk for measles or mumps (eg, students, health care workers, travelers).	Contraindicated in pregnancy and in immunodeficiency states.
Varicella	Adults without a clinical history of varicella, ⊕ titers, or a history of vaccination. Target close contacts of immunocompromised patients and patients at high risk of exposure/transmission (health care/child care workers, institutional staff and residents, college students, women of childbearing age).	Two doses 1–2 months apart.	Contraindicated during pregnancy and in the setting of immunosuppression (including all HIV-infected patients).
Seasonal influenza	All adults ≥ 50 years of age; any adult < 50 years of age with chronic cardiopulmonary disease; health care workers; pregnant women; household contacts or caregivers of young children.	One dose annually.	Healthy, nonpregnant persons 5–49 years of age who are not in contact with immunocompromised patients may receive either **intranasal** or inactivated vaccine. All others should receive inactivated vaccine only.

(continues)

TABLE 2.4. **Adult Immunization Recommendations** *(continued)*

Vaccine	Indications	Schedule	Special Considerations
Pneumococcal (polysaccharide)	All adults ≥ 65 years of age. Adults < 65 years of age with chronic pulmonary disorders (excluding asthma), cardiovascular disease, DM, chronic liver or renal disease, asplenia, or immunosuppression as well as those who are nursing home residents.	One dose for those > 65 years of age at initial vaccination. A second dose at five years is recommended for patients with renal failure, asplenia, or immunosuppression. Give a second dose at 65 years of age (or five years after the first dose) if the first dose was given at < 65 years of age.	The vaccine should be given at least two weeks before elective splenectomy.
Hepatitis A	Chronic liver disease, recipients of clotting factor concentrates, men who have sex with men (MSM), illicit drug users, health care workers in contact with infected individuals, travelers to endemic areas.	Two doses 6–12 months apart.	
Hepatitis B	Renal failure/dialysis, HIV, chronic liver disease, those at risk for STDs (MSM, those not in a long-term, mutually monogamous relationship), health care workers, IV drug users, recipients of factor concentrates, household contacts of HBV-infected individuals.	Three doses (0, 1–2 months, 4–6 months).	Should be offered to any adult seeking protection against HBV.
Meningococcal	Those with asplenia (anatomic or functional) or terminal complement deficiency; college students living in dorms; travelers to endemic areas.	One dose. Consider a second dose at five years for those given polysaccharide vaccine.	

[a]Derived from guidelines established by the Centers for Disease Control and Prevention, 2010.

Obesity and Metabolic Syndrome

OBESITY

Defined as a body mass index (BMI) ≥ 30. Risk factors include gender (female), increasing age, ethnicity (African Americans, Hispanics, Native Americans), and prolonged residency in the United States. Obesity ↑ morbidity and mortality, particularly from complications of hypertension, type 2 DM, hyperlipidemia, CAD, osteoarthritis, sleep apnea, steatohepatitis, and psychosocial disorders.

DIFFERENTIAL

- Hypothyroidism, Cushing's syndrome, polycystic ovarian syndrome, medications (steroids, insulin, atypical antipsychotics).
- Fewer than 1% of obese patients have an identifiable, nonpsychiatric cause of obesity.

DIAGNOSIS

The **BMI** reflects excess adipose tissue and is calculated by dividing measured body weight (kg) by height (meters squared). Definitions are as follows:

- **Normal:** 18.5–24.9.
- **Overweight:** 25.0–29.9.
- **Obesity:** ≥ 30.0–39.9.
- **Extreme obesity:** ≥ 40.

TREATMENT

- **Lifestyle modification and diet:**
  - Weight loss improves type 2 DM, hypertension, cardiovascular risk, and hyperlipidemia (HDL, TG).
  - A multidisciplinary approach combining a reduction in caloric intake, ↑ aerobic exercise, and social support optimizes the maintenance of weight loss.
  - Diets include very low calorie diets (< 800 kcal/day) and low-carbohydrate diets (eg, Atkins). Low-carbohydrate, low-fat diets and calorie-restricted diets have similar outcomes. Although short-term weight loss occurs, the long-term effectiveness of diets is generally poor. Programs that focus on long-term healthy eating habits, rather than short-term solutions, are generally more effective.
- **Medications:**
  - Consider pharmacotherapy in patients with a BMI ≥ 30 or in those with a BMI ≥ 27 with medical complications (hypertension, DM, hyperlipidemia). Avoid sibutramine in the setting of uncontrolled hypertension. Indications for pharmacotherapy are listed in Table 2.5.
  - A course of medication for 6–12 months in conjunction with dietary modification leads to ↑ weight loss when compared to a placebo, but the long-term efficacy of such treatment has not been established.

TABLE 2.5. Commonly Used FDA-Approved Obesity Medications

Drug	Mechanism of Action	Side Effects
Sibutramine	Inhibits the uptake of serotonin and norepinephrine in the CNS (catecholaminergic).	**Adrenergic-like symptoms: Hypertension,** ↑ heart rate, dry mouth, anorexia, constipation, insomnia, dizziness.
Orlistat	Inhibits intestinal lipase; ↓ fat absorption.	**Malabsorption:** Fatty stools, gas, cramping.

KEY FACT

Consider surgery for patients with a BMI ≥ 40 or for those with a BMI ≥ 35 plus obesity-related medical complications.

- Bariatric surgery:
    - Bariatric surgery is more effective than other options for achieving long-term weight loss. Surgery leads to weight reduction and improvement of comorbidities such as DM, hypertension, hyperlipidemia, and sleep apnea.
    - Surgical procedures include gastric banding, gastric bypass (Roux-en-Y), gastroplasty, and duodenal switch procedures.
    - **Indications for bariatric surgery include a BMI ≥ 40 (severe obesity) or a BMI ≥ 35 with obesity-related medical complications.**
    - Perioperative mortality ranges from 0.1% to 1.1% depending on the surgical procedure.
    - Long-term complications of surgery include dumping syndrome, anastomotic stenosis, vitamin B_{12}/iron/vitamin D deficiencies, cholecystitis, and gastritis.

METABOLIC SYNDROME

Present in approximately 60% of obese individuals; confers a threefold risk of CAD. Also associated with an ↑ risk of type 2 DM due to insulin resistance.

DIAGNOSIS

The diagnosis of metabolic syndrome requires three or more of the following:

- **Central or visceral fat:** Elevated abdominal circumference (≥ 40 inches in men, ≥ 35 inches in women) ↑ cardiovascular risk.
- Elevated BP (≥ 130/80).
- Elevated TG (≥ 150 mg/dL or on drug treatment to lower TG).
- Elevated fasting blood glucose (≥ 100 mg/dL).
- Low HDL cholesterol (< 40 mg/dL in men; < 50 mg/dL in women).

TREATMENT

- The goal is to ↓ the risk of clinical atherosclerotic disease and to prevent the onset of type 2 DM.
- Intensive lifestyle change is effective at reducing the rates and complications of metabolic syndrome. Glucophage may ↓ the incidence of developing diabetes but does not appear to be as effective as lifestyle modification.
- Cardiovascular risk factors (lipids, blood glucose, BP) should be closely monitored and well controlled in these patients.

KEY FACT

Intensive lifestyle change, including weight loss, exercise, and a healthy diet, is key to managing metabolic syndrome and preventing clinical atherosclerosis and type 2 DM.

Nutritional and Herbal Supplements

- Vitamin and other nutritional deficiencies are discussed in the Hematology chapter.
- Table 2.6 lists the potential benefits of some common nutritional supplements. Table 2.7 outlines common herbal supplements along with their clinical uses and side effects.
- The level of evidence to support commonly used herbal treatments is poor to fair, and none is currently recommended over FDA-approved medications.
- Because herbs and supplements are not regulated in the same way as prescription drugs, their purity and potency are highly variable.

TABLE 2.6. Effects of Selected Dietary Supplements

Supplement	Clinical Uses	Efficacy
Glucosamine and chondroitin	Osteoarthritis.	Unclear; meta-analyses have shown benefit for pain and function, but the largest randomized clinical trials (RCTs) have not shown improvement over placebo.
Calcium and vitamin D	Prevention and treatment of osteoporosis; prevention of colorectal cancer.	Vitamin D (800 IU/day) ↓ fracture risk. Adequate dietary or supplemental calcium is recommended. The benefits for colorectal cancer are unclear.
Vitamin E	Antioxidant; possible prevention of atherosclerosis; possible slowing of the natural course of Alzheimer's disease.	Ineffective for vascular disease prevention.
Omega-3 fatty acids	Cholesterol lowering; prevention of atherosclerotic disease.	No clear benefit in the prevention of cardiovascular disease, cancer, or overall mortality.
Folic acid	Prevention of neural tube defects; prevention of atherosclerotic disease (through lowering of homocysteine levels).	Doses of 0.4 mg/day or higher are clearly effective in preventing neural tube defects and should be recommended to all women who may become pregnant. Doses of 4 mg/day are recommended for women taking antiepileptic medications during pregnancy. Several trials have shown no benefit in reducing the rate of clinical atherosclerotic disease despite lowered homocysteine levels.
Fiber supplements	Possible prevention of diverticulosis and colon cancer; cholesterol and blood sugar lowering.	Epidemiologic studies suggest a benefit from high-fiber diets, but RCT data are limited.
Soy protein	Relief of menopausal symptoms.	Possibly effective at high doses, especially from dietary sources.

TABLE 2.7. Common Herbal Supplements

Herb	Condition	Efficacy	Side Effects
Ginkgo biloba	Dementia, claudication.	No clear benefit for the prevention of memory decline or for claudication symptoms.	**May have an anticoagulant effect.** Stop this herb one week before surgery.
Echinacea	Prevention and treatment of the common cold.	May ↓ the duration and likelihood of developing URIs.	Rash, pruritus, nausea.
Saw palmetto	BPH.	A recent meta-analysis suggests no improvement in urinary symptoms or flow compared to a placebo.	Mild GI upset, headaches (rare).
St. John's wort	Depression.	May be superior to a placebo and similar to antidepressants in patients with major depression.	**Induces cytochrome P-450,** thus decreasing some drug levels (eg, warfarin, digoxin, OCPs, antiretrovirals). Cannot be combined with prescription antidepressants because of the risk of serotonin syndrome.
Kava	Anxiety, stress, insomnia.	Appears to be efficacious for short-term treatment of anxiety. Longer-term studies are needed.	Sedation, especially in combination with alcohol. There have been several cases of severe hepatotoxicity.
Black cohosh	Menopausal symptoms.	No demonstrated benefit in reducing vasomotor symptoms.	May have estrogenic effects.
Red clover	Menopausal symptoms.	No demonstrated benefit in reducing vasomotor symptoms.	As with other phytoestrogens, red clover should be avoided in patients at ↑ risk for breast cancer.

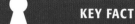

KEY FACT

Hypertrophic cardiomyopathy is the leading cause of sudden cardiac death in young athletes.

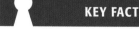

KEY FACT

Commotio cordis, or sudden death due to direct blunt trauma to the chest wall and myocardium, is more common in children and is caused by precipitation of a PVC initiating a tachyarrhythmia.

Athletic Screening for Adolescents

Although rare, sudden death may occur in competitive athletes as a result of **hypertrophic cardiomyopathy** (36%), **coronary anomalies** (19%), LVH, a ruptured aorta (Marfan's syndrome), and other rare congenital or acquired cardiac diseases. Students should be evaluated before they participate in high school and college athletics and every two years during competition. Evaluation should include the following:

- A careful history and physical exam focusing on cardiovascular risk factors, symptoms, and findings.
- An ECG and echocardiogram in the presence of the following:
  - A family history of premature sudden death or cardiovascular disease.
  - Symptoms of chest pain, dyspnea on exercise, syncope, or near-syncope.
  - An elevated BP or abnormalities on cardiac exam (eg, murmur or a history of murmur).
  - Marfan-like appearance (tall stature with long arms/legs/fingers).

Health Care Workers and Disease Exposure/Prevention

A 27-year-old resident physician sustains a needlestick that occurred during a central line placement for a patient who is HIV and HBsAg ⊕. The needlestick occurred two hours ago and penetrated through the resident's latex glove and into his subcutaneous tissue. He rinsed out the wound. What should you advise at this time?

The resident should have his baseline HBV, HCV, and HIV status confirmed. Assuming that he is immune to HBV, all he needs to receive is HIV postexposure prophylaxis with antiretrovirals. If he were not immune to HBV, he would need to receive the HBV vaccine and HBV immunoglobulin immediately.

- TB is commonly transmitted in health care settings. All health care workers should have annual PPD testing and screening for symptoms of active TB.
- Vaccines routinely recommended for health care workers include hepatitis B, MMR, varicella (if not immune from natural infection), influenza, and Tdap.
- Blood-borne viruses—particularly HBV, HCV, and HIV—are the most common infections acquired by needlestick injuries.
- In the event of a needlestick or other percutaneous exposure, urgent assessment is warranted and includes the following measures:
  - Clean the wound thoroughly.
  - Test the exposed worker for HBV (both active infection [HBV surface antigen] and immunity [HBV antibody]), HCV, and HIV.
  - Obtain a history that includes exposure type, the infection status of the source patient (by history and/or laboratory testing), and the vaccination history of the exposed worker.
  - Counsel the worker about the risk of infection and about the risks and benefits of postexposure prophylaxis with antiretrovirals to prevent HIV and/or HBV vaccination/HBIG to prevent HBV if not immune.

KEY FACT

Remember the **"rule of 3's"** for occupational needlestick exposure—the likelihood of needlestick transmission is 30% for HBV, 3% for HCV, and 0.3% for HIV.

Ophthalmology

A 46-year-old woman presents with one day of moderate pain and redness in her right eye. She also has blurry vision, tearing, and photophobia. On exam, her left eye shows conjunctival injection around the cornea, and her acuity is ↓. The cornea is constricted, and intraocular pressure is normal. On slit lamp exam, cells and flares are present in the chamber, and there are deposits on the posterior corneal surface. What is the most appropriate management for this patient?

This patient has anterior uveitis. Although most cases are idiopathic, rheumatologic causes include HLA-B27-associated diseases, trauma, juvenile RA, sarcoidosis, and Behçet's disease. Infections can also cause uveitis. Workup should include CBC, ANA, ESR, Lyme titer, PPD, CXR, and RPR. The patient should be urgently referred to an ophthalmologist.

RED EYE

■ Table 2.8 outlines common causes of red eye, including the following:
  ■ **Conjunctivitis:** The three main etiologies are bacterial, viral, and allergic (see Figures 2.2 and 2.3).

TABLE 2.8. **Common Causes of Red Eye**

	VIRAL CONJUNCTIVITIS	**ALLERGIC CONJUNCTIVITIS**	**BACTERIAL CONJUNCTIVITIS**	**UVEITIS**	**KERATITIS**	**ACUTE ANGLE-CLOSURE GLAUCOMA**
Incidence	Extremely common, especially after URI (adenovirus).	Common.	Common.	Common.	Common.	Uncommon.
Conjunctival injection and discharge	Unilateral or bilateral redness; watery discharge.	Bilateral redness, itching, and tearing; ropy discharge.	Unilateral redness; purulent discharge.	Circumcorneal redness (ciliary flush); no discharge.	Circumcorneal erythema.	Ciliary flush; no discharge.
Pain, photophobia, vision changes	None.	None.	None.	Moderate pain, photophobia, blurred vision.	Pain, tearing, photophobia, ↓ vision. Purulent discharge in bacterial keratitis.	Severe pain, nausea, vomiting, ↓ visual acuity. Systemic symptoms include nausea and headache.
Cornea	Clear.	Clear.	Clear.	Usually clear. Hypopyon or hyphema may be present.	Hazy. Dendritic ulcer in HSV keratitis; punctate corneal lesions in bacterial keratitis.	Hazy or swollen ("steamy").
Pupil	Normal.	Normal.	Normal.	Constricted; possibly irregular; poor light response.	Normal or constricted.	Moderately dilated and fixed; no light response.
Intraocular pressure	Normal.	Normal.	Normal.	Normal.	Normal.	High.
Treatment	Symptomatic; cold compresses.	Cold compresses, antihistamine drops, topical ketorolac (an NSAID), topical mast cell stabilizer.	Erythromycin ointment; polymyxin-trimethoprim drops.	An emergency; refer to an ophthalmologist.	Urgent (viral, HSV) or emergent (bacterial) ophthalmology referral.	An emergency; refer to an ophthalmologist for laser iridectomy. Pupillary constriction (topical pilocarpine), pressure reduction (topical β-blockers, acetazolamide).

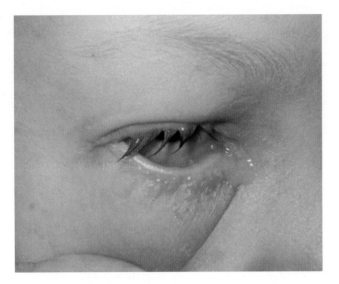

FIGURE 2.2. **Bacterial conjunctivitis.** Note the conjunctival injection and purulent discharge. (Reproduced with permission from USMLERx.com.)

- **Uveitis:** Often associated with systemic disease. The presence of eye pain or ↓ visual acuity should raise suspicion for uveitis in patients presenting with red eye. "**Ciliary flush**" on exam distinguishes this condition from conjunctivitis.
- **Acute angle-closure glaucoma:** Acute onset of pain and vision loss, often associated with headache, nausea, and vomiting. On exam, the pupil is midsized and does not react to light, and the cornea is "steamy" (see Figure 2.4).

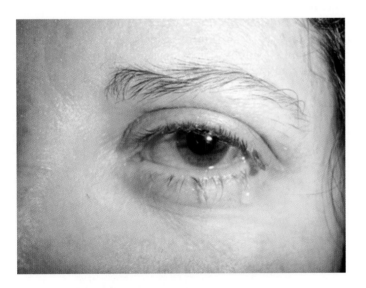

FIGURE 2.3. **Viral conjunctivitis.** Note the conjunctival injection and watery discharge. (Reproduced with permission from USMLERx.com.)

KEY FACT

All patients with a red eye and any of the following should be referred to an ophthalmologist emergently:
- Moderate to severe eye pain
- ↓ visual acuity
- Photophobia
- Pupillary abnormalities
- Ciliary flush (circumcorneal erythema)

KEY FACT

Refer a patient to ophthalmology emergently in the setting of red eye with profound eye pain or visual loss, severe nausea or vomiting and headache (acute-angle glaucoma), or a mid-dilated and fixed pupil.

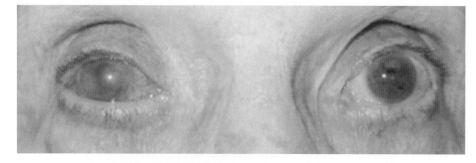

FIGURE 2.4. **Acute angle-closure glaucoma.** Note the firm, red right eye, hazy cornea, and dilated pupil. (Reproduced with permission from USMLERx.com.)

MNEMONIC

Causes of red eye—

GO SUCK

Glaucoma
Orbital disease
Scleritis
Uveitis
Conjunctivitis (viral, bacterial, allergic)
Keratitis (HSV)

KEY FACT

Bacterial keratitis is an important complication of corneal abrasions in contact lens wearers. It is commonly caused by *Pseudomonas* species and has an aggressive course. Contact lens wearers with corneal abrasions should receive prophylactic topical antibiotics and close follow-up.

- **Keratitis:** The most commonly tested etiology of red eye is **HSV keratitis,** which is usually unilateral and suggested by ↓ vision. Branching (dendritic) ulcers on fluorescein stain test are diagnostic.
- Additional etiologies of red eye include the following:
  - **Foreign body:** Characterized by sharp superficial pain. Perform a fluorescein test to rule out corneal abrasion.
  - **Gonorrheal conjunctivitis:** Presents with abrupt onset of redness and purulent discharge in sexually active adults.
  - **Chlamydial conjunctivitis:** Associated with chronic red eye in sexually active adults.
  - **Subconjunctival hemorrhage:** Spares the limbus (see Figure 2.5); common with trauma, prolonged coughing or vomiting, and anticoagulant use. Resolves spontaneously in 2–3 weeks.
  - **Hordeolum (stye):** Infection of Moll's glands along the lash line. Presents with localized erythema, **tenderness,** and swelling. Treat with warm compresses and topical antibiotics.
  - **Chalazion:** Chronic, granulomatous inflammation of the meibomian gland. Presents with hard, **nontender** swelling on the upper or lower lid. Treatment by an ophthalmologist consists of incision and curettage or corticosteroid injection.

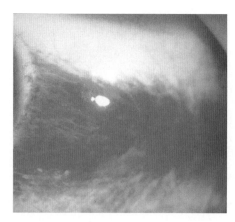

FIGURE 2.5. **Subconjunctival hemorrhage.** Although the sudden appearance of diffuse bright red discoloration is alarming to patients, this condition is benign. (Reproduced with permission from Riordan-Eva P, Whitcher JP. *Vaughan & Asbury's General Ophthalmology,* 17th ed. New York: McGraw-Hill, 2008, Fig. 5-24.)

LOSS OF VISION

A 73-year-old man with hypertension presents to his local urgent-care clinic with two days of sudden vision loss in his right eye. He has no pain. On exam, he can distinguish between light and dark but cannot distinguish movement. Funduscopic exam reveals a pale retina and a cherry-red spot in the macula. An afferent pupillary defect is also detected (paradoxical dilation of the pupil when light is moved from the unaffected eye to the affected eye). What is the diagnosis?

Retinal artery occlusion can present as painless, near-complete, monocular vision loss over seconds, which can be transient (amaurosis fugax) or permanent. This is an ophthalmologic emergency; permanent vision loss can occur without prompt treatment. Embolism is a common cause, as are other states such as atherosclerosis, thrombophilia (eg, OCPs), giant cell arteritis, and collagen vascular disease.

Vision loss is categorized as either acute or chronic.

- The etiologies of **acute loss of vision** include the following:
  - **Retinal artery occlusion:** An emergency characterized by sudden, **painless**, unilateral, near-complete blindness and by a **"cherry-red spot"** in the macula (see Figure 2.6). Can be associated with an afferent pupillary defect. Can be transient (amaurosis fugax, see below) or permanent. Commonly due to an embolus or associated with giant cell (temporal) arteritis.
  - **Amaurosis fugax (transient vision loss):** Most commonly caused by retinal or optic nerve ischemia from carotid thromboembolism. Patients complain that **"a curtain came down over my eye,"** usually for only a few minutes. Evaluate with carotid imaging (ultrasonography or

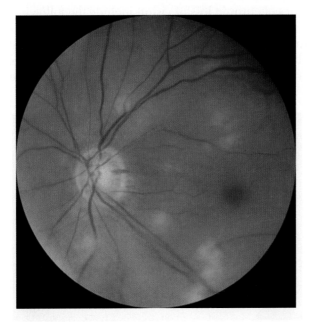

FIGURE 2.6.   Retinal artery occlusion. Color fundus photograph of the left eye demonstrates areas of ischemia ("cotton-wool" spots) and a "cherry-red" spot of the fovea—findings that strongly suggest ischemia to the inner retina, as would be found in a central retinal artery occlusion. (Reproduced with permission from USMLERx.com.)

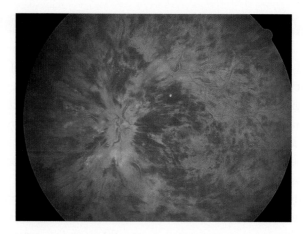

FIGURE 2.7. **Retinal vein occlusion.** Central retinal vein occlusion can produce massive retinal hemorrhage ("blood and thunder"), ischemia, and vision loss. (Reproduced with permission from Fauci AS et al. *Harrison's Principles of Internal Medicine,* 17th ed. New York: McGraw-Hill, 2008, Fig. 29-8.)

MNEMONIC

Cataract causes—

ABCD

Aging
Bang (trauma)
Congenital
Diabetes and other metabolic diseases
(steroids)

MRA), and rule out giant cell arteritis with ESR/CRP in patients ≥ 50 years of age. Consider an echocardiogram and a brain MRI.

- **Retinal vein occlusion:** Subacute and painless with varying degrees of visual loss and intraretinal hemorrhage (see Figure 2.7). Commonly due to hypertension, hyperviscosity syndromes, hypercoagulable states (eg, from OCP use), or Behçet's disease.
- **Vitreous hemorrhage:** Due to vitreous detachment, proliferative diabetic retinopathy, or retinal tears. Visual acuity may be normal or ↓.
- **Retinal detachment:** Unilateral blurred vision that progressively worsens (**floaters or lights in peripheral vision**). May be spontaneous or due to trauma (see Figure 2.8). Considered an emergency. Can also occur postoperatively, particularly after cataract surgery.
- **Optic neuritis:** Unilateral visual loss that develops over several days, often accompanied by pain that improves within 2–3 weeks. Associated with demyelinating diseases, especially MS.
- The etiologies of **chronic loss of vision** include the following:
  - **Age-related macular degeneration (AMD): The most common cause of permanent visual loss in the elderly.** Characterized by rapid or gradual **loss of central vision,** with central scotomas (shadows or distorted vision). "Dry" AMD is characterized by drusen (yellow deposits

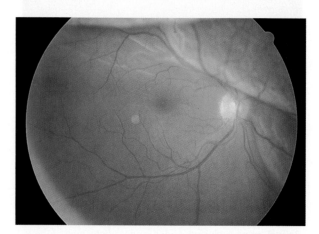

FIGURE 2.8. **Retinal detachment.** Note the elevated sheet of retinal tissue with folds. In this patient, the fovea was spared, so acuity was normal, but a superior detachment produced an inferior scotoma. (Reproduced with permission from Fauci AS et al. *Harrison's Principles of Internal Medicine,* 17th ed. New York: McGraw-Hill, 2008, Fig. 29-14.)

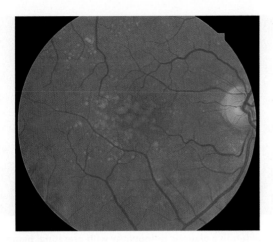

FIGURE 2.9. **Age-related macular degeneration.** Note the accumulation of drusen within the macula, which appear as scattered yellow subretinal deposits. (Reproduced with permission from Fauci AS et al. *Harrison's Principles of Internal Medicine,* 17th ed. New York: McGraw-Hill, 2008, Fig. 29-16.)

in the macula; see Figure 2.9); "wet" AMD is marked by retinal neovascularization. Antioxidants (beta-carotene, vitamins C and E) and zinc supplementation delay progression. Urgent referral is warranted for possible laser treatment.

- **Open-angle glaucoma: Loss of peripheral vision** ("tunnel vision") over years. Characterized by ↑ intraocular pressure and an ↑ cup-to-disk ratio (**"cupping"**). Treatment includes a combination of topical β-blockers, α_2-agonists, and prostaglandin analogs.
- **Cataracts:** Blurred vision occurs over months or years, with visible lens opacities. Treatment consists of surgical lens replacement.
- **Nonproliferative diabetic retinopathy:** The most common cause of legal blindness in adult-onset diabetes. Characterized by dilation of veins, microaneurysms, hard exudates, and retinal hemorrhages (see Figure 2.10). Treat with intensive blood glucose control and laser photocoagulation.

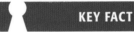

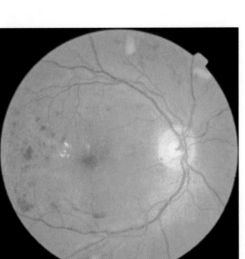

FIGURE 2.10. **Nonproliferative diabetic retinopathy.** Note the microaneurysms, deep hemorrhages, flame-shaped hemorrhage, exudates, and "cotton wool" spots. (Reproduced with permission from Riordan-Eva P, Whitcher JP. *Vaughan & Asbury's General Ophthalmology,* 17th ed. New York: McGraw-Hill, 2008, Fig. 10-6.)

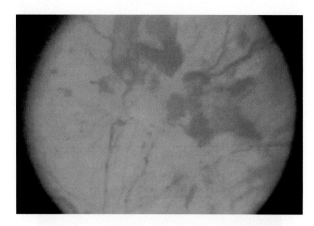

FIGURE 2.11. **Proliferative diabetic retinopathy with preretinal hemorrhage.** (Reproduced with permission from Fuster V et al. *Hurst's the Heart,* 12th ed. New York: McGraw-Hill, 2008, Fig. 12-51.)

- **Proliferative diabetic retinopathy:** Presents with neovascularization; vitreous hemorrhage is a common complication (see Figure 2.11). Treat with laser photocoagulation.

EYE FINDINGS IN SYSTEMIC DISEASES

Uveitis

- Inflammation of the uveal tract, which is made up of the iris, ciliary body, and choroid. May be seen in the following conditions:
  - **Infectious conditions:** Most common are **toxoplasmosis, herpes simplex virus,** and **herpes zoster.** Consider CMV, *Cryptococcus,* and *Candida* if the patient is immunocompromised. Syphilis ("salt and pepper" fundus appearance) and TB are less common but treatable causes.
  - **Immune-mediated conditions:**
    - **Spondyloarthritides and seronegative arthritis-associated conditions:** Reactive arthritis, ankylosing spondylitis, psoriasis, IBD.
    - **Sarcoidosis:** Likely accounts for many "idiopathic" cases of uveitis.
    - **Other:** SLE, Behçet's disease.
  - **Syndromes restricted to the eye.**
  - **Malignancy:** B-cell lymphoma, leukemia.
- **Sx/Exam:** Presents with a painful red eye (anterior uveitis) or painless floaters with ↓ visual acuity (posterior uveitis).
- **Tx:** Refer urgently to ophthalmology and treat the underlying cause; depending on the cause, give topical glucocorticoids initially.

Scleritis

- Localized or diffuse injection of the sclera (connective tissue just below the conjunctival epithelium; see Figure 2.12). Seen in various autoimmune, granulomatous, and infectious diseases.
- **Sx/Exam:** Presents with eye pain and impaired vision.
- **Tx:** Urgent ophthalmology referral is indicated.

Keratoconjunctivitis Sicca (Dry Eye Syndrome)

- A common condition, especially in middle-aged and older women. Hypofunctioning of the lacrimal glands ↓ the aqueous component of tears and leads to dry eyes. Often idiopathic, but may be associated with **Sjögren's syndrome** (check ANA, anti-Ro [SSA], and anti-La [SSB]) and with certain drugs (eg, antihistamines, topical β-blockers).

KEY FACT

Consider Sjögren's syndrome, an autoimmune disease that attacks the exocrine glands that make tears and saliva, in a middle-aged woman who complains of dry eyes.

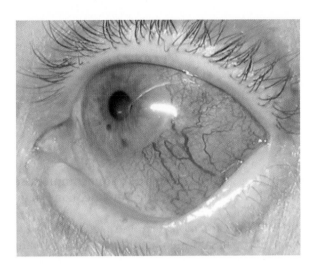

FIGURE 2.12.   Scleritis. Note the injection of scleral vessels and violaceous hue. (Reproduced with permission from USMLERx.com.)

- **Sx/Exam:** Presents with dryness, redness, burning, or a "scratchy" feeling in the eyes.
- **Tx:** Artificial tears (eg, methylcellulose solution).

Ear, Nose, and Throat

BACTERIAL SINUSITIS

 A 54-year-old woman with type 2 DM presents with a cough, nasal congestion, a purulent nasal discharge, and a severe headache for the past month. On exam, she looks unwell and has a low-grade fever, right frontal sinus tenderness, and ↓ vision in the right eye. What are the next most appropriate steps in management?

This patient has symptoms consistent with chronic sinusitis with possible orbital or other intracranial complications, and she should thus undergo an urgent CT scan and referral to a specialist. Her diabetes puts her at risk for mucormycosis, a rare fungal disease that presents as sinusitis but becomes rapidly invasive and requires surgical debridement and amphotericin.

Eighty percent of sinusitis cases are viral. Bacterial sinusitis results from impaired mucociliary clearance and obstruction of the osteomeatal complex. Viral and allergic rhinitis predispose to acute bacterial sinusitis. Etiologies are as follows:

- **Most common causative organisms:** *Streptococcus pneumoniae*, other streptococci, *Haemophilus influenzae*.
- **Less common organisms:** *S aureus* and *Moraxella catarrhalis*.
- Chronic sinusitis may also be caused by *Pseudomonas aeruginosa* and anaerobes.

 KEY FACT

S pneumoniae and *H influenzae* are the most common causes of acute bacterial sinusitis.

SYMPTOMS/EXAM

- Presents with unilateral or bilateral pain over the maxillary or frontal sinus, or with a toothache. Acute sinusitis lasts > 1 week and up to 4 weeks. Chronic sinusitis lasts > 4 weeks.
- Exam reveals purulent nasal discharge and tenderness over the affected sinus.

DIFFERENTIAL

- **Mucormycosis** is a rare but invasive fungal disease that spreads through the blood vessels and primarily affects **immunocompromised** patients, including those with DM, end-stage renal disease, bone marrow transplant, lymphoma, and AIDS.
- It presents as sinusitis with more extreme facial pain accompanied by a **necrotic eschar** of the nasal mucosa and cranial neuropathies in the later stages.
- Treat emergently with amphotericin B and ENT surgical debridement.

DIAGNOSIS

- Generally made through the history and clinical exam.
- Symptoms that last ≥ 7 days and include any of the following are suggestive of bacterial sinusitis:
  - Purulent nasal discharge.
  - Maxillary tooth or facial pain, especially unilateral.
  - Unilateral maxillary sinus tenderness.
  - Symptoms that worsen after initial improvement.
- Imaging is not indicated for uncomplicated acute sinusitis. In cases of chronic sinusitis, refractory sinusitis, or suspected intracranial or orbital complications, a CT scan is more sensitive and cost-effective than x-ray imaging and may identify air-fluid levels or bony abnormalities.
- Abnormal vision, changes in mental status, or periorbital edema may point to intracranial or orbital extension of the infection and warrant urgent referral to a specialist.

TREATMENT

- **Acute bacterial sinusitis:** Amoxicillin or TMP-SMX; amoxicillin-clavulanate in the presence of risk factors for anaerobes or resistant β-lactamase organisms (some strains of *H influenzae* and *M catarrhalis*). Risk factors include DM, immunocompromised states, and recent antibiotic use.
- **Chronic sinusitis:** Amoxicillin-clavulanate for at least 3–4 weeks along with intranasal glucocorticoids.

ACUTE OTITIS MEDIA

Common causative organisms include *S pneumoniae*, *H influenzae*, *M catarrhalis*, *Streptococcus pyogenes*, and viruses.

SYMPTOMS/EXAM

Presents with ear pain, ear fullness, ↓ hearing, and an erythematous, bulging tympanic membrane (see Figure 2.13).

KEY FACT

If sinusitis is chronic and resistant to treatment, consider anatomical sinus obstruction, common variable immunodeficiency, a CF variant, or Wegener's granulomatosis.

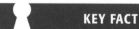

KEY FACT

When used for more than a few days, nasal decongestants such as oxymetazoline can cause rebound nasal congestion and discharge (rhinitis medicamentosa). Do not prescribe for more than 2–3 days at a time.

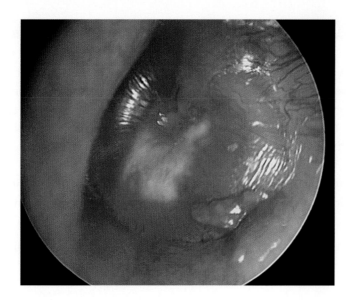

FIGURE 2.13.   Acute otitis media. (Reproduced with permission from Brunicardi FC et al. *Schwartz's Principles of Surgery,* 9th ed. New York: McGraw-Hill, 2010, Fig. 18-1.)

DIFFERENTIAL

Distinguish on exam from serous otitis media, which is characterized by a normal or dull, nonerythematous tympanic membrane with nonpurulent fluid behind it.

TREATMENT

- Amoxicillin × 10–14 days.
- For penicillin-allergic patients, give TMP-SMX or a macrolide (erythromycin, azithromycin, clarithromycin).

OTITIS EXTERNA

Predisposing factors include water exposure or mechanical trauma (eg, Q-tips). Often caused by *S aureus* and gram-⊖ rods (eg, *Pseudomonas, Proteus*). May also be caused by a fungus (eg, *Aspergillus*).

SYMPTOMS/EXAM

Characterized by ear pain that is often accompanied by pruritus and a purulent discharge. Pain is elicited on manipulation of the ear. Erythema and edema of the ear canal with exudate may be seen. A black or white discharge is seen in fungal infections.

TREATMENT

- Avoid moisture and mechanical trauma.
- Give otic drops combining a corticosteroid with either an antibiotic (eg, neomycin sulfate plus polymyxin B sulfate) or acetic acid.
- Clear the canal of cerumen and debris with a curette or hydrogen peroxide; use a cotton wick if blockage is severe.

KEY FACT

Malignant external otitis is seen in diabetics and other immuno-compromised patients. Caused by *Pseudomonas aeruginosa,* the otitis evolves into osteomyelitis and presents with severe ear pain, a foul-smelling discharge, and cranial nerve palsies.

HEARING LOSS (HL)

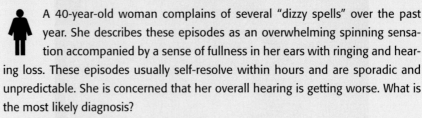

A 40-year-old woman complains of several "dizzy spells" over the past year. She describes these episodes as an overwhelming spinning sensation accompanied by a sense of fullness in her ears with ringing and hearing loss. These episodes usually self-resolve within hours and are sporadic and unpredictable. She is concerned that her overall hearing is getting worse. What is the most likely diagnosis?

Ménière's disease, an idiopathic condition of the inner ear. There is no specific diagnostic test, although patients should have an audiometry evaluation.

Categorized as **conductive** (middle or external ear damage) or **sensorineural** (inner ear—cochlea or auditory nerve).

EXAM

- Differentiate between conductive and sensorineural HL.
    - **Weber test:** With the tuning fork on the forehead, the sound is equally loud in both ears. **In conductive HL, the sound is louder in the affected ear; in sensorineural HL, sound is louder in the normal ear.**
    - **Rinne test:** The tuning fork is first held on the mastoid (bone conduction) and is then held next to the ear (air conduction). In normal conditions and sensorineural HL, air-conducted sound is louder than bone-conducted sound, but with **conductive HL, bone conduction is louder.**
- Conduct an audiology test.

DIFFERENTIAL

Table 2.9 outlines the differential diagnosis of HL.

TREATMENT

- Prevention is the best treatment. Avoid excessive noise.
- Treat the underlying cause with antibiotics, removal of middle or outer ear blockages, repair of the tympanic membrane, or replacement of ossicles (in otosclerosis).
- For persistent sensorineural or conductive HL, consider hearing aids or, in cases of profound HL, cochlear implants.

KEY FACT

Plugging your ear with your finger mimics conductive HL. In the Weber test, sound is louder in the abnormal ear.

TABLE 2.9.   Differential Diagnosis of Hearing Loss

	SENSORINEURAL	CONDUCTIVE
Areas of damage	Inner ear: cochlea or nerve (CN VIII).	Middle or external ear.
Rinne test	Normal (air louder).	Abnormal (bone louder).
Weber test	Sound is louder in the normal ear.	Sound is louder in the abnormal ear.
Causes	Age (presbycusis) is most common; excessive noise exposure, ototoxic drugs, Ménière's disease, acoustic neuroma.	Otitis media, otosclerosis, eustachian tube blockage, perforated tympanic membrane, cerumen.

TINNITUS

Perception of abnormal ear noises, usually due to HL. Although bothersome, it is benign in the absence of other symptoms.

DIFFERENTIAL

- **Ménière's disease** (episodic vertigo, sensorineural HL, tinnitus, and ear pressure).
- Vascular abnormalities such as carotid stenosis, AVMs, and vascular tumors cause **pulsatile tinnitus,** which can often be heard by the examiner.

TREATMENT

Avoid exposure to excessive noise and ototoxic drugs (aminoglycosides, salicylates, loop diuretics, cisplatin). No therapy has been shown to be effective.

PHARYNGITIS

The main concern lies in identifying group A β-hemolytic streptococcal infection (GABHS). Antibiotic treatment of GABHS usually prevents the complications of rheumatic fever and local abscess formation; it does **not** prevent poststreptococcal glomerulonephritis.

SYMPTOMS/EXAM

The four classic features of GABHS (**Centor criteria**) are as follows:

- Fever > 38°C.
- Tender anterior cervical lymphadenopathy.
- The absence of cough.
- Pharyngotonsillar exudate.

KEY FACT

The presence of cough, hoarseness, and rhinorrhea makes GABHS less likely.

DIFFERENTIAL

- **Mononucleosis:** Associated with EBV, and occurs primarily in young adults, accounting for 5–10% of sore throats; characterized by lymphadenopathy, fever, and tonsillar exudates. Symptoms also include severe fatigue, headache, and malaise.
  - Diagnose with a ⊕ heterophile antibody (Monospot) test or a high anti-EBV titer.
  - Complications include hepatitis, a morbilliform rash after **ampicillin** administration, and splenomegaly occurring within the first three weeks.
  - Avoid noncontact sports for 3–4 weeks and contact sports for 4–6 weeks after symptom onset in order to ↓ the risk of splenic rupture.
- **Diphtheria:** Rare in the United States. Presents as sore throat, fever, and malaise with gray pseudomembranes on the tonsils. May be complicated by myocarditis and cranial neuropathies.
- **Viruses:** Viral infection is suggested by rhinorrhea and cough, other upper respiratory tract symptoms, and the absence of tonsillar exudate.
- **STDs:** Gonorrheal and chlamydial pharyngitis should be considered in sexually active patients.

DIAGNOSIS

- **GABHS rapid antigen test:** The **test of choice;** has > 90% sensitivity. Routine cultures are not needed.

- **Clinical algorithm: Count the number of Centor criteria present.**
    - **4 of 4:** Treat empirically without a rapid antigen test.
    - **2–3 of 4:** Test and treat patients with ⊕ results.
    - **0–1 of 4:** No test and no antibiotic treatment.

TREATMENT

- Penicillin × 10 days. Erythromycin for penicillin-allergic patients.
- Antibiotics shorten the symptom course by 1–2 days if begun < 48 hours after symptom onset and also ↓ infectivity (consider if the patient lives with small children).
- **All cases (bacterial, viral):** Symptom relief with acetaminophen or NSAIDs and salt-water gargling.

ACUTE BRONCHITIS

A nonspecific term used to describe patients with normal underlying lungs who develop an acute cough with no clinical evidence of pneumonia. The most common causative organisms are respiratory **viruses** (coronavirus, rhinovirus, influenza, parainfluenza) and, to a lesser extent, atypical bacteria (*Mycoplasma pneumoniae, Chlamydia pneumoniae, Bordetella pertussis*).

SYMPTOMS/EXAM

- Presents with cough (productive or nonproductive) that may persist for 1–3 weeks, often with initial URI symptoms (rhinorrhea, sore throat).
- Exam findings range from clear to wheezes or rhonchi (from bronchospasm).

DIFFERENTIAL

- Community-acquired pneumonia.
- Other URIs.
- *B pertussis* infection (whooping cough) is likely if symptoms persist for ≥ 2 weeks.
    - Presents as a persistent "barking" or paroxysmal cough following typical URI symptoms.
    - A high WBC count with striking lymphocytosis is typical. Throat swab for PCR testing or culture are the diagnostic tests of choice to prevent illness among contacts (especially infants), although sensitivity is low at the time of usual presentation.
    - Treat with erythromycin × 14 days to ↓ shedding.

DIAGNOSIS

Diagnosis is made clinically. CXR is not routinely indicated.

TREATMENT

- **In patients with no underlying pulmonary disease, antibiotics are not indicated** given the common viral etiology.
- Decongestants, expectorants, bronchodilators, and humidified air are used for symptomatic treatment.

TABLE 2.10. **Differential Diagnosis of White Oral Lesions**

	THRUSH	**LEUKOPLAKIA**	**LICHEN PLANUS**
Definition/ epidemiology	Oral candidiasis, often in immunocompromised patients (diabetes, chemotherapy, local radiation, steroids, antibiotics).	Hyperkeratoses due to chronic irritation (dentures, tobacco), but ~2–6% represent dysplasia or early invasive squamous cell carcinoma (SCC).	Common; chronic inflammatory autoimmune disease.
Symptoms	Pain.	None.	Discomfort; often confused with candidiasis, leukoplakia, or SCC.
Exam	Creamy white patches over red mucosa (see Figure 2.14).	**White lesions cannot be rubbed off.**	Reticular or erosive.
Diagnosis	Clinical; can do KOH wet prep (spores).	Biopsy.	Biopsy.
Treatment	Fluconazole × 7–14 days, clotrimazole troches, or nystatin.	Treat if cancer.	Steroids (oral or topical).

ORAL LESIONS

Tables 2.10 and 2.11 outline the differential diagnosis of common oral lesions. See Figures 2.14 through 2.16 for images of oral thrush, aphthous ulcer, and HSV gingivostomatitis, respectively.

TABLE 2.11. **Differential Diagnosis of Common Mouth Ulcers**

	APHTHOUS ULCER (CANKER SORE)	**HERPES STOMATITIS**
Cause	Common; unknown cause (possible association with HHV-6).	Common; HSV.
Symptoms	Pain up to one week; heals within a few weeks.	Initial burning followed by small vesicles and then scabs.
Exam	Shallow, localized ulcers with a grayish base on the buccal and lip mucosa (see Figure 2.15). Smooth border.	Multiple intraoral **vesicular** lesions and erosions with an erythematous base (see Figure 2.16). May coalesce into a larger sore with a **scalloped** border.
Differential	If large or persistent, consider erythema multiforme, HSV, pemphigus, Behçet's disease, IBD, or SCC.	Aphthous ulcer, erythema multiforme, syphilis, cancer.
Treatment	Topical steroids (anti-inflammatory).	Not needed, but oral acyclovir × 7–14 days may shorten the course and mitigate postherpetic pain.
Prognosis	Self-resolves within weeks, but often recurrent.	Resolves quickly; frequent reactivation occurs in immunocompromised patients.

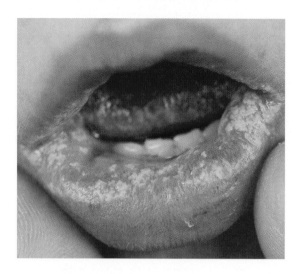

FIGURE 2.14. **Oral candidiasis (thrush).** Note the white, curdlike material on the mucosal surface of the lower lip. (Reproduced with permission from Wolff K, Johnson RA. *Fitzpatrick's Color Atlas & Synopsis of Clinical Dermatology,* 6th ed. New York: McGraw-Hill, 2009, Fig. 25-27.)

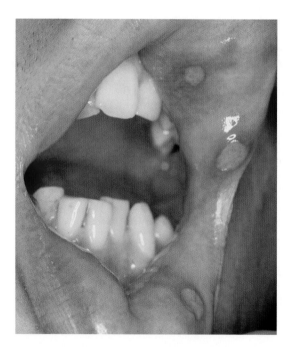

FIGURE 2.15. **Aphthous ulcers.** Multiple painful, gray-based ulcers with erythematous halos are seen on the labial mucosa. (Reproduced with permission from Wolff K, Johnson RA. *Fitzpatrick's Color Atlas & Synopsis of Clinical Dermatology,* 6th ed. New York: McGraw-Hill, 2009, Fig. 34-8.)

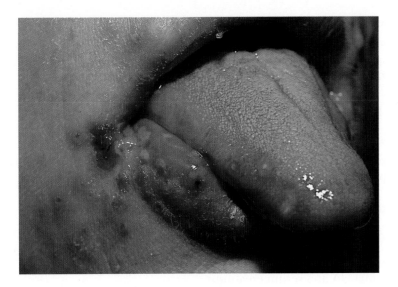

FIGURE 2.16. Herpes simplex primary gingivostomatitis. Note the multiple erosions on the lower perioral skin, lips, and tongue. (Reproduced with permission from Wolff K, Johnson RA. *Fitzpatrick's Color Atlas & Synopsis of Clinical Dermatology,* 6th ed. New York: McGraw-Hill, 2009, Fig. 27-29.)

Urology

URINARY INCONTINENCE

See the Geriatrics chapter for a complete discussion of urinary incontinence, including subtypes, clinical presentation, and treatment.

BENIGN PROSTATIC HYPERPLASIA (BPH)

 A 78-year-old man presents with one year of progressive nocturia and urinary urgency and frequency. He also has difficulty initiating urination and has experienced poor sleep due to frequent awakenings at night. He feels that his symptoms are interfering with his daily activities. What is the most appropriate initial treatment for his BPH?

Watchful waiting and behavior modification are appropriate for mild symptoms, but the severity of this patient's symptoms warrants treatment with an α-blocker such as prazosin or doxazosin, which is first-line therapy for rapid symptomatic relief.

Prevalence ↑ with age; > 90% of men > 80 years of age have an enlarged prostate.

KEY FACT

If symptoms are refractory to an α-blocker alone, add a 5α-reductase inhibitor. 5α-reductase inhibitors may be more effective for patients with severe symptoms and larger prostates, although it may take up to six months for efficacy, whereas α-blockers work immediately.

KEY FACT

Finasteride and dutasteride (5α-reductase inhibitors) can lower PSA levels by 50%. In men who are being screened for prostate cancer and are taking these drugs, the biopsy threshold should be lowered accordingly.

KEY FACT

For BPH, medications are now first line over TURP.

SYMPTOMS

- **Obstructive** symptoms include difficulty initiating a stream, terminal dribbling, and a weak stream.
- **Irritative** symptoms include urgency, frequency, and nocturia.
- DRE may reveal an enlarged, symmetrically firm prostate, but the **size of the prostate correlates poorly with symptom severity.**

DIFFERENTIAL

Prostate cancer, bladder cancer, bladder stones, UTI, interstitial cystitis, prostatitis, prostatodynia, neurogenic bladder.

DIAGNOSIS

- Diagnosed mainly by the history and exam. The American Urological Association symptom score can be useful in evaluating patients and in monitoring response to therapy.
- Obtain a UA and serum creatinine.
- PSA may be elevated in BPH but is not needed for diagnosis.

TREATMENT

- Depending on the severity of symptoms, treatment options include watchful waiting, pharmacologic therapy, and surgery (see also Table 2.12).
  - **Mild:** Watchful waiting with behavior modification.
  - **Moderate to severe:** Initiate treatment with α-blockers for immediate symptomatic relief. If symptoms are severe, combine with a 5α-reductase inhibitor.
- Urology referral and surgery are indicated for severe symptoms or complications of BPH (eg, refractory retention, hydronephrosis, recurrent UTIs, recurrent gross hematuria, renal insufficiency due to BPH, bladder stones, persistent symptoms).
- Surgical options include transurethral resection of the prostate (TURP) and other minimally invasive procedures. Side effects of TURP include the need for transfusion, retrograde ejaculation, impotence (10–40%; operator dependent), urinary incontinence, and hypervolemic hyponatremia.

TABLE 2.12. Medications for BPH

	α₁-BLOCKERS	5α-REDUCTASE INHIBITORS
Drugs	Prazosin, doxazosin, terazosin, **tamsulosin (less hypotension).**	Finasteride, dutasteride.
Mechanism	↓ contractility of the prostate and bladder neck.	Block testosterone conversion to the more potent dihydrotestosterone.
Results	Improve symptoms and urinary flow rates; more effective than 5α-reductase inhibitors for **immediate** symptom relief.	Improve symptoms; ↓ prostate size and ↓ **PSA,** especially in men with larger prostates.
Side effects	**Orthostatic hypotension,** nasal congestion, dizziness, fatigue.	↓ libido, ejaculatory dysfunction, impotence.

ERECTILE DYSFUNCTION (ED)

Defined as an inability to acquire or maintain an erection sufficient for sexual intercourse in > 75% of attempts. Evaluation is directed at distinguishing organic from psychogenic causes (see Table 2.13).

DIAGNOSIS

- **Rule out an organic etiology.** Look for a history of medical conditions associated with ED; perform a physical exam focusing on evidence of endocrine abnormality (gynecomastia, testicle size), GU abnormalities (Peyronie's disease, prostate size), and peripheral neurovascular abnormalities. Screening labs should include glucose, cholesterol, TSH, testosterone, and prolactin.
- If testosterone or prolactin is abnormal, check FSH and LH to rule out a pituitary abnormality.

TREATMENT

- Correct the underlying disorder (testosterone replacement for hypogonadism); eliminate medication- and drug-related causes.
- **Oral phosphodiesterase inhibitors** (sildenafil, vardenafil, tadalafil) are first-line therapy if there is no suspected organic etiology but are **contraindicated with nitrates or active cardiac disease** (can cause hypotension and sudden death). Efficacy is about 70% (less in DM).
- Second-line therapies include intraurethral alprostadil suppositories (especially helpful for neurologic ED), vacuum constrictive pumps, and penile prostheses.

TABLE 2.13.   Medical Conditions Associated with ED

CONDITION	EXAMPLES/COMMENTS
Psychogenic disorders	Performance anxiety, depression, mental stress.
Obesity	
DM	ED is seen in up to 50% of cases.
Peripheral vascular disease	
Endocrine disorders	Hypogonadism, hyperprolactinemia, thyroid abnormalities.
Pelvic surgery	
Spinal cord injury	
Drugs of abuse	Amphetamines, cocaine, marijuana, alcohol, tobacco.
Medications	**Antihypertensives: Thiazides, β-blockers, clonidine, methyldopa.** **Antiandrogens:** Spironolactone, H_2 blockers, finasteride. **Antidepressants:** TCAs, SSRIs. **Other:** Antipsychotics, benzodiazepines, opiates.

KEY FACT

Rapid onset of ED suggests psychogenic causes or medication side effects. More gradual onset is associated with medical conditions. Low libido along with ED suggests a psychogenic, medication-related, or hormonal cause.

KEY FACT

Up to one-quarter of all cases of ED may be related to drug or medication use.

KEY FACT

Oral phosphodiesterase inhibitors are quite effective for all types of ED, including those related to diabetes, psychiatric issues, prostatectomies, and spinal surgeries. Make sure your patient is not concomitantly taking nitrates and does not have unstable cardiac issues.

PROSTATITIS

A 50-year-old man with BPH presents to a clinic with fevers, chills, and dysuria for three days. On exam, his vitals are notable for a temperature of 38°C (100.5°F), a BP of 110/70 mm Hg, and an HR of 80 bpm. He has mild, diffuse tenderness in the lower abdomen without rebound or guarding, and his prostate is very tender. What is the most likely diagnosis and most appropriate management?

This patient likely has acute bacterial prostatitis. A urine culture should be sent, and he should be started on antibiotics that cover gram-⊖ rods, such as TMP-SMX or a fluoroquinolone. If the patient shows signs of hemodynamic instability or inability to take oral meds, he should be hospitalized for IV antibiotics. Once cultures return, oral antibiotics should be adjusted and continued for at least 4–6 weeks.

TABLE 2.14. **Treatment of Prostatitis and Prostatodynia**

	ACUTE BACTERIAL PROSTATITIS	CHRONIC BACTERIAL PROSTATITIS	NONBACTERIAL PROSTATITIS	PROSTATODYNIA
Fever	+	–	–	–
UA	+	–	–	–
Expressed prostatic secretions	Contraindicated.	+	+	–
Bacterial culture	+	+	–	–
Prostate exam	Very tender.	Normal, boggy, or indurated.	Normal, boggy, or indurated.	Usually normal.
Etiology	Gram-⊖ rods (*E coli*); less commonly gram-⊕ organisms (enterococcus).	Gram-⊖ rods; less commonly enterococcus.	Unknown; perhaps *Ureaplasma, Mycoplasma, Chlamydia*. Rarely, fungal or TB.	Varies; includes voiding dysfunction and pelvic floor musculature dysfunction.
Treatment	Broad coverage of gram-⊖ rods, initially with TMP-SMX or a fluoroquinolone until cultures return.	First line: TMP-SMX (diffuses into prostate well). If resistant to TMP-SMX or treatment failure, consider fluoroquinolones. The duration of treatment is controversial: 4–12 weeks.	Erythromycin × 3–6 weeks if response is seen at two weeks.	α-blocking drugs (eg, terazosin) in the setting of urinary symptoms; NSAIDs; benzodiazepines; biofeedback for pelvic floor dysfunction.

(Adapted with permission from McPhee SJ et al. *Current Medical Diagnosis & Treatment 2010.* New York: McGraw-Hill, 2010, Table 23-2.)

The differential includes acute bacterial prostatitis, chronic bacterial prostatitis, nonbacterial prostatitis, and prostatodynia. See Table 2.14 for key features of each.

SYMPTOMS/EXAM

Presents with irritative voiding symptoms and perineal or suprapubic pain. Acute bacterial prostatitis is notable for the presence of fever and an exquisitely tender prostate.

TREATMENT

Table 2.14 outlines the treatment of prostatitis and prostatodynia.

GENITAL LESIONS

Refer to Table 2.15 for the differential diagnosis and treatment of STDs that present as genital lesions. Refer to the Women's Health chapter for a detailed discussion of gonorrheal and chlamydial infections (cervicitis, PID). The diagnosis and treatment of urethritis in men follow the same principles as those of cervicitis in women.

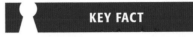

KEY FACT

All patients with genital lesions should be screened for syphilis (serology).

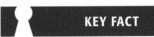

KEY FACT

Chancres are single, painless, clean-based ulcers with painless local lymphadenopathy. *Haemophilus ducreyi* chancroids (not to be confused with syphilis chancres) are painful ulcers that are associated with purulent, painful adenopathy.

TABLE 2.15. Differential Diagnosis of Genital Lesions

	HSV	**GENITAL WARTS (CONDYLOMATA ACUMINATA)**	**1° SYPHILIS**	**CHANCROID**
Cause	HSV-2 > HSV-1.	HPV.	*Treponema pallidum.*	*Haemophilus ducreyi.*
Incubation period/ triggers	**Primary:** +/− asymptomatic; prodrome consists of malaise, genital paresthesias, and fever. **Reactivation:** Most commonly occurs with symptoms; triggers include stress, fever, and infection.	1–6 months; triggers include pregnancy and immuno-suppression.	2–6 weeks.	3–5 days.
Symptoms	Painful, grouped vesicles; tingling, dysesthesia. Asymptomatic shedding is common.	Warty "cauliflower" growths or none.	**Painless,** clean-based ulcer (chancre).	Pustule or pustules erode to form a **painful** ulcer with a necrotic base.
Exam	Groups of multiple, small vesicles.	Warty growths or none.	Ulcer on genitalia; nontender regional lymph nodes.	Usually unilateral, **tender,** fluctuant, matted nodes with overlying erythema.
Diagnosis	Mostly clinical; ⊕ viral culture or DFA or Tzanck smear with ⊕ intranuclear inclusions and multinucleated giant cells.	Clinical if wartlike; 4% acetic acid applied to the lesion turns tissue white with papillae.	**Serology:** RPR ⊕ 1–2 weeks after the 1° lesion is first seen. Immunofluorescence or darkfield microscopy of fluid with treponemes.	Culture of lesion on special media.

(continues)

TABLE 2.15.   **Differential Diagnosis of Genital Lesions** *(continued)*

	HSV	GENITAL WARTS (CONDYLOMATA ACUMINATA)	1° SYPHILIS	CHANCROID
Treatment	**Acute episodes:** Acyclovir 200 mg 5×/day; famciclovir 250 mg TID; valacyclovir 1000 mg BID × 10 days (first episode) or × 5 days (recurrence). **Suppression:** Acyclovir 400 mg BID; famciclovir 250 mg BID; valacyclovir 500 mg BID or 1 g QD.	Trichloroacetic acid; podophyllin (contraindicated in pregnancy); imiquimod.	Benzathine penicillin G IM × 1; doxycycline or tetracycline PO × 2 weeks for penicillin-allergic patients.	Azithromycin 1 g PO × 1 or ceftriaxone 250 mg IM × 1.

Orthopedics

ROTATOR CUFF TENDINITIS OR TEAR

A 45-year-old man presents with three days of right shoulder pain following a recreational softball game. The pain worsens when he attempts to lift his arms above his head and when he lies on his right side at night. On exam, he has pain with active and passive abduction, but his strength is intact. What is the likely diagnosis and the best management plan?

Rotator cuff **tendinitis** caused by repetitive overhead motion. Full strength on exam argues against a rotator cuff **tear;** pain with passive abduction is consistent with impingement. Treatment involves NSAIDs, avoidance of exacerbating activities, corticosteroid injections, and physical therapy with the goal of averting progression to adhesive capsulitis (frozen shoulder). Imaging is not indicated unless there is no improvement with conservative therapy or a full tear is suspected.

The spectrum ranges from subacromial bursitis and rotator cuff tendinitis to partial or full rotator cuff tear. Due to excessive overhead motion (eg, baseball players).

SYMPTOMS

- Presents with nonspecific pain in the anterolateral shoulder with occasional radiation down the lateral arm that worsens at night or with overhead movement, sleeping, or reaching behind (eg, putting on a jacket).
- **Motor weakness with abduction suggests the presence of a tear.**

EXAM

- Exam reveals pain with abduction between 60 and 120 degrees. Tears lead to weakness on abduction ("drop arm test").
- Pain elicited by 60–120 degrees of passive abduction (**impingement sign**) suggests impingement or trapping of an **inflamed rotator cuff** on the overlying acromion.

DIFFERENTIAL

- **Bicipital tendinitis:** Due to repetitive overhead motion (eg, throwing, swimming). Exam reveals tenderness along the biceps tendon or muscle.
- **Degenerative joint disease.**
- **Systemic arthritis:** RA, pseudogout.
- **Referred pain:** May be derived from a pulmonary process (eg, pulmonary embolism, pleural effusion), a subdiaphragmatic process, cervical spine disease, or brachial plexopathy.
- **Adhesive capsulitis (frozen shoulder):** Presents with progressive loss of range of motion (ROM), usually more from stiffness than from pain. Can follow rotator cuff tendinitis; more common in diabetics and older patients.

DIAGNOSIS

- Diagnosis is made by the history and exam.
- An MRI can be obtained if a complete tear is suspected or if no improvement is seen despite conservative therapy and the patient is a surgical candidate.

TREATMENT

- ↓ exacerbating activities; NSAIDs. Also consider steroid injection.
- Physical therapy in the form of ROM exercises and rotator cuff strengthening can be initiated once acute pain has resolved.
- **Refer to orthopedics for possible surgery if there is a complete tear** or if no improvement is seen after several months of conservative therapy.

KNEE PAIN

> A 45-year-old obese woman recently began to exercise regularly as part of a weight loss program. She runs two miles three times per week. For the past month, she has experienced anterior right knee pain with ambulation that worsens when she climbs stairs. What is the most likely diagnosis?
>
> Patellofemoral pain syndrome. This is an "overload" injury that is manifested particularly with knee bending, which exerts pressure between the knee and femur. The typical complaint is anterior knee pain that occurs with activity, especially when the patient walks down steps or hills. Often it also worsens after prolonged sitting ("theater or moviegoer's sign"—pain while getting out of a chair after sitting for a long period). Treatment includes ice, NSAIDs, and exercise.

Table 2.16 outlines the etiologies and clinical characteristics of common knee injuries.

DIAGNOSIS

- **Ottawa Knee Rules:** Obtain an x-ray if any of the following risk factors for fracture are present after acute trauma to the knee (nearly 100% sensitivity):
  - Age ≥ 55 years.
  - Tenderness at the head of the fibula.
  - Isolated patellar tenderness.
  - Inability to bear weight both immediately after trauma and on exam.
  - Inability to flex the knee to 90 degrees.
- **MRI** is most sensitive for soft tissue injuries (eg, meniscal and ligament tears).

KEY FACT

Knee swelling immediately following trauma suggests a ligamentous tear (with hemarthrosis). Swelling that occurs hours to days after trauma suggests a meniscal injury.

TABLE 2.16. Common Knee Injuries

	ILIOTIBIAL BAND SYNDROME	BURSITIS	PATELLOFEMORAL PAIN SYNDROME	MEDIAL MENISCUS TEAR	ACL TEAR
Those affected/ mechanism	Runners.	Runners, obese or deconditioned patients, people who work on their knees.	Runners/ deconditioned patients, often with chondromalacia of the patella. The most common cause of anterior knee pain in the general population, frequently from overuse.	Twisting of the knee while the foot is firmly planted on the ground (soccer, football). Degenerative tears occur in older patients.	Twisting trauma, often in noncontact sports (eg, skiing).
Symptoms	Lateral knee pain or gradual; tightness after running.	Pain with motion and rest. **Prepatellar bursitis:** Pain and swelling over the front of the knee. **Anserine bursitis:** Pain medial and inferior to the knee joint.	Anterior knee pain; often exacerbated by walking up and down stairs/hills.	A pop or tear at the time of injury; severe pain with "locking," "catching," and **swelling that peaks the next day.**	Audible "pop" and giving way; **immediate swelling.**
Exam	Tenderness over the lateral femoral epicondyle.	Exquisite tenderness at the bursa.	Pain on patellar compression while the patient contracts the quadriceps. Exam is often nonspecific.	Medial joint line tenderness; pain on hyperflexion and hyperextension; +/– knee effusion; ⊕ McMurray's test (a pop or clicking sensation along the joint line with tibial rotation).	⊕ anterior drawer sign; ⊕ Lachman's test (↑ anterior movement of the tibia); knee effusion.
Treatment	Rest, NSAIDs, stretching.	Avoid exacerbating activities; physical therapy. Ice/NSAIDs; corticosteroid injection for persistent symptoms.	Activity modification, physical therapy, NSAIDs. Little evidence for corticosteroid injection.	Treat conservatively: RICE (rest, ice, compression, elevation); quadriceps strengthening with physical therapy; surgery only if symptoms persist.	Conservative; RICE. ACL reconstruction if the patient has a high activity level or significant knee instability.

FOOT AND ANKLE PAIN

A common reason for 1° care visits; may be acute or chronic.

DIFFERENTIAL

See Table 2.17 for common causes of foot and ankle pain.

TABLE 2.17.   Common Causes of Foot and Ankle Pain

CAUSE	SEEN IN/ETIOLOGY	SYMPTOMS	DIAGNOSIS	TREATMENT
Plantar fasciitis	Obese patients, prolonged standing, runners, dancers.	Plantar pain, especially with **first steps in morning.**	Tenderness over the insertion of the plantar fascia at the medial heel. **Bone spurs on x-ray are neither sensitive nor specific for plantar fasciitis.**	↓ prolonged standing; arch supports; NSAIDs; stretches. In 80% of cases, symptoms resolve within one year.
Stress fracture	History of prior stress fractures; increasing volume/intensity of physical activity.	Foot pain that worsens with weight bearing.	**Radiographs may miss early fractures.** Obtain a bone scan or an MRI in the setting of high suspicion and when x-ray is ⊖.	**Hard-soled shoe** or walking cast for 3–4 weeks. Avoid exacerbating activities until fully healed.
Metatarsalgia	Seen in those with prolonged pressure on the anterior feet, especially from high heels.	Pain in the area of the metatarsal heads (one or multiple).	A clinical diagnosis; exclude other etiologies.	Avoid offending shoes; NSAIDs.
Morton's neuroma	Entrapment of the interdigital nerve. Affects women more than men.	**Forefoot pain and paresthesias radiating to the toes;** the third web space is classic. Patients feel pain while wearing shoes but not when barefoot.	Usually a clinical diagnosis (tenderness in affected web space); MRI can confirm when surgery is a consideration.	Broad-toed shoes, orthotics, corticosteroid injections. Surgery should be reserved for refractory cases.
Bunions (hallux valgus)	Abnormal foot mechanics and anatomy, joint hypermobility, genetics. May be exacerbated by poor footwear.	Foot pain in the area of the first metatarsal.	**Deformity** of the first MTP joint with valgus deviation of the great toe.	Pain control; shoe modification/orthotics; surgical correction (osteotomy) when pain/functional impairment are severe.
Gout	More common in men. Associated with dietary indiscretion, alcohol, and drugs that affect serum urate levels.	**Sudden onset of exquisite pain in the first MTP** with redness/swelling. Can also present as midfoot or Achilles tenosynovitis.	**Inflammatory signs** at the first MTP. Other joints or risk factors for gout may be present.	NSAIDs, colchicine, oral or intra-articular corticosteroids.

(continues)

TABLE 2.17. **Common Causes of Foot and Ankle Pain** *(continued)*

CAUSE	SEEN IN/ETIOLOGY	SYMPTOMS	DIAGNOSIS	TREATMENT
Achilles tendinitis	Athletes. Consider Achilles tendon tear and spondyloarthropathies in the differential.	Pain with running or jumping that **worsens with dorsiflexion** of the foot.	Tenderness at the Achilles insertion on the calcaneus. Consider an MRI if Achilles tendon tear is suspected.	NSAIDs, stretches, avoidance of offending activity.
Tarsal tunnel syndrome	Entrapment of the posterior tibial nerve under the medial flexor retinaculum. Can be posttraumatic or from chronic overuse.	**Heel/plantar foot pain and paresthesias.** Pain at night and after prolonged weight bearing.	**Tinel's sign:** reproduction of symptoms by tapping the tibial nerve posterior and inferior to the medial malleolus. X-ray is indicated to rule out associated bony abnormalities.	NSAIDs, corticosteroid injections, orthotics.

DIAGNOSIS

In acute ankle or foot pain after trauma, use the **Ottawa Ankle Rules** to determine the need for x-ray imaging (see Figure 2.17).

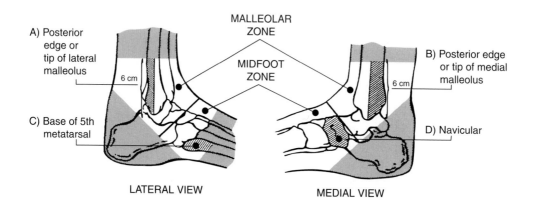

FIGURE 2.17. **Ottawa Ankle Rules for x-rays in ankle/foot trauma.** (Reproduced with permission from Tintinalli JE et al. *Tintinalli's Emergency Medicine: A Comprehensive Study Guide,* 6th ed. New York: McGraw-Hill, 2004, Fig. 276-3.)

LOWER BACK PAIN (LBP)

A 59-year-old man presents to your office with six months of worsening lower back pain that radiates to the left buttock and thigh. The pain worsens with standing and walking downhill and is alleviated by sitting. Sometimes his left leg feels weak after long periods of walking downhill. His physical exam is normal, including 2+ arterial dorsalis pedis pulses. What is the most likely diagnosis, and what diagnostic test should be ordered?

Spinal stenosis; order an MRI. Symptoms typically worsen with standing and back extension and may improve with sitting and flexion. Spinal stenosis ("neurogenic claudication") can be confused with vascular claudication from peripheral vascular disease, but patients with the latter typically have ↓ peripheral pulses.

Extremely common, with up to 80% of the population affected at some time. Three-quarters of LBP patients improve within one month. Most have self-limited, nonspecific mechanical causes of LBP.

EXAM

- **Straight-leg raise test:** ⊕ if passive leg flexion up to 60 degrees while supine or seated causes radicular pain. More sensitive (80%) than specific (40%) for lumbar disk herniation.
- A wide-based gait and a ⊕ Romberg sign are specific signs of spinal stenosis.
- Exam may also localize the origin of the nerve root syndrome (see Table 2.18).

DIFFERENTIAL

- **Serious causes** of back pain and their associated risk factors include the following:
  - **Cancer:** Age > 50, previous cancer history, unexplained weight loss.
  - **Compression fracture:** Age > 50, significant trauma, a history of osteoporosis, corticosteroid use.
  - **Infection (epidural abscess, diskitis, osteomyelitis, or endocarditis):** Fever, recent skin or urinary infection, immunosuppression, **IV drug use.**
  - **Cauda equina syndrome:** Bilateral leg weakness, bowel or bladder incontinence, saddle anesthesia. A surgical emergency.
- **Less urgent causes of back pain** include herniated disk; spinal stenosis (see Table 2.19); sciatica; musculoskeletal strain; and referred pain from a kidney stone, pyelonephritis, an intra-abdominal process, or herpes zoster.

TABLE 2.18. Nerve Root Syndromes (Sciatica)

NERVE ROOT	STRENGTH	SENSORY	REFLEXES
S1	Ankle plantar flexion (toe walking).	Lateral foot.	Achilles.
L5	Great toe dorsiflexion.	Medial forefoot.	None.
L4 (less common)	Ankle dorsiflexion (heel walking).	Medial calf.	Knee jerk.

MNEMONIC

Back pain causes—

DISC MASS

Degeneration (osteoarthritis, osteoporosis, spondylosis)
Infection/**I**njury
Spondylitis
Compression fracture
Multiple myeloma/**M**ets (cancer of the breast, kidney, lung, prostate, or thyroid)
Abdominal pain/**A**neurysm
Skin (herpes zoster), **S**train, **S**coliosis, and lordosis
Slipped disk/**S**pondylolisthesis

KEY FACT

The two most common nerve root impingements are L5 and S1. Test S1 by asking the patient to walk on her toes (think about a ballerina walking on her toes).

KEY FACT

"Red flags" in the history of a patient with new-onset back pain:

- Age > 50
- A history of cancer
- Fever
- Weight loss
- IV drug use
- Osteoporosis
- Lower extremity weakness
- Bowel or bladder dysfunction

TABLE 2.19. **Herniated Disk vs. Spinal Stenosis**

	HERNIATED DISK	**SPINAL STENOSIS**
Etiology	Degeneration of ligaments results in disk prolapse, leading to compression or inflammation of the nerve root. Usually caused by disk herniation into L4–L5 or L5–S1 levels.	Narrowing of the spinal canal from osteophytes at facet joints, bulging disks, or a hypertrophied ligamentum flavum.
Symptoms	Sciatica. **Worsens with sitting (lumbar flexion).**	Neurogenic claudication/pseudoclaudication: pain radiating to the buttocks, thighs, or lower legs. **Worsens with prolonged standing or walking (extension of the spine); improves with sitting or walking uphill (flexion of the spine).**
Exam/diagnosis	See Table 2.18. A ⊕ straight-leg raise (pain at 60 degrees or less) is seen.	May have a ⊕ Romberg sign or wide-based gait. Exam is often unremarkable. MRI confirms the diagnosis (see Figure 2.18).
Treatment	Limited bed rest for < 2 days; ordinary activity; NSAIDs.	Exercise to reduce lumbar lordosis; decompressive laminectomy.

KEY FACT

Do not order imaging on initial evaluation of acute LBP unless severe/ progressive neurologic deficits or other red flags (age, suspicion for underlying malignancy, fever) are present.

DIAGNOSIS

- The history and clinical exam are helpful in identifying the cause.
- A plain x-ray is indicated only if fracture, osteomyelitis, or cancer is being considered. Plain films are insensitive for metastasis, infection, and disk disease.
- Urgent MRI or CT is indicated for suspected cauda equina syndrome, cancer, or infection. For patients with suspected disk disease, imaging is not indicated unless symptoms persist for > 6 weeks or significant neurologic findings are present.

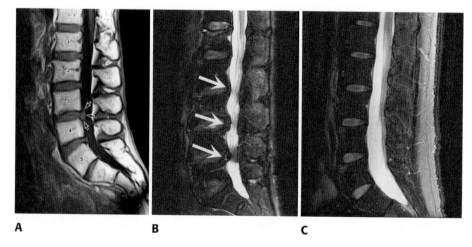

A   B   C

FIGURE 2.18. **Herniated disk vs. lumbar stenosis.** (**A**) An acute disk herniation is outlined by arrows at the L3–L4 level on this sagittal T1-weighted MR image. (**B**) Degenerative changes at multiple levels cause narrowing of the adjacent thecal sac (arrows), which contains CSF (white) on this sagittal fat-suppressed T2-weighted MR image. (**C**) Normal lumbar spine for comparison. (Image A reproduced with permission from Waxman SG. *Clinical Neuroanatomy,* 26th ed. New York: McGraw-Hill, Fig. 6-19. Images B and C reproduced with permission from Fauci AS et al. *Harrison's Principles of Internal Medicine,* 17th ed. New York: McGraw-Hill, 2008, Fig. 16-5.)

TREATMENT

- For mechanical causes of acute LBP, conservative therapy with NSAIDs and muscle relaxants, education, and **early return to ordinary activity** are indicated in the absence of major neurologic deficits or other alarm symptoms, as most cases of LBP resolve within 1–3 months. Bed rest is ineffective. Physical therapy, chiropractor, and acupuncture referrals are effective adjunctive therapies for mechanical LBP.
- Surgery referral is indicated in the setting of suspected cauda equina syndrome, progressive motor weakness or refractory radicular symptoms from nerve root compression (eg, disk herniation), or spinal instability due to tumor or infection. For spinal stenosis, decompressive laminectomy may provide at least short-term symptom improvement.

Cardiovascular Disease

HYPERTENSION

A 60-year-old woman with diet-controlled type 2 DM and hypertension presents to your clinic for routine follow-up. On exam, her BP is 150/90 mm Hg. On her last visit, her BP had been 148/85 mm Hg. She is currently on HCTZ 25 mg PO daily. What is the next step?

In addition to diet and exercise counseling, start a second antihypertensive agent to meet the goal of < 130/80 mm Hg in diabetic patients. An ACEI would be an excellent choice given the patient's coexisting diabetes. Check a chemistry panel prior to initiation of the ACEI, and repeat the panel within one week of starting the medication to rule out acute renal failure and hyperkalemia.

Diagnosed when systolic BP is persistently ≥ 140 **or** diastolic BP is ≥ 90 mm Hg (see Table 2.20). Hypertension is associated with an ↑ risk of MI, heart failure, stroke, and kidney disease.

DIAGNOSIS

- BP should be checked at least every two years starting at age 18.
- Unless acute end-organ damage is present or BP is ≥ 220/115 mm Hg, diagnosis requires multiple BP readings above 140/90 mm Hg on at least two different occasions.

TABLE 2.20. **Blood Pressure Classification**

BP CATEGORY	SYSTOLIC BP (mm Hg)	DIASTOLIC BP (mm Hg)
Normal	< 120	and < 80
Prehypertension	120–139	or 80–89
Stage 1 hypertension	140–159	or 90–99
Stage 2 hypertension	≥ 160	or ≥ 100

 KEY FACT

A DASH diet with 1600 mg of sodium (low salt) leads to an average BP reduction similar to that of single-drug therapy.

KEY FACT

For most hypertensive patients (in the absence of comorbid conditions), thiazide diuretics are the first-line agents of choice. If multiple drugs must be used to control the BP, a diuretic should be included.

 MNEMONIC

Causes of 2° hypertension—

ABCDE

Aldosteronism, obstructive sleep **A**pnea
Bruits (renal artery stenosis), **B**ad kidneys (CKD; most common)
Cushing's syndrome, **C**oarctation, **C**atecholamines (pheochromocytoma)
Drugs (NSAIDs, OCPs, decongestants, cocaine)
Endocrine (thyroid or parathyroid disease), **E**rythropoietin

TABLE 2.21. Lifestyle Modifications for Hypertension

Measure	Comments
Sodium restriction	No added salt or low-sodium diet.
DASH diet (Dietary Approaches to Stop Hypertension)	A diet rich in fruits, vegetables, and low-fat dairy products with ↓ saturated and unsaturated fat.
Weight reduction	If over the ideal BMI.
Aerobic physical activity	
Limitation of alcohol consumption	Limit to < 2 drinks per day for men and < 1 drink per day for women.

KEY FACT

An ↑ in creatinine of 25–30% from baseline is generally considered acceptable when starting an ACEI.

KEY FACT

If patients develop a cough with an ACEI, it is acceptable to try an ARB, which is associated with a lesser risk of cough.

KEY FACT

Special indications:
- **Post-MI:** β-blocker, ACEI.
- **CHF:** β-blocker, ACEI (ARB if intolerant of ACEI). Add aldosterone antagonist if stage C (see the Cardiology chapter).
- **Diabetes:** ACEI or ARB +/− thiazide.
- **CKD:** ACEI or ARB +/− diuretic (thiazide and/or loop).

- The Joint National Committee on Prevention, Detection, Evaluation, and Treatment of High Blood Pressure (JNC 7) identifies three goals of evaluation: (1) to assess lifestyle and other cardiovascular risk factors or other disease that will affect management (diabetes, hyperlipidemia, smoking); (2) to identify 2° causes; and (3) to assess for the presence of target-organ damage and cardiovascular disease (heart, brain, kidney, peripheral vascular disease, retinopathy).
- Consider 2° causes in the setting of severe or refractory hypertension, or if age of onset is ≤ 30 years in non–African American patients without a family history.
- Laboratory workup includes a UA, blood glucose, hematocrit, a lipid panel, potassium/creatinine/calcium levels, and an ECG.

TREATMENT

- The goal of BP management is < **140/90** mm Hg, or < **130/80** in patients with **diabetes, renal disease,** or **cardiovascular disease.**
- Counsel all patients about lifestyle modification (see Table 2.21). If a brief trial of nonpharmacologic therapy fails, medications should be added for those with stage 1 or 2 hypertension (see Table 2.22).
- Other modifiable cardiovascular risk factors (diabetes, hyperlipidemia, smoking) should be screened for and treated in hypertensive individuals.

TABLE 2.22. Antihypertensive Medications

	Thiazides	β-Blockers	ACEIs	Angiotensin II Receptor Blockers (ARBs)	Calcium Channel Blockers (CCBs)
Examples	HCTZ, chlorthalidone.	Atenolol, metoprolol.	Captopril, enalapril, ramipril.	Irbesartan, losartan, valsartan.	**Nondihydropyridines:** Diltiazem, verapamil. **Dihydropyridines:** Amlodipine, felodipine, nifedipine.

(continues)

TABLE 2.22.   Antihypertensive Medications *(continued)*

	THIAZIDES	β-BLOCKERS	ACEIs	ANGIOTENSIN II RECEPTOR BLOCKERS (ARBs)	CALCIUM CHANNEL BLOCKERS (CCBs)
Side effects	Hypokalemia, ED, ↑ insulin resistance, hyperuricemia, ↑ TG. Metabolic side effects are more prominent at doses of > 25 mg/day.	Bronchospasm, bradycardia/AV node blockade, depression, fatigue, ED, ↑ insulin resistance.	**Cough (10%), hyperkalemia, renal failure, angioedema.**	Small chance of cough but likely safe. Less hyperkalemia, renal failure, angioedema.	Conduction defects (nondihydropyridines); lower extremity edema (dihydropyridines).
Indications as first-line drug	Used in most patients as **mono- or combination therapy (stage 1 or 2 hypertension)**, including isolated systolic hypertension in the elderly.	**MI, high CAD risk.**	**DM with micro-albuminuria/ proteinuria; MI with systolic dysfunction or anterior infarct; non-DM-related proteinuria (ie, any type of proteinuria).**	ACEI cough in patients who would otherwise have indications for ACEIs.	Systolic hypertension, advanced age, CAD.
Other indications	Recurrent stroke prevention. May ↓ fracture risk by increasing bone density.	CHF, tachyarrhythmias, migraine.	CHF.	CHF, DM, CKD.	Atrial arrhythmias (nondihydropyridines); isolated systolic hypertension in the elderly (dihydropyridines).
Contra-indications	Gout.	Bronchospasm; high-degree (type II second- or third-degree) heart block.	Pregnancy.	Pregnancy.	High-degree heart block.

SMOKING AND SMOKING CESSATION

Smoking is the leading cause of preventable death in the United States. Treat as follows:

- Apply the **"5 A's" approach** advocated by the National Cancer Institute:
  - **A**sk (about smoking).
  - **A**dvise (all smokers to quit).
  - **A**ssess (readiness to quit).
  - **A**ssist (with pharmacologic and nonpharmacologic measures).
  - **A**rrange (follow-up and support).
- Physician intervention, even if as brief as 1–2 minutes, can ↑ the rate of compliance.
- Offer all patients **pharmacotherapy,** which is **twice as effective** in promoting cessation as behavioral counseling alone (see Table 2.23).

TABLE 2.23.   Smoking Cessation Methods

Method	Mechanism/Use	Side Effects	Contraindications
Nicotine replacement (patch, gum, inhaler, nasal spray)	Apply patch daily. Chew gum or use nasal spray/inhaler PRN cravings.	Skin irritation (patch); mucosal irritation (nasal spray); cough (inhaler).	**Recent MI**, unstable angina, life-threatening arrhythmia, pregnancy (although nicotine replacement may be preferable to continued smoking).
Sustained-release bupropion	Atypical antidepressant. Begin one week prior to quit date; continue three or more months after quitting.	Restlessness/anxiety, tremor, insomnia, GI upset.	**Seizures, head trauma,** heavy alcohol use, history of **eating disorders** (lowers seizure threshold).
Varenicline	Nicotine agonist. Start one week prior to quit date; continue for 12 weeks.	Nausea/vomiting, constipation, **altered dreams, suicidal ideation,** depression, agitation.	Suicidal ideation, unstable psychiatric status.
Behavioral counseling	Individual, group, telephone hotlines.		

- Bupropion may be used in combination with nicotine replacement with additive benefits. Bupropion alone is more effective than a nicotine patch alone.
- Varenicline may be more efficacious than bupropion or nicotine replacement. However, it can cause GI upset and has been associated with neuropsychiatric symptoms such as suicidal ideation, agitation, and depressive behavior.

Common Symptoms

VERTIGO

An 85-year-old woman with CAD, hypertension, and DM presents with two months of vertigo. The vertigo is episodic and is associated with blurry vision and slightly slurred speech. On exam, she has vertical nystagmus. What is the most likely diagnosis?

Central vertigo from vertebrobasilar insufficiency.

Can originate in the peripheral (labyrinth/inner ear) or central vestibular system. The most common peripheral causes of vertigo are benign paroxysmal positional vertigo (BPPV), Ménière's disease, and acute labyrinthitis. Other forms of dizziness include the following:

- **Presyncope:** A feeling of impending loss of consciousness or near-syncope. Usually due to postural changes rather than to arrhythmia or structural heart disease. See the Cardiology chapter for further details.
- **Disequilibrium:** Unsteadiness with standing or walking. Common in older patients; often multifactorial.
- **Lightheadedness:** Anxiety.

KEY FACT

Peripheral vertigo is often more severe than central vertigo but should not have any associated neurologic symptoms.

SYMPTOMS

- Presents with a sensation of exaggerated motion when there is little or no motion.
- Peripheral vertigo is often accompanied by nausea and vomiting; central vertigo often occurs in conjunction with other posterior circulation findings.
- Ipsilateral facial numbness/weakness or limb ataxia suggests a lesion of the cerebellopontine angle.

EXAM

- Orthostatics.
- **Dix-Hallpike maneuver (positional testing):** Quickly bring the patient from a sitting to a supine position with one ear turned toward the table; repeat on the other side. A ⊕ test is defined as the presence of fatigable (10- to 20-second) nystagmus with or without vertigo. ⊕ in approximately 50% of patients with BPPV.

DIAGNOSIS/TREATMENT

Differentiate between central and peripheral vertigo as indicated in Tables 2.24 and 2.25.

UNINTENTIONAL WEIGHT LOSS

Defined as an unintended weight loss of > 5% of usual body weight over 6–12 months. Associated with excess morbidity and mortality; idiopathic in up to one-third of cases. Other etiologies are as follows:

- **Cancer** and **GI disorders** (malabsorption, pancreatic insufficiency) and **psychiatric disorders** (depression, anxiety, dementia, anorexia nervosa) account for up to two-thirds of cases.
- Other causes include hyperthyroidism, DM, chronic diseases, and infections. Difficulty with food preparation or intake from any cause (eg, social isolation with inability to shop/cook, ill-fitting dentures, dysphagia) should always be considered.

KEY FACT

Ménière's disease, which is characterized by unilateral or bilateral tinnitus, lower-frequency hearing loss, ear fullness, and episodic vertigo, develops in early to mid-adulthood and may improve with a ↓ in salt, caffeine, alcohol, and nicotine.

KEY FACT

Acute labyrinthitis can be distinguished from vestibular neuronitis because the vertigo occurs after a URI and can be associated with hearing loss.

TABLE 2.24. Causes of Central Vertigo

	ACOUSTIC NEUROMA (CN VIII SCHWANNOMA)	**BRAINSTEM ISCHEMIA**	**BASILAR MIGRAINE**	**MULTIPLE SCLEROSIS**
Symptoms	Unilateral hearing loss with tinnitus and vertigo.	**Symptoms of vertebrobasilar insufficiency: diplopia, dysarthria,** numbness.	Occipital **headache, visual disturbances,** sensory symptoms.	Chronic imbalance.
Duration	Continuous.	Varies.	Varies.	Fluctuating.
Exam/diagnosis	MRI.	MRI, angiogram.	Diagnosis of exclusion.	MRI.
Treatment	Surgery.	Stroke treatment.	β-blockers, ergots.	See the Neurology chapter.

TABLE 2.25. **Causes of Peripheral Vertigo**

	BPPV	MÉNIÈRE'S DISEASE	VESTIBULAR NEURONITIS/ ACUTE LABYRINTHITIS	POSTTRAUMATIC
Symptoms	Onset is a few seconds **following head motion;** nausea/vomiting.	Has four repeated, classic symptoms: episodic vertigo, **sensorineural hearing loss, tinnitus, and ear fullness.**	May be preceded by URI; **sudden, continuous.**	
Duration	**Up to one minute.**	One to several hours.	A few days to one week.	A few days to one month.
Diagnosis	⊕ **Dix-Hallpike.**	**Clinical; MRI to rule out acoustic neuroma.**	Clinical.	Clinical. CT if concerned about basilar skull fracture.
Etiology	Dislodging of otolith into the semicircular canal.	Distention of the endolymphatic compartment of the inner ear.	Unknown; often occurs after URI.	Post–head trauma.
Treatment	**Epley maneuver** (canalith repositioning); **habituation exercises.**	Bed rest; **avoid triggers (caffeine, salt, EtOH, nicotine) +/– diuretics;** symptomatic treatment with antihistamines, anticholinergics, and benzodiazepines.	Symptomatic (meclizine or benzodiazepines).	Symptomatic.

DIAGNOSIS

- The history and exam often provide clues.
- CBC, TSH, electrolytes, UA, CXR, and age-appropriate cancer screening tests.
- If initial testing is ⊖, observe the patient over time. If the symptoms/exam are suggestive, pursue further cancer screening or GI evaluation.

TREATMENT

- Treat the underlying disorder.
- Set caloric intake goals; give caloric supplementation.
- Appetite stimulants (megestrol acetate, dronabinol) are sometimes used in the presence of low appetite, usually in patients with conditions such as cancer and HIV/AIDS.

FATIGUE

A common symptom and nonspecific complaint with many causes. Consider **chronic fatigue syndrome** (CFS) if a patient has fatigue lasting at least six months that is not alleviated by rest and that interferes with daily activities, in combination with four or more of the following: impaired memory or concentration, sore throat, tender cervical or axillary lymph nodes, muscle pain, polyarthralgias, new headaches, unrefreshing sleep, and postexertion malaise.

- Can be mistaken for chronic EBV syndrome.
- A clinical diagnosis; no specific labs are required. Consider sending labs for EBV, ANA, RF, and Lyme titers in endemic areas.
- Treatment requires a multidisciplinary approach that includes antidepressants if applicable (SSRIs, TCAs), cognitive-behavioral therapy, graded exercises, and supportive patient-physician relationships. **Graded aerobic exercise** improves fatigue and physical functioning. Also consider concomitant antidepressants, which can help with sleep or fibromyalgia-like symptoms.

CHRONIC COUGH

Defined as a cough lasting > 8 weeks. The **"big three"** causes are as follows:

- **Postnasal drip:** Presents with a boggy nasal mucosa and a "cobblestone" oropharynx.
- **Cough-variant asthma:** Cough worsens at night, and wheezes are exacerbated by seasonal allergies, exercise, and cold weather.
- **GERD:** May present with heartburn and with cough that worsens at night, but asymptomatic in 75% of cases.

Additional causes include post-URI cough (may persist for two months), *B pertussis*, chronic bronchitis, and **ACEI** use (may last for a few weeks after cessation).

DIAGNOSIS

- Start with empiric treatment if one of the "big three" causes is suspected (see below).
- If empiric therapy fails, consider CXR, PFTs (+/– methacholine challenge) for suspected asthma, esophageal pH monitoring for GERD, ENT referral, or a sinus CT for postnasal drip.

TREATMENT

- Empirically treat the "big three" with nasal corticosteroids (postnasal drip), bronchodilators +/– inhaled steroids (asthma), or acid suppressants (GERD).
- Maximal therapy for the suspected condition for 2–4 weeks is recommended prior to further diagnostic testing.

MNEMONIC

Causes of chronic cough—

GASPS AND COUgh

GERD
Asthma
Smoking, chronic bronchitis
Postinfection
Sinusitis, postnasal drip
ACEIs
Neoplasm
Diverticulum
CHF
Outer ear disease
Upper airway obstruction

INSOMNIA

The most common of all sleep disorders, affecting roughly 15% of patients at some point, with ↑ prevalence associated with lower SES, recent stress, and drug/alcohol abuse. **Chronic insomnia** is defined as > 3 weeks of difficulty falling or staying asleep, frequent awakenings during the night, and a feeling of insufficient sleep (daytime fatigue, forgetfulness, irritability). Exacerbating factors include stress, pain, caffeine, daytime napping, early bedtimes, drug withdrawal (alcohol, benzodiazepines, opiates), and alcoholism.

DIFFERENTIAL

Restless leg syndrome (RLS), periodic limb movement disorder (PLMD). See Table 2.26 for further details.

TABLE 2.26.   Differential Diagnosis of Insomnia

	RESTLESS LEG SYNDROME	PERIODIC LIMB MOVEMENT DISORDER	INSOMNIA
Symptoms	Spontaneous leg movements associated with paresthesias that occur at rest and improve with leg movement.	Intermittent limb movements during non-REM sleep; seen in > 75% of patients with RLS.	Difficulty initiating or maintaining sleep with impairment in daytime function.
Disease associations	**Iron deficiency** (even in the absence of anemia), end-stage renal disease, DM; idiopathic in most cases.	Uremia, TCAs, MAOIs.	Depression, anxiety, stimulants, chronic pain, alcohol.
Pathophysiology	Unknown; may involve abnormal dopamine transmission.		Unknown or disease specific.
Treatment	Correct the underlying disorder (eg, iron supplementation); give dopaminergic agonists (carbidopa/levodopa, pramipexole) or benzodiazepines if dopaminergic agonists fail.	Same as that for RLS.	Correct the underlying disorder; sleep hygiene; medications.

DIAGNOSIS

- Diagnosis is mainly clinical.
- Rule out psychiatric and medical conditions—eg, depression, PTSD, delirium, chronic pain, medication side effects, GERD, and nocturia from BPH or DM.
- Labs for RLS include CBC, ferritin, and BUN/creatinine.
- Polysomnography may help diagnose PLMD and RLS and may also rule out other sleep-related disorders (eg, sleep apnea).

TREATMENT

- Treat the underlying disorder.
- Sleep hygiene and relaxation techniques are effective treatments for chronic insomnia.
- Benzodiazepines and benzodiazepine receptor agonists (zolpidem, zaleplon) are FDA approved for the treatment of short-term insomnia (7–10 days). Only eszopiclone, a longer-acting benzodiazepine receptor agonist, is FDA approved for the treatment of chronic insomnia. Antidepressants such as trazodone are commonly used off-label for this indication despite a lack of evidence for their safety or efficacy.

CHRONIC LOWER EXTREMITY EDEMA

The differential for chronic **bilateral lower extremity edema** includes the following (see also Table 2.27):

- **Venous insufficiency:** The most important risk factor for venous insufficiency is prior DVT or phlebitis. Other risk factors include obesity, age, injury, and a history of pregnancy. Varicose veins may be the only finding in the early stages. Edema, skin changes, and ulcerations (medial ankle) are later findings.
- **Lymphedema:** Can be idiopathic (due to a congenital abnormality of the lymphatic system) or 2° to lymphatic obstruction (eg, from tumor, filari-

TABLE 2.27.   Causes of Chronic Bilateral Lower Extremity Edema

MECHANISM	CAUSES
Elevated capillary hydrostatic pressure	**Venous insufficiency:** A heavy, achy feeling that worsens as the day progresses; brawny edema. CHF, constrictive pericarditis. **IVC compression:** Tumor, clot, lymph nodes. Pregnancy. **Filariasis:** Lymph node obstruction by *Wuchereria bancrofti* and *Brugia malayi.* **Drugs:** NSAIDs, glucocorticoids, estrogen.
↑ capillary permeability	Hypothyroid myxedema, drugs (CCBs, hydralazine), vasculitis.
↓ oncotic pressure	Nephrotic syndrome, protein-losing enteropathy, cirrhosis, malnutrition.

asis, lymph node dissection, or radiation). The dorsum of the foot is commonly affected. Late changes include a nonpitting "peau d'orange" appearance.

- **Varicose veins:** May occur with or without chronic venous insufficiency.
- **Right-sided heart failure.**
- **Low albumin states:** Nephrotic syndrome; protein-losing enteropathy.
- **Inferior vena cava obstruction.**

The differential for **unilateral lower extremity edema** is as follows:

- **Venous insufficiency:** Post–vein graft for CABG, prior DVT, leg injury.
- **Complex regional pain syndrome:** Hyperesthesia and hyperhidrosis that occur a few weeks after trauma; trophic skin changes and pain out of proportion to the exam (see below).
- **DVT:** Usually acute edema.
- **Infection:** Cellulitis or fasciitis.
- **Inflammation:** Gout; ruptured Baker's cyst (posterior knee).

DIAGNOSIS

- The etiology can often be determined without diagnostic testing.
- Depending on the history and exam, consider an echocardiogram, a UA for protein, liver enzymes, and abdominal/pelvic imaging to rule out systemic causes of edema or venous obstruction.
- Lower extremity ultrasound with Doppler can rule out DVT and demonstrate venous incompetence.
- Radionuclide lymphoscintigraphy is the gold-standard test for lymphedema.

TREATMENT

- Treat the underlying causes, including discontinuation of contributing medications.
- Compression stockings. Below-knee stockings ↓ postthrombotic syndrome in proximal DVT.
- Lifestyle modification (↓ salt) and leg elevation.
- Surgery and sclerotherapy are options for advanced varicosities.
- Meticulous skin care, gradient pressure stockings, massage therapy, and external pneumatic compression are modalities used to treat lymphedema. Avoid diuretics in light of the concern for intravascular volume depletion.

COMPLEX REGIONAL PAIN SYNDROME (CRPS)

A 32-year-old right-handed man presents with eight months of burning pain in his right arm. The pain started when he sustained an injury while waiting tables at a restaurant. He initially had a burning and painful sensation in his arm, which also had periods of being warm and then cool. Exam reveals brawny edema and excess sweat in the arm as well as ↑ muscle tone. What is the most likely diagnosis and workup?

No tests can diagnose CRPS definitively, but an x-ray of the affected limb may show osteopenia from disuse, and a bone scan may be helpful. Treatment is aimed at decreasing the pain and preventing atrophy with physical therapy. Neuropathic pain medications such as TCAs and gabapentin may be helpful. An oral steroid taper and regional nerve blocks are also options.

A rare condition characterized by autonomic and vasomotor instability in the affected extremity. Previously known as reflex sympathetic dystrophy, the syndrome is usually **preceded by direct physical trauma,** which may be minor. Surgery on the affected limb may also precede the development of CRPS. Most commonly affects the **hand.**

SYMPTOMS

- Presents as:
    - Diffuse pain of the affected extremity that is often burning, intense, and worsened by light touch.
    - Swelling.
    - Disturbances of color and temperature.
    - Dystrophic changes of affected skin and nails.
    - Limited ROM.
- The shoulder-hand variant presents with hand symptoms along with limited ROM at the ipsilateral shoulder. May occur after MI or neck/shoulder injury.

DIAGNOSIS

- No specific diagnostic tests are available, but **bone scan** is sensitive and reveals ↑ uptake in the affected extremity. MRI may also be helpful.
- Later in the course, x-rays reveal generalized **osteopenia.**

TREATMENT/PREVENTION

- Early mobilization and physical therapy after injury/surgery/MI ↓ the chance of developing CRPS and improves the prognosis once it has occurred.
- TCAs are first-line pharmacologic therapy; neuropathic pain medications (gabapentin, topical lidocaine), local steroid injections, oral glucocorticoids, bisphosphonates, and calcitonin may also be used.
- Regional nerve blocks and dorsal column stimulation are helpful as well.

Medical Ethics

Based on a group of fundamental principles that should guide the best practice (see Table 2.28).

DECISION MAKING

- Decisions about medical care should be **shared** between the patient (or surrogate) and the provider.
- **Informed consent** can be verbal but should be put in writing for high-risk treatments.
- Patients can give informed consent provided that they demonstrate **decision-making capacity** by:
  - Understanding their medical condition and the treatment being proposed.
  - Communicating their understanding about potential risks, benefits, and alternatives.
  - Making decisions that are rational and consistent over time and with their values.
  - Demonstrating that they are not influenced by delirium.
- If a patient lacks the capacity to make decisions, his or her advance directive or assigned surrogate should guide decisions.

CONFIDENTIALITY

- **HIPAA,** the Health Insurance Portability and Accountability Act of 1996, provides specific guidelines governing when and how the sharing of confidential patient information is acceptable.
- Exceptions to the rule of confidentiality include the following:
  - Child or elder abuse or domestic violence.
  - Reportable diseases (eg, STDs, conditions that could impair driving).
  - Threats by the patient to others' lives.
- When confidentiality must be broken, physicians should, when possible, discuss the need for disclosure with the patient in advance.

KEY FACT

Exceptions to the requirement for informed consent include life-threatening emergencies or circumstances in which patients waive their right to participate in the decision-making process.

KEY FACT

A diagnosis of dementia does not necessarily imply that the patient lacks capacity to make decisions as long as the patient can satisfy the requirements of decision-making capacity.

TABLE 2.28. Guiding Principles in Biomedical Ethics

PRINCIPLE	EXPLANATION	EXAMPLE
Beneficence	Act in patients' best interest.	A physician counsels a hyperlipidemic patient on lifestyle modifications.
Nonmaleficence	Do no harm to your patient.	A physician advises against epidural steroid injection for chronic back pain due to spinal stenosis because it is unlikely to benefit the patient.
Justice	The equitable distribution of resources within a population.	Organ transplantation.
Autonomy	The right of patients to make their own decisions about their health care.	A patient gives informed consent for (or refuses) surgery.
Fidelity	Truthful disclosure to patients.	A physician informs a patient that pneumothorax occurred during thoracentesis.

ERROR REPORTING

Patients who have been injured, even if no error occurred, should be informed promptly and completely about what has happened.

IMPAIRED PHYSICIANS

- Physicians who are impaired must not take on patient care responsibilities that they may not be able to perform safely and effectively.
- Causes include substance use (alcohol, other drugs), psychiatric illness, advanced dementia, or physical illness that interferes with the cognitive and/or motor skills needed to deliver care.
- Physicians have an ethical responsibility to protect patients from other physicians they know to be impaired. Legal reporting requirements vary.

FUTILE CARE

- Physicians are not obliged to provide care that they believe is futile.
- Futility is difficult to define quantitatively, but generally accepted futile conditions are as follows:
  - CPR in a patient who fails maximal life-support measures (eg, a patient who suffers cardiac arrest due to hypotension refractory to multiple vasopressors).
  - An intervention that has already been tried and failed (eg, if cancer worsened despite a complete course of chemotherapy, there would be no obligation to provide another course of the same therapy).
  - Treatment with no physiologic basis (eg, plasmapheresis for septic shock).
- Ethical "gray zones" in futility include withdrawing life-sustaining support because the chance of success is small or because the patient's best outcome would be a low quality of life. Ethics consultations are often required to sort through these complex situations.

RESOURCE ALLOCATION

- Physicians should use health resources judiciously and appropriately (ie, they should avoid unnecessary tests, medications, procedures, and consults).
- A physician's 1° responsibility is to his/her patient, and larger resource allocation decisions should be made at the societal, policy level.

Gay and Lesbian Health

Sexual practices, not orientation, determine the risk of infections and cancers. Patients in same-sex relationships may have had opposite-sex relationships in the past (and vice versa), and specific high-risk practices (eg, receptive anal intercourse) may occur in patients who self-identify as either "gay" or "straight."

RISKS

- There is an ↑ risk of anal cancer (caused by HPV) in men who have sex with men (MSM), particularly in those who are HIV ⊕.
- There may be a somewhat ↓ risk of cervical cancer and HPV among women who have sex with women; however, many women who self-identify as lesbian have had sex with men, and rates of HPV infection are significant in this population.
- There is a ↓ risk of gonorrhea, syphilis, and chlamydia among women not having sex with men.
- HIV, gonorrhea, chlamydia, syphilis, hepatitis A, and hepatitis B are ↑ among MSM.

SCREENING

- **In MSM:**
  - Screen for HIV and HBV, **urethritis** (*Neisseria gonorrhoeae, Chlamydia trachomatis*), and proctitis (*N gonorrhoeae, C trachomatis,* HSV, syphilis).
  - Offer HBV and HAV vaccines.
  - **Anal Pap smear:** In HIV-⊕ MSM, this test has characteristics similar to those of the cervical Pap smear.
- **In women who have sex with women,** cervical cancer screening should proceed according to standard guidelines (see the discussion of cancer screening above) even if patients have never had heterosexual contact.

Evidence-Based Medicine

MAJOR STUDY TYPES

Table 2.29 outlines the major types of studies seen in the medical literature.

TEST PARAMETERS

Test parameters measure the clinical usefulness of a test. These include the following:

- **Sensitivity (Sn) ("PID"—Positive in Disease):** The probability that a given test will be ⊕ in someone who has the disease in question.
- **Specificity of a test (Sp) ("NIH"—Negative in Health):** The probability that a given test will be ⊖ in someone who does not have the disease in question.
- **Positive predictive value (PPV):** The probability that a disease is present in a person with a ⊕ test result.
- **Negative predictive value (NPV):** The probability that a disease is absent in a person with a ⊖ test result.
- **Likelihood ratio (LR):** The proportion of patients **with** a disease who have a certain test result divided by the proportion of patients **without** the disease in question who have the same test result ("**WOWO**"—With Over WithOut). **Example:** A high-probability V/Q scan has an LR of 14. This means that a high-probability V/Q scan is 14 times more likely to be seen in patients **with** pulmonary embolism than in patients **without** pulmonary embolism.

KEY FACT

A highly **Se**nsitive test, when **N**egative, rules **out** the disease (**SnNout**).

KEY FACT

A highly **Sp**ecific test, when **P**ositive, rules **in** the disease (**SpPin**).

KEY FACT

Sensitivity and specificity are characteristics of the diagnostic test itself. They do not depend on the population being tested or on disease prevalence.

KEY FACT

Unlike sensitivity and specificity, the PPV and NPV of a test vary depending on the prevalence of the disease in the population being tested.

TABLE 2.29. Statistical Study Types

Study Type	Explanation	Example	Advantages	Disadvantages
Randomized controlled trial	Assigns exposure to subjects and observes disease outcome.	Assigning patients with hypertension to one of two treatments: diuretics or ACEIs.	True experiment erases unforeseen confounders. The optimal study type for assessing the effects of a particular intervention/exposure.	Expensive. The study population may be homogeneous, limiting the ability to generalize the results to the overall population. Small sample sizes limit the power to detect small but potentially important differences between groups.
Cohort study	Identifies exposure subjects first and **then follows** for disease outcomes.	Identifying obese adults and following them for development of hypertension.	The most robust observational study type; evaluates multiple exposures.	May take a long time to develop disease. Confounding and unmeasured variables may lead to incorrect conclusions.
Case-control study	Identifies cases and noncases of the disease outcome **before** determining exposure.	Identifying children born with a rare birth defect and looking at possible in utero exposures.	Inexpensive; fast; good for rare diseases and for generating hypotheses to subject to more rigorous study.	Prone to biases.
Cross-sectional study	Identifies exposure and outcome **at the same time** for each subject within a specified population.	Determining how many patients hospitalized with an upper GI bleed have a history of recent NSAID use.	Often survey data.	No ability to detect temporal relationship between exposure and outcome.
Systematic review	Summarizes the results of multiple individual trials addressing the same (or similar) research questions.	Qualitative review of all trials of omega-3 fatty acids for the prevention of cardiovascular disease.	Sets forth rigorous criteria to determine which studies will be included or excluded from the review. This helps limit bias in the summary conclusions.	Studies are often too small or too heterogeneous to apply rigorous statistical methods to the summary analysis. Qualitative summary conclusions are substituted for numeric data.
Meta-analysis	A subset of systematic reviews. Quantitative compilation of data from multiple small studies to generate a pooled result.	Cochrane review of all randomized trials comparing glucosamine with placebo or other treatments for patients with osteoarthritis.	Provides an estimate of treatment effect, including magnitude of effect, when individual studies are too small to derive robust conclusions.	Uses a variety of statistical methods. Different meta-analyses of the same data can produce different results. When component studies are heterogeneous, it is difficult to interpret/use a pooled result.

TABLE 2.30. Calculating PPV and NPV

	DISEASE PRESENT	**DISEASE ABSENT**
Test ⊕	True ⊕ **a**	False ⊕ **b**
Test ⊖	**c** False ⊖	**d** True ⊖

Calculating PPV, NPV, and LRs

Creating a 2 × 2 table of test results and disease status allows one to calculate PPV and NPV, as well as ⊕ and ⊖ LRs, when sensitivity and specificity are known (see Table 2.30):

- Sensitivity = a / a + c.
- Specificity = d / b + d.
- PPV = a / a + b.
- NPV = d / c + d.
- LR (+) = (sensitivity) / (1 – specificity).
- LR (–) = (1 – sensitivity) / (specificity).

An illustrative example of how to calculate PPV, NPV, and LRs, and how they depend on disease prevalence, is outlined below.

- For a given disease, the diagnostic test under consideration has the following characteristics:
    - Sensitivity = 90%
    - Specificity = 95%
- For this test, then, the **likelihood ratios** of ⊕ and ⊖ results are as follows:
    - LR (+) = 0.90 / (1 – 0.95) = 18.
    - LR (–) = (1 – 0.90) / 0.95 = 0.105.
- Since the LRs are far from 1, this test appears to be useful both for ruling disease in and for ruling it out. However, disease prevalence in the population has a crucial effect on test performance, as seen below.

Example:

- Suppose the disease prevalence in the population in question is 20%. Given a total population of 1000 individuals, the 2 × 2 table of disease status/test result can be constructed as shown in Table 2.31.

KEY FACT

Although there is no formal cutoff point, a ⊕ LR between 1 and 3 indicates a diagnostic test that is not very useful in ruling in disease. A ⊕ LR > 10 is generally accepted as a highly valuable diagnostic test.

KEY FACT

LRs are applied to pretest probabilities (the likelihood, before performing a diagnostic test, that the patient has the disease in question) to either ↑ (⊕ test) or ↓ (⊖ test) the likelihood that disease is present.

TABLE 2.31. 2 × 2 Table, Assuming 20% Disease Prevalence

	DISEASE PRESENT	**DISEASE ABSENT**	**TOTALS**
Test ⊕	180 a	40 b	220
Test ⊖	c 20	d 760	780
Totals	200	800	1000

- From this table, one can calculate PPV and NPV:
    - PPV = a / a + b = 180/220 = 81.8%.
    - NPV = d / c + d = 760/780 = 97.4%.
- In this population, 81.8% of ⊕ results occur in people who truly do have the disease (true ⊕s), while 97.4% of ⊖ results occur in people who truly do not have the disease (true ⊖s).
- For the same diagnostic test with the same sensitivity and specificity, **if the disease prevalence were 2%, the values in the 2 × 2 table would change** (see Table 2.32). In this population, the PPV and NPV are different:
    - PPV = a / a + b = 18/67 = 26.9%.
    - NPV = d / c + d = 931/933 = 99.8%.
- In this population, only 26.9% of ⊕ results occur in people who truly have the disease; 99.8% of ⊖ results occur in people who truly do not have the disease.
- This example illustrates that when a disease is rare in the population being tested, even a fairly sensitive and specific test will have a low PPV. False ⊕s will be far more common than true ⊕s in this population.

Number Needed to Treat (NNT)

Defined as the number of patients who must receive the treatment in question in order to achieve one additional favorable outcome (or avoid one additional adverse outcome) compared to the control treatment. The lower the NNT, the more effective the treatment. **NNT = 1 / absolute risk reduction.**

- A randomized trial finds that subjects treated with a placebo have a 25% incidence of adverse outcome X. Subjects treated with drug A have a 14% incidence of the same adverse outcome.
- The absolute reduction in risk for adverse outcome X with drug A vs. placebo is 25% – 14% = 11%. Thus, NNT = 1/0.11 = 9.09.
- This means that approximately nine patients would have to be treated with drug A instead of the placebo to prevent one case of adverse outcome X.

TABLE 2.32. **2 × 2 Table, Assuming 2% Disease Prevalence**

	DISEASE PRESENT	DISEASE ABSENT	TOTALS
Test ⊕	18 a	49 b	67
Test ⊖	c 2	d 931	933
Totals	20	980	1000

TABLE 2.33.   **Threats to the Validity of Statistical Studies**

	EXPLANATION	EXAMPLES
Confounding	Another variable (confounding factor) is associated with the predictor variable and the outcome variable without being in the causal pathway.	Coffee drinking is associated with a risk of MI. This does not mean that coffee causes MI; rather, coffee drinking (the confounder) is associated with smoking (the true predictor variable), and smoking causes MI.
Measurement (misclassification) biases	When the method of measuring an exposure or outcome misclassifies subjects either at random or in a systematic way. **Random misclassification:** When participants are placed in the wrong group (either with or without exposure/disease) in a random fashion. This biases the results to the null. **Nonrandom misclassification:** When placement into the correct vs. incorrect exposure group is dependent on disease status. Recall bias is a common type of nonrandom misclassification. **Recall bias:** Self-reporting by study subjects is influenced by knowledge of the study hypothesis, or knowledge of subjects' own disease status.	Misclassification bias occurs if subjects provide inaccurate information. For example, subjects may underreport behaviors perceived as socially unacceptable, such as heavy alcohol use. If the likelihood of underreporting alcohol intake is independent of disease status, random misclassification of subjects occurs. Recall bias: In a case-control study, cancer patients may think harder than healthy controls about past toxic exposures, are more likely to recall them, and are thus more likely to be categorized as "exposed."
Selection bias	Study subjects are selected into (or drop out of) a study in a way that misleadingly changes the degree of association.	Subjects recruited into a study from a subspecialty referral center are more likely to have severe forms of illness than those from a broader community-based sample. Subjects who drop out of a study after recruitment may have different disease characteristics or associations than those who continue the study.

THREATS TO VALIDITY

Table 2.33 and the discussion below delineate factors that can adversely affect the outcome of a statistical study.

- **Lead-time bias:** The time by which a screening test advances the date of diagnosis from the usual symptomatic phase to an earlier, presymptomatic phase. It occurs because the time between diagnosis and death will always ↑ by the amount of lead time (see Figure 2.19).
    - **Example:** A new screening test for pancreatic cancer is able to detect disease in a presymptomatic stage.
    - Unfortunately, the poor overall prognosis for the disease remains the same. Screened patients know about their diagnosis sooner and live with the disease longer because of this knowledge, but their death is not truly postponed because no treatment exists to alter the outcome for patients diagnosed earlier in the course of illness.
- **Length-time bias:** Because cases vary in the lengths of their presymptomatic phase, screening will overdetect cases of slowly progressing disease

 KEY FACT

Screen-detected patients will always live longer than clinically detected patients even if early detection and treatment confer no benefit. This is due to lead-time and length-time biases.

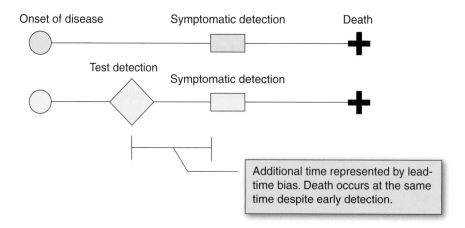

FIGURE 2.19.   Lead-time bias.

(longer duration in the asymptomatic phase) and will miss rapidly progressing cases.

- **Example:** In Figure 2.20, mammography is able to detect two cases of slowly growing breast cancer because of the long period between disease onset and symptoms, but two cases with rapid progression from onset to symptoms are missed. This type of bias occurs with every screening test.
- Because more slowly progressive cases are more likely to be detected by the screening test, patients with screen-detected disease appear to have better outcomes than those with inherently aggressive disease diagnosed because of symptoms.

HYPOTHESIS TESTING

- **_p_-value:** A quantitative estimate of the probability that a particular study result could occur by chance alone if in fact there is no difference between groups or no treatment effect.
    - A result with a $p < 0.05$ signifies that the probability of the results occurring by chance is < 1 in 20 and is considered to be "statistically significant."

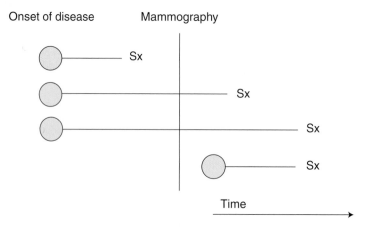

FIGURE 2.20.   Length-time bias. Two cases of breast cancer with brief time between disease onset and symptom appearance (top and bottom cases) are missed by routine mammography. Two other cases, with longer presymptomatic phases, are detected by mammography.

- **Example:** A study finds that treatment A, compared to placebo, causes a 20% reduction in the chance of outcome B, with a p-value < 0.05. This means that there is less than a 5% chance that the difference in treatment effect between the two drugs is due to chance alone.
- **Confidence interval (CI):** If a given study were repeated 100 times, the range into which results would be expected to fall in x% of trials is the x% CI. In the medical literature, the 95% CI is generally used (ie, the range into which results would fall in 95 out of 100 repeats of the study in question).
  - **Example:** A study finds that the LR of a diagnostic test is 6.7.
  - The 95% confidence interval for this result is $5.0 - 8.2$. This finding is abbreviated as LR $= 6.7$ (95% CI, $5.0 - 8.2$).

KEY FACT

A narrower CI around a result indicates a more precise result. Larger studies generally produce narrower CIs.

NOTES

CHAPTER 3

Cardiovascular Disease

Anuj Gaggar, MD, PhD
Sanjiv Shah, MD

Cardiac Diagnosis and Testing

You should know this topic well, as it is an extremely high-yield area for boards testing.

THE PHYSICAL EXAM

Arterial Pulsations

Know these examples of abnormal arterial pulsations and the disorders with which they are commonly associated (see also Figure 3.1):

- **Asymmetric pulses:** Aortic dissection (good pulses in the upper extremities vs. absent or diminished pulses in the lower extremities).
- **Carotid pulsations:**
  - **Pulsus tardus** (delayed upstroke): Aortic **stenosis.**
  - **Bisferiens pulse:** Two palpable peaks during systole; occurs in aortic **regurgitation** (with or without aortic stenosis) and hypertrophic cardiomyopathy.
- **Peripheral pulses:**
  - **Corrigan (water-hammer) pulse:** Occurs in chronic, hemodynamically significant aortic regurgitation. Characterized by a rapid rise and fall of the radial pulse accentuated by wrist elevation.
  - **Pulsus paradoxus:** Defined as a ↓ **in BP of > 10 mm Hg** during normal inspiration. Occurs in cardiac tamponade, constrictive pericarditis, severe asthma, and COPD.
  - **Pulsus alternans:** Alternation of amplitude with every other heartbeat. Occurs in severe systolic heart failure.

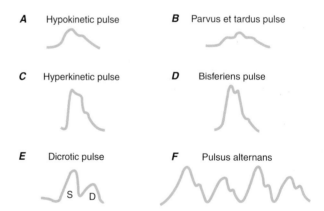

FIGURE 3.1. **Arterial pulse waveforms.** (Adapted with permission from Fuster V et al. *Hurst's the Heart,* 12th ed. New York: McGraw-Hill, 2008, Fig. 12-43.)

Venous Pulsations

A 37-year-old man with a bicuspid aortic valve is admitted to the hospital for endocarditis. On hospital day 3 he is noted to have ↑ fatigue, and examination of his jugular vein reveals occasional prominent a waves. What is his ECG likely to show?

Complete heart block. This patient likely has aortic endocarditis given his bicuspid aortic valve, which predisposes him to aortic disease. The finding of prominent a waves likely refers to cannon a waves, which are often found with complete heart block. Inasmuch as progression to heart block is a known sequela of aortic valve endocarditis, this is the most likely ECG finding in this patient.

The following are examples of **normal jugular venous pulsations** (see also Figure 3.2). These are testable, so know them well.

- **a wave:** Right atrial contraction.
- **x descent:** Atrial relaxation.
- **v wave:** Ventricular systole (with passive venous filling of the atrium).
- **y descent:** Opening of the tricuspid valve with rapid emptying of the right atrium.
- **Jugular venous pressure (JVP):** During inspiration, the JVP declines.

Abnormal patterns of jugular venous pulsations include the following (see also Figure 3.3):

- **Cannon a waves:** Atrioventricular (AV) dissociation (the atrium contracts against a closed tricuspid valve).
- **Large a wave:** Tricuspid stenosis, pulmonary hypertension, pulmonary stenosis.
- **Absent a waves:** Atrial fibrillation (AF).
- **Large v wave:** Tricuspid regurgitation.
- **Prominent x descent:** Cardiac tamponade; constrictive pericarditis.
- **Rapid y descent:** Constrictive pericarditis; restrictive cardiomyopathy.
- **Blunted y descent:** Tricuspid stenosis; right atrial myxoma (obstruction of right atrial emptying).
- **Absent y descent:** Cardiac tamponade.
- **Kussmaul's sign:** An ↑ in JVP during inspiration. Seen in chronic constrictive pericarditis; occasionally seen in tricuspid stenosis and CHF.

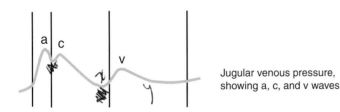

Jugular venous pressure, showing a, c, and v waves

FIGURE 3.2. **Normal jugular venous pulse waveforms.**

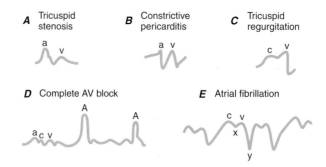

FIGURE 3.3. **Abnormal jugular venous pulse waveforms.** a—a positive wave due to contraction of the right atrium. c—a positive deflection due to bulging of the tricuspid valve toward the atria at the onset of ventricular contraction. x—a negative deflection due to atrial relaxation. v—a positive deflection due to filling of the right atrium against the closed tricuspid valve during ventricular contraction. y—a negative deflection due to emptying of the right atrium upon ventricular relaxation. (Adapted with permission from Fuster V et al. *Hurst's the Heart,* 12th ed. New York: McGraw-Hill, 2008, Fig. 12-46.)

Heart Murmurs

Table 3.1 illustrates the differential diagnosis of valvular heart disease. Table 3.2 differentiates systolic murmurs on the basis of their response to various physiologic maneuvers. Further distinctions are as follows:

- In general, right-sided murmurs and heart sounds are louder during inspiration, whereas left-sided murmurs are louder during expiration.
- Squatting and straight-leg raising ↑ cardiac filling, causing murmurs to get louder (with the exception of mitral valve prolapse [MVP] and hypertrophic obstructive cardiomyopathy [HOCM]). Standing and Valsalva maneuvers ↓ cardiac filling, causing murmurs to ↓ (with the exception of MVP and HOCM).
- Handgrip ↑ vascular resistance and can help distinguish MVP from HOCM; MVP murmurs get louder, whereas HOCM murmurs diminish.

> **KEY FACT**
>
> Inspiration (↑ venous return to the right atrium) ↑ right-sided murmurs but ↓ left-sided murmurs.

TABLE 3.1. **Differential Diagnosis of Valvular Heart Disease**

	MITRAL STENOSIS	**MITRAL REGURGITATION**	**AORTIC STENOSIS**	**AORTIC REGURGITATION**	**TRICUSPID STENOSIS**	**TRICUSPID REGURGITATION**
Inspection	Malar flush.	Prominent apical impulse to the left of the midclavicular line (MCL). "Water-hammer" pulse.	Sustained point of maximal impulse (PMI).	Hyperdynamic PMI to the left of the MCL. Wide pulse pressure with a diastolic pressure of < 60 mm Hg.	**Giant a wave** in jugular pulse. Olive-colored skin (mixed jaundice and local cyanosis).	**Large v wave** in jugular pulse.
Heart sounds	**Opening snap** in early diastole.	Prominent S3. Midsystolic **clicks** may be present.	**Paradoxic splitting of S2.** Prominent S4.	—	—	—

(continues)

TABLE 3.1. Differential Diagnosis of Valvular Heart Disease *(continued)*

	MITRAL STENOSIS	MITRAL REGURGITATION	AORTIC STENOSIS	AORTIC REGURGITATION	TRICUSPID STENOSIS	TRICUSPID REGURGITATION
Murmurs	Diastolic low-pitched, rumbling murmur. Rarely, short diastolic (Graham Steell) murmur along the lower left sternal border.	Pansystolic blowing murmur.	Midsystolic harsh murmur.	Diastolic blowing murmur. May be associated with a low-pitched mid-diastolic murmur at the apex (Austin Flint murmur).	Diastolic.	Systolic.
Optimum auscultatory conditions (louder murmur)	After exercise, left lateral recumbency.	After exercise. In prolapse, findings are most prominent while standing.	Patient resting, leaning forward; breath held in full expiration.	Patient leaning forward; breath held in expiration.	Murmur is usually louder and at a peak during inspiration. Patient is recumbent.	Murmur usually becomes louder during inspiration.
X-ray	Straight left heart border. Large left atrium sharply indenting the esophagus.	Enlarged left ventricle and left atrium.	Prominent ascending aorta; small knob. Calcified valve is common.	Moderate to severe left ventricular enlargement. Prominent aortic knob.	Enlarged right atrium only.	Enlarged right atrium and ventricle.
ECG	LAE.	LVH.	LVH.	LVH.	—	—

(Adapted with permission from McPhee SJ et al. *Current Medical Diagnosis & Treatment 2010.* New York: McGraw-Hill, 2010, Table 10-2.)

Heart Sounds

The following are examples of abnormal and normal heart sounds:

- **S1:**
  - Heard when the mitral and tricuspid valves close.
  - ↓ with severe left ventricular systolic dysfunction, mitral regurgitation, and a long PR interval.
  - ↑ with mitral stenosis (the mitral valve slams shut) and a short PR interval.
- **S2:**
  - Heard when the aortic (A2) and pulmonic (P2) valves close.
  - In normal hearts, A2 comes before P2.
  - A2 is ↓ in severe aortic stenosis.
  - **Physiologic splitting:** The time between A2 and P2 widens during inspiration.
  - **Variable/wide splitting:** All causes of right ventricular overload—eg, pulmonic stenosis, ventricular septal defect (VSD), mitral regurgitation, and right bundle branch block (RBBB).

TABLE 3.2. Differential Diagnosis of Systolic Murmurs Based on Response to Various Maneuvers[a]

Maneuver	Innocent Flow Murmur	Tricuspid Regurgitation	Aortic Stenosis	Mitral Regurgitation/ VSD	Mitral Valve Prolapse	Hypertrophic Obstructive Cardiomyopathy
Inspiration	– or ↑	↑	–	–	–	–
Standing	↓	–	–	–	↑	↑
Squatting	↑	–	–	–	↓	↓
Valsalva	↓	↓	↓	↓	↑	↑
Handgrip/ transient arterial occlusion	↓	–	–	↑	↑	↓
Post-PVC	↑	–	↑	–	–	↑

[a]↑ or ↓ = change in intensity of murmur; – = no consistent change.
(Reproduced with permission from Crawford MH. *Current Diagnosis & Treatment: Cardiology,* 3rd ed. New York: McGraw-Hill, 2009, Table 1-2.)

- **Fixed splitting:** Atrial septal defect (ASD).
- **Paradoxical splitting:** ↑ splitting **with expiration.** Etiologies include aortic stenosis, left bundle branch block (LBBB), paced rhythm, and left ventricular systolic dysfunction.
- S3:
  - A low-pitched sound heard in diastole just after S2. Usually best heard at the apex.
  - Occurs as a result of sudden limitation of blood flow during ventricular filling.
  - Can be a normal finding in healthy young adults.
  - Abnormal in older adults; suggests ↑ filling pressures. Associated with enlargement of the ventricle and typically due to systolic dysfunction (but can be seen in diastolic dysfunction). Hemodynamically significant mitral regurgitation is another cause.
  - **A strong predictor of perioperative cardiovascular events.**
- S4:
  - A low-pitched sound heard in diastole just before S1.
  - Coincides with atrial systole ("atrial kick").
  - Occurs as a result of a stiff left ventricle with ↑ ventricular filling during atrial systole.
  - A normal finding with advancing age due to loss of ventricular compliance.
  - Pathologic causes include long-standing hypertension, aortic stenosis, hypertrophic cardiomyopathy, and other causes of a stiff left ventricle.
  - Absent in AF.
- Additional diastolic sounds:
  - **Opening snap:** A high-frequency, early diastolic sound most frequently caused by **mitral stenosis.**
  - **Pericardial knock:** A high-pitched sound due to abrupt termination of ventricular filling in early diastole in the setting of constrictive pericarditis. Pericardial knock occurs earlier in diastole and has a higher pitch than an S3.

NONINVASIVE CARDIAC TESTING

Electrocardiography (ECG)

A 62-year-old man presents with chest pain and is noted to have ECG changes consistent with an old MI. After acute coronary syndrome is ruled out, he undergoes a dipyridamole nuclear stress test, which shows a perfusion defect in the anterior wall during stress that does not improve with rest. What should the next step be?

Medical management. Given that the area of perfusion deficit did not improve with rest, it is likely to represent a myocardial scar rather than an area of viable but at-risk tissue. Coronary angiography with stent placement is not likely to improve this perfusion defect, so the patient should be managed with ASA and should be evaluated for the appropriateness of β-blockers, ACEIs, and HMG-CoA inhibitors.

The following are fundamentals of ECG interpretation:

- **Dimensions (one small box):** Height: 0.1 mV = 1 mm; duration: 40 msec = 1 mm. *[handwritten: 0.04 sec]*
- **Rate:** The normal heart rate is 60–100 bpm (300 ÷ number of large boxes = rate).
- **QRS axis:** A normal axis is –30° to +90°. An axis less than –30° is left axis deviation; an axis more than +90° is right axis deviation. Use QRS in leads I and II to determine axis. Upright in I and II = normal axis; upright in I and downward in II = left axis deviation; downward in I and upright in II = right axis deviation; downward in I and II = extreme axis deviation. *[handwritten: I, aVF]*
- **Intervals:**
  - **PR:** Normal 120–200 msec (3–5 small boxes).
  - **QRS:** Abnormal > 120 msec (> 3 small boxes).
  - **QT:** Normal < 1/2 RR interval (rule of thumb).
  - **QTc:** Abnormal > 440 msec. *[handwritten: $QT_c = \frac{QT}{\sqrt{R-R}}$, should not exceed >500ms c QT- prolonging meds]*
- **Right atrial abnormality (only one criterion is needed):**
  - **Lead II:** P > 2.5 mm (P-wave height > 2.5 small boxes).
  - **Lead V₁:** P > 1.5 mm (P-wave height > 1.5 small boxes).
- **Left atrial abnormality (only one criterion is needed):**
  - **Lead II:** P > 120 msec with notches separated by at least one small box.
  - **Lead V₁:** P wave has a ⊖ terminal deflection that is ≥ 40 msec by 1 mm (one small box by one small box).
- **Left ventricular hypertrophy (LVH):** There are numerous criteria for LVH, three of which are listed below. All are specific but insensitive, so fulfillment of one criterion is sufficient for LVH in patients > 35 years of age. There is ↓ specificity in younger patients (those < 35 years of age).
  - $RaVL > 9$ mm in women and > 11 mm in men.
  - $RaVL + SV_3 > 20$ mm in women and > 25 mm in men.
  - $SV_1 + (RV_5 \text{ or } RV_6) > 35$ mm.
- **Right ventricular hypertrophy (RVH):** The following findings suggest RVH (there are several others):
  - Right axis deviation.
  - $RV_1 + SV_6 > 11$ mm (or simply look for a deep S wave in V_6).
  - R:S ratio > 1 in V_1 (in the absence of RBBB or posterior MI).

- **RBBB** (see Figure 3.4):
  - QRS > 120 msec.
  - Wide S wave in I, V_5, and V_6.
  - Second R wave (R′) in right precordial leads, with R′ greater than the initial R (look for "rabbit ears" in V_1 and V_2).
- **LBBB** (see Figure 3.4):
  - QRS > 120 msec, broad R wave in I and V_6, broad S wave in V_1, and a normal axis **or**
  - QRS > 120 msec, broad R wave in I, broad S wave in V_1, RS in V_6, and left axis deviation.
- **Left anterior fascicular block:** There are several sets of criteria for left anterior fascicular block:
  - The axis is more ⊖ than −45°.
  - Q in aVL; time from onset of QRS to the peak of the R wave > 0.05 sec.
  - Also look for Q in lead I and S in lead III.
- **Left posterior fascicular block: Must exclude anterolateral MI, RVH, and RBBB.** Axis > 100° and Q in lead III; S in lead I.
- Figure 3.5 illustrates the appearance on ECG of a range of medical conditions and drug effects. Figure 3.6 illustrates wide-complex tachycardia.

Exercise Treadmill Testing

A screening test for patients with symptoms suggestive of CAD **who have a normal resting ECG** and the ability to undergo vigorous exercise testing.

- Exercise ↑ myocardial O_2 demand and unmasks ↓ coronary flow reserve in patients with hemodynamically significant coronary stenoses.
- ST-segment depression (especially if horizontal or downsloping > 0.1 mV and lasting > 0.08 sec) has very high sensitivity and specificity for CAD if peak heart rate is at least **85%** of the maximum predicted rate (220 – age).

KEY FACT

Inferior MI is an important cause of new left axis deviation.

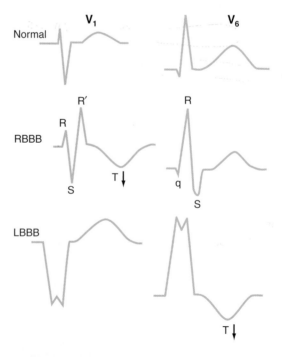

FIGURE 3.4. **Bundle branch blocks.** (Reproduced with permission from Fauci AS et al. *Harrison's Principles of Internal Medicine,* 17th ed. New York: McGraw-Hill, 2008, Fig. 221-10.)

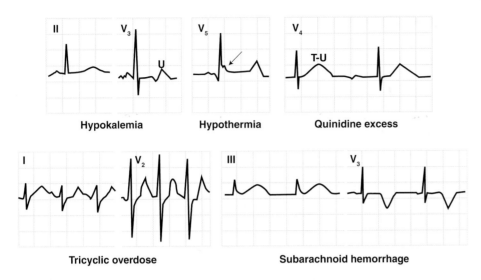

FIGURE 3.5. **ECG manifestations of various medical conditions and drug effects.**

- False ⊕s are more common in women and in those with atypical chest pain, no chest pain, and anemia.
- False ⊖s are more common in patients with preexisting CAD.
- An abnormal resting ECG (eg, digoxin or LVH) may also ↓ the sensitivity and specificity of results.

ECG criteria that favor ventricular tachycardia:

1. AV dissociation
2. QRS width: > 0.14 sec with RBBB configuration
   > 0.16 sec with LBBB configuration
3. QRS axis: Left axis deviation with RBBB morphology
   Extreme left axis deviation (northwest axis) with LBBB morphology
4. Concordance of QRS in precordial leads
5. Morphologic patterns of the QRS complex
   RBBB: Mono- or biphasic complex in V_1
   RS (*only with left axis deviation*) or QS in V_6

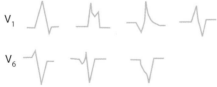

LBBB: Broad R wave in V_1 or V_2 ≥ 0.04 sec
Onset of QRS to nadir of S wave in V_1 or V_2 of ≥ 0.07 sec
Notched downslope of S wave in V_1 and V_2
Q wave in V_6

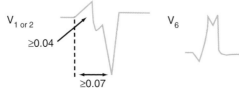

FIGURE 3.6. **Wide-complex tachycardia.** (Reproduced with permission from Kasper DL et al. *Harrison's Principles of Internal Medicine,* 16th ed. New York: McGraw-Hill, 2005: 1352.)

Echocardiography

A noninvasive ultrasound imaging modality used to identify anatomic abnormalities of the heart and great vessels, to assess the size and function of cardiac chambers, and to evaluate valvular function.

- **Resting** regional left ventricular wall motion abnormalities (hypokinesis, akinesis) are highly suggestive of ischemic heart disease but can also be seen in nonischemic dilated cardiomyopathy. The distribution of wall motion abnormalities suggests the culprit coronary artery.
- **Stress echocardiography:** Used to determine regional wall motion abnormalities in patients with a relatively normal resting echocardiogram and signs or symptoms of ischemic heart disease. Stress with exercise or dobutamine. **Contraindications** for using dobutamine include uncontrolled hypertension or recent clinically significant arrhythmia.
- **Doppler:** Used to investigate blood flow in the heart and great vessels. Very useful for detecting stenotic or regurgitant blood flow across the valves as well as any abnormal communications within the heart. Doppler velocities across a valve can be converted to pressure gradients.
- **Bubble study:** Injection of agitated normal saline to diagnose right-to-left shunts. Consider patent foramen ovale or ASD if bubbles flow directly from the right to the left atrium; consider intrapulmonary shunt with delayed appearance of bubbles in the left atrium.
- **Transesophageal echocardiography (TEE):** A small ultrasound probe placed into the esophagus that allows for higher-resolution images, especially of **posterior** cardiac structures (because the esophagus is just posterior to the heart). Common indications include the detection of left atrial thrombi, valvular vegetations, and thoracic aortic dissection.

Myocardial Perfusion Imaging

A nuclear medicine study that looks for the presence and distribution of areas of myocardial ischemia on the basis of differences in myocardial perfusion.

- Exercise or pharmacologic stress (dipyridamole or adenosine) is used to induce coronary vasodilation, which ↑ flow to the myocardium perfused by healthy coronary arteries but fails to ↑ flow in the distribution of a hemodynamically significant stenosis. A contraindication to the use of either dipyridamole or adenosine is COPD, as both agents cause bronchoconstriction.
- Perfusion images show defects in areas where blood flow is relatively ↓. If a perfusion defect on the initial (stress) imaging improves on repeat (rest) imaging after 3–24 hours, the area is presumably still viable (ie, it is a reversible defect).
- A fixed defect suggests myocardial scar tissue (or hibernating myocardium). Redistribution images can be performed after 24 hours to look for additional areas of viable myocardium.

Other Noninvasive Tests

- **Coronary CT angiography:** Currently investigational.
- **Cardiac MRI:** A useful adjunctive test for assessing left and right ventricular morphology and function, myocardial viability, CAD, valvular heart disease, nonischemic cardiomyopathy, cardiac masses, congenital heart disease, and pericardial disease in selected patients.

CARDIAC CATHETERIZATION AND CORONARY ANGIOGRAPHY

Cardiac Catheterization Indications

Indications for cardiac catheterization include evaluation of acute and chronic CAD, cardiogenic shock, heart failure, pulmonary hypertension, suspected valvular disease, and congenital heart disease. It is also performed to assess the severity of disease and to guide further therapy.

Coronary Angiography Indications

- **Elective (diagnostic):** For patients with known or suspected CAD who are candidates for coronary revascularization.
- **1°:** Initial reperfusion therapy for acute ST-segment-elevation MI (STEMI).
- **Rescue:** After failed thrombolysis (if there is ongoing chest pain and/or a ↓ of < 50% in ST-segment elevation 60–90 minutes after thrombolysis).

Coronary Stents

An 85-year-old man undergoes coronary angiography and has drug-eluting stents placed into his left circumflex artery. On day 2 postangiography, he is noted on routine labs to have an ↑ creatinine level and a normal WBC count (50% neutrophils, 20% eosinophils). Exam reveals cold toes with a slight bluish discoloration. Is this a complication of the procedure?

Yes. This patient likely has atheroembolic disease stemming from catheterization, which is manifesting with typical symptoms of renal failure, eosinophilia, and emboli to the distal digits. Although renal failure is more commonly associated with contrast nephropathy, the remaining findings make atheroembolic disease more likely. Treatment is largely supportive.

- Patients treated with coronary stents must be treated with **ASA and clopidogrel** for at least four weeks for bare-metal stents and for at least six months for drug-eluting stents (newer guidelines suggest treating with clopidogrel for > 1 year to prevent life-threatening stent thrombosis). If there are no contraindications, the continuation of clopidogrel for one year following stenting ↓ the risk of death and MI.
- Some believe that preprocedural loading with clopidogrel should be avoided if there is a chance that the patient will undergo coronary artery bypass grafting (CABG) in the next 5–7 days (associated with ↑ bleeding complications).
- Drug-eluting stents ↓ the incidence of restenosis with the use of antiproliferative agents (eg, sirolimus and paclitaxel) but require more prolonged treatment with clopidogrel.

Indications for CABG

- Left main stenosis.
- Symptomatic two-vessel disease with proximal LAD disease and a ↓ ejection fraction (EF) or ischemia on noninvasive imaging.
- Symptomatic three-vessel CAD.

Complications During Percutaneous Coronary Intervention (PCI)

- **Coronary arterial complications** include the following:
  - Distal microembolization of the coronary artery (5%).
  - Vessel perforation or dissection (1%).
  - **Abrupt closure (< 1% with stenting):** Of all cases, 75% occur within minutes of angioplasty and 25% within 24 hours. Usually due to dissection or thrombosis. One-third have major ischemic complications requiring emergent revascularization.
  - **Subacute thrombotic occlusion of coronary stent (1–4%) within 2–14 days:** Often results in MI or death.
  - **Gradual restenosis:** Defined as ≥ 50% narrowing of the luminal diameter within 1–6 months. There is a ↓ risk of in-stent restenosis with drug-eluting stents.
- **Other complications** are as follows:
  - Retroperitoneal bleeding.
  - Femoral artery hematoma, pseudoaneurysm, or fistula formation.
  - **Contrast nephropathy:** Usually occurs 24–48 hours after contrast load. Diabetes and preexisting renal insufficiency are the most important risk factors. Prevent with pre- and postprocedural hydration. Acetylcysteine, ↓ volume of contrast, and low osmolar contrast are other preventive measures.
  - **Atheroembolic kidney disease:** Look for eosinophilia, eosinophiluria, hypocomplementemia, and distal embolic complications ("blue toes").
  - **Anaphylaxis or allergic reaction to contrast media:** In the presence of known contrast allergy, premedicate with diphenhydramine and steroids.
  - **Hyperthyroidism in patients with known (or unknown) Graves' disease or toxic thyroid nodule:** Can present weeks to months after iodinated contrast load.

Coronary Artery Disease (CAD)

ACUTE CORONARY SYNDROMES

Acute coronary syndromes encompass STEMI, non-ST-segment-elevation MI (NSTEMI), and unstable angina. Etiologies include unstable plaques with nonocclusive thrombosis (unstable angina and NSTEMI) and thrombotic occlusion of an epicardial coronary artery (STEMI).

SYMPTOMS

Ischemic chest pain is often described as dull or squeezing substernal pain or left-sided discomfort associated with dyspnea and diaphoresis, with radiation down the left arm or into the neck or jaw.

EXAM

Acute ischemia may be associated with an S4. Ischemic systolic dysfunction can cause pulmonary edema and an S3. Elevation of JVP is uncommon in the absence of right ventricular involvement or a prior history of CHF.

DIFFERENTIAL

Aortic dissection, pulmonary embolism, acute pericarditis, tension pneumothorax.

DIAGNOSIS

- Based primarily on **risk factors** and **initial ECG during chest pain** (see Figure 3.7).
- In patients with chest pain, the initial goal is to rule out STEMI that requires immediate reperfusion therapy.
- In patients without ST-segment elevation, cardiac enzymes will determine if patients have NSTEMI or unstable angina.

TREATMENT

- **Immediate reperfusion is the goal for STEMI.**
    - 1° PCI is generally preferred if it is available.
    - Pharmacologic thrombolysis is also considered first-line therapy if it is administered **within 12 hours** of chest pain onset (especially at medical facilities that do not have access to 24-hour PCI).
- **Absolute contraindications to thrombolysis** are as follows:
    - Active internal bleeding.
    - A history of hemorrhagic stroke.
    - Other strokes within the past year.
    - A known CNS neoplasm.
    - A BP of > 180/110 mm Hg despite antihypertensive therapy.
    - Suspected aortic dissection.
- **Medical therapy for NSTEMI and unstable angina** includes the following:
    - ASA, β-blockers, ACEIs, and low-molecular-weight or unfractionated heparin. The addition of clopidogrel and glycoprotein IIB/IIIA inhibitors should be considered for high-risk patients.

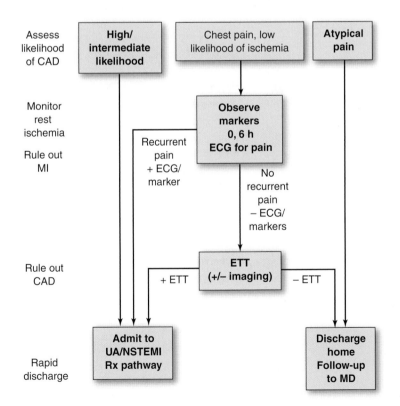

FIGURE 3.7.   Evaluation of patients presenting with suspected unstable angina/NSTEMI.
ETT = exercise tolerance test.

- If pain persists despite medical therapy or there is an ↑ in the troponin level, the patient is at higher risk of an event within six weeks and should proceed to coronary angiography.
- Increasing evidence supports an early aggressive strategy (cardiac catheterization within 48 hours) for moderate- to high-risk patients who present with acute coronary syndromes. Patients with recurrent angina, ↑ cardiac biomarkers, or ST-segment depression should be considered for early coronary angiography.

COMPLICATIONS

- **Delayed therapy:** Ischemic arrhythmias (VT/VF); extension of infarction resulting in chronic heart failure.
- **Complications of thrombolysis and aggressive anticoagulation/antiplatelet regimens:** Hemorrhagic stroke, GI bleeding, retroperitoneal bleeding.
- **Hemodynamic complications of acute MI:** See Table 3.3.

TABLE 3.3. Hemodynamic Complications of Acute MI

CONDITION	CARDIAC INDEX ([L/MIN]/m²)	PCWP[a] (mm Hg)	SYSTOLIC BP (mm Hg)	TREATMENT
Uncomplicated	> 2.5	≤ 18	> 100	
Hypovolemia	< 2.5	< 15	< 100	Successive boluses of normal saline. In the setting of inferior wall MI, consider right ventricular infarction (especially if right atrial pressure is > 10 mm Hg).
Volume overload	> 2.5	> 20	> 100	Diuretics (eg, furosemide 10–20 mg IV). Nitroglycerin, topical paste or IV.
Left ventricular failure	< 2.5	> 20	> 100	Diuretics (eg, furosemide 10–20 mg IV). IV nitroglycerin (or, if the patient is hypertensive, IV nitroprusside).
Severe left ventricular failure	< 2.5	> 20	< 100	**If BP is ≥ 90 mm Hg:** IV dobutamine +/− IV nitroglycerin or sodium nitroprusside. **If BP is < 90 mm Hg:** IV dopamine. **If accompanied by pulmonary edema:** Attempt diuresis with IV furosemide; may be limited by hypotension. In the presence of a new systolic murmur, consider acute VSD or mitral regurgitation.
Cardiogenic shock	< 1.8	> 20	< 90 with oliguria and confusion	IV dopamine. Intra-aortic balloon pump. Coronary angiography may be life-saving.

[a]PCWP = pulmonary capillary wedge pressure.

(Reproduced with permission from Kasper DL et al. *Harrison's Manual of Medicine*, 16th ed. New York: McGraw-Hill, 2005: 628.)

COMPLICATIONS OF ACUTE MYOCARDIAL INFARCTION

Ventricular Septal Defect (VSD)

- Affects 1–2% of patients with acute MI; occurs 3–7 days after MI.
- Risk factors include large infarcts, single-vessel disease, poor collateral circulation, first infarct, and diabetes. Older women are also at ↑ risk.
- Sx/Exam:
    - Presents as acute CHF symptoms with a new systolic murmur and thrill.
    - Exam reveals a holosystolic murmur that radiates from left to right over the precordium, heard loudest over the left lower sternal border.
- **Dx:** Echocardiography; right heart catheterization (with a Swan-Ganz catheter) to look for an ↑ in O_2 saturation in the right ventricle compared with the right atrium, IVC, and SVC.
- **Tx:** Vasodilators and surgical correction. If the patient is hypotensive, an intra-aortic balloon pump (IABP) can serve as a bridge until surgical intervention can be performed.

Papillary Muscle Rupture

- Affects 1% of patients with acute MI; occurs 2–7 days after MI. Risk factors include inferior MI and VSD.
- Sx/Exam:
    - Presents as sudden acute pulmonary edema.
    - Exam reveals a new systolic murmur, heard loudest at the apex, that radiates to the axilla. The intensity of the murmur does not correlate with the severity of mitral regurgitation.
- **Dx:** Echocardiography; right heart catheterization.
- **Tx:** Vasodilators and surgical correction. If the patient is hypotensive, an IABP can serve as a bridge until surgical intervention can be performed.

Left Ventricular Free Wall Rupture

- Affects < 1% of patients with acute MI; accounts for up to 15% of early MI deaths. Occurs 5–14 days after MI or earlier in patients who receive thrombolysis.
- Risk factors include transmural MI, first MI, single-vessel disease, lack of collaterals, and female gender.
- Sx/Exam:
    - The classic presentation is that of nausea followed by hypotension, shock, and death.
    - Exam reveals acute decompensation related to cardiac tamponade (↑ JVP, pulsus paradoxus, diminished heart sounds).
- **Dx:** Echocardiography; right heart catheterization.
- **Tx:** Urgent pericardiocentesis and thoracotomy. **Cardiac rupture is a cardiothoracic surgical emergency.**

Cardiogenic Shock

- Risk factors include anterior MI, diabetes, and older age.
- **Exam:** Look for signs of heart failure with associated hypotension. ↓ urine output is common.
- **Dx:** CXR, echocardiography, right heart catheterization.
- **Tx:** Revascularization, ventilatory support, dopamine/dobutamine. IABP and left ventricular assist device for severe cases.

Left Ventricular Aneurysm

- Affects 10–30% of patients after acute MI; incidence is decreasing in the era of PCI. Can occur acutely, but most cases are chronic and persist for > 6 weeks after MI. Anterior MI is a risk factor.
- **Exam:** Exam reveals a large, diffuse PMI; S3 may be present.
- **Dx:** ECG (Q waves in V_{1-3} with persistent ST-segment elevation), echocardiography, cardiac MRI.
- **Tx:**
  - **Acute:** Treat associated cardiogenic shock.
  - **Chronic:** Anticoagulate with heparin/warfarin if mural thrombus is present; consider a defibrillator if the left ventricular EF is < 35% or there are documented ventricular arrhythmias.
- **Prevention:** Early revascularization.

Early Pericarditis

- Affects 10% of patients with acute MI; occurs 1–4 days after MI. Transmural MI is a risk factor.
- **Sx:** Pain worsens when patients are supine and radiates to the trapezius ridge.
- **Exam:** Presents with a pericardial friction rub.
- **Dx:** ECG may show evidence of pericarditis; echocardiography may reveal pericardial effusion.
- **Tx:** ASA. Avoid NSAIDs and corticosteroids, which may interfere with the healing of infarcted myocardium. Avoid heparin to ↓ the risk of pericardial hemorrhagic transformation.

Late Pericarditis (Dressler's Syndrome)

> A 52-year-old man presents to the hospital two weeks after having been admitted for an MI with new chest pain and fever. The pain worsens when he is supine and is unrelenting. On exam, he is found to be mildly tachycardic with a normal BP. Labs show a WBC count of 12,000/mL and a low troponin level, and a bedside echocardiogram reveals a small pericardial effusion. What is the treatment of choice for this patient?
>
> ASA. This patient likely has Dressler's syndrome, a late-onset pericarditis that follows acute MI. Although pericarditis normally responds well to NSAIDs, the potential effect of NSAIDs on wound healing makes them an unfavorable choice (as is the case with steroids). A left ventricular free wall rupture would also be characterized by a pericardial effusion, but the patient would more likely be hypotensive, obtunded, or near death.

- Affects 1–3% of patients with acute MI; thought to be 2° to immune-mediated injury. Occurs 1–8 weeks after MI.
- **Exam:** Presents with a pericardial rub and with fever.
- **Dx:** ECG may show evidence of pericarditis; echocardiography may show pericardial effusion.
- **Tx:** ASA. If > 4 weeks have elapsed since the MI, NSAIDs and/or corticosteroids can be used.

Arrhythmias

- Can occur at any time post-MI. Reperfusion arrhythmias within 24–48 hours of MI generally do not mandate aggressive therapy.

- **Dx:** ECG, telemetry. **Routine electrophysiologic or signal-average ECG testing is not recommended.**
- **Tx:** If ventricular arrhythmias persist for > 48 hours post-MI and are symptomatic or hemodynamically significant, implantation of a defibrillator is more effective than antiarrhythmics.

Ischemic Complications

- Infarct extension, postinfarction angina, or reinfarction.
- **Dx/Tx:** Cardiac catheterization with PCI when indicated.

Embolic Complications

- Nonhemorrhagic stroke occurs in approximately 1% of patients post-MI, typically within 10 days after MI.
- Risk factors include anterior MI, large MI, and left ventricular aneurysm.
- **Exam:** Depends on the site of embolization. Look for signs of stroke or of limb or intestinal ischemia.
- **Tx:** Anticoagulation with heparin/warfarin.

CARDIOGENIC SHOCK

Occurs in approximately 5–7% of patients with acute MI and is the **leading cause of death related to acute MI.** Etiologies are as follows:

- **Left ventricular systolic dysfunction:** The most common cause of cardiogenic shock (75% of patients).
- **STEMI:** Causes cardiogenic shock more frequently than does NSTEMI.
- **Acute, severe valvular insufficiency:** Most often due to acute mitral regurgitation.
- Cardiac tamponade.
- Left ventricular free wall rupture.
- Ventricular septal rupture.
- **Left ventricular outflow tract obstruction:** Aortic stenosis; hypertrophic cardiomyopathy.
- **Obstruction to left ventricular filling:** Mitral stenosis; left atrial myxoma.
- **Acute or acute-on-chronic right ventricular failure:** Acute right ventricular MI, decompensated pulmonary hypertension, acute pulmonary embolism.

Symptoms/Exam

- Hypotension (systolic BP < 90 mm Hg) or relative hypotension (a large ↓ in systolic BP in a chronically hypertensive patient). Note that some patients with severe end-stage heart failure will have chronically low BP; look for evidence of hypoperfusion in these patients.
- Tachycardia.
- Hypoperfusion (cyanosis, poor peripheral pulses) despite adequate filling pressures.
- Dyspnea.
- Altered mental status (acute delirium).
- ↓ urine output.

Treatment

- If the underlying etiology is ischemic, proceed immediately to revascularization (PCI or CABG).
- Urgent revascularization is superior to medical management (thrombolysis) alone.

- **Supportive care** includes vasopressors, mechanical ventilation, and IABP.
  - Vasopressor therapy usually consists of dopamine and dobutamine. Norepinephrine can also be used in cases of refractory hypotension.
  - Placement of an IABP ↓ afterload and improves coronary perfusion in diastole. It is contraindicated in patients with severe peripheral vascular disease and hemodynamically significant aortic insufficiency.
- For ischemia-induced cardiogenic shock, nitrates and nitroprusside can be used, but only with extreme caution. Nitroprusside can cause coronary steal phenomenon and exacerbate ischemia. IABP is a more effective therapy for coronary ischemia in these patients and is the treatment of choice.
- Ventricular assist devices can serve as a bridge to cardiac transplantation.

CHRONIC STABLE ANGINA

The hallmark is chronic, reproducible, exercise-induced chest discomfort that is relieved by rest and nitroglycerin. Unlike unstable angina and MI, stable angina is thought to involve a **fixed** coronary stenosis that limits myocardial O_2 delivery; angina results when demand outstrips supply. The most important CAD risk factors are diabetes, smoking, hyperlipidemia, hypertension, age, and a family history of premature CAD.

SYMPTOMS

Ischemic chest pain is often described as dull or squeezing substernal or left-sided discomfort associated with dyspnea and diaphoresis, with radiation down the left arm or into the neck.

EXAM

No specific exam findings can rule in or rule out CAD as a cause of chest pain.

DIFFERENTIAL

GERD, esophageal spasm, herpes zoster, chest wall pain, costochondritis, coronary vasospasm.

DIAGNOSIS

- Noninvasive stress testing with or without imaging (nuclear imaging or echocardiography).
- Invasive cardiac catheterization (angiography) is the gold standard.

TREATMENT

- **Risk factor reduction:** Includes smoking cessation and aggressive treatment of hypertension, hyperlipidemia, and diabetes (see the Ambulatory Medicine chapter).
- **Antianginal medical therapy:** Nitrates, β-blockers, calcium channel blockers (CCBs).
- **2° prevention:** ASA, statins, and ACEIs have been shown to reduce cardiovascular events in patients with chronic CAD.
- **Revascularization:** PCI or CABG.
- **Enhanced external counterpulsation:** Used in patients whose angina is refractory to medical therapy and in whom revascularization is not possible.

COMPLICATIONS

Reduction in quality of life; limitation of activities of daily living.

KEY FACT

Flow-limiting stenoses that are responsible for stable angina are less likely to rupture and cause acute coronary syndromes than nonocclusive unstable plaques.

DIAGNOSTIC STRATEGIES AND RISK STRATIFICATION FOR CHEST PAIN

Evaluation of Patients with Chest Pain

- The most important single test in the initial evaluation of patients with chest pain is the **ECG**, which should be obtained and interpreted within the first five minutes of presentation.
- The history, physical exam, and initial laboratory and radiographic assessment should focus on **excluding life-threatening causes of chest pain** (acute ischemic heart disease, aortic dissection, acute pericarditis, pulmonary embolism, tension pneumothorax, esophageal rupture).
- Troponins and CK-MB biomarkers typically become elevated **6–8 hours** after the onset of chest pain. Troponins remain elevated for several days; therefore, in patients with a recent MI, checking CK-MB can be useful to look for recurrent MI.

Acute Treatment

- All patients with chest pain should receive O_2, and an IV should be placed.
- Unless contraindicated, all patients with chest pain presumed to be ischemic in etiology should receive ASA, β-blockers, nitrates, and heparin during the initial evaluation.

Risk Stratification

- All patients who present with chest pain should be risk stratified according to the presence or absence of coronary **risk factors** (eg, older age, hypertension, DM, hyperlipidemia, smoking, a family history of premature CAD, CKD).
- As the number of risk factors ↑, the likelihood that the patient's chest pain is ischemic in origin ↑ as well (even if the chest pain is atypical).
- Guidelines for stress testing are as follows:
  - High-risk patients with chest pain (eg, ST-segment elevation on ECG or the presence of heart failure in the setting of ischemia) should proceed directly to cardiac catheterization.
  - Lower-risk patients with a high likelihood of ischemia (as determined primarily by the presence of coronary risk factors, a history of CAD, ECG findings, or a ⊕ troponin result) should undergo cardiac stress testing (ideally prior to discharge from the hospital).
  - Patients with an ↑ troponin level and two or more high-risk prognostic variables (age ≥ 65 years, three or more traditional CAD risk factors, documented CAD with ≥ 50% stenosis, ST-segment deviation, two or more anginal episodes within the last 24 hours, ⊕ biomarkers, or ASA use within the past week) should undergo cardiac catheterization within 24 hours.

MANAGEMENT OF CORONARY ARTERY DISEASE

Risk Factor Reduction

- **Modifiable CAD risk factors** such as DM, hypertension, hyperlipidemia, and smoking should be aggressively treated.
- Other risk factors (eg, CKD, cocaine use) should also be addressed.

KEY FACT

DM is now considered a CAD equivalent.

Pharmacologic Therapy

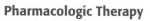

- **ASA:** ↓ mortality. Give 81 mg daily. If ASA is absolutely contraindicated, clopidogrel can be used effectively.
- **Clopidogrel:** ↓ mortality in patients who have had recent acute coronary syndromes or who have had a coronary stent placed.
- **Statins:** ↓ mortality and the risk of acute cardiac events. The goal LDL should be < 70 mg/dL in patients with a history of CAD.
- **β-blockers:** ↓ mortality. **All patients with CAD** should be on β-blockers unless there are absolute contraindications to their use. In patients with reactive airway disease, cardioselective β-blockers should be tried and discontinued only if bronchospasm occurs. **DM is not a contraindication to β-blocker use.**
- **ACEIs:** ↓ mortality and the risk of MI and stroke. If they are not well tolerated, an angiotensin receptor blocker (ARB) should be prescribed.

Indications For Elective Revascularization

- Chronic stable angina with three-vessel disease.
- Two-vessel disease with proximal LAD involvement.
- One- or two-vessel disease with high-risk features on noninvasive testing.
- Significant left main CAD (> 50% stenosis).
- Refractory symptoms of chronic angina.

Congestive Heart Failure (CHF)

Table 3.4 and the discussion that follows outline the stages, types, and clinical characteristics of CHF. These stages have goal-directed therapy at each stage. The New York Heart Association (NYHA) also classifies heart failure into four categories (class I–IV), from no limitation in physical activity to symptoms at rest.

SYSTOLIC VS. DIASTOLIC HEART FAILURE

Heart Failure with Reduced EF (Systolic Heart Failure)

- Clinically defined as evidence of a ↓ EF (typically < 40%) in the setting of symptoms and signs of heart failure.
- Affects all ages; more common in males. CAD is present in approximately 70% of patients with a ↓ EF.
- **Exam:** S3 is present.
- **Dx:** Echocardiography shows a ↓ EF (≤ 40%). The left ventricle is typically dilated, and wall motion abnormalities may be present in both ischemic and nonischemic cases.

Heart Failure with Preserved EF (Diastolic Heart Failure)

- Clinically defined as a normal EF (> 50%) in the setting of symptoms and signs of heart failure.
- Affects elderly patients; occurs more often in females. Comorbidities include hypertension, DM, obesity, obstructive sleep apnea, and CKD.
- Most patients will have diastolic dysfunction as the primary underlying pathophysiology.
- **Exam:** S4 is present (S3 may be present in patients with significantly elevated left ventricular filling pressures).
- **Dx:** Echocardiogram shows a normal or near-normal EF (> 50%); LVH is common.

TABLE 3.4. Stages of Heart Failure

STAGE	DESCRIPTION	TREATMENT
A	Patients who are at risk of developing heart failure because of comorbidities strongly associated with the development of heart failure (eg, hypertension, CAD, DM). No structural or functional abnormalities of the valves or ventricles.	ACEIs/ARBs; treat the underlying condition (eg, hypertension, CAD).
B	Patients who have structural heart disease that is strongly associated with the development of heart failure but no symptoms or history of heart failure (eg, LVH; enlarged, dilated left ventricle; asymptomatic severe valvular heart disease; previous MI).	ACEIs/ARBs, β-blockers, implantable defibrillator if EF is low (< 35%) despite medical therapy.
C	Patients who have current or prior symptoms of heart failure associated with underlying structural heart disease. Represents the largest group of patients with clinical evidence of heart failure.	As in stage B. Salt restriction, diuretics. Selected patients may be given nitrates/hydralazine, digoxin, aldosterone antagonists, or cardiac resynchronization therapy.
D	Patients who have marked symptoms of heart failure at rest despite maximal medical therapy and who require specialized interventions. Examples include patients with recurrent hospitalizations as well as those who are in hospital awaiting heart transplantation, on continuous IV support for symptom relief, on a mechanical circulatory assist device, or in hospice.	As in stage C. Consider mechanical support, experimental surgery/drugs, transplantation, or hospice.

(Adapted with permission from Fuster V et al. *Hurst's the Heart,* 12th ed. New York: McGraw-Hill, 2008, Table 26-1.)

Diastolic Dysfunction

Very common. Often coexists with systolic dysfunction; frequently associated with hypertension and ischemic heart disease. Diastolic dysfunction (based on echocardiographic findings) does not equal diastolic heart failure. Many patients have asymptomatic diastolic dysfunction (which is a risk factor for future morbidity and mortality), but diastolic heart failure denotes symptomatic heart failure in the setting of diastolic dysfunction. Etiologies are as follows:

- **Myocardial:** Impaired relaxation (ischemia, hypertrophy, cardiomyopathies, hypothyroidism, aging); ↑ passive stiffness (diffuse fibrosis, scarring, hypertrophy, infiltrative).
- **Pericardial:** Constrictive pericarditis; cardiac tamponade.
- **Other:** Volume overload of the right ventricle; extrinsic compression (eg, tumor).

SYMPTOMS

Indistinguishable from systolic dysfunction on the basis of symptoms. May be asymptomatic, although patients have higher mortality when compared to controls.

KEY FACT

In patients with isolated diastolic dysfunction, always consider underlying myocardial or pericardial causes of a stiff left ventricle (eg, infiltrative diseases, constrictive pericarditis, restrictive cardiomyopathies).

EXAM

- Look for evidence of heart failure (elevated jugular venous pulsations, crackles on lung exam, lower extremity edema).
- On cardiac exam, listen for an S4. **An S3 can be present when left ventricular filling pressures are severely ↑** (the presence or absence of S3 and/or S4 cannot be used to distinguish systolic from diastolic dysfunction).

DIAGNOSIS

- Echocardiography shows a **normal EF** in the setting of signs and symptoms of heart failure.
- Also look for other clues of diastolic dysfunction (abnormal mitral inflow pattern, LVH, RVH/enlargement, left atrial enlargement) or causes of diastolic dysfunction (pericarditis, infiltrative diseases).

TREATMENT

See below.

TREATMENT OF CONGESTIVE HEART FAILURE

Systolic Heart Failure

KEY FACT

Even with maximal medical therapy (eg, ACEIs, β-blockers), patients with an EF of < 30% still have a ↓ in the incidence of sudden death with placement of an implantable cardioverter-defibrillator (ICD).

- **Diuretics:** Acutely used to ↓ symptoms of pulmonary edema; confer **no mortality benefit.**
- **ACEIs:** Have a proven **mortality benefit.** If ACEIs are not tolerated because of cough, switch to an ARB.
- **Hydralazine with nitrates:** Useful in an acute setting to ↓ pulmonary edema by decreasing preload and afterload. Associated with a **mortality benefit** when used, but confers less benefit than ACEIs. In African American patients, a greater mortality benefit is gained than that provided by ACEI/ARB therapy.
- **Spironolactone:** Yields a **mortality benefit** in class III–IV heart failure.
- **β-blockers:** Confer a **mortality benefit** in all classes of heart failure. However, they should not be initiated in the setting of acutely decompensated heart failure. Proven benefit is limited to carvedilol, bisoprolol, and long-acting metoprolol.
- **B-type natriuretic peptide (nesiritide):** Acts primarily as a vasodilator. Can be considered in severe heart failure requiring vasodilator therapy when nitroprusside and nitroglycerin are contraindicated. May provide additional improvement in symptoms, but may be associated with ↑ renal dysfunction and possibly ↑ mortality.
- **Mechanical therapy:** For severe heart failure due to ischemia, consider an IABP. For very poor cardiac output, consider a ventricular assist device as a bridge to cardiac transplantation.
- **Cardiac resynchronization:** Confers a **mortality benefit.** Pacemaker-based therapy (with leads in the right atrium, the right ventricle, and a branch of the coronary sinus to pace the left ventricle) is used in patients with systolic heart failure (NYHA Class II–IV), an EF of < 35%, and a wide QRS (> 120 msec) on ECG. Improves ventricular synchrony and cardiac output.
- **Cardiac transplantation:** See Table 3.5.

KEY FACT

Patients who have had an MI with CHF (EF < 40%) will derive a mortality benefit from the addition of eplerenone, an aldosterone antagonist.

Diastolic Heart Failure

- **No treatment has been convincingly shown to ↓ mortality in patients with diastolic heart failure.**

TABLE 3.5. Indications for and Contraindications to Cardiac Transplantation

VARIABLE	CRITERIA
Indications	1. End-stage heart disease that limits the prognosis for survival > 2 years or severely limits daily quality of life despite optimal medical and other surgical therapy. 2. No 2° exclusion criteria. 3. A suitable psychosocial profile and social support system. 4. A suitable physiologic/chronologic age.
Exclusion criteria	1. Active infectious process. 2. Recent pulmonary infarction. 3. Insulin-requiring diabetes with evidence of end-organ damage. 4. Irreversible pulmonary hypertension (pulmonary vascular resistance [PVR] poorly responsive to nitroprusside with a PVR > 2 or a pulmonary systolic pressure of > 50 mm Hg at peak dose or at a mean arterial pressure of 65–70 mm Hg). 5. Presence of circulating cytotoxic antibodies. 6. Presence of active PUD. 7. Active or recent malignancy. 8. Presence of severe COPD or chronic bronchitis. 9. Substance or alcohol abuse. 10. Presence of peripheral or cerebrovascular disease. 11. Other systemic diseases that would jeopardize rehabilitation posttransplant.

(Adapted with permission from Braunwald E et al. *Harrison's Principles of Internal Medicine,* 15th ed. New York: McGraw-Hill, 2001.)

- **Avoid exacerbating factors** such as AF, tachycardia, ischemia, hypertension, fluid overload, and anemia. **Aggressively control hypertension.**
- ACEIs and ARBs may aid in cardiac remodeling.
- **Diuresis and slowing the heart rate:** β-blockers and nondihydropyridine CCBs (eg, diltiazem, verapamil) may help symptoms but have not been proven to ↓ mortality. Use caution in patients with advanced diastolic heart failure, who may need preload and/or chronotropy (relatively high heart rates) to maintain cardiac output.

Cardiomyopathies and Myocarditis

Tables 3.6 and 3.7 and the discussion below outline the etiologies, classification, and evaluation of cardiomyopathies.

TABLE 3.6. Clinical Classification of Cardiomyopathies

CATEGORY	CHARACTERISTICS
Dilated	Left and/or right ventricular enlargement, impaired systolic function, CHF, arrhythmias, emboli.
Restrictive	Endomyocardial scarring or myocardial infiltration resulting in restriction to left and/or right ventricular filling.
Hypertrophic	Disproportionate LVH, typically involving the septum more than the free wall, with or without an intraventricular systolic pressure gradient; usually of a nondilated left ventricular cavity.

(Adapted with permission from Kasper DL et al. *Harrison's Principles of Internal Medicine,* 16th ed. New York: McGraw-Hill, 2005: 1408.)

TABLE 3.7. Evaluation of Cardiomyopathies

	SUBTYPE		
MODALITY	**DILATED**	**RESTRICTIVE**	**HYPERTROPHIC**
CXR	Moderate to marked cardiac silhouette enlargement; pulmonary venous hypertension.	Mild cardiac silhouette enlargement. Usually normal.	Mild to moderate cardiac silhouette enlargement.
ECG	ST-segment and T-wave abnormalities.	Low voltage; conduction defects.	ST-segment and T-wave abnormalities; LVH; abnormal Q waves.
Echocardiogram	Left ventricular dilatation and dysfunction.	$\downarrow$ left ventricular wall thickness; normal or mildly $\downarrow$ systolic function.	Asymmetric septal hypertrophy; systolic anterior motion of the mitral valve.
Radionuclide studies	Left ventricular dilatation and dysfunction (RVG).[a]	Normal or mildly $\downarrow$ systolic function (RVG).	Vigorous systolic function (RVG); perfusion defect (^{201}Tl).[a]
Cardiac catheterization	Left ventricular dilatation and dysfunction; $\uparrow$ left- and often right-sided filling pressures; $\downarrow$ cardiac output.	Normal or mildly $\downarrow$ systolic function; $\uparrow$ left- and right-sided filling pressures.	Vigorous systolic function; dynamic left ventricular outflow obstruction; $\uparrow$ left- and right-sided filling pressures.

[a]RVG = radionuclide ventriculogram; ^{201}Tl = thallium 201.

(Reproduced with permission from Kasper DL et al. *Harrison's Principles of Internal Medicine,* 16th ed. New York: McGraw-Hill, 2005: 1409.)

RESTRICTIVE CARDIOMYOPATHY

A 47-year-old man presents to the ER with shortness of breath. On evaluation, he is found to have mild hypotension and tachycardia but is afebrile. Exam reveals an elevated JVP that $\uparrow$ with inspiration and an ECG that is notable for no ST- or T-wave changes, a prolonged PR interval, and low voltages. Labs showed nephrotic-range proteinuria. What test is most likely to lead to a diagnosis in this patient?

Fat pad biopsy. This patient's hypotension, tachycardia, Kussmaul's sign, and low voltages on ECG point to an infiltrative process that has resulted in restrictive cardiomyopathy. The presence of nephrotic-range proteinuria limits the differential but makes amyloidosis a possible diagnosis. In this case, the diagnostic test of choice would be a fat pad biopsy to assess for amyloid deposition.

Infiltration or fibrosis of the myocardium causing impaired ventricular filling with preserved systolic function. In end-stage disease, systolic dysfunction may develop. Causes include amyloidosis, sarcoidosis, hemochromatosis, scleroderma, and radiation.

SYMPTOMS

Patients present with dyspnea, fatigue, and peripheral edema.

EXAM

Exam reveals an elevated JVP that ↑ with inspiration (**Kussmaul's sign**) and a normal left ventricular impulse; hepatosplenomegaly and ascites are seen in advanced disease.

DIFFERENTIAL

- **Hypertrophic cardiomyopathy.**
- **Dilated cardiomyopathy.**
- **Constrictive pericarditis:** Clinical presentation and physical exam may yield findings identical to those of restrictive cardiomyopathy. MRI shows pericardial thickening (> 5 mm), and right heart catheterization demonstrates equalization of diastolic pressures in constrictive pericarditis. See Table 3.8 for differentiating features of constrictive pericarditis and restrictive cardiomyopathy.

DIAGNOSIS

- **ECG:** Shows conduction system disease, low QRS voltage, and nonspecific ST/T-wave changes.
- **Echocardiography:** Demonstrates a restrictive filling pattern with a preserved EF and biatrial enlargement. Infiltrative causes can present with the characteristic granular appearance of myocardium.
- **Right heart catheterization:** Dip-and-plateau ventricular filling pressure ("**square root**" **sign**), pulmonary hypertension, respiratory concordance of the right and left ventricles.
- **Myocardial biopsy:** Detects infiltrative diseases such as amyloidosis.

TREATMENT

- **Treat the underlying disease process** (eg, amyloidosis, sarcoidosis).
- **Diuretics:** ↓ symptoms from venous congestion, but **overdiuresis can lead to ↓ cardiac output due to preload dependence.**
- **β-blockers/CCBs:** May improve diastolic function early in the disease process by slowing heart rate and increasing ventricular filling time. Caution should be used in administration, as this may result in a fall in cardiac output in patients with more advanced disease, who are dependent on heart rate to ↑ cardiac output in the setting of a fixed stroke volume. **Avoid CCBs in amyloid heart disease, as they can cause significant ⊖ chronotropy.**
- **Cardiac transplantation:** Remains an option for patients with intractable heart failure without severe systemic disease.

HYPERTROPHIC CARDIOMYOPATHY (HCM)

An autosomal dominant disorder of myocardial structural proteins that causes premature, severe LVH. A subset of hypertrophic cardiomyopathy cases may have asymmetric septal hypertrophy and dynamic outflow tract obstruction.

SYMPTOMS

Presents with dyspnea, chest pain, and syncope.

EXAM

- The obstructive form presents with a systolic crescendo-decrescendo murmur that **intensifies with a ↓ in left ventricular volume** (eg, **standing, Valsalva maneuver**) and **diminishes with an ↑ in left ventricular volume** (eg, **hand grip** or **raising the legs when the patient is in a supine position**).

TABLE 3.8. Constrictive Pericarditis vs. Restrictive Cardiomyopathy and Cardiac Tamponade

VARIABLE	CONSTRICTIVE PERICARDITIS	RESTRICTIVE CARDIOMYOPATHY	CARDIAC TAMPONADE
History	TB, cardiac surgery, radiation therapy, collagen vascular disease, trauma, prior pericarditis.	Amyloidosis, hemochromatosis, sarcoidosis.	Prior pericardial effusion, cardiac surgery, malignancy (eg, breast cancer), recent MI.
Physical exam			
Pulsus paradoxus	May be present.	Rare.	Frequent.
JVP	Prominent x and y descents; Kussmaul's sign may be present.	Prominent x and y descents; Kussmaul's sign may be present.	Absent or diminished y descent.
Heart sounds	Pericardial knock.	Prominent S4.	Muffled.
Murmurs	Not typically present.	Mitral and tricuspid regurgitation are often present.	Not typically present.
ECG	Nonspecific.	Right or left atrial enlargement; AV conduction delay; bundle branch block.	Low voltage; electrical alternans.
CXR	Pericardial calcification.	Nonspecific.	Enlarged cardiac silhouette.
Echocardiography	Pericardial thickening; pericardial effusion may be present; ventricular septal flattening with inspiration.	Atrial enlargement; moderate or severe diastolic dysfunction.	Pericardial effusion present; right ventricular collapse during diastole.
Hemodynamics			
Equalization of diastolic pressures	Present.	Left-sided pressures are often higher than right-sided pressures.	Present.
Dip-and-plateau sign ("square root" sign)	Present.	Present.	Not typically present.
Respiratory variation in left/ right ventricular pressure tracings	Discordant peak right and left ventricular pressures.	Concordant peak right and left ventricular pressures.	Variable.

- An S4 and a sustained apical impulse are characteristic.
- Carotid upstrokes are **bifid** owing to midsystolic obstruction.

DIFFERENTIAL

- **Valvular aortic stenosis:** The murmur of aortic stenosis radiates to the neck. Aortic stenosis also has weak and delayed carotid upstrokes (parvus et tardus).
- **Hypertensive heart disease:** Not typically associated with asymmetric septal hypertrophy or outflow tract obstruction.

DIAGNOSIS

- **ECG:** Shows LVH and left atrial enlargement along with a broad, deep Q wave in leads I and II and in the left precordial leads (pseudoinfarction pattern). The apical form of the disease can have giant anterior T-wave inversions.
- **Echocardiogram:** Demonstrates LVH with systolic anterior motion of the mitral valve and left ventricular outflow tract obstruction. The pattern of hypertrophy varies. In the classic obstructive phenotype, the septum is asymmetrically hypertrophied. The left ventricular cavity is small and hypercontractile, often with diastolic dysfunction.
- **Holter monitor:** Detects ventricular arrhythmias as the cause of syncope.
- **Genetic testing:** Not routinely done, but has the potential to identify the genotype (which has prognostic value) and screen family members.

TREATMENT

- **Avoid strenuous exercise.**
- **β-blockers or verapamil:** Improve symptoms by negative inotropy, which ↓ the outflow tract gradient and slows heart rate to ↑ filling time.
- **Electrophysiologic study and ICD placement:** Indicated for patients with syncope or a family history of sudden cardiac death.
- **Surgical myectomy:** Removes tissue from hypertrophic septum and relieves outflow tract obstruction. Improves symptoms but does not ↓ the rate of sudden cardiac death.
- **Percutaneous alcohol septal ablation:** Has the same objective as surgical myectomy by injection of alcohol into a hypertrophic septum, causing local infarction.
- **Endocarditis prophylaxis:** Patients with dynamic outflow obstruction or mitral regurgitation should receive endocarditis prophylaxis.

KEY FACT

The following HCM patients should undergo risk stratification (electrophysiologic testing) and possible ICD placement: those with a family history of sudden death, syncope (especially if recurrent or exertional), nonsustained VT on Holter monitoring, > 3 cm thickness of the interventricular septum, or ↓ BP with exercise.

KEY FACT

Agents that ↓ left ventricular volume, such as nitrates and diuretics, ↑ the outflow tract gradient and ↑ murmur intensity and are thus contraindicated in patients with hypertrophic cardiomyopathy.

DILATED CARDIOMYOPATHY

Most commonly occurs in the setting of ischemic heart disease. *Idiopathic dilated cardiomyopathy* is a term used to describe a dilated left ventricle with a ↓ EF in the absence of systemic hypertension, CAD, chronic alcoholism, congenital heart disease, or other systemic diseases known to cause dilated cardiomyopathy. Etiologies are as follows:

- **Idiopathic:** A genetic predisposition may exist.
- **2° to a known etiologic agent:**
    - **Acute myocarditis:** Infectious, toxic, or immune mediated.
    - **Drugs/toxins:** Anthracyclines, cocaine, amphetamines, alcohol.
    - **Nutritional:** Thiamine, carnitine deficiency.
    - **Collagen vascular disease** (eg, Churg-Strauss syndrome).
    - **Chronic viral infections:** HIV.
    - **Endocrine:** Thyroid disorders, hypocalcemia, hypophosphatemia.
    - **Late-stage hemochromatosis.**
    - **X-linked muscular dystrophies.**

SYMPTOMS

Exertional dyspnea, fatigue, syncope, ↓ exercise tolerance, and edema.

EXAM

Exam reveals an ↑ JVP, a diffuse PMI, S3, S4, a holosystolic murmur of mitral regurgitation, evidence of fluid overload (eg, crackles on lung exam, lower extremity edema, ascites), and evidence of AF or other arrhythmias.

DIAGNOSIS

- **ECG:** Can be normal. If abnormal, look for evidence of left ventricular enlargement, conduction disorders (wide QRS, LBBB), or arrhythmias (AF, nonsustained VT).
- **Echocardiogram:** ↓ EF; dilated left ventricle.
- **Laboratory evaluation:** Can be helpful in diagnosing specific etiologies (eg, HIV).
- **Coronary angiography:** Excludes ischemic heart disease.
- **Endomyocardial biopsy: Not routinely recommended and generally low yield.**

TREATMENT

- Similar to that of systolic heart failure.
- **Revascularization:** Appropriate for patients with ischemic dilated cardiomyopathy.
- **Neurohormonal blockade:** β-blockers, **ACEIs** (or ARBs), spironolactone (for patients with stage III or IV heart failure).
- **Symptom control:** Diuretics, nitrates.
- **Anticoagulation: Controversial;** generally used only in patients with a history of systemic thromboembolism, AF, or evidence of an intracardiac thrombus.
- **Other:** Hemofiltration (for patients with oliguria or renal dysfunction refractory to diuretics), cardiac resynchronization (biventricular pacing), ventricular assist devices, cardiac transplantation, ICDs for ↓ EF (< 35%) or malignant arrhythmias (eg, VT).

ACUTE MYOCARDITIS

A common cause of "idiopathic" dilated cardiomyopathy. Patients are typically young and healthy, and many present after a viral upper respiratory illness. Can be a cause of sudden cardiac death. Etiologies are as follows:

- **Infectious: Most commonly viral** (coxsackievirus, HIV), but can be caused by numerous pathogens, including *Trypanosoma cruzi* (Chagas' disease).
- **Immune mediated:** Allergic reaction to medications, sarcoidosis, scleroderma, SLE, and others.
- **Toxic:** Medications (anthracyclines), alcohol, heavy metals, and others.

SYMPTOMS

Can be nonspecific. Look for flulike symptoms, fever, arthralgias, and malaise. In more severe cases, patients can present with chest pain, dyspnea, and symptoms of heart failure (eg, orthopnea, edema, ↓ exercise tolerance).

EXAM

Exam can be normal. If abnormal, look for evidence of heart failure.

DIFFERENTIAL

CAD, aortic dissection, pericarditis, pulmonary embolism, pulmonary and GI illnesses.

DIAGNOSIS

- The gold standard is **endomyocardial biopsy,** but because of patchy involvement of the myocardium, yield is not great and the test can be insensitive. By the time most patients seek medical care, fibrosis is the only finding on biopsy.

- **ECG:** Can be abnormal but is neither sensitive nor specific.
- **Cardiac biomarkers:** Elevated in the acute phase.
- **Echocardiography:** Can be helpful to look for focal wall motion abnormalities and ↓ EF, but findings are nonspecific.
- **Cardiac catheterization:** To exclude CAD.

TREATMENT

- No specific therapy. Steroids have not been shown to be helpful.
- Treat heart failure.
- Cardiac transplantation for severe cases.

Pericardial Disease

ACUTE PERICARDITIS

Pericardial inflammation that results in chest pain, a pericardial friction rub, and diffuse ST-segment elevation. Common etiologies are viral illness, connective tissue disease, and post-MI. May also be idiopathic.

SYMPTOMS

- Classically described as sharp, pleuritic chest discomfort that **worsens while supine and eases while leaning forward.** Dull pain similar in quality to angina pectoris is also possible.
- A prodrome of flulike symptoms with fever and myalgias is often present in patients with viral pericarditis.

EXAM

A pericardial **friction rub** is the hallmark. Classically described as having three components: atrial contraction, ventricular contraction, and ventricular filling.

DIFFERENTIAL

- **Acute myocardial ischemia/infarction:** Reciprocal ST-segment depressions and absence of PR depression are key to distinguishing the ECG changes of STEMI from those of pericarditis.
- **Aortic dissection.**
- **Pneumothorax.**
- **Early repolarization:** A normal variant pattern of ST-segment elevation, usually with a "fishhook" configuration of the J point.
- **Costochondritis:** A diagnosis of exclusion.

DIAGNOSIS

- Diagnosed by the following:
  - A consistent history of chest pain typical of acute pericarditis.
  - The presence of friction rub on exam (may not have the classic three components described above).
  - The presence of typical ECG changes (diffuse ST-segment elevation, PR-segment depression) **not compatible with a single coronary distribution** (see Figure 3.8 and Table 3.9); PR-segment elevation in aVR.
- Echocardiography is useful for excluding a large pericardial effusion and for evaluating other causes of chest pain, but many patients will have only a small effusion or a normal echocardiogram.

KEY FACT

Consider the diagnosis of myocarditis in young patients who present after a viral illness. They commonly have no coronary risk factors and have ⊕ cardiac enzymes but normal coronary arteries on cardiac catheterization.

KEY FACT

In acute pericarditis, the atrial current of injury is reflected in aVR as PR-segment elevation, also known as the "knuckle sign" (the PR segment appears as if a knuckle is pushing it up).

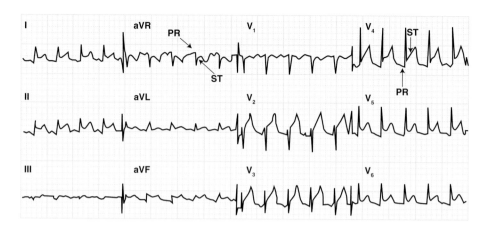

FIGURE 3.8. **Acute pericarditis on ECG.** (Adapted with permission from Kasper DL et al. *Harrison's Principles of Internal Medicine*, 17th ed. New York: McGraw-Hill, 2008, Fig. 232-1.)

TREATMENT

- NSAIDs.
- Colchicine can be useful for patients with multiple recurrent episodes.
- Steroids are often used as a last resort when patients do not respond to other therapies.

COMPLICATIONS

- Anticoagulation should be avoided, but conversion to hemorrhagic pericarditis is rare.
- Echocardiography to rule out tamponade in patients with hypotension and ↑ JVP.

PERICARDIAL EFFUSION

Slowly developing effusions can be asymptomatic. Rapidly developing effusions can lead to tamponade, causing severe chest pain and dyspnea. Etiologies include pericarditis, infections, uremia, malignancy, myxedema, nephrotic syndrome, cirrhosis, status post–cardiac surgery, and medications.

TABLE 3.9. **ECG in Acute Pericarditis vs. Acute ST-Elevation MI**

PATHOLOGY	ST-SEGMENT ELEVATION	ECG LEAD INVOLVEMENT	EVOLUTION OF ST AND T WAVES	PR-SEGMENT DEPRESSION
Pericarditis	Concave upward.	All leads involved except aVR and V_1.	ST remains elevated for several days; after ST returns to baseline, T waves invert.	Yes, in the majority of cases.
Acute MI	Convex upward.	ST elevation over the infarcted region only; reciprocal ST depression in opposite leads.	T waves invert within hours, while ST is still elevated; followed by Q-wave development.	No.

(Reproduced with permission from Kasper DL et al. *Harrison's Manual of Medicine*, 16th ed. New York: McGraw-Hill, 2005: 613.)

EXAM

A pericardial friction rub may be present. However, there may be a lack of findings in small effusions. Larger effusions can cause muffled heart sounds and ↑ jugular venous pulsations. Rapidly evolving effusions can cause symptoms of cardiac tamponade.

DIAGNOSIS

- **ECG:** Low voltage; electrical alternans (beat-to-beat variation in the height of the QRS complex).
- **CXR:** Cardiomegaly with a characteristic "boot-shaped" or "water-bottle" heart (see Figure 3.9).
- **Echocardiography:** Useful for visually detecting the effusion as well as for ruling out tamponade physiology.
- **Pericardiocentesis:** Can help diagnose the underlying cause of the effusion (eg, transudate vs. exudate).

TREATMENT

- If the patient is unstable, follow guidelines for the treatment of **cardiac tamponade.**
- Drainage of fluid via pericardiocentesis or pericardial window may be necessary in slowly evolving effusions that become symptomatic.

CONSTRICTIVE PERICARDITIS

Impaired ventricular filling due to thickening and scarring of pericardium. Commonly associated with recurrent episodes of acute pericarditis, prior radiation therapy, tuberculosis, collagen vascular disease, and status post–cardiac surgery.

SYMPTOMS

Presents with insidious onset of systemic venous congestion (and, less commonly, pulmonary congestion) as well as with ↓ cardiac output (fatigue, dyspnea, peripheral edema).

KEY FACT

If fluid from a bloody pericardial effusion clots on drainage, the fluid is likely coming from an acute or subacute ruptured myocardium or blood vessel. In other forms of bloody pericardial fluid (eg, renal failure or malignancy), the fluid does not clot.

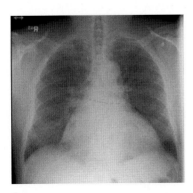
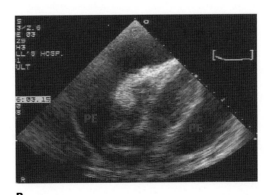

A   **B**

FIGURE 3.9. **Pericardial effusion and tamponade.** (A) Frontal CXR shows enlargement of the cardiac silhouette with a "water-bottle heart" configuration in a patient with a pericardial effusion. (B) Apical four-chamber transthoracic echocardiogram shows a large pericardial effusion (PE) with collapse of the right atrium and right ventricle in early diastole in a patient with cardiac tamponade. (Image A reproduced with permission from USMLERx.com. Image B reproduced with permission from Hall JB et al. *Principles of Critical Care,* 3rd ed. New York: McGraw-Hill, 2005, Fig. 28-7A.)

EXAM

- ↑ JVP with prominent y descent and **Kussmaul's sign** (↑ JVP during inspiration).
- There are prominent x and y descents on jugular venous pulsation exam, leading to an M-shaped contour. Pulsus paradoxus may be present.
- A pericardial knock (a high-pitched third heart sound heard shortly after A2) may be heard following S2, representing rapid cessation of early diastolic filling.

DIFFERENTIAL

- **Restrictive cardiomyopathy:** A similar presentation that may require MRI and/or myocardial biopsy to distinguish. On hemodynamic study, right and left ventricular pressures are concordant with respiration in restriction and discordant in constriction.
- **Cardiac tamponade:** Blunted y descent on right atrial pressure tracing, absence of Kussmaul's sign, and more frequent presence of pulsus paradoxus. Right heart catheterization shows diastolic equalization of pressures in both disorders, but a dip-and-plateau pattern is seen only in constriction (and restriction). Table 3.9 further outlines the distinctions between tamponade and pericardial restriction.
- **Cirrhosis:** Patients with hepatic congestion and ascites due to constriction can be incorrectly diagnosed as having cryptogenic cirrhosis.

DIAGNOSIS

- **ECG:** No specific findings, but low voltage may be present.
- **CXR:** Shows pericardial calcifications (on lateral view) in approximately 25% of patients; bilateral pleural effusions are often present.
- **Echocardiogram:** Demonstrates pericardial thickening and adhesions, septal bounce, and a plethoric IVC without inspiratory collapse.
- **Right heart catheterization:** Equalization of diastolic pressures and dip-and-plateau pattern ("**square root**" sign) that reflects early diastolic filling followed by constraint from fixed pericardial volume. Interventricular discordance is specific for pericardial constriction.
- **MRI:** The most sensitive imaging modality for measuring abnormal pericardial thickness (see Figure 3.10).

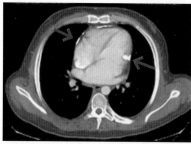

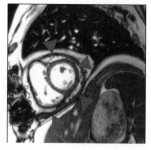

A   **B**

FIGURE 3.10. **Constrictive pericarditis.** (**A**) Transaxial image from a contrast-enhanced CT demonstrates calcification of the pericardium (arrows) in a patient with constrictive pericarditis. (**B**) Short-axis image from a cine-MRI demonstrates a thickened pericardium (arrowheads) in a patient with constrictive pericarditis. (Image A reproduced with permission from Fauci AS et al. *Harrison's Principles of Internal Medicine,* 17th ed. New York: McGraw-Hill, 2008, Fig. 222-9. Image B reproduced with permission from Fuster V et al. *Hurst's the Heart,* 12th ed. New York: McGraw-Hill, 2008, Fig. 21-25A.)

TREATMENT

Surgical pericardectomy is the treatment of choice, but mortality ranges from 5% to 12%, and symptom relief may not occur for several months following the procedure.

CARDIAC TAMPONADE

An accumulation of pericardial fluid under pressure that impedes ventricular filling. Most commonly associated with malignancy, trauma, idiopathic factors, and ventricular rupture following MI.

SYMPTOMS

Presents with dyspnea, chest pain, and lightheadedness.

EXAM

Tachycardia and hypotension with diminished heart sounds and clear lungs; ↑ JVP with blunting or absence of the y descent. Pulsus paradoxus is > 10 mm Hg.

DIFFERENTIAL

- **Constrictive pericarditis:** Has a slow, insidious onset. Kussmaul's sign is usually present. Echocardiogram shows pericardial thickening without large effusion.
- **Tension pneumothorax:** Can also present with tachycardia, hypotension, and elevated neck veins with **pulsus paradoxus.** ↑ ventilator pressures and loss of unilateral breath sounds are clues.

DIAGNOSIS

- **ECG:** Low voltage and/or electrical alternans.
- **Echocardiogram:** Pericardial effusion with right atrial and right ventricular collapse; a plethoric IVC that does not collapse with inspiration. An ↑ respiratory variation of mitral and tricuspid inflow patterns (the echo equivalent of pulsus paradoxus) is also seen.
- **Cardiac catheterization:** Equalization of diastolic pressures (right atrial, right ventricular, pulmonary arterial, PCWP).

TREATMENT

- **IV fluids:** ↑ preload and improve ventricular filling.
- **Dopamine:** Can improve cardiac output in preparation for pericardiocentesis.
- **Pericardiocentesis:** Usually performed with echocardiographic or fluoroscopic guidance to drain pericardial fluid.
- **Pericardial window:** Surgically placed or via balloon pericardiotomy to prevent reaccumulation of fluid.

KEY FACT

Cardiac tamponade is more closely related to the rate of pericardial fluid accumulation than to the size of the effusion. A small effusion may cause tamponade if it is acute.

Electrophysiology

VENTRICULAR TACHYCARDIA (VT) AND VENTRICULAR FIBRILLATION (VF)

A 55-year-old man is brought to the ER by ambulance after he collapsed while at work. He is found to be in monomorphic VT and is successfully cardioverted. He has no acute lesions on coronary angiography, and cardiac imaging reveals an area of nonreversible perfusion defect laterally. His EF on echocardiography is 35%. What intervention is likely to have the greatest effect on his subsequent survival?

Placement of an ICD. This patient has a high chance of recurrence given that he likely had monomorphic VT from his associated scar from a prior MI. Inasmuch as this is a nonreversible lesion, an ICD is likely to be the most life-saving intervention, especially in the setting of a low EF.

Commonly caused by ischemia/infarction, cardiomyopathy, electrolytes, and drug toxicity. Types of VT are as follows (see also Figure 3.11):

- **Monomorphic:** Characterized by a uniform QRS pattern; most commonly associated with myocardial scar.
- **Polymorphic:** Bizarre and changing QRS morphology as seen in torsades de pointes; may be precipitated by myocardial ischemia. Torsades is most

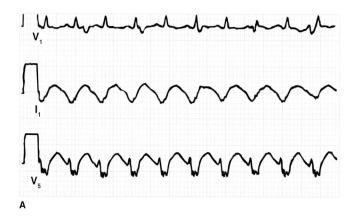

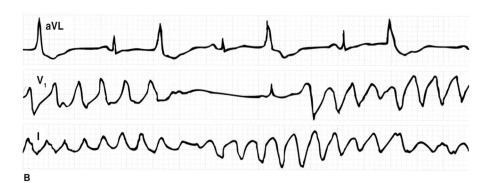

FIGURE 3.11. Ventricular tachycardia. (A) Monomorphic VT with AV dissociation. P waves are dissociated from the underlying wide-complex rhythm (best seen on lead V₁). **(B)** Polymorphic VT associated with a prolonged QT interval. (Adapted with permission from Kasper DL et al. *Harrison's Principles of Internal Medicine,* 16th ed. New York: McGraw-Hill, 2005: 1352, 1353.)

often associated with medications and electrolyte abnormalities that prolong the QT interval, such as type IC and type III antiarrhythmics, hypomagnesemia, hypocalcemia, and hypokalemia.

SYMPTOMS

Chest pain, dyspnea, and syncope due to poor systemic perfusion are common. The initial manifestation of VT/VF in many patients is sudden cardiac death.

EXAM

Cannon A waves on jugular venous pulsation are seen during VT as a result of AV dissociation.

DIFFERENTIAL

Supraventricular tachycardia (SVT) with aberrant conduction.

DIAGNOSIS

- **For unstable patients, always assume VT until proven otherwise.**
- For stable patients, the Brugada criteria can be used to distinguish SVT with aberrancy from VT. Major criteria are as follows:
  - **AV dissociation is always VT.**
  - The absence of RS complexes in all precordial leads is VT.
  - Complexes not typical of LBBB or RBBB are usually VT.

TREATMENT

- **Electrical cardioversion** is the treatment of choice for unstable patients.
- IV therapy with amiodarone is now first-line therapy for stable VT.
- Polymorphic VT (including torsades de pointes) can be treated with rapid magnesium infusion and overdrive pacing.
- **ICD placement is indicated for patients whose etiologies are not thought to be transient or reversible.**

COMPLICATIONS

Sudden cardiac death, hypoxic encephalopathy, demand cardiac ischemia/MI.

KEY FACT

Rule out myocardial ischemia in cases of polymorphic VT with a normal QT interval on baseline ECG.

ATRIAL FIBRILLATION (AF)

A 64-year-old man with a history of alcoholism presents with AF and is found to have dilated cardiomyopathy with an EF of 40%. His echocardiogram shows left atrial enlargement, chamber dilation, and no obvious intracardiac thrombus. What would be the optimal treatment for his condition?

Amiodarone or digoxin and warfarin. The patient is unlikely to benefit from cardioversion, as the duration of his AF is unknown, and he already has structural heart disease that will likely lead to a recurrence of AF. This patient's CHADS2 score (one point for age and one point for CHF) indicates that warfarin and not ASA would be appropriate anticoagulation for this patient. Given his ↓ EF, either digoxin or amiodarone should be used as rate control.

The most common arrhythmia in the general population. Prevalence ↑ with age (10% of individuals > 80 years of age have AF). Etiologies are as follows:

- **Most common:** Hypertension, valvular heart disease, heart failure, CAD.
- **Other causes:** Pulmonary disease (COPD, pulmonary embolism), ischemia, rheumatic heart disease (rheumatic mitral stenosis), hyperthyroidism, sepsis, alcoholism, Wolff-Parkinson-White (WPW) syndrome, cardiac surgery.
- **Lone AF:** Normal echo; no risk factors (ie, no hypertension, age < 65 years).

SYMPTOMS/EXAM

Can be asymptomatic or manifest as palpitations, fatigue, dyspnea, dizziness, diaphoresis, and/or symptoms of heart failure.

DIFFERENTIAL

- **Irregular tachycardias:** AF, atrial flutter with variable block, multifocal atrial tachycardia, frequent premature atrial contractions.
- **Regular tachycardias:** Sinus tachycardia, atrial tachycardia (AT), AV nodal reentrant tachycardia (AVNRT), AV reentrant tachycardia (AVRT), accelerated junctional tachycardia.

DIAGNOSIS

- **ECG:** AF is the most common cause of an irregularly irregular rhythm on ECG (see Figure 3.12). **Look for the absence of P waves.**
- **Echocardiogram:** Used to predict stroke risk (look for structural abnormalities such as LVH, left atrial enlargement, mitral stenosis, and ↓ EF). TEE can be used to visualize thrombus in the left atrium.

> **KEY FACT**
>
> In patients > 65 years of age, maintaining sinus rhythm with antiarrhythmics is no more effective than rate control and anticoagulation in reducing the incidence of stroke or mortality.

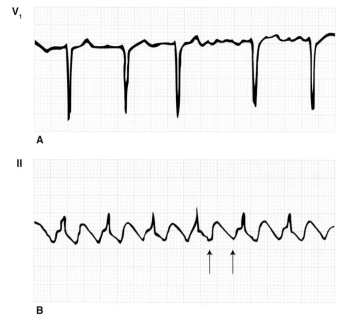

FIGURE 3.12. **Atrial fibrillation and atrial flutter.** (A) Lead V_1 demonstrates an irregular ventricular rhythm associated with poorly defined irregular atrial activity consistent with AF. (B) Lead II demonstrates atrial flutter, identified by the regular "sawtooth-like" activity (arrows) at an atrial rate of 300 bpm with 2:1 ventricular response. (Adapted with permission from Kasper DL et al. *Harrison's Principles of Internal Medicine,* 16th ed. New York: McGraw-Hill, 2005: 1345.)

TREATMENT

- Unstable patients: Proceed directly to cardioversion (biphasic is preferable to monophasic).
- **Rate control:** β-blockers or centrally acting nondihydropyridine CCBs (diltiazem, verapamil) are first line. For a ↓ EF, use amiodarone or digoxin.
- **Rhythm control:** Guidelines suggest flecainide, propafenone, or sotalol as first-line therapy in patients without heart disease. Patients with CHF can be started on amiodarone or dofetilide; for those with CAD, sotalol is first line. Patients with hypertension and LVH should be started on amiodarone (those with hypertension and no LVH can be treated with flecainide or propafenone).
- **Anticoagulation:** Warfarin (with a goal INR of 2–3) or ASA.
- **Patients with a score of 2 or greater by the CHADS2 criteria** (1 point for CHF, Hypertension, Age > 60, Diabetes; 2 points for prior Stroke or TIA) should be anticoagulated with **warfarin** as opposed to ASA alone to **prevent stroke.**
  - If the CHADS2 score is < 2, warfarin or ASA can be used.
  - **Lone AF** should be treated with **ASA alone.**
  - Anticoagulation is unnecessary if AF is new onset and the duration is < 48 hours.
  - If AF is > 48 hours or if < 48 hours and associated with rheumatic mitral valve disease, anticoagulate with warfarin for 3–4 weeks prior to cardioversion (goal INR 2–3).
- **TEE-guided cardioversion:** Trials of TEE-guided cardioversion used anticoagulation for 24 hours prior to cardioversion and anticoagulated following cardioversion.
- **Postcardioversion:** Anticoagulate with warfarin for four weeks.
- **Rate control vs. rhythm control:** Studies have demonstrated that rate control with anticoagulation has the same outcome as rhythm control and may also be safer.
- **Post–cardiac surgery AF:** Most common after mitral valve surgery; occurs on postoperative days 2–3. Cardioversion is the most effective therapy. If AF recurs after cardioversion, treat with rate control and anticoagulation. Prophylaxis includes perioperative β-blockers or amiodarone.
- **WPW patients who present in AF with rapid ventricular response:** If baseline ECG shows a delta wave or if the current ECG shows wide, bizarre QRS complexes during AF, **avoid AV nodal blocking agents** (β-blockers, CCBs, adenosine, digoxin). The treatment of choice is IV procainamide, which slows conduction in the entire atrium. **If AV nodal blocking agents are given in this situation, the atrial impulses in rapid AF can proceed down the accessory pathway and cause VF and death.**

ATRIAL FLUTTER

After AF, atrial flutter is the most common atrial arrhythmia. It is usually caused by a macro-reentrant circuit within the **right atrium.**

SYMPTOMS/EXAM

May be asymptomatic. When symptoms occur, patients generally complain of palpitations, an irregular or fast heartbeat, lightheadedness, dyspnea, or ↓ exercise tolerance.

DIAGNOSIS

- **Always consider the diagnosis of atrial flutter in patients who have a heart rate of ~ 150 bpm,** since atrial flutter usually presents with a 2:1 AV block.
- May be typical or atypical.
  - **Typical flutter:** The most common type of atrial flutter. ECG will generally show a **sawtooth pattern in the inferior leads** (II, III, aVF; see Figure 3.12). Look for discrete, upright, P-wave-like deflections in lead V_1 (the P-wave rate should be approximately 300 bpm).
  - **Atypical flutter:** Look for continuous, regular atrial activity at a rate of 250–350 bpm without typical flutter morphology. If a sawtooth pattern is present but not in inferior leads and rhythm is irregular, it is most likely AF and not atrial flutter.

TREATMENT

- In the acute setting, three treatment options exist for the restoration of sinus rhythm:
  - **Antiarrhythmic drugs:** Ibutilide, flecainide, propafenone. Ibutilide is approximately 60% effective in restoring sinus rhythm but carries the risk of torsades de pointes due to QT prolongation.
  - **Cardioversion:** Useful in cases of hemodynamic instability.
  - **Rapid atrial pacing:** Overdrive pacing.
- Rate control can be achieved with centrally acting CCBs, β-blockers, or digoxin.
- **Long-term treatment:**
  - Radiofrequency ablation is highly effective.
  - Alternative treatments include antiarrhythmic drugs or antitachycardia pacemakers.
  - These treatments generally require long-term anticoagulation with warfarin to ↓ the risk of thromboembolism.

KEY FACT

When using ibutilide for chemical cardioversion of atrial flutter, monitor the QT interval closely. Torsades de pointes can occur, treatment for which consists of IV magnesium and cardioversion.

PAROXYSMAL SUPRAVENTRICULAR TACHYCARDIA (PSVT)

The most common type of PSVT is AVNRT. Other forms are AT and AVRT. Mechanisms for PSVT are as follows:

- **AT:** Tachycardia arising from an ectopic atrial focus (↑ automaticity).
- **AVRT:** Reentry via an AV bypass tract (WPW syndrome if a delta wave is present on ECG).
- **AVNRT:** Reentry within the AV node.

SYMPTOMS

Presents with palpitations, lightheadedness, and occasionally chest discomfort. Paroxysms usually begin in young adulthood and ↑ with age. Attacks begin and end suddenly and may last a few seconds or persist for hours.

EXAM

- Not usually associated with structural heart disease.
- There are no specific exam findings except for cannon A waves in the jugular venous pulsation during AVNRT due to atrial contraction against a closed tricuspid valve.

DIFFERENTIAL

Based on the ECG:

- **If QRS is narrow:** AVRT, AVNRT.
- **If QRS is wide:** PSVT with aberrancy vs. VT.
- **If QRS is wide and the rhythm is irregular with bizarre QRS complexes:**
  AF conducting via an accessory pathway.

DIAGNOSIS

- ECG (see Figure 3.13).
  - AVRT is a macro-reentrant circuit with retrograde P waves.
  - AVNRT is a micro-reentrant circuit with P waves buried in QRS.
  - AT has a "long RP" relationship, with P waves preceding each QRS.
- Holter or event monitoring is essential if episodes are not documented on
  a 12-lead ECG.
- An electrophysiologic study can be used for diagnosis and ablative therapy.

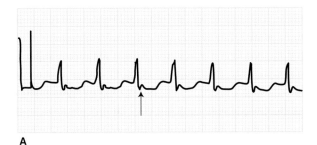

A

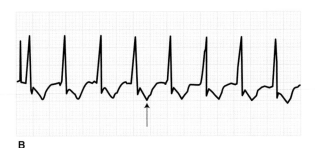

B

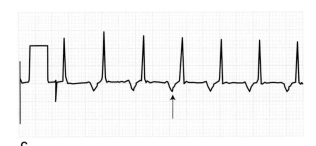

C

FIGURE 3.13. **Examples of supraventricular tachycardia.** Arrows indicate P waves. **(A)** AV nodal reentry. Upright P waves are visible at the end of the QRS complex. **(B)** AV reentry using a concealed bypass tract. Inverted retrograde P waves are superimposed on the T waves. **(C)** Automatic atrial tachycardia. Inverted P waves follow the T waves and precede the QRS complex. (Adapted with permission from Kasper DL et al. *Harrison's Principles of Internal Medicine,* 16th ed. New York: McGraw-Hill, 2005: 1349.)

TREATMENT

- Acute termination can occur with carotid massage or rapid administration of adenosine.
- Medical management consists of AV nodal blocking agents (eg, β-blockers).
- Curative therapy consists of catheter-based ablation.

COMPLICATIONS

- Rapid rates in older patients can cause demand ischemia and MI.
- The treatment of AF conducting via an accessory pathway with AV nodal blockade can cause rapid bypass tract conduction, leading to VF.

WOLFF-PARKINSON-WHITE (WPW) SYNDROME

A 63-year-old woman presents to the hospital with palpitations and is found to have AF with a rate of 145 bpm. She is hemodynamically stable, and her ECG is notable for AF with rapid ventricular response and prominent delta waves. What is the appropriate therapy for this patient?

IV procainamide. Because the patient is hemodynamically stable, she does not need urgent cardioversion. The presence of delta waves implies a bypass tract, which may be indicative of WPW syndrome. Treatment with β-blockers or CCBs may ↑ through the bypass tract, and therefore IV procainamide is the treatment of choice.

In patients with WPW syndrome, an accessory pathway exists between the atria and ventricles as a result of a defect in the separation of the atria and ventricles during fetal development. WPW syndrome may be found incidentally on routine ECG. However, patients with WPW syndrome are at risk for tachyarrhythmias and even sudden cardiac death.

DIAGNOSIS

- If the accessory pathway allows **anterograde conduction**, electrical impulses from the atria can conduct down the accessory pathway into the ventricles, causing ventricular preexcitation with a short PR interval and **classic delta waves on ECG** (slurring of the upstroke on the QRS, best seen in lead V_4; see Figure 3.14).
- Some patients with WPW syndrome have accessory pathways that allow only **retrograde conduction** from the ventricles to the atria. In these patients, the resting ECG will not show a delta wave. These patients have a so-called concealed bypass tract, and though they may have a normal resting ECG, they are still prone to the development of an AVNRT.

TREATMENT

Electrophysiologic study and catheter ablation of the bypass tracts is the treatment of choice for patients with WPW syndrome.

COMPLICATIONS

- **AF** is the 1° complication of WPW syndrome.
- If the patient has a concealed bypass tract (ie, no evidence of a delta wave or other evidence of WPW syndrome on baseline ECG), the standard treatment for AF (or any tachycardia) is safe.

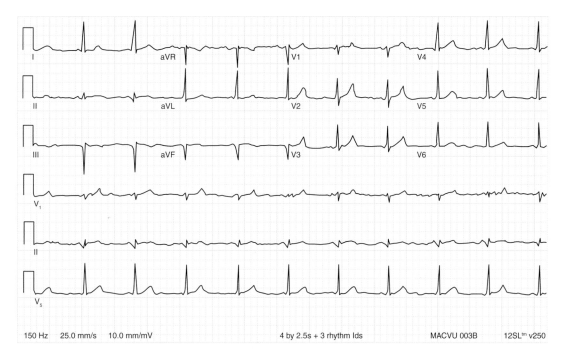

150 Hz   25.0 mm/s   10.0 mm/mV   4 by 2.5s + 3 rhythm lds   MACVU 003B   12SL^{tm} v250

FIGURE 3.14. **Classic Wolff-Parkinson-White ECG.** Note the short PR interval and classic delta waves on ECG (slurring of the upstroke of the QRS best seen in V$_4$).

- If the patient has evidence of a bypass tract on ECG (a delta wave) or if the patient is in AF with bizarre, aberrantly conducted complexes, this represents an emergency situation. **Do not give such patients AV nodal blocking agents,** as doing so can allow for 1:1 conduction of AF via the bypass tract, leading to VF and cardiac arrest. The treatment of choice for these patients is procainamide or cardioversion.

CARDIAC SYNCOPE

Cardiac syncope can be due to structural heart disease or arrhythmias. It classically presents either with exertion (structural) or suddenly and without warning (arrhythmic). Overall causes are as follows:

- **Cardiac:** 18%.
- **Neurologic:** 10%.
- **Vasovagal:** 24%.
- **Orthostatic:** 8%.
- **Medications:** 3%.
- **Unknown:** 37%.

SYMPTOMS/EXAM

- Causes may be structural or arrhythmic.
- **Common structural causes:**
  - **Aortic stenosis:** Usually occurs with exertion; look for associated angina or heart failure.

- **Hypertrophic obstructive cardiomyopathy:** Can occur in all ages; may be dynamic in nature (ie, may manifest in the setting of ↓ preload, such as postexercise). Syncope may also occur in a nonobstructive form as a result of ventricular arrhythmias.
  - **Less common structural causes:** Pulmonary embolism, aortic dissection, cardiac tamponade.
  - **Uncommon structural causes:** Pulmonary hypertension, atrial myxoma, subclavian steal.
- **Arrhythmic causes:**
  - **Bradycardia:**
    - **Sinus bradycardia:** Sick sinus syndrome, medications (eg, β-blockers, CCBs).
    - **AV block (second, third degree):** Usually due to age-related conduction disease, medications, and/or ischemia.
    - **Carotid sinus hypersensitivity.**
  - **Tachycardia:**
    - **SVT:** A rare cause of syncope.
    - **VT:** Most often due to structural and/or ischemic heart disease.

DIAGNOSIS

- **ECG:** Look for evidence of ischemia, arrhythmia, new bundle branch block, or a prolonged QT interval.
- **Echocardiogram:** Look for structural heart disease. Consider in patients with syncope and a history of heart disease, those with an abnormality on physical exam (eg, murmur) or ECG, or elderly patients.
- **Holter monitoring:** Use when the patient has symptoms that suggest arrhythmia (eg, a cluster of spells, sudden loss of consciousness, palpitations, use of medications associated with arrhythmia, known heart disease, an abnormal ECG).
- **Tilt-table testing:** Use in patients with normal hearts and relatively infrequent syncope, nondiagnostic Holter monitoring, or symptoms that suggest vasovagal spells (eg, warmth, nausea) but lack an obvious precipitating event.

TREATMENT

Guidelines for hospital admission are as follows:

- Evidence of MI, stroke, or arrhythmia.
- **Definite admission:** Chest pain; a history of CAD, heart failure, or ventricular arrhythmia; evidence of heart failure or valvular disease; focal neurologic deficits on physical exam; new ECG abnormalities.
- **Possible admission:** Patients > 70 years of age; those with exertional or frequent syncope, orthostasis, or injury due to a syncopal episode.

BRADYCARDIA

Incidence ↑ with age. Etiologies are as follows:

- **Intrinsic causes:** Idiopathic senile degeneration; ischemia (usually involving the inferior wall); infectious processes (endocarditis, Chagas' disease, Lyme disease); infiltrative diseases (sarcoidosis, amyloidosis, hemochromatosis); autoimmune disease (SLE, RA, scleroderma); iatrogenic factors (heart transplant, surgery); inherited/congenital disease (myotonic muscular dystrophy); conditioned heart (trained athletes).
- **Extrinsic causes:** Autonomic (neurocardiac, carotid sinus hypersensitivity, situational), medications (β-blockers, CCBs, clonidine, digoxin, antiar-

rhythmics), metabolic (electrolyte abnormalities, hypothyroidism, hypothermia), neurologic (↑ ICP, obstructive sleep apnea).

SYMPTOMS

Patients may be asymptomatic or may present with dizziness, weakness, fatigue, heart failure, or loss of consciousness (syncope). Symptoms can also be related to the underlying cause of the bradycardia.

EXAM

Look for evidence of ↓ pulse rate and evidence of the underlying cause of bradycardia. Look for **cannon A** waves in cases of complete AV dissociation (complete heart block).

DIAGNOSIS

- **ECG:** Look for the origin of the rhythm and whether dropped beats or AV dissociation is present (evidence of AV block; see Table 3.10).
- **Telemetry,** event monitors, tilt-table testing, and electrophysiologic studies can also be helpful.

TREATMENT

- If the patient is **unstable,** follow ACLS protocols.
- If possible, treat the underlying cause (eg, endocarditis).
- **Medications:** Atropine, **glucagon** (for β-blocker overdose), calcium (for CCB overdose). Note that calcium is **contraindicated** in digoxin toxicity.
- **Transcutaneous or transvenous pacing:** Appropriate if medical therapy is ineffective.
- **Indication for permanent pacemakers:** Documented symptomatic bradycardia. If the patient is asymptomatic, pacemakers may be considered in patients with third-degree AV block with > 3 seconds of asystole or a heart rate < 40 bpm while the patient is awake. In second-degree type II AV block, pacemakers have a class II indication (there is conflicting evidence and opinion regarding the need for permanent pacing).

INDICATIONS FOR PERMANENT PACING

Indications for permanent cardiac pacing, based on expert guidelines, are classified as follows: I (definite indications), II (indications with conflicting evidence or opinion), or III (not indicated or harmful). **All indications assume that transient causes such as drugs, electrolytes, and ischemia have been corrected or excluded.**

> **KEY FACT**
>
> If left untreated, Lyme disease can cause varying degrees of AV conduction block at any time in the course of the disease.

TABLE 3.10. **ECG Findings with AV Block**

TYPE OF BLOCK	ECG FINDINGS
First degree	Prolonged PR interval (> 200 msec).
Second degree type I (Wenckebach)	Progressive prolongation of the PR interval until there is a dropped QRS. Progressive shortening of the RR interval and a constant PP interval are other signs.
Second degree type II	Regularly dropped QRS (eg, every third QRS complex is dropped). Constant PR interval (no prolongation). Usually associated with bundle branch blocks.
Third degree	Complete dissociation of P waves and QRS complexes (P-wave rate > QRS rate).

Class I

- **Third-degree AV block** and advanced second-degree AV block associated with the following:
    - Symptomatic bradycardia.
    - Arrhythmias or other conditions requiring medications that result in symptomatic bradycardia.
    - Documented asystole of > 3 seconds or escape rates of < 40 bpm in **awake,** asymptomatic patients.
    - After AV junction ablation.
    - Post–cardiac surgery when AV block is not expected to resolve.
    - Neuromuscular diseases with AV block due to the unpredictable progression of AV conduction disease in these patients.
- **Second-degree AV block** (regardless of type) associated with symptomatic bradycardia.

Class IIA

- Asymptomatic third-degree AV block with **awake** escape rates of > 40 bpm.
- Asymptomatic type II second-degree block with narrow QRS (with wide QRS, it becomes a class I indication).
- Asymptomatic type I second-degree block with intra- or infra-His levels found on an electrophysiologic study done for another indication.
- First- and second-degree AV block with symptoms suggestive of pacemaker syndrome.

Class IIB

- Marked first-degree AV block (PR > 300 msec) in patients with left ventricular dysfunction.
- Neuromuscular diseases with any level of AV block due to the unpredictable progression of block in these patients.

Class III

- Asymptomatic first-degree AV block.
- Asymptomatic type I second-degree AV block not known to be due to a problem within or below the bundle of His.
- AV block that is expected to resolve and/or is not likely to recur.

SUDDEN CARDIAC DEATH

Approximately 450,000 sudden cardiac deaths occur annually in the United States. Etiologies include CAD, MI, pulmonary embolism, aortic dissection, cardiac tamponade, and other acute cardiopulmonary insults. Seventy-five percent of patients do not survive cardiac arrest.

Causes in Young Athletes

- In young athletes, the causes of sudden cardiac death differ from those in the overall population. Causes in this population include the following (in order of decreasing incidence):
    - Hypertrophic cardiomyopathy.
    - Commotio cordis (a sudden blow to the precordium causing ventricular arrhythmia).
    - Coronary artery anomalies.
    - Myocarditis.

- Ruptured aortic aneurysm (eg, due to Marfan's syndrome or Ehlers-Danlos syndrome).
- Arrhythmogenic right ventricular dysplasia, in which the right ventricle is replaced by fat and fibrosis, causing an ↑ frequency of ventricular arrhythmias.
- Aortic stenosis.
- Myocardial bridge causing coronary ischemia during ventricular contraction.
- Atherosclerotic CAD.
- Coronary artery vasospasm.
- Brugada syndrome, which is caused by a sodium channel defect that predisposes to VF. The baseline ECG shows incomplete RBBB and ST-segment elevation in the precordial leads.
- Long QT syndrome.
- **Noncardiac precipitants** of sudden cardiac death in young athletes include asthma, illicit drug use (eg, cocaine, ephedra, amphetamines), and heat stroke.

Screening in Young Athletes

- It is difficult to assess patients for risk factors of sudden cardiac death because these conditions are rare and because millions of young athletes need to be screened.
- Although screening usually involves history taking and physical examination, these measures alone lack the sensitivity to detect even the most common causes of sudden cardiac death in athletes (eg, hypertrophic cardiomyopathy).
- In patients with a suggestive history or physical examination, further workup with ECG and echocardiography is warranted.

Implantable Cardioverter-Defibrillators (ICDs)

RISK FACTORS FOR VENTRICULAR ARRHYTHMIAS

Include dilated cardiomyopathy (with a ↓ EF), hypertension, hyperlipidemia, tobacco, diabetes, a family history of sudden cardiac death, myocardial ischemia and reperfusion, and toxins (eg, cocaine).

2° PREVENTION

- **Goal:** To prevent recurrent sudden cardiac death in patients with a history of VT or VF.
- **Drugs:** Antiarrhythmic drugs have been disappointing in the 2° prevention of sudden cardiac death, especially in the large group of patients who are post-MI. Standard therapies for CAD alone (especially β-blockers) play a significant role in decreasing sudden cardiac death in these patients.
- **Devices: ICDs** are superior to amiodarone in patients with CAD who have survived cardiac arrest and have a **low** EF.
- ICDs do not have a survival advantage over amiodarone in patients who have an EF of > 35%.

1° PREVENTION

- **Goal:** To prevent sudden cardiac death in patients who have no history of VT and/or VF.
- Studies have shown that in patients with a history of MI who have an EF of < 30%, ICD therapy improves mortality and is superior to antiarrhythmic therapy.

INDICATIONS FOR *ICD* USE

- **Etiology of heart failure:** Recent studies indicate that ICD therapy appears effective for **both** ischemic and nonischemic cardiomyopathy.
- **Severity of heart failure:** Consider ICDs in patients with an EF of < 35%.
- **Noninvasive testing:**
  - **T-wave alternans:** Microfluctuations in the morphology of T waves on ECG may indicate an ↑ risk of sudden cardiac death (requires specialized testing).
  - **Heart rate variability:** ↓ heart rate variability corresponds to worsening heart failure and may be associated with an ↑ risk of sudden cardiac death.

Valvular Heart Disease

AORTIC STENOSIS

The most common causes are senile calcific aortic stenosis and congenital bicuspid aortic valve. Rheumatic aortic stenosis is usually not hemodynamically significant and **almost always occurs in the presence of mitral valve disease.**

SYMPTOMS

Presents with a long asymptomatic period followed by the development of the classic triad of **angina, syncope, and heart failure.** The normal valve area is 3 cm^2, and symptoms usually do not develop until the area is < 1 cm^2.

EXAM

- A crescendo-decrescendo systolic murmur is heard at the base of the heart with radiation to the carotid arteries. Late-peaking murmurs signify more severe stenosis.
- Diminished and delayed carotid upstrokes (parvus et tardus) and a sustained PMI due to LVH may be present.
- A systolic ejection click can occur in patients with a bicuspid aortic valve. A2 diminishes in intensity, and S2 may be single.

DIFFERENTIAL

- **Sub- or supravalvular stenosis:** Due to left ventricular outflow tract membrane or fibromuscular ring (rare).
- **Hypertrophic obstructive cardiomyopathy:** Murmur accentuated with Valsalva or standing and ↓ by hand grip.

DIAGNOSIS

- **Echocardiography:** A modified Bernoulli equation is used to derive the pressure gradient across the aortic valve. The aortic valve area is derived by the continuity equation. The severity of aortic stenosis can be classified as follows:
  - **Mild disease:** A valve area < 1.5 cm^2, mean gradient < 25 mm Hg.
  - **Moderate disease:** A valve area 1.0–1.5 cm^2, mean gradient 25–40 mm Hg.
  - **Severe disease:** A valve area < 1 cm^2, mean gradient > 40 mm Hg.
- **Follow-up echocardiography:** Recommended every year for severe aortic stenosis; every 1–2 years for moderate aortic stenosis; and every 3–5 years for mild aortic stenosis.

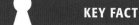

KEY FACT

In aortic stenosis, aortic valve replacement should be performed as soon as symptoms develop to prevent cardiac death.

KEY FACT

Aortic stenosis has been associated with an ↑ risk of GI bleeding, which is now thought to be due to acquired von Willebrand's disease from disruption of von Willebrand factor multimers as they pass through the stenotic aortic valve.

- **Cardiac catheterization:** Required to exclude significant coronary stenoses in symptomatic patients who are scheduled for surgery and are at risk for CAD. Also needed to confirm the severity of aortic stenosis when there is a discrepancy between clinical and noninvasive data.
- **Dobutamine stress testing:** Used in cases of low-gradient aortic stenosis (severe aortic stenosis by valve area, but mean gradient < 40 mm Hg) to distinguish true stenosis from pseudostenosis caused by ↓ systolic function. If true aortic stenosis is present, the gradient will ↑ and the valve area will remain unchanged. If pseudostenosis is present, the valve area will ↑.
- **CT/MRI:** Imaging of the aorta is important in patients with bicuspid aortic valve, as these patients have a higher likelihood of aortic root and proximal aortic dilatation, and there is an association between aortic coarctation and bicuspid aortic valve. Echocardiography can also diagnose proximal aortic dilatation and aortic coarctation.

TREATMENT

- **Aortic valve replacement:** The only therapy for **symptomatic** aortic stenosis. Older patients do quite well after aortic valve replacement and should not be disqualified on the basis of age alone. Patients who are unlikely to outlive a bioprothesis can be spared the lifelong anticoagulation that is required for mechanical valves.
- **Antibiotic prophylaxis against subacute bacterial endocarditis:** Indicated for **all patients.**
- **Aortic valvuloplasty:** May be effective in young adults with congenital aortic stenosis. **Less effective in patients with degenerative aortic stenosis, and should be considered palliative therapy or a bridge to surgery.**

COMPLICATIONS

- Sudden death may occur but is uncommon (< 1% per year) in patients with severe asymptomatic aortic stenosis.
- **If left untreated, the average time to death is as follows:**
  - **After onset of syncope:** 2.5–3.0 years.
  - **After onset of angina:** 3 years.
  - **After onset of dyspnea:** 2 years.
  - **After onset of CHF:** 1.5 years.

AORTIC REGURGITATION

Can be caused by destruction or malfunction of the valve leaflets (infective endocarditis, bicuspid aortic valve, rheumatic valve disease) or dilatation of the aortic root such that the leaflets no longer coapt (Marfan's syndrome, aortic dissection).

SYMPTOMS

- **Acute aortic regurgitation:** Presents with rapid onset of cardiogenic shock.
- **Chronic aortic regurgitation:** A long asymptomatic period followed by progressive dyspnea on exertion and other signs of heart failure.

EXAM

- Exam reveals a soft S1 (usually due to a long PR interval) and a soft or absent A2 with a decrescendo blowing diastolic murmur at the base.
- A wide pulse pressure with water-hammer peripheral pulses is also seen.

- Other peripheral signs include a bruit over the femoral artery (Duroziez's sign); nail-bed pulsations (Quincke's pulse); and a popliteal-brachial BP difference of > 20 mm Hg (Hill's sign).
- In acute aortic regurgitation, these signs are usually not present, and the only clues may be ↓ intensity of S1 and a short, blowing diastolic murmur.

DIFFERENTIAL

Other causes of diastolic murmurs include mitral stenosis, tricuspid stenosis, pulmonic insufficiency, and atrial myxoma.

DIAGNOSIS

- **Echocardiography:** Essential for determining left ventricular size and function as well as the structure of the aortic valve. TEE is often necessary to rule out endocarditis in acute aortic regurgitation.
- **Cardiac catheterization:** Aortography can be used to estimate the degree of regurgitation if noninvasive studies are inconclusive. Coronary angiography is indicated to exclude CAD in patients at risk prior to surgery.

TREATMENT

- In asymptomatic patients with normal left ventricular function, afterload reduction may be considered, but evidence supporting its benefit is lacking. ACEIs or other vasodilators may ↓ left ventricular volume overload and slow progression to heart failure.
- **Aortic valve replacement:** Should be considered in symptomatic patients or in those without symptoms who develop worsening left ventricular dilatation and systolic failure.
- **Acute aortic regurgitation:** Surgery is the definitive therapy, since mortality is high in this setting. IV vasodilators may be used as a bridge to surgery.
- **Endocarditis prophylaxis:** Consider in all patients.

COMPLICATIONS

Irreversible left ventricular systolic dysfunction if valve replacement is delayed.

MITRAL STENOSIS

A 43-year-old woman from Vietnam presents with shortness of breath. On exam, she is noted to have an ↑ JVP, a loud P2, and an apical diastolic rumble following an opening snap. Her ECG shows right-axis deviation, RVH, and biatrial enlargement. What is the diagnosis?

Rheumatic mitral valve disease. This patient likely has mitral stenosis, as indicated by her exam findings of an apical diastolic rumble and an opening snap. This is likely long-standing mitral stenosis that has led to pulmonary hypertension, resulting in RVH and a loud P2. Given that she grew up in Asia, rheumatic heart disease is the most likely etiology.

Almost exclusively due to **rheumatic heart disease,** with rare cases due to congenital lesions and calcification of the mitral annulus. The normal mitral valve area is 4–6 cm². Severe mitral stenosis occurs when the valve area is < 1 cm².

SYMPTOMS

- Characterized by a long asymptomatic period followed by gradual onset of dyspnea on exertion and findings of right heart failure and pulmonary hypertension.
- Hemoptysis and thromboembolic stroke are late findings.

EXAM

- Exam reveals a loud S1 and an opening snap of stenotic leaflets after S2 followed by an apical diastolic rumble.
- Signs of pulmonary hypertension (a loud P2) and right heart failure (↑ JVP and hepatic congestion) are present in advanced disease.

DIFFERENTIAL

- **Left atrial myxoma:** Causes obstruction of mitral inflow.
- **Cor triatriatum:** Left atrial septations/membrane can mimic mitral stenosis clinically.
- **Aortic insufficiency:** Can mimic the murmur of mitral stenosis (Flint murmur) due to restriction of mitral valve leaflet motion by regurgitant blood from the aortic valve, but no opening snap is present.

DIAGNOSIS

- **Echocardiography:** Used to estimate valve area and to measure the transmitral pressure gradient. Mitral valve morphology on echocardiography determines a patient's suitability for percutaneous valvuloplasty.
- **TEE:** Indicated to exclude left atrial thrombus in patients scheduled for balloon valvuloplasty.
- **Cardiac catheterization:** Can be used to directly measure the valve gradient through simultaneous recording of PCWP and left ventricular diastolic pressure. Rarely needed for diagnosis; performed prior to percutaneous balloon valvuloplasty.

TREATMENT

- **Percutaneous mitral balloon valvotomy:** Unlike aortic valvuloplasty, balloon dilatation of the mitral valve has proven to be a successful strategy in patients without concomitant mitral regurgitation.
  - Consider this intervention in symptomatic patients with isolated mitral stenosis and an effective valve area of < 1.0 cm^2.
  - This is the appropriate intervention in pregnant women for whom medical therapy has failed.
  - Severe annular calcification, severe mitral regurgitation, and atrial thrombus are all contraindications to balloon valvuloplasty.
- **Mitral valve replacement:** For patients who are not candidates for valvuloplasty.
- Endocarditis prophylaxis is indicated for all patients.

COMPLICATIONS

- Left atrial enlargement and AF with resultant stasis is common and can result in left atrial thrombus formation and embolic stroke.
- Pulmonary hypertension and 2° tricuspid regurgitation.

KEY FACT

Patients with rheumatic heart disease typically have involvement of the mitral valve. Isolated involvement of the aortic or tricuspid valve with sparing of the mitral valve is exceedingly rare in patients with rheumatic heart disease.

MITRAL REGURGITATION

Common causes of mitral regurgitation include mitral valve prolapse, myxomatous (degenerative) mitral valve disease, dilated cardiomyopathy (which causes functional mitral regurgitation due to dilatation of the mitral valve annulus), rheumatic heart disease (acute mitral valvulitis produces the Carey Coombs murmur of acute rheumatic fever), acute ischemia (due to rupture of a papillary muscle), mitral valve endocarditis, and trauma to the mitral valve.

SYMPTOMS

- **Acute mitral regurgitation:** Abrupt onset of dyspnea due to pulmonary edema.
- **Chronic mitral regurgitation:** Can be asymptomatic. In severe cases, can present with dyspnea and symptoms of heart failure.

EXAM

- Exam reveals a soft S1 and a holosystolic, blowing murmur heard best at the apex with radiation to the axilla. S3 can be due to mitral regurgitation alone (in the absence of systolic heart failure), and its presence suggests severe mitral regurgitation.
- Acute mitral regurgitation can be associated with hypotension and pulmonary edema; murmur may be early systolic.
- The intensity of the murmur does not generally correlate with mitral regurgitation severity as documented by echocardiogram.

DIFFERENTIAL

- **Aortic stenosis:** Can mimic the murmur of mitral regurgitation (Gallavardin phenomenon).
- **Tricuspid regurgitation:** Characterized by a holosystolic murmur best heard at the left sternal border; ↑ in intensity with inspiration.

DIAGNOSIS

- **Early detection of mitral regurgitation is essential because treatment should be initiated before symptoms occur.**
- **Exercise stress testing:** Document exercise limitation before symptoms occur at rest.
- **Echocardiography:** Transthoracic echocardiography (TTE) is important for diagnosis as well as for grading the severity of mitral regurgitation. TEE is useful in patients who may need surgical repair or mitral valve replacement.
  - Echocardiography should be performed every 2–5 years in mild to moderate mitral regurgitation with a normal end-systolic diameter and an EF of > 65%.
  - Echocardiography should be performed every 6–12 months in patients with severe mitral regurgitation, an end-systolic diameter of > 4.0 cm, or an EF of < 65%.
- **Catheterization:** To exclude CAD prior to surgery.

TREATMENT

- **Medications:** ACEIs are useful only in patients with left ventricular dysfunction or hypertension.
- **Surgical intervention:**
  - **Indications for surgery** include symptoms related to mitral regurgitation, left ventricular dysfunction, AF, or pulmonary hypertension.

KEY FACT

In patients with mitral regurgitation, the intensity of the murmur on physical exam does not correlate with disease severity. In patients with acute myocardial ischemia, even a low-intensity murmur of mitral regurgitation should alert the physician to the possibility of papillary muscle rupture.

- **Optimal timing of surgery is early in the course of the disease,** when patients progress from a chronic, compensated state to symptomatic mitral regurgitation.
  - Surgical outcomes are best in patients who have an EF of > 60% and a left ventricular end-systolic diameter of < 4.5 cm.
- **Mitral valve repair:** Associated with better outcomes than mitral valve replacement. Repair is most successful when mitral regurgitation is due to prolapse of the posterior mitral valve leaflet.
- **Mitral valve replacement:** For symptomatic patients with an EF of > 30% when the mitral valve is not technically repairable.
- **Patients with EF < 30%:** Medical therapy is the mainstay of treatment. In refractory cases associated with severe symptoms, surgical repair or valve replacement has variable success; therefore, left ventricular assist devices and cardiac transplantation are the treatment options.

MITRAL VALVE PROLAPSE

Defined by a displaced and abnormally thickened, redundant mitral valve leaflet that projects into the left atrium during systole. Most recent studies demonstrate a prevalence of approximately 0.5–2.5% in the general population, with men and women affected equally. Mitral valve prolapse may be complicated by chordal rupture or endocarditis, both of which can lead to severe mitral regurgitation. Etiologies are as follows:

- 1°: Familial, sporadic, Marfan's syndrome, connective tissue disease.
- 2°: CAD, rheumatic heart disease, "flail leaflet," ↓ left ventricular dimension (hypertrophic cardiomyopathy, pulmonary hypertension, dehydration).

SYMPTOMS

Most patients have no symptoms, and the diagnosis is often found incidentally on physical exam or echocardiography. However, some patients may present with atypical chest pain, palpitations, or TIAs.

EXAM

- Exam reveals a midsystolic click followed by a midsystolic murmur with characteristic response to maneuvers.
- In more severe cases, listen for the holosystolic murmur of mitral regurgitation.

DIAGNOSIS

Echocardiography should be used for initial assessment; then follow every 3–5 years unless symptomatic or associated with mitral regurgitation (check echocardiogram yearly).

TREATMENT

- **ASA:** After a TIA and for patients < 65 years of age with lone AF.
- **Warfarin:** After a stroke and for those < 65 years of age with coexistent AF, hypertension, mitral regurgitation, or heart failure.
- β-blockers and electrophysiologic testing for control of arrhythmias.
- Surgery for cases of severe mitral regurgitation.

 KEY FACT

Endocarditis prophylaxis is not needed for mitral valve prolapse unless patients have evidence of mitral regurgitation, thickened mitral valve leaflets, or an audible systolic murmur associated with the midsystolic click.

PROSTHETIC VALVES

Indications for Placement

- **Bioprosthetic valves:** Older patients or those who cannot take long-term anticoagulant therapy (eg, bleeding diathesis, high risk for trauma, poor compliance).
- **Mechanical valves:** Young patients; patients with a prolonged life expectancy of > 20 years or with other indications for chronic anticoagulation (eg, AF). Note that newer bioprosthetic valves last longer, and future percutaneous valve replacement options may ↓ the need to use mechanical valves even in young patients.

Repair vs. Replacement

- **Repair:** Mitral valve prolapse, ischemic mitral regurgitation, bicuspid aortic valve with prolapse, mitral or tricuspid annular dilatation with normal leaflets.
- **Replacement:** Rheumatic heart disease, endocarditis, a heavily calcified valve, restricted leaflet motion, extensive leaflet destruction.

Anticoagulation

- No anticoagulation is needed for porcine valves after **three months** of warfarin therapy. ASA can be used in high-risk patients.
- For patients with mechanical valves, the level of anticoagulation depends on the location and type of valve (valves in the mitral and tricuspid position and older **caged-ball valves are most prone to thrombosis**).
- Risk factors for thromboembolic complications include AF, previous systemic emboli, left atrial thrombus, and severe left ventricular dysfunction.

Complications of Prosthetic Valves

- AF.
- Conduction disturbances.
- Endocarditis:
  - **Early prosthetic valve endocarditis:** Occurs during the first 60 days after valve replacement, most commonly due to *Staphylococcus epidermidis*; often fulminant and associated with high mortality rates.
  - **Late prosthetic valve endocarditis:** Most often occurs in patients with multiple valves or bioprosthetic valves. Microbiology is similar to that of native valve endocarditis.
- **Hemolysis:** Look for schistocytes on peripheral smear. Usually occurs in the presence of a perivalvular leak.
- **Thrombosis:**
  - At highest risk are those with mitral location of the valve and inadequate anticoagulation.
  - Presents clinically as heart failure, poor systemic perfusion, or systemic embolization.
  - Often presents acutely with hemodynamic instability.
  - Diagnose with echocardiography.
  - For small thrombi (< 5 mm) that are nonobstructive, IV heparin should be tried initially. For large thrombi (> 5 mm), use more aggressive therapy such as fibrinolysis or valve replacement.
- **Perivalvular leak:** Rare. In severe cases, look for hemolytic anemia and valvular insufficiency causing heart failure.
- **Emboli:** Typically present as stroke, but can present as intestinal or limb ischemia.
- **1° valve failure:** Most common with bioprosthetic valves; usually occurs after 10 years, but newer valves may last > 20 years.

Adult Congenital Heart Disease

Congenital heart disease comprises 2% of adult heart disease. Only the most common noncyanotic heart defects will be presented here. Table 3.11 outlines the extent to which patients with congenital cardiac malformations can tolerate pregnancy. Examples of adult congenital heart disease follow.

ATRIAL SEPTAL DEFECT (ASD)

There are three major types: ostium secundum (most common), ostium primum, and sinus venosus.

SYMPTOMS

Most cases are asymptomatic and are either diagnosed incidentally on echocardiography or found during workup of paradoxical emboli. Large shunts can cause dyspnea on exertion and orthopnea.

EXAM

- Characterized by a **fixed wide splitting of S2** with a loud P2 as pulmonary hypertension develops.
- Exam reveals a systolic flow murmur (usually best heard at the left upper sternal border) due to ↑ flow across the pulmonic valve, and occasionally a diastolic rumble across the tricuspid valve due to ↑ flow.

DIAGNOSIS

- **ECG:** Shows incomplete RBBB with right axis deviation in ostium secundum ASD. Left axis deviation suggests ostium primum ASD; RVH may be present in all forms.
- **CXR:** Shows a prominent pulmonary artery, an enlarged right atrium, and an enlarged right ventricle.
- **Echocardiography with agitated saline bubble study:** Can be used to visualize the intracardiac shunt and to determine the ratio of pulmonary-to-systemic blood flow (Q_p/Q_s).

TABLE 3.11. Tolerance of Pregnancy in Patients with Congenital Cardiac Malformations

WELL TOLERATED	INTERMEDIATE EFFECT	POORLY TOLERATED
NYHA class I	NYHA class II–III	NHYA class IV
Left-to-right shunts without pulmonary hypertension	Repaired transposition of the great arteries	Right-to-left shunt; unrepaired cyanotic heart disease
Aortic or mitral valvular regurgitation (mild to moderate)	Fontan repairs	Pulmonary hypertension and/or pulmonary vascular disease (eg, Eisenmenger's syndrome, 1° pulmonary hypertension)
Pulmonic or tricuspid regurgitation (if low pressure, even severe)	Aortic or mitral stenosis (moderate) Ebstein's anomaly	
Pulmonic stenosis (mild to moderate)		Aortic or mitral stenosis (severe)
Well-repaired tetralogy of Fallot		Pulmonic stenosis (severe)
		Marfan's syndrome or aortic coarctation

(Reproduced with permission from Kasper DL et al. *Harrison's Principles of Internal Medicine*, 16th ed. New York: McGraw-Hill, 2005: 1383.)

- **TEE:** Extremely useful for documenting the location and size of the defect and for excluding associated lesions.
- **Cardiac catheterization** documenting an ↑ in O_2 saturation between the SVC and the right atrium is the gold standard.

TREATMENT

- Percutaneous device closure is the treatment of choice for ostium secundum ASDs.
- Surgical correction is indicated for very large defects as well as for ostium primum and sinus venosus defects.
- Endocarditis prophylaxis is not indicated for isolated uncorrected ASDs but is indicated for six months after closure by device or surgery.

COMPLICATIONS

- Paradoxical embolization leading to TIAs and strokes.
- AF and atrial flutter.
- Pulmonary hypertension and **Eisenmenger's syndrome.**
- Endocarditis is rare in patients with secundum ASD but can occur in other types.

COARCTATION OF THE AORTA

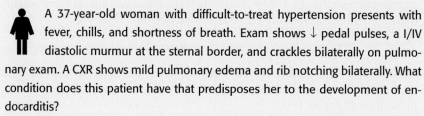

A 37-year-old woman with difficult-to-treat hypertension presents with fever, chills, and shortness of breath. Exam shows ↓ pedal pulses, a I/IV diastolic murmur at the sternal border, and crackles bilaterally on pulmonary exam. A CXR shows mild pulmonary edema and rib notching bilaterally. What condition does this patient have that predisposes her to the development of endocarditis?

Bicuspid aortic valve. This patient has a diastolic murmur suggestive of aortic regurgitation and also has fevers and chills, making aortic endocarditis likely. Patients with rib notching, difficult-to-treat hypertension, and ↓ pedal pulses may have undiagnosed aortic coarctation, which is often associated with a bicuspid aortic valve.

Proximal narrowing of the descending aorta just beyond the left subclavian artery with development of collateral circulation involving the internal mammary, intercostal, and axillary arteries. A bicuspid aortic valve is present in > 50% of patients with coarctation of the aorta. More common in males than in females.

SYMPTOMS

Presents with headache, dyspnea, fatigue, and leg claudication.

EXAM

Exam reveals diminished femoral pulses with a radial-to-femoral-pulse delay and a continuous scapular murmur due to collateral flow.

DIFFERENTIAL

- Other causes of 2° hypertension, including renal artery stenosis.
- Peripheral arterial disease leads to diminished femoral pulses and claudication.

DIAGNOSIS

- **CXR:** Reveals rib notching from enlarged collaterals.
- **ECG:** Shows LVH.
- **Echocardiography:** To look for bicuspid aortic valve; can also document the severity of coarctation.
- **Cardiac catheterization with aortography:** Can define stenosis and measure gradient.
- **MRI/MRA:** Offer excellent visualization of the location and extent of coarctation along with collateral circulation (see Figure 3.15).

TREATMENT

- Medical treatment of hypertension.
- Surgical correction is appropriate for patients < 20 years of age and in older patients with upper extremity hypertension and a gradient of ≥ 20 mm Hg.
- Balloon dilatation with or without stent placement is an alternative for native or recurrent coarctation.
- Requires prophylaxis for endocarditis during dental procedures in which there may be perforation of the oral mucosa.

COMPLICATIONS

- LVH due to ↑ afterload.
- Severe hypertension.
- Aortic dissection or rupture.
- SAH due to rupture of aneurysms of the circle of Willis (rare).
- Premature CAD.

> **KEY FACT**
>
> Coarctation of the aorta is commonly associated with congenital bicuspid aortic valve.

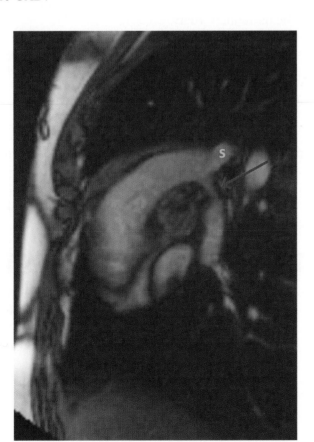

FIGURE 3.15. Aortic coarctation. Parasagittal cine-MRI sequence showing a coarctation of the aorta (arrow) just distal to the origin of the left subclavian artery (S). (Reproduced with permission from USMLERx.com.)

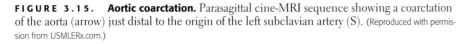

PATENT DUCTUS ARTERIOSUS (PDA)

Uncommon in adults. Risk factors include premature birth and exposure to rubella virus in the first trimester.

Symptoms

Usually asymptomatic, but moderate to large shunts can cause dyspnea, fatigue, and left ventricular overload (due to ↑ pulmonary blood flow). In late stages, large shunts can cause signs and symptoms of pulmonary hypertension and right heart failure (Eisenmenger's syndrome).

Exam

- Exam reveals a continuous "machinery-like" murmur at the left upper sternal border and bounding peripheral pulses due to rapid aortic runoff to the pulmonary artery.
- In the presence of pulmonary hypertension (Eisenmenger's syndrome), the murmur is absent or soft, and there is differential cyanosis involving the lower extremities and sparing the upper extremities.

Differential

Other shunts, including ASDs and VSDs.

Diagnosis

- **ECG:** Nonspecific; LVH and left atrial enlargement can be seen.
- **Echocardiography:** Can be used to calculate the shunt fraction and to estimate pulmonary artery systolic pressure. Abnormal ductal flow can be visualized in the pulmonary artery.
- **Cardiac catheterization:** Can be used to document an ↑ in O_2 saturation from the right ventricle to the pulmonary artery. Aortography can be used to look for communication between the aorta and the pulmonary artery.
- **Cardiac MRI:** The gold-standard test with which to diagnose PDA (cardiac CT can also be used to visualize PDA).

Treatment

Endocarditis prophylaxis, transcatheter coil closure, surgical correction.

Complications

Eisenmenger's syndrome with pulmonary hypertension and shunt reversal; infective endocarditis.

KEY FACT

Differential cyanosis of the fingers (pink) and toes (blue and clubbed) is pathognomonic for Eisenmenger's syndrome caused by an uncorrected PDA.

VENTRICULAR SEPTAL DEFECT (VSD)

Most VSDs occur in close proximity to the membranous portion of the intraventricular septum, but muscular, supracristal, inlet, and outlet VSDs can also occur.

Symptoms

Most patients diagnosed in adulthood are asymptomatic, but insidious dyspnea on exertion and orthopnea may develop.

Exam

- A holosystolic murmur is heard at the left lower sternal border with a right ventricular heave and prolonged splitting of S2.

- As pulmonary arterial pressure ↑, a loud P2 and tricuspid regurgitation can also be appreciated.
- Cyanosis, clubbing, and signs of right heart failure can appear with the development of Eisenmenger's syndrome.

DIFFERENTIAL

Other shunts, including ASD and PDA.

DIAGNOSIS

- Echocardiography with an agitated saline bubble study can be used to visualize the intracardiac shunt, determine size, and ascertain Q_p/Q_s.
- Cardiac catheterization documenting an ↑ in O_2 saturation between the right atrium and right ventricle is the gold standard.
- **ECG:** Nonspecific; LVH and left atrial enlargement in the absence of pulmonary hypertension can be seen. Right atrial enlargement, RVH, and RBBB can develop with the development of pulmonary hypertension.
- **CXR:** Cardiomegaly and enlarged pulmonary arteries.

TREATMENT

- Endocarditis prophylaxis for a VSD of any size.
- Diuretics and vasodilators to ↓ left-to-right shunt and symptoms of right heart failure.
- Surgical correction is appropriate for patients with significant shunt (Q_p/Q_s > 1.7:1).
- Once pulmonary hypertension occurs, mortality is high.

COMPLICATIONS

- **Eisenmenger's syndrome:**
  - Long-standing left-to-right shunting causes pulmonary vascular hyperplasia, resulting in pulmonary arterial hypertension and shunt reversal (development of right-to-left shunt).
  - Symptoms include dyspnea, chest pain, syncope, and hemoptysis.
- **Other:** Paradoxical embolism leading to TIAs or stroke; infective endocarditis.

KEY FACT

Surgical closure is contraindicated once Eisenmenger's syndrome develops because it can ↑ pulmonary hypertension and precipitate right heart failure.

Other Topics

AORTIC DISSECTION

Approximately 2000 cases are diagnosed each year in the United States. Aortic dissection is associated with uncontrolled hypertension, medial degeneration of the aorta (Marfan's syndrome, Ehlers-Danlos syndrome), cocaine use, coarctation, congenital bicuspid valve, trauma, cardiac surgery, pregnancy, and syphilitic aortitis. **Type A = proximal dissection; type B = distal dissection** (the dissection flap originates distal to the left subclavian artery).

SYMPTOMS

- Classically presents as a sudden-onset "tearing" or "ripping" sensation originating in the chest and radiating to the back, but symptoms may not be classic.
- Unlike MI, pain is maximal at the onset and is not gradual in nature.

- Can present with organ hypoperfusion due to occlusion of arteries by the dissection flap (eg, coronary ischemia, stroke, intestinal ischemia, renal failure, limb ischemia).
- Other presentations include cardiac tamponade, aortic insufficiency, and acute MI (typically due to involvement of the right coronary artery) in cases of proximal aortic dissection.

EXAM

- BP is ↑ (although hypotension can be seen with proximal dissections associated with tamponade).
- In proximal dissection, listen for the diastolic murmur of aortic insufficiency.
- Exam reveals pulse deficits or unequal pulses between the right and left arms.
- Can present with focal neurologic deficits (from associated cerebrovascular infarct) or with paraplegia (from associated anterior spinal artery compromise).

DIFFERENTIAL

Acute MI, cardiac tamponade, thoracic or abdominal aortic aneurysm, pulmonary embolism, tension pneumothorax, esophageal rupture.

DIAGNOSIS

- Three major clinical predictors are sudden, tearing chest pain; differential pulses or BPs between the right and left arms; and abnormal aortic or mediastinal contour on CXR. If all three are present, the positive likelihood ratio is 0.66. The negative likelihood ratio if all three are absent is 0.07.
- **CXR:** Look for a widened mediastinum (occurs in approximately 60% of all aortic dissections; see Figure 3.16).

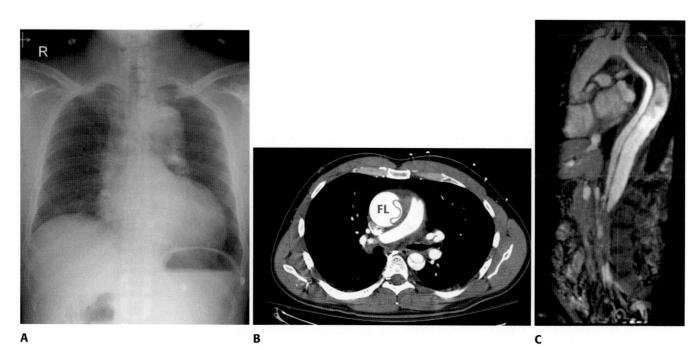

A   B   C

FIGURE 3.16.   Aortic dissection. (A) Frontal CXR showing a widened mediastinum in a patient with an aortic dissection. **(B)** Transaxial contrast-enhanced CT showing a dissection involving the ascending and descending aorta (FL = false lumen). **(C)** Sagittal MRA image showing a dissection involving the descending aorta, with a thrombus (T) in the false lumen. (Images A and C reproduced with permission from USMLERx.com. Image B reproduced with permission from Doherty GM. *Current Diagnosis & Treatment: Surgery,* 13th ed. New York: McGraw-Hill, 2010, Fig. 19-17.)

- **TEE:** The fastest and most portable method for unstable patients, but may not be available at all hospitals. Sensitivity is 98% and specificity 95%.
- **Chest CT:** Has a sensitivity and specificity up to 98%.
- **MRI:** Highly sensitive (98%) and specific (98%), but the test is slow and may not be available at many hospitals. Good for following patients with type B dissections.
- **Aortography:** Not ideal given the invasive nature of the test and the associated delay in initiating definitive surgical therapy.

TREATMENT

- **Type A:** Surgical repair.
- **Type B:** Admit to the ICU for medical management of hypertension. Treat first with IV β-blockers (esmolol, labetalol) and then with IV nitroprusside. Avoid anticoagulation. Surgery is indicated for complications of dissection, end-organ damage, or failure to control hypertension.

COMPLICATIONS

- Acute MI from occlusion of the right coronary artery by the dissection flap or dissection of the coronary artery.
- Acute aortic insufficiency, which can present as hemodynamic instability and heart failure.
- Cardiac tamponade due to dissection into the pericardium.
- Cardiac arrest.
- Cerebrovascular accident (due to concomitant carotid artery dissection).
- Occlusion of distal arteries can lead to end-organ damage (eg, paraplegia, renal failure, intestinal ischemia, limb ischemia).

KEY FACT

Proximal (type A) aortic dissection can present as acute paraplegia due to occlusion of the anterior spinal artery.

PERIPHERAL VASCULAR DISEASE

Atherosclerosis of the peripheral arterial system is associated with the same clinical risk factors as coronary disease (smoking, diabetes, hypertension, and hyperlipidemia).

SYMPTOMS

Intermittent claudication is reproducible pain in the lower extremity muscles that is brought on by exercise and relieved by rest; however, most peripheral vascular disease is asymptomatic.

EXAM

Presents with poor distal pulses, femoral bruits, loss of hair in the legs and feet, slow capillary refill, and poor wound healing (chronic ulceration).

DIFFERENTIAL

- Nearly all peripheral vascular disease is caused by atherosclerosis. Less common causes include coarctation, fibrodysplasia, retroperitoneal fibrosis, and radiation.
- Nonarterial causes of limb pain include spinal stenosis (pseudoclaudication), deep venous thrombosis, and peripheral neuropathy (often coexists with peripheral vascular disease in diabetics).

DIAGNOSIS

- **Ankle-brachial index (ABI) < 0.90** (the highest ankle systolic pressure measured by Doppler divided by the highest brachial systolic pressure).

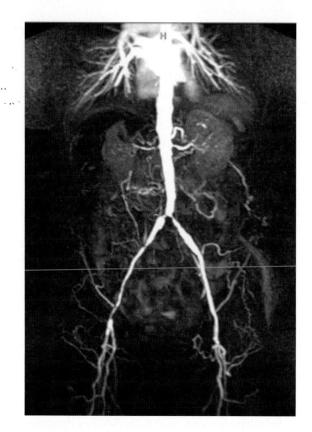

FIGURE 3.17. **Peripheral arterial disease.** Coronal contrast-enhanced MRA shows multi-focal atherosclerotic disease that is most severe at the origins of the common iliac (arrows) and right renal (arrowhead) arteries. (Reproduced with permission from USMLERx.com.)

- **MR and CT angiography of the lower extremities** are useful noninvasive diagnostic tests (see Figure 3.17).
- Lower extremity **angiography** is the gold standard.

TREATMENT

- Aggressive cardiac risk factor reduction, including control of smoking, hypertension, and hyperlipidemia.
- Initiate a structured exercise rehabilitation program.
- Pharmacotherapy:
    - **Antiplatelet agents:** ASA is first-line therapy for overall cardiovascular event reduction, but data also support the use of ticlopidine, clopidogrel, and dipyridamole in peripheral vascular disease.
    - **ACEIs.**
    - **Pentoxifylline:** ↑ RBC deformability to ↑ capillary flow.
    - **Cilostazol:** Inhibits platelet aggregation and promotes lower arterial vasodilation.
- **Surgery:** Percutaneous transluminal angioplasty and lower extremity revascularization bypass surgery should be used only for severe symptoms such as resting pain/ischemia or threatened limb. Thrombolytic therapy is appropriate for acute limb ischemia.

COMPLICATIONS

- Critical leg ischemia leading to limb amputation.
- Even asymptomatic peripheral vascular disease is a major risk factor for adverse cardiovascular events.

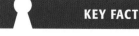
KEY FACT

If defined as an ABI of < 0.90, most peripheral vascular disease is asymptomatic but still confers a high risk of adverse cardiovascular events and death.

CHAPTER 4

Critical Care

Christina A. Lee, MD
Christian A. Merlo, MD, MPH

Review: Vent management
Factors affecting CVP
asthma & rests
Pressors
Sedation

Swens & measurements

Acute Respiratory Distress Syndrome (ARDS)

Acute **hypoxemic** respiratory failure with bilateral pulmonary infiltrates that is not heart failure. Commonly associated with pneumonia, aspiration, sepsis, trauma, acute pancreatitis, cardiopulmonary bypass, transfusion of blood products, inhalation injury, and reperfusion injury following lung transplantation.

SYMPTOMS/EXAM

- Presents with rapid onset of dyspnea, tachypnea, and diffuse crackles.
- Reduced single-breath DL_{CO} is the most common pulmonary function abnormality in survivors.

DIFFERENTIAL

Cardiogenic pulmonary edema, pneumonia, diffuse alveolar hemorrhage.

DIAGNOSIS

- Look for bilateral alveolar infiltrates on CXR with no evidence of left heart failure (if measured, pulmonary artery wedge pressure is < 18 mm Hg). See Figure 4.1.
- ARDS = the above plus a Pao_2/Fio_2 ratio of < 200, or
- **Acute lung injury** = a Pao_2/Fio_2 ratio of < 300. A less severe form of ARDS.

TREATMENT

- Search for and treat the underlying cause. A bronchoalveolar lavage (BAL) may narrow the etiology and help tailor antibiotic therapy in the event of pneumonia.
- Most patients with ARDS require mechanical ventilation.
- **Low tidal volumes of 6 cc per kilogram of predicted body weight** ↓ mortality.

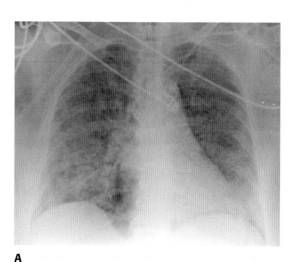

A

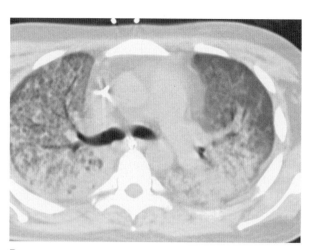

B

FIGURE 4.1. **Acute respiratory distress syndrome.** (A) Frontal CXR showing patchy areas of airspace consolidation in a patient with ARDS. (B) Transaxial CT showing ground-glass opacity anteriorly and consolidations dependently in a patient with exudative-phase ARDS.
(Reproduced with permission from Fauci AS et al. *Harrison's Principles of Internal Medicine,* 17th ed. New York: McGraw-Hill, 2008, Figs. 262-2 and 262-4.)

- Positive end-expiratory pressure (PEEP) can help improve oxygenation and ↓ high levels of inspired O_2. A low PEEP strategy is recommended to ↓ barotrauma risk.
- Keep **plateau pressure** ≤ **30 cm H_2O** to prevent barotrauma (see the discussion of ventilator management). Plateau pressure is measured by occluding the expiratory port at end inspiration and reflects the static compliance of the lungs and chest wall.
- A conservative fluid management strategy is associated with a shorter duration of mechanical ventilation and a ↓ length of ICU stay.
- There is no definitive evidence for corticosteroids in the prevention and treatment of ARDS.

Acute Respiratory Failure

Failure in oxygenation (hypoxemia), ventilation (hypercarbia), or both.

SYMPTOMS/EXAM

- Dyspnea, tachypnea, respiratory alkalosis, and hypoxemia suggest hypoxic respiratory failure.
- ↓ respiratory rate and somnolence suggest hypercarbic respiratory failure.

DIFFERENTIAL

The differential of acute respiratory failure is outlined in Tables 4.1 and 4.2.

TREATMENT

Treatment depends on the etiology. Provide sufficient O_2 through supplemental oxygen and adequate ventilation (noninvasive or invasive; see below).

KEY FACT

To improve mortality in mechanically ventilated patients with ARDS, target a tidal volume of **6 cc per kilogram** of predicted body weight.

KEY FACT

Good chest compressions are the most important component of CPR.

KEY FACT

Updates to the AHA's CPR guidelines: It's no longer A-B-C; it's C-A-B. First do **C**ompressions; then focus on **A**irway and **B**reathing. Second, do AED shocks only one at a time, with two minutes of CPR in between.

TABLE 4.1.   Etiologies of Hypoxemic Respiratory Failure (more intrinsic lung factors)

CAUSE	MECHANISM	DISEASE STATES	COMMENTS
↓ Fio_2 or low total O_2	O_2 is replaced by other gases (enclosed spaces, fire), or low O_2 from high altitudes and air travel results in ↓ Pao_2.		
Diffusion abnormality	Reduction in diffusion capacity leads to a low Pao_2.	Pulmonary alveolar proteinosis.	An uncommon cause of hypoxemic respiratory failure.
Hypoventilation	↓ minute ventilation results in ↑ $Paco_2$ and ↓ Pao_2.	See Table 4.2.	**Normal** alveolar-arterial (A-a) gradient.
Ventilation-perfusion (V/Q) mismatch	Altered ratio of perfusion to ventilation.	Pulmonary embolus, pulmonary hypertension, COPD, asthma.	↑ A-a gradient; Pao_2 corrects with supplemental O_2.
Shunt	Perfusion to the nonventilated lung or a communication between the arterial and venous systems.	ARDS, pneumonia, pulmonary AVM, congenital heart disease, patent foramen ovale with right-to-left flow.	↑ A-a gradient; Pao_2 does **not** correct with supplemental O_2.

TABLE 4.2.   **Etiologies of Hypercarbic Respiratory Failure** (more emphasic factors)

CAUSE	MECHANISM	DISEASE STATES
CNS disorders/↓ ventilatory drive	↓ minute ventilation leads to ↑ $Paco_2$.	Drug overdose, CNS lesion/infarction, central sleep apnea, hypothyroidism.
Peripheral nerve disorders	Same as above.	Guillain-Barré syndrome, ALS, poliomyelitis, West Nile virus, ICU-acquired paresis.
Neuromuscular junction disorders	Same as above.	Myasthenia gravis, botulism.
Muscle disorders	Same as above.	Muscular dystrophy, glycogen storage disease, ICU-acquired paresis.
Lung disorders	↓ alveolar ventilation due to obstructive lung disease leads to ↑ $Paco_2$.	COPD, asthma, CF.
Chest wall disorders	Chest wall mechanics are altered, leading to ↓ alveolar ventilation and ↑ $Paco_2$.	Kyphoscoliosis, massive obesity.

Ventilator Management

There are two types of mechanical ventilation: noninvasive ventilation and invasive mechanical ventilation.

- **Noninvasive positive pressure ventilation (NPPV):**
    - Refers to positive pressure ventilation delivered via a mask rather than by endotracheal or tracheostomy tube. Can deliver pressure support as continuous positive airway pressure (CPAP) or bilevel positive airway pressure (BiPAP).
    - **Indications:** Hypercapnic COPD exacerbations, acute CHF, acute respiratory failure in immunosuppressed patients. **Early use of NPPV in these patients ↓ intubation rates.**
    - **Contraindications:** Severe acidemia, inability to protect the airway, inability to comply, impending cardiac or respiratory arrest, upper GI bleeding, recent facial/upper airway, GI surgery.
    - **Common uses:** CPAP is used for acute CHF or obstructive sleep apnea; BiPAP is used for COPD as well as for acute CHF.
- **Invasive mechanical ventilation:** Invasive ventilatory support is provided through an endotracheal tube or a tracheostomy tube. The main indications for mechanical ventilation are acute respiratory failure and airway protection.

MODE

Full ventilatory support can be provided in a number of ways. Common ways include the following:

- **Assist control (AC):** Delivers a **preset tidal volume** (TV) with a **minimum mandatory respiratory rate** (RR). Spontaneous breaths above the minimum RR trigger the same TV as mandatory breaths. AC is a good first choice in most clinical situations and is the most common ventilator mode used in the ICU and for ARDS.

> **KEY FACT**
>
> Coma or impending cardiac or respiratory arrest warrants immediate intubation. Do not use NPPV to delay intubation if the patient is in severe respiratory distress.

> **KEY FACT**
>
> Use CPAP for CHF and BiPAP for COPD. Check an ABG 1–2 hours after NPPV is initiated. If no improvement is seen on ABG, intubate.

- **Synchronized intermittent mandatory ventilation:** Delivers a preset TV with a minimum mandatory RR. Spontaneous breaths above the minimum rate trigger variable TV. The spontaneous breaths and mandatory breaths are synchronized to reduce breath stacking.
- **Pressure support:** Provides inspiratory pressure support to ↓ the work of breathing for each breath. All breaths are spontaneous. The patient's lung mechanics determine TV and RR, so close monitoring is required.

SETTINGS AND MEASUREMENTS

Table 4.3 outlines the differential for patients with ventilator crises.

- **Respiratory rate:** The minute ventilation (MV) needs prior to intubation should be approximated. $MV = RR \times TV$. Rates up to 35 are generally acceptable unless the patient cannot fully exhale at such rapid rates (eg, in status asthmaticus).
- **Tidal volume:** Low tidal volumes ↓ mortality in ARDS and may ↓ the risk of ventilator-induced lung injury.
- **Fio$_2$:** Start with 100% Fio$_2$ and then titrate the levels down to a goal Pao$_2$ ≥ 60 mm Hg or an arterial oxygen saturation of > 90% (or 88% in ARDS).
- **PEEP:** A small amount (5 cm H$_2$O) is typically used. ↑ levels are used in ARDS to improve oxygenation and possibly to prevent further lung injury. Higher levels of PEEP may also be used in cardiogenic pulmonary edema to improve oxygenation and to ↓ preload and afterload.

TABLE 4.3. Etiologies of Ventilator Crises

↑ Peak Airway Pressure/Normal Plateau Pressure	↑ Peak Airway Pressure/High Plateau Pressure	↓ O$_2$ Saturation	Rising Partial Pressure of CO$_2$	Patient Distress
Endotracheal tube obstruction, kink, or malposition. **Airway obstruction:** Bronchospasm, mucous plug. **Patient effort/ agitation:** Coughing, biting, fighting.	**Reduced lung compliance:** Pulmonary edema, pneumonia. **Reduced chest wall/abdominal compliance:** Pneumothorax, abdominal distention.	Ventilator/mixer malfunction. Endotracheal tube malposition/leak. **New lung derangement:** Atelectasis, aspiration, edema. **New cardiovascular derangement:** Shock, pulmonary embolism, decreases in hemoglobin concentration. ↑ oxygen consumption. Changes in body position, increasing shunt.	Ventilator malfunction. Endotracheal tube malfunction/leak. **New patient mechanical derangement:** Bronchospasm, edema. ↑ dead space. ↑ CO$_2$ production.	Pain/discomfort unrelated to the ventilator or respiratory system (eg, myocardial ischemia). Endotracheal tube malposition. Increasing work of breathing. Rising partial pressure of CO$_2$. Oxyhemoglobin desaturation. Shock/pulmonary embolism. Inadequate sedation. Alcohol or drug withdrawal.

(Adapted with permission from Hall JB et al. *Principles of Critical Care*, 3rd ed. New York: McGraw-Hill, 2005, Table 36-4.)

- **Auto-PEEP:** Measured by covering the expiratory port on the ventilator at end expiration. Caused by delayed emptying of the lungs and subsequent initiation of a new breath before the lungs have fully emptied. Common in mechanically ventilated patients with COPD and asthma. Can be treated by decreasing RR or TV or by increasing expiratory time.

SEDATION MANAGEMENT AND WEANING

- Administer both anxiolytic and analgesic medications while patients are receiving mechanical ventilation through an endotracheal tube.
- Daily interruption of sedative infusions ↓ the duration of mechanical ventilation and ICU stays.
- Once the patient is awake, attempt a spontaneous breathing trial to determine readiness for extubation. Also evaluate the strength of cough, secretions, and upper airway patency prior to extubation. Weigh the benefits of early extubation (preventing pneumonia, GI bleeding, venous thromboembolism) against the effects of premature extubation (reintubation, which ↑ mortality).

Shock

A 68-year-old woman is brought into the ER by family members after they noted that the woman had become increasingly lethargic over the past five days. Her temperature is 39.5°C (103.1°F), BP 75/40 mm Hg, heart rate 130 bpm, respiratory rate 24, and O_2 saturation 89% on room air. Her skin is warm on exam. Her WBC count is 15, and her UA is ⊕ for nitrites and leukocyte esterase. After the infusion of 3 L of IV normal saline, her BP is 80/45 mm Hg. What is the most appropriate initial vasopressor to use to treat her hypotension?

Norepinephrine or dopamine for septic shock. Also consider use of phenylephrine or vasopressin as second-line agents.

A physiologic state characterized by ↓ tissue perfusion and subsequent tissue hypoxia. Prolonged tissue hypoxia often leads to cell death, organ damage, multiorgan system failure, and eventual death.

SYMPTOMS/EXAM

Varies depending on the underlying cause of shock (see Table 4.4). Most patients are hypotensive.

DIAGNOSIS

See Table 4.4 for the four categories of shock. If the type of shock is still unclear after physical exam, additional information can be obtained through use of invasive monitoring devices.

- **Echocardiography:** Distinguishes poor cardiac function from hypovolemia; confirms pericardial tamponade or significant pulmonary hypertension.
- **Central venous catheter:** Estimates right heart filling pressures.
- **Pulmonary artery catheter:** Measures cardiac output and pulmonary capillary occlusion pressure (PCOP, also known as "wedge pressure"), and

TABLE 4.4.   **Categories of Shock**

	PHYSICAL EXAM	CARDIAC OUTPUT	SVR	PCOP ("WEDGE PRESSURE")	EXAMPLES
Distributive	Warm extremities; rapid capillary refill.	↑	↓	↓	Sepsis, anaphylaxis.
Cardiogenic	Cool, clammy extremities; delayed capillary refill; elevated JVP.	↓	↑	↑ (except in RV infarct)	Acute MI, CHF.
Hypovolemic	Cool extremities; flat JVP.	↓	↑	↓	Trauma, bleeding.
Obstructive	Cool extremities; variable JVP.	↓	↑	↑ (tamponade) or ↓ (pulmonary embolism)	Tamponade, pulmonary embolism, tension pneumothorax.

calculates SVR to differentiate the type of shock. Has not been shown to improve patient outcomes compared to central venous catheters.

TREATMENT

Focus on resuscitation and improving end-organ perfusion.

- Aggressive IV fluid hydration (normal saline is first line) should be given to patients with hypovolemic or distributive shock. Blood products should be administered in cases of trauma or acute bleeding.
- Broad-spectrum antibiotics should be given empirically if infection is suspected.
- If a patient remains in shock despite the restoration of intravascular volume, use vasopressors.

KEY FACT

Adrenal insufficiency and severe hypo- or hyperthyroidism may present clinically as shock. These diagnoses should be considered when patients fail to respond to fluid resuscitation.

Sepsis

A clinical syndrome associated with severe infection that arises from systemic inflammation and uncontrolled release of proinflammatory mediators, leading to extensive tissue injury. Associated with high mortality and morbidity. See Table 4.5 for details on the spectrum of disease.

SYMPTOMS/EXAM

- Variable; patients with systemic inflammatory response syndrome (SIRS) may have bounding pulses, warm extremities, and rapid capillary refill.
- Patients with severe sepsis and those with septic shock may have weak pulses, cool extremities, and slow capillary refill.

DIFFERENTIAL

Cardiogenic, obstructive, or hypovolemic shock; fulminant hepatic failure; drug overdose; adrenal insufficiency; pancreatitis.

DIAGNOSIS/TREATMENT

- Always obtain appropriate cultures, including blood cultures, before starting antibiotic therapy.
- IV antibiotic therapy geared toward suspected pathogens should be initiated within the first hour of severe sepsis.

TABLE 4.5. Conditions Associated with Sepsis

CONDITION	DEFINITION
SIRS	A clinical syndrome recognized by the presence of two or more of the following: ■ Temperature > 38°C or < 36°C. ■ HR > 90 bpm. ■ RR > 20 breaths per minute or a $Paco_2$ < 32 mm Hg. ■ WBC > 12,000 cells/mm³, < 4000 cells/mm³, or > 10% bands.
Sepsis	SIRS with known or suspected infection.
Severe sepsis	Sepsis with organ dysfunction and hypoperfusion.
Septic shock	Sepsis with hypotension despite adequate fluid resuscitation combined with altered mental status, oliguria, and/or lactic acidosis.

MNEMONIC

Treating patients with severe sepsis is as easy as ABCDE:

Antibiotics/**A**RDS–low tidal volume ventilation
Blood sugar control
Corticosteroids
Drotrecogin alfa (activated)
Early goal-directed therapy

■ Start early and aggressive volume resuscitation first (↓ mortality) before vasopressors. The goal is a mean arterial pressure of > 65 mm Hg and a central venous pressure of 8–12 mm Hg.

■ Use vasopressors in patients who are volume repleted but still hypotensive. Norepinephrine and dopamine are first-line agents for septic shock. Vasopressin and phenylephrine may be considered after failure of fluids and conventional vasopressors.

■ Treatment should **not** include low-dose dopamine for renal protection.

■ Empiric corticosteroids do **not** improve survival in patients with septic shock. In the setting of profound, refractory shock, perform a cosyntropin stimulation test (see the Endocrine chapter), and then give corticosteroids while awaiting results.

Recombinant human activated protein C or drotrecogin alfa (activated) is recommended for patients with a high risk of death and no absolute contraindication related to bleeding risk.

■ Consider the following interventions in all critically ill patients:
  ■ ↓ catheter-related bloodstream infections via handwashing, cleaning the skin with chlorhexidine, avoiding the femoral vein, using full-barrier precautions during catheter insertion, and removing unnecessary catheters.
  ■ Intensive insulin therapy targeting a blood glucose level of 80–110 mg/dL may ↑ mortality in sepsis. Thus, the goal blood glucose level should be < 150 mg/dL.
  ■ Once hypoperfusion has resolved, blood transfusion should occur only at a hemoglobin level of ≤ 7 **g/dL** unless the patient is suffering from cardiac ischemia, lactic acidosis, or acute hemorrhage.

■ Sepsis is one of the most common causes of ARDS, and low tidal volume ventilation (**6 cc per kilogram of predicted body weight**) should be initiated if the patient develops this condition.

■ All patients in the ICU should receive DVT and GI prophylaxis.

Fever in the ICU

Defined as a temperature of ≥ 38.3°C (≥ 101°F). Both infectious and noninfectious sources are common causes of fever in the ICU.

SYMPTOMS/EXAM

Review the patient's history and medications and perform a thorough physical exam, including skin.

DIFFERENTIAL

See the mnemonics **PAID WOMAN** and **VW CARS**.

DIAGNOSIS/TREATMENT

- Obtain blood cultures as well as other cultures (wound, urine, stool, endotracheal aspirate).
- If an obvious source of infection is identified, start antibiotics. If there is no obvious source of infection and fever is ≤ 39°C (≤ 102°F), evaluate for the noninfectious causes listed in the mnemonic **PAID WOMAN.** If fever is > 39°C (> 102°F), remove old central lines and culture the catheter tip at the same time as a peripheral blood culture.
- An NG tube should be removed and replaced with an orogastric tube, and a CXR should be reviewed for any new infiltrates. Start empiric antibiotics if fever persists.

Ventilator-Associated Pneumonia (VAP)

Defined as pneumonia that develops ≥ 48 hours after intubation. Up to 25% of mechanically ventilated patients develop VAP. The most common etiologic agents are *S aureus, Pseudomonas aeruginosa,* and Enterobacteriaceae (eg, *Enterobacter cloacae*).

SYMPTOMS/EXAM

- Presents with fever, worsening hypoxia, and ↑ purulent secretions from the endotracheal tube.
- Chronic lung disease, length of mechanical ventilation, aspiration, head-of-bed level, use of NG tubes, and delayed extubation can all ↑ the risk of VAP.

DIAGNOSIS

Clinical, radiographic, and airway sampling are all frequently used, but controversy exists as to which diagnostic strategy is best.

- **Clinical criteria:** VAP is suggested by fever ≥ 48 hours after intubation, new pulmonary infiltrate, leukocytosis, and ↑ secretions.
- **Radiographic criteria:** New infiltrate on CXR.
- **Airway sampling:** Via bronchoscopy, mini-BAL (lavage of lower airways), or tracheal aspirate. There is no clear benefit to any method.

MNEMONIC

Noninfectious causes of fever in the ICU—

PAID WOMAN

Pancreatitis/**P**ulmonary embolism
Adrenal insufficiency
Ischemic bowel
Drug reaction/**D**VT
Withdrawal (eg, from prior prolonged usage of opioids)
Other
Myocardial infarction
Acalculous cholecystitis
Neoplasm

MNEMONIC

Infectious causes of fever in the ICU—

VW CARS

Ventilator-associated pneumonia
Wound infection
C *difficile* colitis
Abdominal abscess
Related to catheter
Sepsis/**S**inusitis

KEY FACT

If fever continues despite empiric broad-spectrum antibiotics, consider abdominal imaging and antifungal coverage.

The most common etiologic agents of VAP are *S aureus, P aeruginosa,* and Enterobacteriaceae (eg, *E cloacae*).

Keeping patients in a semirecumbent position (30–45 degrees) rather than supine is an easy intervention to help prevent VAP.

TREATMENT

Appropriate initial antibiotic coverage is the most important factor in determining patient outcomes. Narrow antibiotics as cultures become available to prevent the development of bacterial resistance. Guidelines are as follows:

- Patients should initially receive broad-spectrum antibiotics to cover *S aureus, Pseudomonas,* and Enterobacteriaceae. Antibiotics should be based on local resistance patterns and should be rapidly narrowed on the basis of respiratory cultures.
- An eight-day course of antibiotics is recommended for VAP patients who have elicited a good clinical response and in whom no *Pseudomonas* has been isolated (*Pseudomonas* needs a longer course).

PREVENTION

Four easy interventions can be used to prevent VAP:

- Keep the head of the bed elevated to at least **30 degrees.**
- Use universal and barrier precautions in the setting of multiple-drug-resistant organisms, including washing hands and wearing special gowns.
- Remove the NG tube and convert to orogastric tube placement.
- ↓ the amount of mechanical ventilation time by interrupting sedation daily, using weaning protocols, and using noninvasive mechanical ventilation if applicable.

CHAPTER 5

Dermatology

Miten Vasa, MD
Siegrid S. Yu, MD

Common Skin Disorders

ACNE

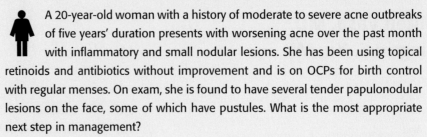

A 20-year-old woman with a history of moderate to severe acne outbreaks of five years' duration presents with worsening acne over the past month with inflammatory and small nodular lesions. She has been using topical retinoids and antibiotics without improvement and is on OCPs for birth control with regular menses. On exam, she is found to have several tender papulonodular lesions on the face, some of which have pustules. What is the most appropriate next step in management?

Oral tetracycline for at least 6–8 weeks along with a topical retinoid for moderate to severe inflammatory acne (topical antibiotics are not usually used in conjunction with oral antibiotics).

Due to excess sebum, abnormal follicular keratinization, and proliferation of *Propionibacterium acnes*. Medications that exacerbate acne include glucocorticoids, anabolic steroids, lithium, some antiepileptics, OCPs with androgenic potential, and iodides. **Dietary factors do not play a significant role.**

TREATMENT

The therapeutic ladder is as follows:

- **Milder cases (comedonal acne with blackheads/whiteheads but no inflammatory lesions): Topical** retinoid + benzoyl peroxide or a **topical** antibiotic.
- **More severe/inflammatory cases: Systemic** antibiotics, oral isotretinoin, antiandrogens, or spironolactone.

ROSACEA

A 40-year-old woman presents with a facial rash of two months' duration involving her cheeks and nose. She has no fatigue, ulcers, or joint pain, and the rash worsens after she eats spicy food. Exam reveals an erythematous rash with discrete papules and pustules limited to the cheeks, nasolabial folds, and nose. Her CBC, chemistry, TSH, and ANA are all normal. What is the most likely diagnosis?

Rosacea, an inflammatory dermatitis that affects the central face, including the nasolabial folds, and is associated with triggers, including spicy foods. In contrast, the malar rash of SLE is photosensitive and spares the nasolabial folds and areas below the nares and lower lip. The classic patchy, flushed discoloration of rosacea mimics sunburn. Rhinophyma, or the presentation of a bulbous, red nose, is a variant of this condition.

A chronic inflammatory **facial** disorder affecting middle-aged to older adults.

SYMPTOMS

- Presents with episodic flushing and facial erythema.
- **Triggers** include hot liquids, spicy food, alcohol, sun, and heat.

KEY FACT

Isotretinoin is teratogenic and is contraindicated in pregnancy. Side effects include dry skin, cheilitis, transaminase elevation, and hypertriglyceridemia. Depression has also been associated with its use.

KEY FACT

In recalcitrant cases of acne, signs such as hirsutism and irregular menses may point to possible endocrine disorders (congenital adrenal hyperplasia, PCOS, Cushing's disease).

KEY FACT

Think rosacea when the story is a chronic, waxing-and-waning facial rash that involves the cheeks and nose and is triggered by hot and spicy things or by alcohol.

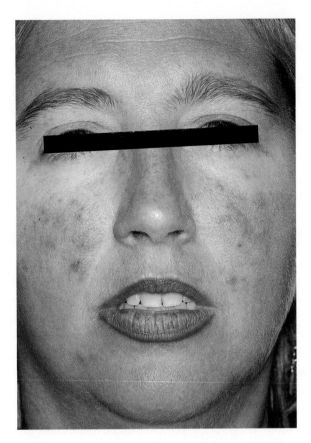

FIGURE 5.1. **Rosacea.** Papules, pustules, and telangiectasias are seen on the central face. Note the lack of comedones. (Reproduced with permission from Wolff K, Johnson RA. *Fitzpatrick's Color Atlas & Synopsis of Clinical Dermatology,* 6th ed. New York: McGraw-Hill, 2009, Fig. 1-7.)

EXAM

- **No comedones are seen.** Exam reveals diffuse erythema and telangiectasias along with occasional erythematous papules and pustules (see Figure 5.1).
- Symmetric **central facial** involvement is also characteristic (malar cheeks, nose, chin, forehead).
- **Rhinophyma**—also known as **"Santa Claus nose"** — is most often seen in men with long-standing disease.

TREATMENT

- **Avoidance of triggers;** sunscreen use.
- The therapeutic ladder is as follows: topical antibiotic (eg, metronidazole gel) → oral antibiotic (eg, tetracycline) → oral isotretinoin for severe disease.

SEBORRHEIC DERMATITIS

An inflammatory reaction to *Malassezia globosa* (formerly *Pityrosporum ovale*) yeast. Disease associations include **AIDS, Parkinson's disease, stroke, and any acute illness.**

KEY FACT

If it looks like rosacea but the patient has been taking topical steroids, think of steroid-induced dermatitis and stop the steroids.

KEY FACT

Rosacea keratitis is uncommon but may lead to blindness.

KEY FACT

Severe, recalcitrant seborrheic dermatitis may be a clue pointing to underlying HIV infection or Parkinson's disease.

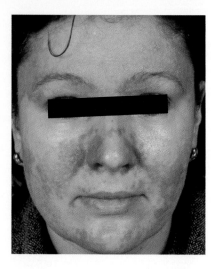

FIGURE 5.2. **Seborrheic dermatitis.** Note the yellow, "greasy" scales on an erythematous base, localized to the central face. (Reproduced with permission from Wolff K et al. *Fitzpatrick's Color Atlas & Synopsis of Clinical Dermatology*, 5th ed. New York: McGraw-Hill, 2005: 51.)

SYMPTOMS/EXAM

- Exam reveals dry or "greasy," yellow, sharply demarcated scales on an erythematous base (see Figure 5.2). The greasy appearance and scalp involvement distinguish this condition from rosacea.
- Generally localized to the **scalp, postauricular region, central facial area** (especially the eyebrows and nasolabial folds), and flexural areas.
- Usually improves during the summer and worsens in the fall and winter.

TREATMENT

- **Scalp:** Shampoos containing tar, zinc, selenium, or ketoconazole.
- **Face:** Ketoconazole 2% cream +/– topical steroids.

PSORIASIS

 A 45-year-old man presents with a rash on the extensor surfaces of his elbows and knees that has occurred episodically ever since he was a teenager. He has derived no relief from OTC topical hydrocortisone. Exam reveals sharply demarcated, erythematous plaques with silvery-white scales on the back of his elbows and front of knees, but covering < 3% of the total body area. His CBC, chemistry, and UA are normal. What is the diagnosis, and what is the most appropriate next step in management?

Psoriasis with typical lesions. The next step involves high-potency topical corticosteroids for about two weeks, which can then be rotated with topical therapies such as vitamin D analogs, retinoids, anthralin, and tar preparations. Topical coal tar can be used as a corticosteroid-sparing drug in resistant cases and is highly effective when combined with UVB phototherapy. Phototherapy is generally used when the patient is resistant to topical therapy or when large areas of the body are involved and topical therapy is impractical.

A T-cell immune-mediated inflammatory disease that has a genetic predisposition and is characterized by a bimodal peak incidence at 27 and 55 years of age. It has several distinct clinical presentations.

SYMPTOMS

- Usually asymptomatic, although itching may be present.
- **Koebner's phenomenon**—psoriatic lesions induced at sites of injury or irritation to normal skin—may also be seen.
- **Triggers** include trauma, stress, and **medications** (lithium, β-blockers, prednisone taper, antimalarials, ACEIs, interferons).
- A severe form is seen in **HIV** infection.

EXAM

- Nail pitting (fine "ice-pick" stippling) is common.
- Subtypes are as follows:
    - **Localized plaque type:** Most common. Presents with sharply demarcated, erythematous plaques with silvery-white scales, often symmetrically distributed on the elbows, knees, scalp, palms, and soles. **Gluteal pinking and umbilical skin involvement are pathognomonic** (see Figure 5.3).
    - **Guttate ("droplike"):** Occurs in young adults **following strep throat.** Characterized by numerous small, discrete plaques that are widely distributed.

 KEY FACT

Consider HIV in a patient with severe psoriasis.

 KEY FACT

Nail pitting and distal finger (DIP) arthritis are manifestations of psoriasis.

KEY FACT

Think of guttate psoriasis if you see widespread plaques after a sore throat.

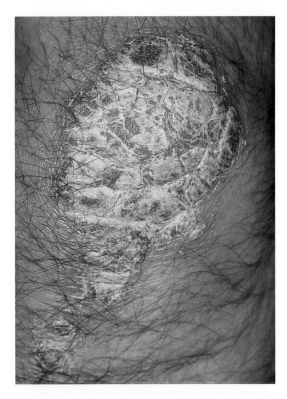

FIGURE 5.3.   Psoriasis vulgaris (elbow). Note the well-demarcated erythematous plaque with thick white scale. (Reproduced with permission from Wolff K et al. *Fitzpatrick's Color Atlas & Synopsis of Clinical Dermatology,* 5th ed. New York: McGraw-Hill, 2005: 57.)

- **Generalized pustular or erythrodermic:** Rare, life-threatening variants.
- **Inverse variant:** Involves the flexural surfaces (axillae, groin).

DIAGNOSIS

- Diagnosed by clinical findings; biopsy is rarely performed.
- In **guttate psoriasis,** consider obtaining an ASO titer and/or a throat culture for group A β-hemolytic streptococcal infection.

TREATMENT

- **Limited plaque disease: Topical therapies** such as potent topical steroids, steroid-sparing vitamin D analogs (calcipotriene), retinoids, coal tar, and anthralin.
- **Generalized disease:** UVB light, oral retinoids, PUVA (psoralen and UVA light).
- **Refractory disease or psoriatic arthritis:** Methotrexate, cyclosporine, sulfasalazine, biologics (eg, alefacept, efalizumab, etanercept).
- **Guttate psoriasis:** Penicillin VK or erythromycin to treat strep throat +/– topical therapies or UVB.

COMPLICATIONS

Psoriatic arthritis (affects < 10% of psoriasis patients) affects the **DIP joints** of the hands and may cause **sacroiliitis.** See the Rheumatology chapter for a more detailed discussion.

KEY FACT

Day treatment with crude coal tar and UVB is associated with disease remission in > 80% of cases.

KEY FACT

Boards questions will focus on the recognition of psoriasis (classic plaques on the flexural surfaces and guttate variety); stepwise treatment based on the severity of disease; and associations with HIV, steroids, and psoriatic arthritis.

KEY FACT

Systemic corticosteroids are contraindicated in the treatment of psoriasis because of the risk of inducing pustular psoriasis and severe disease rebound on withdrawal of medication.

KEY FACT

Consider pityriasis rosea if you see a mildly itchy rash in a Christmas tree distribution with a herald patch.

KEY FACT

Tinea corporis (ringworm) is often mistaken for pityriasis rosea, but tinea corporis has scaly skin at the advancing border, which does not occur with pityriasis.

KEY FACT

Although seborrheic keratoses are benign, if multiple lesions appear suddenly, consider the presence of an internal malignancy.

PITYRIASIS ROSEA

Most often occurs in young adult **women.** Caused by human herpesvirus 6 and 7 (HHV-6 and -7).

SYMPTOMS

A larger **"herald patch"** often precedes the generalized trunk eruption by 1–2 weeks. Mild pruritus is common.

EXAM

- Exam reveals dull pink "salmon-colored" plaques up to 2 cm in diameter with a "cigarette paper" (wrinkled) appearance, a silver **collarette of scale,** and a well-demarcated erythematous base (see Figure 5.4).
- Lesions are characterized by a **"Christmas tree"** distribution, with the long axis of lesions following lines of cleavage.
- Involves the trunk and proximal extremities; **spares the face.**

TREATMENT

A **self-limited** illness that shows spontaneous resolution within about two months.

SEBORRHEIC KERATOSIS

- The most common benign epidermal growth; probably has an autosomal dominant inheritance.
- Sx/Exam:
  - Asymptomatic; occasionally pruritic.
  - Has a **"stuck-on"** appearance.
- Tx: No treatment is necessary.

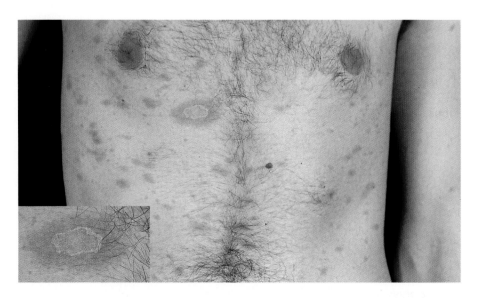

FIGURE 5.4. **Pityriasis rosea.** Pink plaques with an oval configuration are seen that follow the lines of cleavage. Inset: herald patch. The collarette of scale is more obvious on this magnification. (Reproduced with permission from Wolff K, Johnson RA. *Fitzpatrick's Color Atlas & Synopsis of Clinical Dermatology,* 6th ed. New York: McGraw-Hill, 2009, Fig. 7-1A and B.)

Cutaneous Infections

IMPETIGO

A superficial infection of the epidermis that is **contagious** and **autoinoculable.** Caused by *Staphylococcus*, group A streptococcal infection, or both. Infection may occur as a 1° event or as a 2° superinfection of an underlying dermatitis.

SYMPTOMS/EXAM

1° lesions are vesicles or pustules that most often affect the **face,** often with an overlying **honey-colored crust** (see Figure 5.5).

DIAGNOSIS

Gram stain and culture can confirm clinical suspicion if the diagnosis is in doubt.

TREATMENT

Mupirocin ointment for limited disease; systemic antibiotics for more severe involvement.

KEY FACT

Bullous impetigo is usually caused by *S aureus.*

KEY FACT

Recurrent impetigo suggests *S aureus* nasal carriage. Treat with intranasal mupirocin +/− oral rifampin plus another antistaphylococcal antibiotic.

ERYSIPELAS

Acute cellulitis usually affecting the **central face** and due to **group A streptococci.** Elderly and immunocompromised patients are at greater risk than the general population.

SYMPTOMS

- Patients are **systemically ill** with fevers, chills, and malaise.
- Lesions are hot, painful, and **rapidly advancing.**

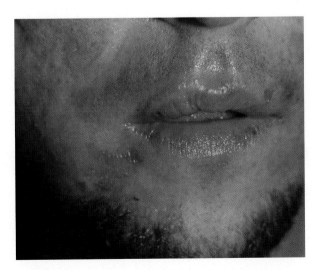

FIGURE 5.5. **Impetigo.** Crusted erosions that may be due to *Streptococcus* or *S aureus*, including MRSA, are seen on the face of a 22-year-old diabetic. (Reproduced with permission from Wolff K, Johnson RA. *Fitzpatrick's Color Atlas & Synopsis of Clinical Dermatology*, 6th ed. New York: McGraw-Hill, 2009, Fig. 24-12.)

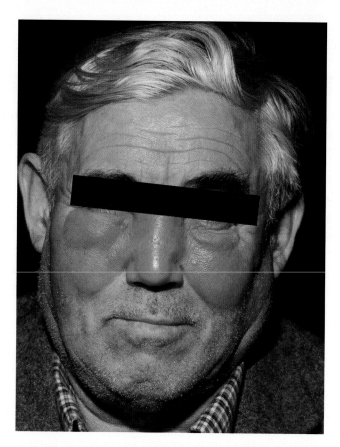

FIGURE 5.6. **Erysipelas of the face.** Painful, well-defined, shiny, erythematous, edematous plaques caused by group A streptococcus. (Reproduced with permission from Wolff K, Johnson RA. *Fitzpatrick's Color Atlas & Synopsis of Clinical Dermatology,* 6th ed. New York: McGraw-Hill, 2009, Fig. 24-22.)

Exam

Exam reveals **brightly erythematous,** smooth, indurated edematous plaques with raised, **sharply demarcated** margins (see Figure 5.6).

Treatment

Prompt administration of **IV antibiotics** with activity against β-hemolytic streptococci.

Complications

If the condition is left untreated, bacteremia and sepsis may develop.

ANTHRAX

Caused by *Bacillus anthracis,* a gram-⊕, spore-forming aerobic rod; transmitted through the skin or mucous membranes or by inhalation via contaminated soil, animals, animal products, or **biological warfare. Ninety-five percent of anthrax cases worldwide are cutaneous.**

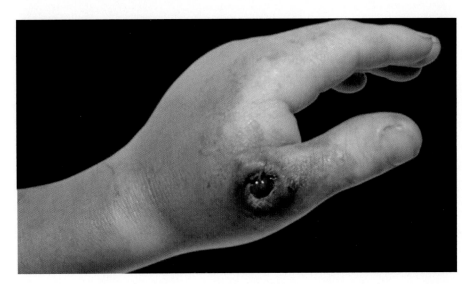

FIGURE 5.7.   Cutaneous anthrax. A painless black eschar is seen at the site of inoculation with a central hemorrhagic ulceration on the thumb associated with massive edema of the hand. (Reproduced with permission from Wolff K, Johnson RA. *Fitzpatrick's Color Atlas & Synopsis of Clinical Dermatology,* 6th ed. New York: McGraw-Hill, 2009, Fig. 24-45A.)

SYMPTOMS

- Has three clinical manifestations: cutaneous, GI, and pulmonary (wool-sorters' disease).
- A two- to seven-day incubation period is followed by the development of characteristically evolving lesions (see below).

EXAM

- The 1° lesion is a small, **nontender,** pruritic, erythematous macule that evolves into a papule with **vesicles,** significant erythema, and edema (see Figure 5.7).
- One to three days later, the papule ulcerates, leaving the characteristic black **necrotic eschar** that usually resolves over six weeks.

DIAGNOSIS

Smear or culture will confirm the gram-⊕ organism.

TREATMENT

Oral ciprofloxacin or doxycycline may be effective for mild, localized cutaneous disease; give these agents IV in bioterrorism-associated anthrax. Treatment duration is 60 days.

DERMATOPHYTOSIS (TINEA)

A superficial fungal infection of the skin, hair follicles, and/or nails that is transmitted from person to person via **fomites.** Scalp infection is seen mainly in children. Predisposing factors include atopic dermatitis, immunosuppression, sweating, and occlusion.

SYMPTOMS/EXAM

- **Tinea pedis:** Presents with dry scales, maceration, and/or fissuring of the web spaces and scaling in a "moccasin" or "ballet slipper" distribution; vesicles and bullae may occur.

KEY FACT

Most cutaneous cases of anthrax resolve spontaneously without significant sequelae, but 10–20% of untreated cutaneous cases may result in death.

KEY FACT

Tinea pedis affecting the web spaces is the most common inciting factor for cellulitis in otherwise healthy patients.

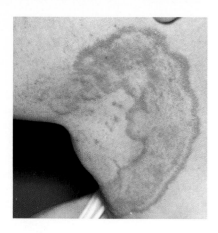

FIGURE 5.8. Tinea corporis. A typical "ringworm-like" configuration can be seen. (Reproduced with permission from Wolff K et al. *Fitzpatrick's Dermatology in General Medicine,* 7th ed. New York: McGraw-Hill, 2008, Fig. 188-11.)

KEY FACT

Griseofulvin is the treatment of choice for tinea capitis. Topicals are ineffective.

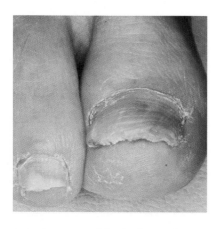

FIGURE 5.9. Distal subungual onychomycosis. (Reproduced with permission from Wolff K et al. *Fitzpatrick's Dermatology in General Medicine,* 7th ed. New York: McGraw-Hill, 2008, Fig. 188-18.)

- **Tinea cruris (groin):** Characterized by erythematous, well-demarcated plaques with **clear centers** and active, advancing, scaly, **sharp borders.** Usually begins unilaterally; more common in men. The differential includes intertrigo and erythrasma.
- **Tinea corporis:** Involves the face, trunk, and extremities. The size and degree of inflammation can vary, with scaly skin at the advancing border (see Figure 5.8).
- **Tinea barbae (beard):** Often accompanied by folliculitis and pseudofolliculitis (ingrown hairs).
- **Tinea capitis:** Commonly affects the scalp, eyebrows, and eyelashes. Lesions generally show evidence of active infection with exudate, inflamed crusts, matted hair, and even debris. In severe cases, it can develop into a patch with hair loss and scarring alopecia.
- **Tinea unguium/onychomycosis:** Yellowing and thickening of the nail with subungual debris; frequently associated with chronic tinea pedis (see Figure 5.9).

DIAGNOSIS

- KOH of skin scraping to identify hyphae +/– fungal culture.
- Infected hairs in tinea capitis fluoresce in "black" UV light (Wood's light).

TREATMENT

- Maintain good hygiene; keep affected areas dry.
- Topical antifungals; oral antifungals in refractory cases. Treatment of any of the tinea infections requires administration of topical creams twice daily for at least two weeks, with continuation of therapy at least one week after resolution of the lesions.
- **Topical therapy is usually ineffective for onychomycosis.** The risks and benefits of oral antifungal therapy should be considered. Terbinafine has the highest cure rate, followed by itraconazole and then griseofulvin.

PITYRIASIS (TINEA) VERSICOLOR

A 40-year-old woman presents with one month of a nonpruritic, nonpainful spreading rash from which she has derived no relief with an OTC corticosteroid cream. Exam shows hypopigmented macules on the chest, abdomen, and shoulders. Direct microscopic exam of a scale with 10% KOH shows large, blunt hyphae and thick-walled budding spores in a "spaghetti and meatballs" pattern. Her LFTs are normal. What is the most likely diagnosis and the most appropriate treatment?

Pityriasis (tinea) versicolor, a superficial mycotic infection, is effectively treated with ketoconazole shampoo or pill. Patients usually notice the infection because involved areas do not tan, resulting in hypopigmentation. The infection commonly recurs, and prophylaxis and/or periodic courses of treatment may be necessary.

A mild superficial infection caused by a nondermatophyte fungus (***Malassezia globosa,* formerly named *Pityrosporum ovale***) and facilitated by high humidity and sebum production. It commonly affects young and middle-aged adults.

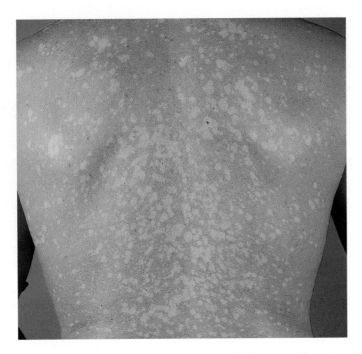

FIGURE 5.10. **Tinea versicolor.** Note the multiple, well-demarcated hypopigmented macules. (Reproduced with permission from Wolff K, Johnson RA. *Fitzpatrick's Color Atlas & Synopsis of Clinical Dermatology,* 6th ed. New York: McGraw-Hill, 2009, Fig. 13-13A.)

SYMPTOMS/EXAM

- Exam reveals numerous round or oval, sharply demarcated macules that may be tan, brown, pink, or white (see Figure 5.10).
- Often presents in a seborrheic distribution involving the upper trunk and shoulders.

DIAGNOSIS

KOH of skin scraping to identify hyphae and budding spores ("**spaghetti and meatballs**" appearance) (see Figure 5.11).

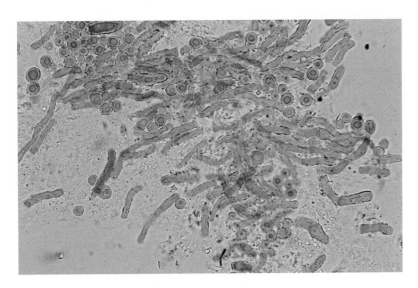

FIGURE 5.11. **Tinea versicolor on KOH prep.** Note the "spaghetti and meatballs" appearance of *Malassezia* on microscopy. (Reproduced with permission from Wolff K et al. *Fitzpatrick's Dermatology in General Medicine,* 7th ed. New York: McGraw-Hill, 2008, Fig. 189-11.)

KEY FACT

If a patient with tinea pedis develops pruritic vesicles on the hands, it may represent an **id reaction**— a hypersensitivity reaction to a tinea infection on a distant body site.

KEY FACT

Tinea lesions that are painful suggest a 2° bacterial infection.

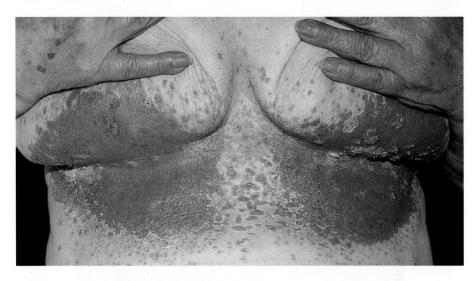

FIGURE 5.12. **Cutaneous candidiasis: intertrigo.** Confluent bright red papules with "satellite" pustules are seen. (Reproduced with permission from Wolff K et al. *Fitzpatrick's Color Atlas & Synopsis of Clinical Dermatology*, 5th ed. New York: McGraw-Hill, 2005: 719.)

TREATMENT

Ketoconazole shampoo and oral ketoconazole are both highly effective. **A single oral dose of ketoconazole 400 mg results in short-term cure in 90% of cases.**

CANDIDIASIS

Risk factors include DM, obesity, sweating, heat, maceration, systemic and topical steroid use, and chronic debilitation. Antibiotics and OCP use may also be contributory.

SYMPTOMS/EXAM

- Favors moist intertriginous areas.
- **Brightly erythematous,** sharply demarcated plaques are seen with scalloped borders (see Figure 5.12).
- **Satellite lesions** (pustular lesions at the periphery) may coalesce and extend into larger lesions.

DIAGNOSIS

Usually a clinical diagnosis, supported by KOH with pseudohyphae and yeast forms or culture (see Figure 5.13).

TREATMENT

Keep dry and use topical antifungals.

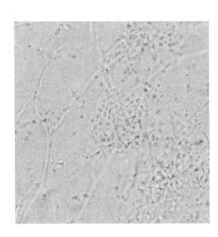

FIGURE 5.13. *Candida* **on KOH prep.** Note the pseudomycelia in clusters of grapelike yeast cells. (Reproduced with permission from Wolff K et al. *Fitzpatrick's Dermatology in General Medicine*, 7th ed. New York: McGraw-Hill, 2008, Fig. 189-1.)

HERPES SIMPLEX (HSV)

A 40-year-old woman with culture-proven HSV infection of the face presents with progression of the infection despite high-dose IV acyclovir. She has a history of recurrent herpes labialis infections since childhood, underwent hematopoietic stem cell transplantation four months ago for acute myeloid leukemia (AML), and is currently on high-dose immunosuppressive drugs. Exam reveals umbilicated vesicular lesions with raised, nonpustular, erythematous edges on her right cheek. Her labs show leukopenia and a creatinine level of 2.0 mg/dL. What is the most appropriate antiviral treatment?

Foscarnet for acyclovir-resistant HSV infection. Because administration of foscarnet can cause significant electrolyte abnormalities, routine lab studies are indicated before this drug is initiated. Cidofovir is another option but causes renal toxicity.

Morbidity results from recurrent outbreaks. Transmission occurs through direct contact with mucosal surfaces. **Asymptomatic viral shedding** occurs in 60–80% of infected patients.

Symptoms/Exam

Presents with small, grouped vesicles/vesiculoulcerative lesions with serpiginous borders and with satellite vesicles on an erythematous base that crust, most commonly affecting the vermilion border of the lips, the genitals (often with enlarged inguinal lymph nodes), and the buttocks.

Diagnosis

Direct fluorescent antibody, viral culture, PCR (most sensitive, but costly), or evidence of viropathic changes on biopsy.

Treatment

- Lesions spontaneously heal within one week.
- Immediate treatment with oral antiviral agents may ↓ the duration of the outbreak by 12–24 hours.
- Immunosuppressed patients may require parenteral acyclovir.
- Acyclovir-resistant cases are treated with foscarnet or cidofovir.

Complications

- Disseminated cutaneous disease in patients with underlying dermatitis (eczema herpeticum; see Figure 5.14).
- Immunosuppressed patients are at risk for potentially life-threatening systemic disease involving the lungs, liver, and CNS.

KEY FACT

Consider suppressive treatment with low-dose antivirals for patients with frequent or severe outbreaks, as such treatment can ↓ outbreaks by 85% and viral shedding by 90%.

KEY FACT

Oral valacyclovir is the most appropriate antiviral agent for genital HSV infection without systemic complications (meningitis, encephalitis, urinary retention). Oral famciclovir and acyclovir are other options.

KEY FACT

HSV is the most common cause of recurrent erythema multiforme.

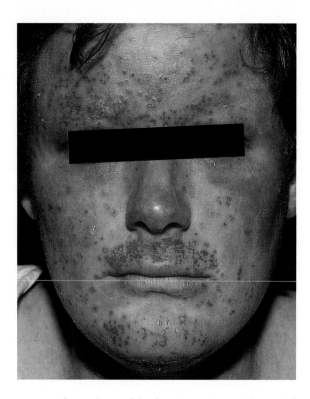

FIGURE 5.14. **Eczema herpeticum of the face in a patient with HSV infection.** Confluent and discrete crusted erosions associated with erythema and edema are seen in a patient with atopic dermatitis. (Reproduced with permission from Wolff K, Johnson RA. *Fitzpatrick's Color Atlas & Synopsis of Clinical Dermatology,* 6th ed. New York: McGraw-Hill, 2009, Fig. 27-35.)

HERPES ZOSTER

 A 65-year-old woman presents two months after an episode in which she had a painful rash on her left trunk for a week. Acetaminophen with codeine has not proven effective, and she continues to feel sharp pains, especially when she tries to sleep. Exam reveals scattered areas of hypopigmentation in a dermatomal distribution with tingling and pain on light touch. What is the most likely diagnosis and the most appropriate treatment?

Postherpetic neuralgia (PHN) from herpes zoster causing pain after the rash has healed. Treat with gabapentin, which has been shown to ↓ pain and improve sleep. Spontaneous resolution of PHN is common, particularly during the first six months of the episode, but treatment may be indicated for pain that interferes with functioning or sleep. Other treatment options are capsaicin, amitriptyline, and regional nerve blocks.

Varicella-zoster virus (VZV) is the agent of the 1° infection **varicella** (chickenpox) and is also responsible for its reactivation in the form of **herpes zoster** (shingles). There is a 10–20% lifetime incidence of herpes zoster in those who have had chickenpox, and incidence ↑ with age. The risk of zoster is also greater in immunosuppressed adults (eg, those with HIV infection and malignancy).

SYMPTOMS

Presents with unilateral **dermatomal pain** followed by skin lesions.

KEY FACT

Disseminated zoster or zoster in apparently healthy patients < 40 years of age should raise suspicion for HIV disease.

EXAM

- Exam reveals clustered vesicular lesions, most commonly on the trunk or face (see Figure 5.15).
- **Herpes zoster ophthalmicus** accounts for approximately 7–10% of all zoster cases. Lesions on the eye, eyelid, and forehead indicate CN V involvement. Vesicles occurring on either the tip or the side of the nose (**Hutchinson's sign**) are more likely indicative of infection in the deep structures of the eye.

DIAGNOSIS

Direct fluorescent antibody, viral culture, PCR, or evidence of viropathic changes on biopsy.

TREATMENT

- Antivirals (famciclovir and valacyclovir) are recommended to ↓ pain, vesicle formation, viral shedding, and ocular involvement in patients with HIV disease, those > 50 years of age, and those presenting within 72 hours of symptom onset.
- Early treatment with oral corticosteroids should be reserved for severe cases but can speed healing and significantly resolve acute neuralgia, leading to more rapid return to normal function, undisturbed sleep, and cessation of analgesics.
- Treatment is always indicated in the presence of ocular involvement as well as for immunosuppressed and debilitated patients with extensive cutaneous involvement. Use IV antivirals for ocular and disseminated disease.

COMPLICATIONS

There is an ↑ risk of PHN in the **elderly** and following **trigeminal** zoster. Treatment is typically with gabapentin. Other options include capsaicin, amitriptyline, opioids, and regional nerve blocks.

KEY FACT

Consider disseminated zoster if lesions involve multiple dermatomes or are bilateral. Treatment requires IV antivirals.

KEY FACT

The pain of zoster may precede skin lesions by several days and may mimic that of angina, pleurisy, cholecystitis, appendicitis, or hepatitis.

KEY FACT

Antiviral therapy within 72 hours may ↓ the duration and severity of PHN. This is especially important in the elderly, a population that is at ↑ risk for the development of this complication.

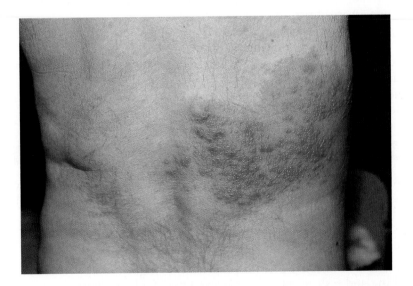

FIGURE 5.15. **Herpes zoster in T8–T10 dermatomes in a patient with VZV infection.** Grouped vesicles and pustules are seen on a base of erythema and edema involving the posterior chest wall. (Reproduced with permission from Wolff K et al. *Fitzpatrick's Color Atlas & Synopsis of Clinical Dermatology,* 5th ed. New York: McGraw-Hill, 2005: 823.)

SMALLPOX

Caused by variola, a double-stranded DNA poxvirus transmitted via viral implantation on the oropharyngeal or respiratory mucosa.

SYMPTOMS

- A 12-day incubation period is followed by the **sudden onset** of fever, headache, malaise, and vomiting.
- A centrifugally spreading rash appears after the cessation of constitutional symptoms.

EXAM

- Erythematous macules evolve synchronously into vesicles and pustules. Lesions crust over in approximately two weeks and heal with characteristic pitted scarring.
- The rash in smallpox occurs after fever and is most prominent on the face and extremities, palms, and soles, and lesions are all at the same stage (eg, all papules or all macules). By contrast, chickenpox lesions occur with fever, are at different stages, and are most prominent on the trunk, sparing the palms and soles.

DIAGNOSIS

Electron microscopy (staining for poxvirus particles), PCR, IgM-specific antibody, or cell culture.

TREATMENT

- Supportive. Give antibiotics if 2° bacterial infection is suspected.
- **Vaccination is controversial** because of **vaccine-related complications:**
  - **Generalized vaccinia:** Infection with vaccinia virus 4–10 days after vaccination; can be due to autoinoculation upon contact with the vaccination site. Immunosuppressed patients (chemotherapy, HIV, pregnancy) are at risk.
  - **Eczema vaccinatum:** Vaccinia virus superinfects the skin of patients with eczema or atopic dermatitis.
- Vaccinia immune globulin may be used for the treatment of eczema vaccinatum and severe generalized vaccinia.
- **The case fatality rate is 20–30%** and usually results from bacterial superinfection or severe inflammatory response.

SCABIES

Skin infestation by the mite *Sarcoptes scabiei.* The female adult burrows and lays eggs in the stratum corneum. Highly **contagious;** spreads through prolonged contact with an infected host.

SYMPTOMS

- Presents with **intense pruritus,** especially at night.
- Itching and rash result from a delayed type IV hypersensitivity reaction to the mites, their eggs, or their feces, resulting in a two- to four-week delay between infection and onset of symptoms.
- Crusted (or "Norwegian") scabies occurs in immunocompromised and institutionalized patients.

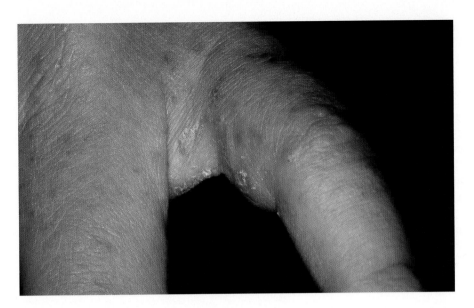

FIGURE 5.16. **Scabies.** Papules and burrows are seen in typical locations on the finger web. (Reproduced with permission from Wolff K, Johnson RA. *Fitzpatrick's Color Atlas & Synopsis of Clinical Dermatology*, 6th ed. New York: McGraw-Hill, 2009, Fig. 28-16.)

EXAM

- Exam reveals small pruritic vesicles, pustules, excoriations, and **burrows;** look in the **webbed spaces** of the fingers (see Figure 5.16), volar wrists, elbows, **axillae,** belt line, feet, scrotum, and areolae.
- **The face is usually spared.**
- A generalized **hypersensitivity rash** may develop at distant sites.
- In crusted scabies, lesions are hyperkeratotic and crusted, covering large areas. Associated scalp lesions and nail dystrophy are also seen.

DIAGNOSIS

Examine **skin scrapings** with light microscopy to identify mites, ova, or fecal pellets (see Figure 5.17).

TREATMENT

- Apply **permethrin 5%** cream below the neck; leave on for eight hours and shower off. Treatment may be repeated in one week. Wash linens and clothing in hot water. Note that permethrin 1% as a shampoo is used for head lice (pediculosis).
- **Ivermectin** may be needed to treat crusted scabies, conventional cases refractory to topical therapy, epidemics in institutions, or superinfected scabies.

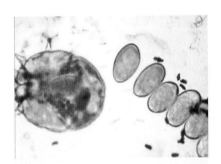

FIGURE 5.17. **Scabies on skin scraping.** Microscopic examination of a mineral oil preparation after scraping a burrow reveals a gravid female mite with oval, gray eggs and fecal pellets. (Reproduced with permission from Wolff K et al. *Fitzpatrick's Dermatology in General Medicine,* 7th ed. New York: McGraw-Hill, 2008, Fig. 208-5.)

> **KEY FACT**

Itching and rash 2° to hypersensitivity reactions may persist for weeks or months despite effectively treated scabies infection.

Dermatologic Manifestations of Systemic Diseases

CARDIOVASCULAR

Infective Endocarditis

Dermatologic findings associated with infective endocarditis are outlined in Table 5.1.

TABLE 5.1. Dermatologic Manifestations of Infective Endocarditis

CLINICAL FINDINGS	CHARACTERISTICS
Petechiae	
Splinter hemorrhages	Subungual, dark red linear macules (see Figure 5.18).
Roth's spots	Oval retinal hemorrhages with a clear, pale center.
Janeway lesions	Small, slightly papular red/violaceous hemorrhages on the palmar and plantar surfaces (see Figure 5.19A). Most commonly seen in acute endocarditis.
Osler's nodes	Small, **tender** violaceous papules on the pads of the digits (**O**sler = **O**uch) (see Figure 5.19B).
Clubbing	
Peripheral emboli	

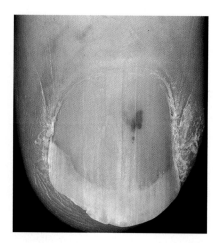

FIGURE 5.18. Splinter hemorrhage. A subungual hemorrhage in the midportion of the fingernail bed is seen in a woman with endocarditis. These may also be seen in cholesterol emboli or following nail trauma. (Reproduced with permission from Wolff K, Johnson RA. *Fitzpatrick's Color Atlas & Synopsis of Clinical Dermatology*, 6th ed. New York: McGraw-Hill, 2009, Fig. 33-28.)

KEY FACT

Livedo reticularis is a clinical reaction pattern resulting from vascular obstruction or hyperviscosity. Some cases may be caused by drugs such as corticosteroids, amantadine, or epinephrine.

Livedo Reticularis

A 65-year-old woman with a history of CAD and hypertension presents with abdominal pain, a low-grade fever, myalgias, nausea, generalized weakness, and acute renal failure (ARF) with a creatinine level of 5 mg/dL (baseline 1.2 mg/dL). About one week ago she was hospitalized with chest pain and had a cardiac catheterization, and a stent was placed. Her exam reveals a temperature of 37.8°C (100°F), a left carotid bruit, nonpalpable distal pulses with her left great toe cool and cyanotic, pretibial edema, and a netlike violaceous rash visible over her legs. Her labs reveal a leukocyte count of 7000/µL with 60% neutrophils, 30% lymphocytes, and 10% eosinophils; a low C3 and a normal C4 level; and a UA that shows 1+ blood, 5–10 erythrocytes/hpf, 1+ protein, and 3–5 leukocytes/hpf. What is the most likely diagnosis?

Atheroembolic disease, or cholesterol emboli syndrome. This condition is a rare sequela of recent cardiac catheterization and can mimic vasculitis. It results in ARF, livedo reticularis of the lower extremities, cyanotic toes, low C3 levels, and peripheral eosinophilia. Funduscopy can show a Hollenhorst plaque (cholesterol emboli in the vessels of the retina).

Obstruction of arteriolar flow from vasospasm, obstruction, hyperviscosity, or obstruction of venous outflow. May be idiopathic. 2° etiologies include the following:

- Atheroemboli (postangiography/post–cardiac catheterization) and cholesterol emboli syndrome (see the Rheumatology chapter).
- Antiphospholipid antibody syndrome.
- SLE.
- Cryoglobulins.
- Medications (eg, prednisone, amantadine, epinephrine).
- Other hypercoagulable states and vasculitides.

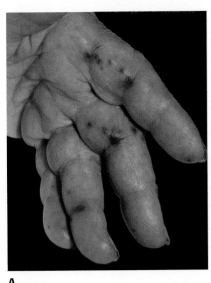

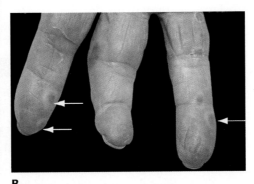

A   **B**

FIGURE 5.19.   Cutaneous manifestations of infective endocarditis. (A) Janeway lesions. Note the hemorrhagic, infarcted papules on the volar fingers in a patient with *S aureus* endocarditis. **(B)** Osler's nodes (arrows). (Image A reproduced with permission from Wolff K, Johnson RA. *Fitzpatrick's Color Atlas & Synopsis of Clinical Dermatology*, 6th ed. New York: McGraw-Hill, 2009, Fig. 24-46. Image B reproduced with permission from Wolff K et al. *Fitzpatrick's Dermatology in General Medicine*, 7th ed. New York: McGraw-Hill, 2008, Fig. 151-11.)

SYMPTOMS/EXAM

- Symmetric; involves the extremities. More prominent with exposure to cold.
- Presents with a mottled or **netlike bluish** (livid) discoloration of the skin (see Figure 5.20).

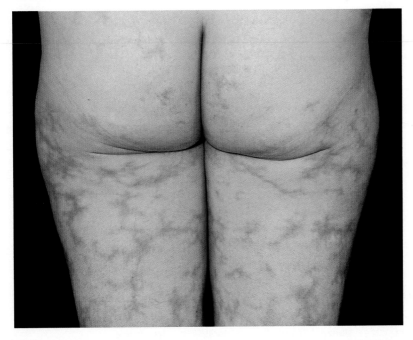

FIGURE 5.20.   Symptomatic livedo reticularis. A bluish, netlike, arborizing pattern is seen on the posterior thighs and buttocks. (Reproduced with permission from Wolff K, Johnson RA. *Fitzpatrick's Color Atlas & Synopsis of Clinical Dermatology*, 6th ed. New York: McGraw-Hill, 2009, Fig. 14-19.)

DIAGNOSIS

Test for underlying disease with coagulation studies, ANA, RF, antiphospholipid antibodies, and cryoglobulins.

TREATMENT

- Treat the underlying disease.
- Pentoxifylline 400 mg PO TID and low-dose ASA may be helpful.

GASTROINTESTINAL

A 45-year-old man, formerly an IV drug user, presents with several months of a lower extremity rash. Physical exam reveals palpable purpura on the lower extremities. Labs show an AST of 70 U/L, an ALT of 90 U/L, an alkaline phosphatase level of 80 U/L, ⊕ anti-HCV antibody, ⊕ anti-HBs antibody, and ⊖ HBsAg. What diagnostic test should be done next?

Serum cryoglobulins to test for cryoglobulinemia associated with HCV. The skin lesions are characteristic of vasculitis. Measuring serum and urine porphyrin levels is not indicated because although porphyria cutanea tarda (PCT) is also associated with HCV, the lesions in PCT are characterized by plaques in sun-exposed areas such as the dorsa of the hands.

> **KEY FACT**
>
> A ⊕ test for RF is often seen in cryoglobulinemia.

Table 5.2 outlines the dermatologic manifestations of common GI disorders.

TABLE 5.2. Dermatologic Manifestations of GI Disorders

DISORDER	ETIOLOGY	SKIN MANIFESTATIONS	MOST COMMON DISEASE ASSOCIATIONS
Porphyria cutanea tarda	↓ activity of uroporphyrinogen decarboxylase, an enzyme in the heme biosynthetic pathway. May be inherited or acquired.	**Painless** vesicles and bullae on the face and dorsa of the hands (**light-exposed areas**). Facial hypertrichosis.	HCV (85%). **Medications: NSAIDs, estrogens, tetracyclines.**
Cryoglobulinemia	Cryoglobulins are immunoglobulins that precipitate on cold exposure, causing vessel occlusion or immune complex vasculitis.	Palpable purpura, livedo reticularis.	**HCV; lymphoproliferative disorders (lymphoma, myeloma).**
Lichen planus	Idiopathic.	Flat-topped purple, polygonal, pruritic papules (see Figure 5.21). Affect the flexor wrist, lumbar region, shins, and penis. Mucous membrane lesions are found in 40–50% of cases.	**Chronic HBV and HCV;** 1° biliary cirrhosis. **Medications:** Streptomycin, tetracycline, NSAIDs, HCTZ, antimalarials.
Dermatitis herpetiformis	Likely immune complexes of IgA and epidermal tissue transglutaminase. The cutaneous manifestation of gluten sensitivity.	**Extremely pruritic,** grouped vesicles symmetrically distributed over the elbows, forearms, back, buttocks, and knees (see Figure 5.22).	**Gluten-sensitive enteropathy; celiac disease.** ↑ risk of GI lymphoma.
Pyoderma gangrenosum	Unknown; an underlying immunologic abnormality is favored.	Painful, rapidly advancing deep ulcer (see Figure 5.23).	**Ulcerative colitis > Crohn's disease.**

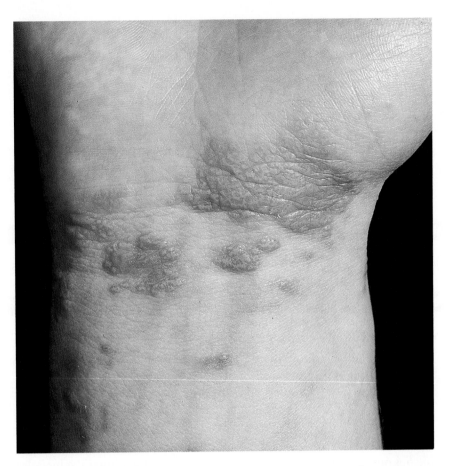

FIGURE 5.21. **Lichen planus.** Flat-topped, polygonal, sharply defined, shiny, violaceous papules are seen. (Reproduced with permission from Wolff K, Johnson RA. *Fitzpatrick's Color Atlas & Synopsis of Clinical Dermatology*, 6th ed. New York: McGraw-Hill, 2009, Fig. 7-4A.)

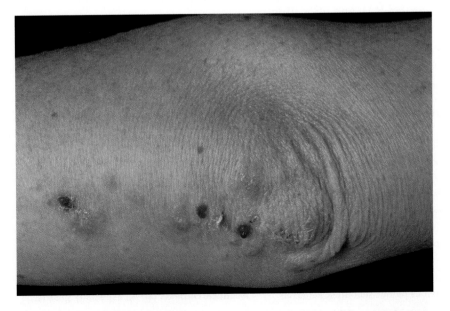

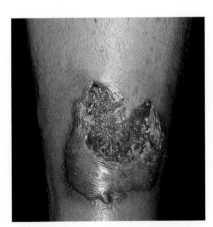

FIGURE 5.23. **Pyoderma gangrenosum.** A painful ulcer is seen with a dusky-red peripheral rim and an undermined border. (Reproduced with permission from Wolff K et al. *Fitzpatrick's Color Atlas & Synopsis of Clinical Dermatology*, 5th ed. New York: McGraw-Hill, 2005: 153.)

FIGURE 5.22. **Dermatitis herpetiformis.** The classic early lesions of dermatitis herpetiformis are seen, including papules, urticarial plaques, small grouped vesicles, and crusts on the elbow. (Reproduced with permission from Wolff K, Johnson RA. *Fitzpatrick's Color Atlas & Synopsis of Clinical Dermatology*, 6th ed. New York: McGraw-Hill, 2009, Fig. 6-16.)

TABLE 5.3.   **Dermatologic Manifestations of Hematologic Disease**

Disorder	Skin Manifestations	Most Common Disease Associations
1° AL amyloidosis	Blood vessel fragility leads to "raccoon eyes" and "pinch purpura" (purpura due to mild trauma). Macroglossia.	Multiple myeloma; Waldenström's macroglobulinemia.
Mastocytosis	Solitary mastocytoma or generalized urticaria. A ⊕ Darier's sign (pruritus and wheal) is elicited by stroking.	Lymphoma, leukemia.

HEMATOLOGIC

Table 5.3 outlines the dermatologic manifestations of hematologic disorders.

ONCOLOGIC

Posttransplant Skin Malignancy

- Squamous cell carcinomas are more common than basal cell carcinomas in posttransplant patients.
- The incidence of malignancy ↑ with the duration of immunosuppressive therapy.

Paraneoplastic Disease

Table 5.4 outlines the dermatologic manifestations of common paraneoplastic disorders.

Sweet's Syndrome

A **neutrophilic dermatosis** that can be subdivided into five groups: paraneoplastic (most commonly associated with **AML** and lymphomas), drug induced, pregnancy related, associated with inflammatory or autoimmune disorders (eg, RA), and idiopathic.

TABLE 5.4.   **Dermatologic Manifestations of Neoplastic Disease**

Disorder	Skin Manifestations	Commonly Associated Malignancy
Glucagonoma	Necrolytic migratory erythema, glossitis, angular cheilitis.	Glucagon-secreting tumors of the pancreas.
Dermatomyositis	Heliotrope rash, Gottron's papules (violaceous papules overlying the finger joints), photodistributed eruption.	**Ovarian cancer;** other solid tumors.
Extramammary Paget's disease	Erythematous plaques with scales, erosion, and exudate. Affects the anogenital region.	Underlying vulvar or penile adenocarcinomas and regional internal malignancies.
Leukocytoclastic vasculitis	Small vessel vasculitis; palpable purpura (see Figure 5.24).	Lymphoproliferative neoplasms; solid tumors.
Sign of Leser-Trélat	Abrupt eruption of numerous pruritic seborrheic keratoses.	**Adenocarcinomas (60%), especially gastric.**

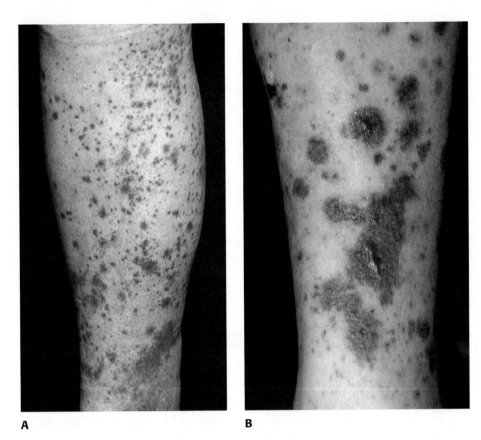

A   **B**

FIGURE 5.24. **Hypersensitivity vasculitis.** (**A**) Cutaneous vasculitis presents clinically as palpable purpura on the lower extremities. The lesions shown here have central puncta that are darker red and do not blanch with a glass slide, indicating hemorrhage. (**B**) A more advanced stage in which lesions have progressed to hemorrhagic bullae and some have become necrotic. (Reproduced with permission from Wolff K, Johnson RA. *Fitzpatrick's Color Atlas & Synopsis of Clinical Dermatology,* 6th ed. New York: McGraw-Hill, 2009, Fig. 14-34.)

DIAGNOSIS

Two major and two minor criteria are required for diagnosis:

- **Major:**
  1. Abrupt onset of tender, erythematous plaques. Lesions are often described as "pseudovesicular" in that they look like vesicles or bullae but are firm on palpation.
  2. Histopathology consistent with Sweet's syndrome.
- **Minor:**
  1. Fever and constitutional symptoms.
  2. Leukocytosis.
  3. Preceded by associated infection (eg, streptococcus or yersiniosis) or associated with malignancy, inflammatory disorders, or pregnancy.
  4. **Excellent response to corticosteroids.**

TREATMENT

First-line treatment is systemic corticosteroids. Alternative treatments are dapsone, colchicine, and potassium iodide.

 KEY FACT

If a patient with AML or an autoimmune disorder (eg, RA) abruptly develops tender red plaques associated with fevers and an ↑ WBC count, consider Sweet's syndrome. Biopsy demonstrates an abundance of PMNs, and the condition responds well to steroids.

TABLE 5.5.   **Dermatologic Manifestations of Endocrine and Metabolic Disease**

Disorder	Skin Manifestations	Most Common Disease Associations
Acanthosis nigricans	Velvety, dirty hyperpigmentation; affects the axillae, groin, and neck (see Figure 5.25). Insidious; asymptomatic.	**Insulin resistance:** DM, obesity, Cushing's disease. **Medications:** Nicotinic acid, glucocorticoid therapy, OCPs, growth hormone therapy. **Paraneoplastic:** Gastric adenocarcinoma.
Necrobiosis lipoidica	Waxy plaques with an elevated border. Affects the lower legs (> 80% pretibial). Lesions have a brownish-red color and an atrophic yellow center (see Figure 5.26).	DM.
Xanthoma	Crops of small, discrete, dome-shaped, yellow-orange papules. Affects the eyelids and tendons (classically involving the Achilles tendon) (see Figure 5.27).	Hyperlipidemia; familial combined hypertriglyceridemia (triglyceride level > 1000 mg/dL; 1° biliary cirrhosis.

ENDOCRINE AND METABOLIC

A 40-year-old woman presents with two years of progressive fatigue but no other symptoms. Exam reveals xanthomas on the extensor surfaces and mild hepatomegaly. Labs reveal a normal CBC, AST, and ALT; an alkaline phosphatase level of 600 U/L; and a total bilirubin of 3.2 mg/dL. What is the most likely diagnosis, and what studies would help establish this diagnosis?

1° biliary cirrhosis is most likely. Up to 80% of patients report fatigue. Xanthomas and an elevated serum alkaline phosphatase are also characteristic. An antimitochondrial antibody titer should be determined next, because titers of > 1:40 occur in > 90% of patients with 1° biliary cirrhosis.

Table 5.5 outlines the dermatologic manifestations of endocrine and metabolic disorders.

RENAL

Cutaneous signs associated with end-stage renal disease (ESRD) are as follows:

- **Nephrogenic systemic fibrosis:** A complication usually seen 2–4 weeks after exposure to gadolinium contrast (eg, from MRI) in patients with ESRD. Presents as a scleroderma-like, progressive skin hardening that leads to marked reduction in quality of life and mobility and occasionally causes fibrosis of visceral organs (see Figure 5.28).
- **Calcinosis cutis:** Calcified subcutaneous nodules or masses that are painless and do not ulcerate.
- **Calciphylaxis:** Calcific uremic arteriolopathy. Progressive calcification of vessels leads to ischemic necrosis of surrounding skin and soft tissues. Lesions present as painful violaceous nodules on the trunk, proximal extremities, and buttocks (see Figure 5.29). Risk factors include use of warfarin, vitamin D analogs, or calcium-based phosphate binders; an elevated calcium-phosphorus product (> 55); protein S or C deficiency; obesity; and female gender.

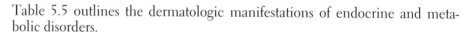

FIGURE 5.25.   Acanthosis nigricans. Note the velvety, dark brown epidermal thickening of the armpit. (Reproduced with permission from Wolff K, Johnson RA. *Fitzpatrick's Color Atlas & Synopsis of Clinical Dermatology*, 6th ed. New York: McGraw-Hill, 2009, Fig. 5-1.)

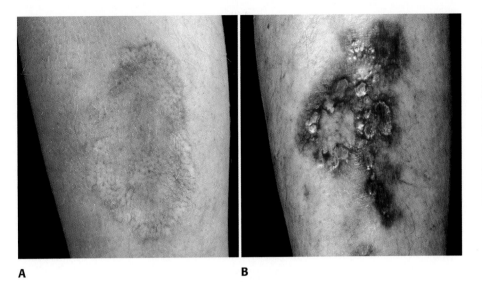

A

B

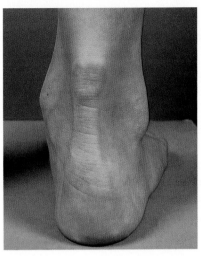

FIGURE 5.27. Tendon xanthomata typical of heterozygous familial hypercholesterolemia. (Reproduced with permission from Wolff K et al. *Fitzpatrick's Dermatology in General Medicine,* 7th ed. New York: McGraw-Hill, 2008, Fig. 135-4.)

FIGURE 5.26. Necrobiosis lipoidica diabeticorum. (A) A large, symmetric plaque with an active tan-pink, well-demarcated, raised, firm border and a yellow center in the pretibial region of a diabetic female. The central parts of the lesion are depressed with atrophic changes of epidermal thinning and telangiectasis against a yellow background. **(B)** An extensive plaque of necrobiosis lipoidica on the lower leg of a diabetic female, representing a late lesion after a healed ulceration. Apart from the features of necrobiosis lipoidica, there is extensive scarring and atrophic depressed scars. (Reproduced with permission from Wolff K, Johnson RA. *Fitzpatrick's Color Atlas & Synopsis of Clinical Dermatology,* 6th ed. New York: McGraw-Hill, 2009, Fig. 15-6.)

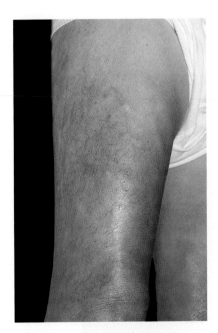

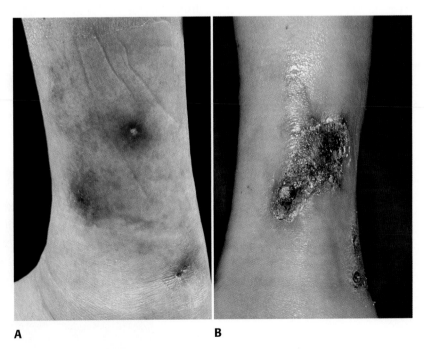

A

B

FIGURE 5.28. Nephrogenic fibrosing dermopathy. A brawny, platelike induration bound down on palpation, with an uneven surface on the legs. This patient had end-stage chronic kidney disease and was on hemodialysis. Gadolinium contrast MRI scans are a risk factor for this condition in patients with chronic kidney disease. (Reproduced with permission from Wolff K, Johnson RA. *Fitzpatrick's Color Atlas & Synopsis of Clinical Dermatology,* 6th ed. New York: McGraw-Hill, 2009, Fig. 17-3.)

FIGURE 5.29. Calciphylaxis. (A) Early stage. An area of mottled erythema is seen with two small ulcerations. The patient has chronic kidney disease and is on hemodialysis. **(B)** A more advanced lesion showing an area of jagged necrosis on the lower leg of a hemodialysis patient with diabetes and chronic kidney disease. The surrounding skin is indurated and represents a platelike subcutaneous mass that is appreciated only on palpation. (Reproduced with permission from Wolff K, Johnson RA. *Fitzpatrick's Color Atlas & Synopsis of Clinical Dermatology,* 6th ed. New York: McGraw-Hill, 2009, Fig. 17-1.)

TABLE 5.6. **Important Mucocutaneous Findings Associated with HIV Infection**

MUCOCUTANEOUS FINDING	ASSOCIATION WITH HIV INFECTION
Acute retroviral syndrome Kaposi's sarcoma Oral hairy leukoplakia (see Figure 5.30) Bacillary angiomatosis Any STD Skin findings of IV drug use	High—serotesting is always indicated.
Herpes zoster Molluscum contagiosum—multiple facial in an adult (see Figure 5.31) Candidiasis—oropharyngeal, esophageal, or recurrent vulvovaginal	Moderate—serotesting may be indicated.
Generalized lymphadenopathy Seborrheic dermatitis Aphthous ulcers (recurrent, refractory to therapy) (see Figure 5.32)	Possible—serotesting may be indicated.

(Adapted with permission from Wolff K, Johnson RA. *Fitzpatrick's Color Atlas & Synopsis of Clinical Dermatology*, 6th ed. New York: McGraw-Hill, 2009, Table 31-2.)

- **Pruritus:** Can be severe, leading to lichen simplex chronicus (hyperpigmented, leathery plaques) or prurigo nodularis (hard, keratotic nodules) from chronic rubbing and scratching.
- **Uremic frost:** Very rare.
- **Xerosis:** Dry skin.

HIV DISEASE

In HIV-infected patients, **seborrheic dermatitis** is the **most common** cutaneous condition, usually developing early and increasing in severity with de-

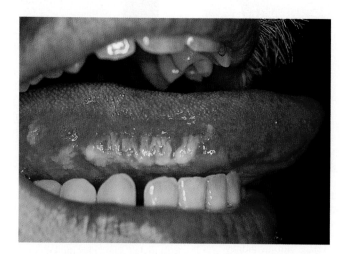

FIGURE 5.30. **Oral hairy leukoplakia.** White plaques with vertical corrugations are seen on the inferolateral aspect of the tongue. The lesions are fixed, unlike those of thrush, which can be brushed off with a gauze pad. The condition is pathognomonic for HIV infection. (Reproduced with permission from Wolff K et al. *Fitzpatrick's Dermatology in General Medicine,* 7th ed. New York: McGraw-Hill, 2008, Fig. 198-5.)

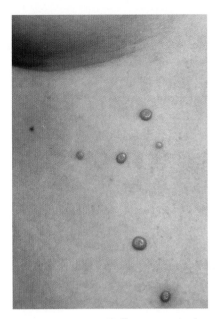

FIGURE 5.31. Molluscum contagiosum. Note the umbilicated center. The condition is more common among HIV-infected patients. (Reproduced with permission from Wolff K et al. *Fitzpatrick's Dermatology in General Medicine,* 7th ed. New York: McGraw-Hill, 2008, Fig. 195-12A.)

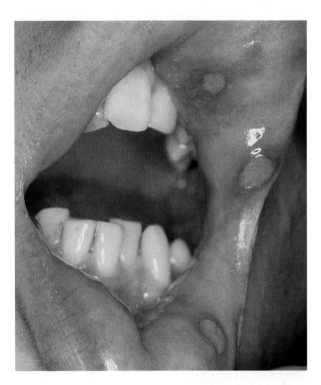

FIGURE 5.32. Aphthous ulcers. Multiple painful, gray-based ulcers with erythematous halos are seen on the labial mucosa. (Reproduced with permission from Wolff K, Johnson RA. *Fitzpatrick's Color Atlas & Synopsis of Clinical Dermatology,* 6th ed. New York: McGraw-Hill, 2009, Fig. 34-8.)

creasing CD4 counts. Common mucocutaneous findings and skin disorders associated with HIV are outlined in Tables 5.6 and 5.7 and in the sections that follow.

TABLE 5.7. Common Skin Disorders Found in HIV-Infected Patients

CD4 > 200	CD4 < 200	CD4 < 50
Seborrheic dermatitis	**Infection:**	**Unusual opportunistic infections:**
Psoriasis	■ Chronic HSV	■ Chronic HSV
Reiter's syndrome	■ Molluscum contagiosum	■ Refractory molluscum contagiosum
Atopic dermatitis	■ Bacillary angiomatosis	■ Chronic VZV
Herpes zoster	■ Systemic fungal infection	■ Atypical mycobacteria
Rosacea	■ Mycobacterial infection	■ Crusted scabies
Oral hairy leukoplakia	■ KS	■ KS
Warts	**Inflammatory:**	
S aureus folliculitis	■ Eosinophilic folliculitis	
Mucocutaneous candidiasis	■ Drug reactions	
KS	■ Photodermatitis	
	■ Prurigo nodularis	

Kaposi's Sarcoma (KS)

> A 40-year-old man with a five-year history of HIV (last CD4 count 400/µL; HIV RNA viral load 20,000–30,000 copies/mL) presents with a new lesion on his left arm that he first noticed a month ago. He has never received antiretroviral therapy and has been asymptomatic until now. Exam reveals a small, raised, nontender, violaceous lesion on his left arm. Labs show no significant change in his CD4 count or in his HIV RNA. CBC, chemistry, LFTs, and CXR are all normal. Excisional biopsy of the lesion shows spindle cells and other features consistent with KS. What is the most appropriate treatment?
>
> Start highly active antiretroviral therapy (HAART) and defer systemic chemotherapy unless visceral or extensive skin involvement develops. This patient does not have extensive cutaneous or mucosal disease or visceral (lung or GI tract) involvement, so systemic chemotherapy is not needed at this time. However, KS is an AIDS-related complication, so HAART should be started immediately.

A **vascular** neoplasm linked to infection with **HHV-8. Often confused with bacillary angiomatosis,** the skin lesions of *Bartonella* infection. KS almost exclusively affects men who have sex with men.

Symptoms/Exam

- Presents with asymptomatic mucocutaneous lesions that may bleed easily or ulcerate and cause pain.
- Less commonly involves the respiratory tract (nodules or hemoptysis) or the GI tract (GI bleed).

Diagnosis

Diagnosed by skin biopsy of characteristic lesions (see Figure 5.33).

Treatment

- HAART. KS frequently regresses and sometimes resolves completely when HAART proves successful.
- Local measures include intralesional chemotherapy, irradiation, laser surgery, and excision.

Complications

Larger or ulcerated lesions may bleed, cause functional disturbance, or obstruct lymphatic drainage.

HIV-Associated Lipodystrophy

Lipodystrophy is part of a metabolic syndrome that includes hyperlipidemia, insulin resistance, and type 2 DM. Protease inhibitors are frequently implicated, most commonly **ritonavir/saquinavir,** followed by indinavir, nelfinavir, and the nucleoside analog stavudine. However, lipodystrophy can also occur in HIV-infected patients who are not on protease inhibitors.

KEY FACT

More than 90% of patients with pulmonary KS will have mucocutaneous KS. Inspect the skin and hard palate!

KEY FACT

A new violaceous skin lesion in a patient with HIV is either KS or bacillary angiomatosis.

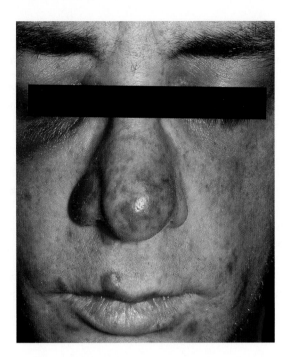

FIGURE 5.33.   HIV-associated Kaposi's sarcoma. Multiple bruise-like purplish and brownish macules, papules, and nodules can be seen. (Reproduced with permission from Wolff K, Johnson RA. *Fitzpatrick's Color Atlas & Synopsis of Clinical Dermatology*, 6th ed. New York: McGraw-Hill, 2009, Fig. 20-19.)

SYMPTOMS/EXAM

Clinical features include the following:

 Facial and peripheral fat wasting.
 Dorsothoracic fat pad hypertrophy.
■ ↑ abdominal girth (**central adiposity**) 2° to accumulation of intra-abdominal fat.

TREATMENT

Substitution of a non–protease inhibitor may be beneficial.

Autoimmune Diseases with Prominent Cutaneous Features

Table 5.8 lists the dermatologic manifestations of common autoimmune disorders, including SLE, dermatomyositis, and scleroderma.

TABLE 5.8. Cutaneous Manifestations of Autoimmune Diseases

DISORDER	CUTANEOUS MANIFESTATIONS	SYSTEMIC ASSOCIATIONS
SLE	**Acute cutaneous:** Malar ("butterfly") rash (see Figure 5.34); photodistribution. **Other:** Discoid plaques, periungual telangiectasias, alopecia, lupus panniculitis.	See the Rheumatology chapter for details on the diagnosis and management of SLE.
Dermatomyositis	Heliotrope rash (a violaceous rash over the eyelids) is nearly pathognomonic. Gottron's papules (flat-topped violaceous papules) over bony prominences, especially the MCP joints. "Shawl sign" (erythema over the upper back and chest).	↑ **risk of malignancy (ovary; other solid tumors [breast, lung, stomach, colon, uterus]).**
Scleroderma	**Extremities:** Raynaud's phenomenon, sclerodactyly, periungual telangiectasias, sclerosis, calcinosis (see Figure 5.35). **Face:** Telangiectasias; masklike facies. **Other:** Cutaneous calcification.	See the Rheumatology chapter for a discussion of the systemic manifestations of scleroderma.
Morphea (localized scleroderma of unknown etiology)	Asymptomatic, with violaceous and then ivory-colored plaques.	Associated with *Borrelia burgdorferi* infection in Europe only; also occurs post–radiation therapy.

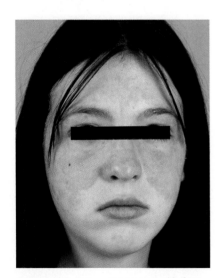

FIGURE 5.34. Acute systemic lupus erythematosus. A typical "malar rash" is seen with red, sharply defined erythema in a "butterfly" pattern on the face. (Reproduced with permission from Wolff K et al. *Fitzpatrick's Color Atlas & Synopsis of Clinical Dermatology,* 5th ed. New York: McGraw-Hill, 2005: 385.)

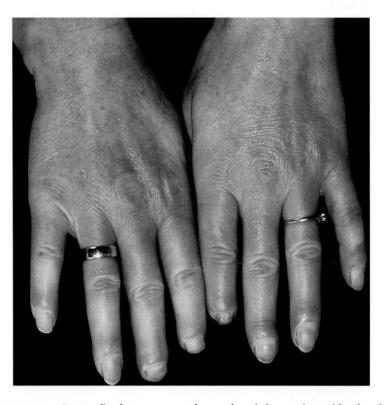

FIGURE 5.35. Raynaud's phenomenon and acrosclerosis in a patient with scleroderma. (Reproduced with permission from Wolff K et al. *Fitzpatrick's Color Atlas & Synopsis of Clinical Dermatology,* 5th ed. New York: McGraw-Hill, 2005: 399.)

Cutaneous Reaction Patterns

ERYTHEMA NODOSUM

An immunologic reaction in the panniculus (fat) triggered by infection, medications, and benign and malignant systemic diseases. The cause is often undetermined. See Table 5.9 for etiologies.

TABLE 5.9. Cutaneous Reaction Patterns and Their Associated Diseases

REACTION PATTERN	DEFINITION	SIGNS AND SYMPTOMS	ASSOCIATED DISEASES
Erythema nodosum	Inflammatory/ immunologic reaction pattern of the panniculus.	**Tender bumps on the anterior shins.** Appear as red, ill-defined erythematous lesions, but palpated as deep-seated nodules. Fever, malaise, arthralgias (50%).	**Infection:** ▪ Streptococcal ▪ TB ▪ Other bacteria, fungi, viruses **Medications:** ▪ Sulfonamides ▪ **OCPs** **Other:** ▪ **Sarcoidosis** (Löfgren's syndrome) ▪ Ulcerative colitis > Crohn's disease ▪ Leukemia ▪ Behçet's disease
Urticaria		Transient wheals, pruritus, dermatographism (see Figure 5.36).	**Acute urticaria** (< 30 days): ▪ **Medications** ▪ Foods ▪ Parasites ▪ Arthropod bites **Chronic urticaria** (> 30 days): ▪ **Idiopathic (80%)** ▪ Autoimmune ▪ Malignancy
Erythema multiforme (EM)	Reaction pattern of dermal blood vessels and 2° epidermal changes.	**Target lesion** (see Figure 5.37): ▪ Palms and soles, face, genitals ▪ Bilateral, symmetric **EM minor:** ▪ Little or no mucous membrane involvement ▪ No systemic symptoms **EM major:** ▪ ⊕ **Nikolsky's sign** ▪ Systemic (pulmonary, eyes)	**Recurrent EM minor:** ▪ **HSV (the cause in 90% of cases)** **EM major:** ▪ Medications (sulfonamides, NSAIDs, anticonvulsants [phenytoin]) ▪ *Mycoplasma pneumoniae* **Idiopathic: 50%**

SYMPTOMS/EXAM

- Presents with erythematous, tender nodules that are most commonly located on the anterior shins.
- Fever, malaise, and arthralgias are seen with onset of new lesions.

TREATMENT

- Spontaneous resolution is seen in 3–6 weeks without scarring.
- NSAIDs, prednisone, potassium iodide.

URTICARIA

A 20-year-old man has episodes of large, raised red welts and intense itching all over his body that last for 48 hours and then disappear. He has had about three such episodes a week for the past two months with no obvious trigger and has derived no relief from hydroxyzine and fexofenadine. His temperature is 37.9°C (100.3°F), and exam reveals discrete, dark wheal-and-flare lesions consistent with urticaria on both arms and legs and on his trunk and back. Some lesions look like purpura. UA shows erythrocytes and erythrocyte casts. What measure will most likely establish the diagnosis?

A skin biopsy, as urticaria that does not respond to usual treatment should prompt a workup for urticarial vasculitis, including ESR, CBC, and skin biopsy from the edge of the wheal. Histopathologic evidence of vascular damage, nuclear debris, or erythrocyte extravasation is diagnostic.

A vascular reaction of the skin characterized by localized cutaneous edema (wheals) and severe itching or stinging. It is categorized as acute (resolution within six weeks of onset) and chronic (daily episodes lasting > 6 weeks.) Etiologies are numerous, and the **cause is often undetermined.** For common etiologies, see Table 5.9.

SYMPTOMS/EXAM

Presents with erythematous, pruritic wheals that remain for < 24 hours (see Figure 5.36). Individual lesions that persist **for > 24 hours suggest urticarial vasculitis** and require a biopsy.

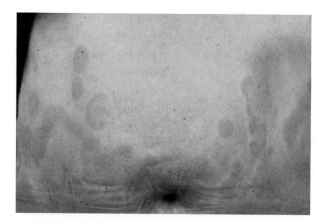

FIGURE 5.36. Urticaria. Pruritic wheals have a white to light pink color centrally and are accompanied by peripheral erythema. (Reproduced with permission from Wolff K et al. *Fitzpatrick's Color Atlas & Synopsis of Clinical Dermatology,* 5th ed. New York: McGraw-Hill, 2005: 363.)

TREATMENT

Antihistamines are the mainstay of treatment.

COMPLICATIONS

Urticarial vasculitis, a form of leukocytoclastic vasculitis that is often limited to the skin. Most cases are idiopathic, but the condition can also be medication induced, related to rheumatic diseases such as SLE, or caused by viral infection. Treatment is dictated by the underlying cause; if no cause can be identified, a trial of anti-inflammatory or immunomodulating medications is indicated.

ERYTHEMA MULTIFORME (EM)

Also known as erythema multiforme minor or herpes simplex–associated erythema multiforme (HAEM), EM is an immunologic reaction pattern of dermal blood vessels with 2° epidermal change. Ninety percent of cases of EM minor are associated with HSV infection. EM major, or Stevens-Johnson syndrome, is more commonly caused by *Mycoplasma pneumoniae* or medications (eg, sulfonamides, NSAIDs, anticonvulsants).

SYMPTOMS/EXAM

- Target lesions present with a dusky-purple central zone (or, later, with a crust, blister, or erosion) with an outer concentric red zone (see Figure 5.37).
- Symmetric and bilateral involvement of the **palms, soles,** faces, and genitalia is seen.
- Subtypes can be further distinguished as follows:
  - **EM minor:** No mucosal involvement; no systemic symptoms.
  - **EM major:** Presents with bullae; involves two mucosal surfaces; shows systemic involvement of the eyes and lungs.

KEY FACT

Ninety percent of cases of EM minor are due to HSV infection. By contrast, EM major is more frequently due to medications and to *Mycoplasma* infection.

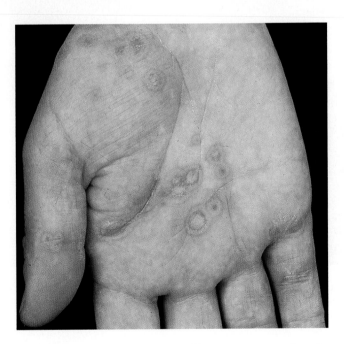

FIGURE 5.37. **Erythema multiforme.** Targetoid lesions are seen on the palms. (Reproduced with permission from Wolff K et al. *Fitzpatrick's Dermatology in General Medicine,* 7th ed. New York: McGraw-Hill, 2008, Fig. 38-2.)

TREATMENT

- **EM minor:** Self-limited; consider acyclovir prophylaxis for recurrent episodes.
- **EM major:** Hospitalization (often to a burn unit in light of fluid/electrolyte imbalances); stop the offending drug. Supportive care, ophthalmology consult, and physical therapy.

BLISTERING DISORDERS

Bullous pemphigoid and **pemphigus vulgaris** are **autoimmune blistering disorders** of the skin and mucous membranes resulting from the loss of epidermal cell-to-cell adhesion (see Figures 5.38 and 5.39). Table 5.10 distinguishes these disorders in terms of their clinical presentation.

DIAGNOSIS

- Submit skin biopsy for histology and direct immunofluorescence.
- In bullous pemphigoid, indirect immunofluorescence reveals circulating anti–basement membrane antibodies in the sera of 70% of patients.

TREATMENT

Topical high-potency steroids for localized disease; prednisone +/– other immunosuppressants for diffuse disease.

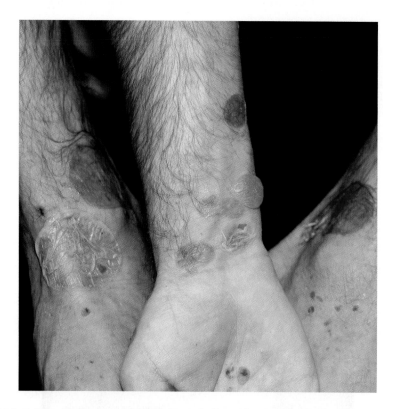

FIGURE 5.38. **Bullous pemphigoid.** Tense bullae with serous fluid are seen. (Reproduced with permission from Wolff K, Johnson RA. *Fitzpatrick's Color Atlas & Synopsis of Clinical Dermatology*, 6th ed. New York: McGraw-Hill, 2009, Fig. 6e-BP-2.)

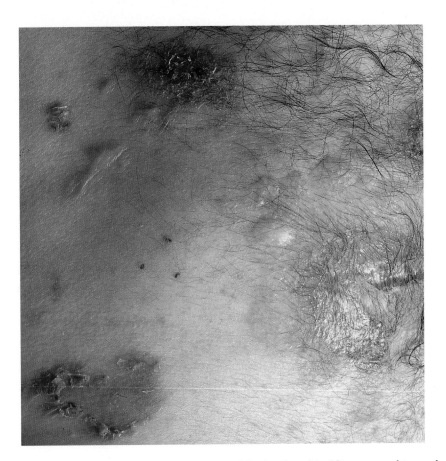

FIGURE 5.39. **Pemphigus vulgaris.** Because of the fragility of the blisters, pemphigus vulgaris presents as erosions. (Reproduced with permission from Wolff K et al. *Fitzpatrick's Color Atlas & Synopsis of Clinical Dermatology,* 5th ed. New York: McGraw-Hill, 2005: 104.)

TABLE 5.10. Bullous Pemphigoid vs. Pemphigus Vulgaris

	BULLOUS PEMPHIGOID	**PEMPHIGUS VULGARIS**
Site of blistering	Subepidermal.	Intraepidermal.
Epidemiology	Age > 60. The most common autoimmune blistering disease.	Age 40–60.
Pruritus	Severe.	Not prominent.
Nikolsky's sign (superficial separation of skin with pressure)	⊖	⊕
Oral mucosal lesions	Minority (< 30%).	Majority (> 50%).
Blisters and bullae	Intact, tense (see Figure 5.38).	Rupture easily; flaccid (see Figure 5.39).
Subtypes	None.	Drug induced (penicillamine and ACEIs), paraneoplastic.

Cutaneous Drug Reactions

In the **hospital**, two-thirds of all cutaneous reactions are due to **penicillins/β-lactams, sulfonamides,** and **blood products. In ambulatory settings, antibiotics, NSAIDs,** and **anticonvulsants** are the most common culprits. The most frequent drug eruptions are as follows:

- **Morbilliform** (30–50% of cases).
- **Fixed.**
- **Urticaria** +/– angioedema.

See Tables 5.11 and 5.12 and Figures 5.40 and 5.41 for the pathophysiology and clinical patterns of various drug eruptions.

DIAGNOSIS

- Clinical features favoring medication as a cause of skin reactions include the following:
  - Previous experience with a given drug.
  - Lack of alternative explanations (eg, worsening of preexisting disease, infection).
  - **Timing:** Most drug reactions occur **within two weeks. Hypersensitivity reactions may be delayed up to eight weeks.**
  - **Discontinuation:** Reaction should abate within three weeks.
  - **Rechallenge:** Allows for a definitive diagnosis, although usually impractical.

TABLE 5.11. Nonimmunologic Drug Reactions

MECHANISM	EXAMPLE
Expected adverse effects	Chemotherapy-induced alopecia.
Ecologic disturbance	Candidiasis and antibiotics.
Overdosage	Warfarin purpura.
Drug interaction	Barbiturates and warfarin (purpura).
Cumulative	Argyria (silver nitrate), antimalarial pigmentation.
Idiosyncratic causes	Drug-induced lupus in response to procainamide.
Altered metabolism	Warfarin necrosis and lack of protein C.
Exacerbation of underlying disorder	Lithium, β-blockers, ASA, ibuprofen, amoxicillin, antimalarials, interferons (psoriasis).
Phototoxicity	↑ sensitivity to sun caused by toxic photoproducts of different drugs (tetracyclines).
Direct release of mast cell mediators	ASA, NSAIDs, radiographic contrast material.
Jarisch-Herxheimer phenomenon	Penicillin therapy for syphilis; antifungal therapy for dermatophyte. Manifested by fever, chills, headache, myalgias, and exacerbation of skin lesions.

(Adapted with permission from Kerdel FA, Jimenez-Acosta F. *Dermatology: Just the Facts.* New York: McGraw-Hill, 2003: 36.)

TABLE 5.12. **Clinical Features of Severe Cutaneous Reactions Often Induced by Drugs**

DIAGNOSIS	TYPICAL SKIN LESIONS	COMMON SIGNS AND SYMPTOMS	OTHER CAUSES NOT RELATED TO MEDICATIONS	DRUGS MOST OFTEN IMPLICATED
Stevens-Johnson syndrome (SJS)	Small blisters on dusky purpuric macules or atypical targets (see Figure 5.40). Rare areas of confluence. Detachment of ≤ 10% of body surface area.	Some 10–30% present with fever.	*Mycoplasma* or HSV (rare).	NSAIDs, sulfa drugs, antiepileptics (phenytoin, carbamazepine), penicillin, allopurinol.
Toxic epidermal necrolysis (TEN)	Individual lesions are like those seen in SJS (see Figure 5.41).	Fever is nearly universal. "Acute skin failure"; leukopenia. Confluent erythema. The outer layer of the epidermis readily separates from the basal layer with lateral pressure **(Nikolsky's sign).** Large sheet of necrotic epidermis. Detachment of > 30% of body surface area.	Viral infections, immunization, chemicals, *Mycoplasma* pneumonia.	Same as above.
Anticonvulsant hypersensitivity syndrome	Severe exanthem (may become purpuric). Exfoliative dermatitis.	Some 30–50% of cases present with fever, lymphadenopathy, **hepatitis, nephritis,** and **eosinophilia.**	Cutaneous lymphoma.	Anticonvulsants.
Anticoagulant-induced necrosis	Purpura and necrosis.	Pain in affected areas.	DIC.	Warfarin, especially in the setting of low protein C or S.
Angioedema	Urticaria or swelling of the central part of the face.	Respiratory distress, cardiovascular collapse.	Insect stings, foods.	NSAIDs, ACEIs, penicillin.

(Adapted with permission from Kasper DL et al. *Harrison's Principles of Internal Medicine,* 16th ed. New York: McGraw-Hill, 2005: 323.)

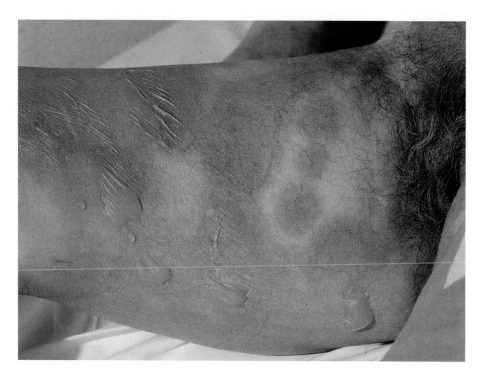

FIGURE 5.40. **Stevens-Johnson syndrome.** Generalized eruption of initially targetlike lesions that become confluent, brightly erythematous, and bullous. (Reproduced with permission from Wolff K et al. *Fitzpatrick's Color Atlas & Synopsis of Clinical Dermatology,* 5th ed. New York: McGraw-Hill, 2005: 145.)

- Consider drug levels for dose-dependent reactions.
- Skin biopsy is helpful in determining the reaction pattern but cannot identify the specific agent.
- Peripheral **eosinophilia** is suggestive of drug sensitivity.

TREATMENT

The treatment of drug reactions is dependent on the cause.

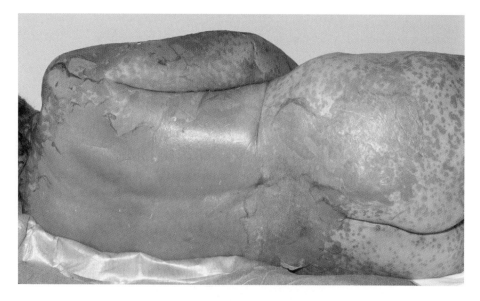

FIGURE 5.41. **Toxic epidermal necrolysis.** Bulla formation with rapid desquamation. (Reproduced with permission from Wolff K et al. *Fitzpatrick's Color Atlas & Synopsis of Clinical Dermatology,* 5th ed. New York: McGraw-Hill, 2005: 147.)

Cutaneous Oncology

MELANOMA

A malignancy of melanocytes that may occur on any skin or mucosal surface. It is the **sixth most common cancer** in the United States. Risk factors are expressed in the mnemonic **MMRISK.**

SYMPTOMS

- Look for a **changing mole** (see the mnemonic "the ABCDEs").
- **Superficial spreading** malignant melanomas are most common (responsible for 70% of all melanomas in Caucasians), arising on sun-exposed regions of older patients (see Figure 5.42).

EXAM

Physical findings are expressed in the mnemonic "**the ABCDEs.**"

DIAGNOSIS

- **Tumor thickness** (Breslow's classification) and lymph node status are the most important prognostic factors. Melanomas < **1 mm** in thickness are considered **lower risk,** and **staging workup is typically not indicated in these cases.** Regional spread is stage III and metastasis is stage IV.
- Additional significant prognostic indicators include site, specific histologic features, and gender (men are at higher risk than women).

TREATMENT

Wide reexcision with appropriate margins. Sentinel lymph node biopsy is recommended for malignant melanomas > 1 mm thick and is also essential in medical decision making with regard to adjuvant therapy.

COMPLICATIONS

Metastasis usually occurs in the following sequence: local recurrence, regional lymph nodes, distant metastasis (liver, lung, bone, brain). Five-year survival rates with lymph node involvement and distant metastasis are 30% and 10%, respectively.

BASAL CELL CARCINOMA (BCC)

Represents **80% of all skin cancers.** Lesions occur in sun-exposed areas. The mean age at diagnosis is 62 years.

SYMPTOMS/EXAM

- **Head and neck:** Presents with papules or nodules with telangiectasias and a "pearly" or translucent quality. A central erosion or crust (noduloulcerative type) is often seen (see Figure 5.43).
- **Chest, back, and extremities:** A scaly erythematous plaque (superficial type) is seen that may resemble a plaque of eczema.

DIAGNOSIS

Shave biopsy.

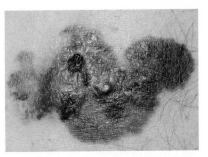

FIGURE 5.42.   Superficial spreading melanoma. A highly characteristic lesion is seen with an irregular pigmentary pattern and scalloped borders. (Reproduced with permission from Wolff K et al. *Fitzpatrick's Color Atlas & Synopsis of Clinical Dermatology,* 5th ed. New York: McGraw-Hill, 2005: 318.)

MNEMONIC

Malignant melanoma risk—

MMRISK

Moles: atypical
Moles: total number > 50
Red hair and freckling
Inability to tan: skin phototypes I and II
Severe sunburn, especially in childhood
Kindred: first-degree relative

MNEMONIC

Melanoma—

The ABCDEs

Asymmetry
Borders: irregular
Color: variegated
Diameter > 6 mm
Evolution: lesion changes over time

KEY FACT

Patients with numerous atypical nevi (atypical nevus syndrome or dysplastic nevus syndrome) and with two first-degree relatives with a history of melanoma have a lifetime risk of melanoma approaching 100%.

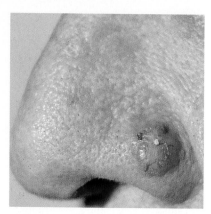

FIGURE 5.43. Nodular basal cell carcinoma. Note the smooth, pearly nodule with telangiectasias. (Reproduced with permission from Wolff K et al. *Fitzpatrick's Color Atlas & Synopsis of Clinical Dermatology,* 5th ed. New York: McGraw-Hill, 2005: 283.)

KEY FACT

Avoiding direct sunlight, especially during peak hours, is associated with a ↓ risk for squamous cell carcinoma and malignant melanoma.

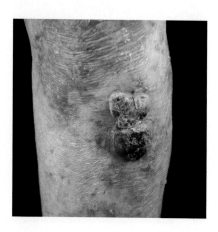

FIGURE 5.44. Squamous cell carcinoma. A hyperkeratotic nodule with ulceration. (Reproduced with permission from Wolff K et al. *Fitzpatrick's Color Atlas & Synopsis of Clinical Dermatology,* 5th ed. New York: McGraw-Hill, 2005: 279.)

TREATMENT

Treatment is dependent on the individual tumor and on patient characteristics. Both surgical and nonsurgical techniques are employed. Sun avoidance and patient education are key components of management.

COMPLICATIONS

Metastatic spread is uncommon (< 0.1%).

SQUAMOUS CELL CARCINOMA (SCC)

Represents 20% of all skin cancers; typically affects patients > 55 years of age. SCC in situ, also known as Bowen's disease, is confined to the epidermis; invasive SCC invades into the dermis. SCCs may arise within **actinic keratoses** or within HPV-induced lesions (see Figure 5.44).

DIAGNOSIS

Skin biopsy.

TREATMENT

- Treatment of invasive disease is primarily **surgical.**
- Prevention with sun avoidance and patient education are key components of disease management.

COMPLICATIONS

The overall five-year recurrence and metastatic rates are 8% and 5%, respectively.

CUTANEOUS T-CELL LYMPHOMA (CTCL)

Also known as mycosis fungoides, CTCL is an indolent malignancy of mature CD4 helper T lymphocytes. Average age of onset is 50 years (range 5–70); men are affected twice as often as women. CTCL is divided into patch, plaque, and tumor stages (see Figure 5.45).

SYMPTOMS/EXAM

- Presents with scaly, **pruritic, erythematous patches and plaques** most commonly located in a "bathing trunk" distribution.
- Erythroderma with Sézary syndrome is rare.

TREATMENT

Topical corticosteroids, UV light, or nitrogen mustard for patch/plaque stages; systemic therapy for nonresponsive or more advanced disease.

COMPLICATIONS

Sézary syndrome is the leukemic form of CTCL and consists of erythroderma, lymphadenopathy, and circulating Sézary cells. Without therapy, its course is progressive, and patients succumb to opportunistic infections. Therapy includes treatment for CTCL as well as supportive measures for erythroderma.

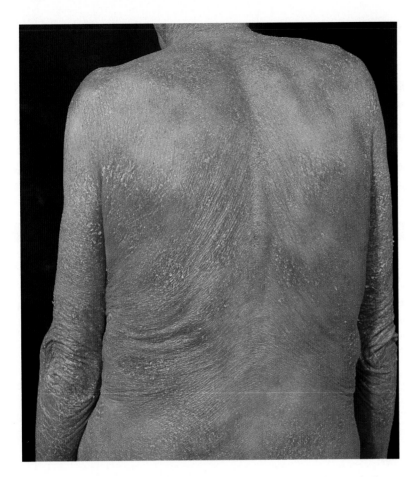

FIGURE 5.45. **Cutaneous T-cell lymphoma.** Note the universal erythema, thickening, and scaling. (Reproduced with permission from Wolff K, Johnson RA. *Fitzpatrick's Color Atlas & Synopsis of Clinical Dermatology,* 6th ed. New York: McGraw-Hill, 2009, Fig. 8-3.)

Miscellaneous

PIGMENTARY DISORDERS

Tables 5.13 and 5.14 outline disorders associated with hyper- and hypopigmentation.

TABLE 5.13.   **Disorders of Hyperpigmentation**

DISORDER	ASSOCIATED DISEASE
Pigmented nevi, freckles, lentigines	Peutz-Jeghers syndrome (intestinal polyps with oral mucosa and cutaneous hyperpigmented freckles).
Melasma	Estrogen effect; often seen in pregnancy.
Café-au-lait spots, axillary freckling	Neurofibromatosis.

TABLE 5.14. **Disorders of Hypopigmentation**

DISORDER	ASSOCIATED DISEASE
Vitiligo (melanocytes destroyed) (see Figure 5.46)	Hypothyroidism, hyperthyroidism, pernicious anemia, DM, Addison's disease.
Albinism	The eye and vision are often affected.
Piebaldism	Autosomal dominant; neurologic dysfunction.

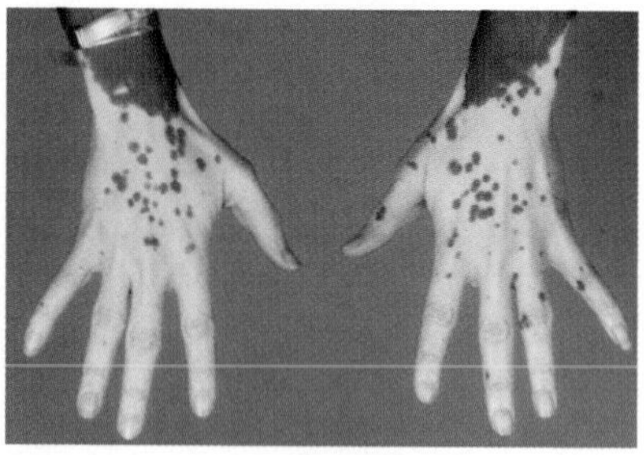

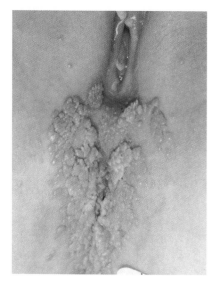

FIGURE 5.46. **Vitiligo.** Note the typical acral distribution demonstrating striking cutaneous depigmentation as a result of loss of melanocytes. (Reproduced with permission from Fauci AS et al. *Harrison's Principles of Internal Medicine,* 17th ed. New York: McGraw-Hill, 2008, Fig. 52-12.)

VERRUCA AND CONDYLOMA

HPV causes clinical lesions that vary according to subtype. More than 150 types of HPV have been identified.

- **Verruca vulgaris,** the common wart (70% of all warts), occurs primarily on the extremities.
- **Condylomata acuminata,** warts in the **anogenital** region (see Figure 5.47), are the most commonly diagnosed STD.
  - Genital HPV types (**types 16 and 18**) play an important role in the malignant transformation of benign verrucae into **cervical and anogenital cancer.**
  - ↑ incidence and more widespread disease are seen in **immunocompromised** patients.

TREATMENT

- In immunocompetent patients, lesions usually **resolve spontaneously** over 1–2 years.
- Treatment modalities include mechanical destruction (cryotherapy, laser therapy) or stimulation of the immune system (topical imiquimod; application of sensitizing agents).

COMPLICATIONS

Malignant transformation to SCC may occur in certain subtypes.

FIGURE 5.47. **Human papillomavirus.** Anogenital warts are lesions produced by human papillomavirus and in this patient are seen as multiple verrucous papules coalescing into plaques. (Reproduced with permission from Fauci AS et al. *Harrison's Principles of Internal Medicine,* 17th ed. New York: McGraw-Hill, 2008, Fig. 178-1.)

CHAPTER 6

Endocrinology

Christina A. Lee, MD
Diana M. Antoniucci, MD, MAS
Karen Earle, MD
Melissa Weinberg, MD

Pituitary and Hypothalamic Disorders

Under hypothalamic regulation, the anterior pituitary produces and releases ACTH, TSH, FSH, LH, GH, and prolactin (see Figure 6.1). The posterior pituitary stores and releases ADH and oxytocin.

PITUITARY TUMORS

 A 63-year-old man on warfarin for atrial fibrillation (AF) presents to the ER with an excruciating headache, nausea, vomiting, vertigo, and altered mental status. He has a history of a pituitary adenoma. On exam, he is found to have meningismus. His BP is 65/35 mm Hg. What is the most likely diagnosis?

While you should rule out a hemorrhagic stroke and ruptured aneurysm, pituitary apoplexy must also be considered. Pituitary apoplexy is a complication that occurs when a pituitary mass spontaneously hemorrhages or outgrows its blood supply, leading to panhypopituitarism. CT/MRI may show a high-density mass in the sella. Corticosteroids are required to treat acute adrenal insufficiency (AI), which usually manifests as hypotension.

Microadenomas are < 1 cm; **macroadenomas** are > 1 cm. The risk of panhypopituitarism and visual loss ↑ with tumor size.

SYMPTOMS/EXAM

- **Neurologic symptoms:** Headache; visual field cuts, especially "tunnel vision"; diplopia.

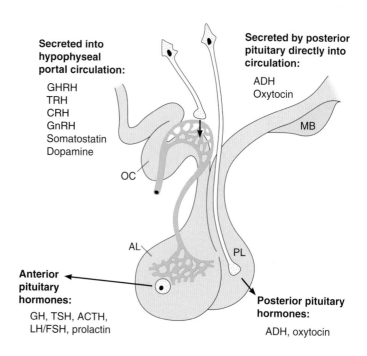

Secreted into hypophyseal portal circulation:

GHRH
TRH
CRH
GnRH
Somatostatin
Dopamine

Secreted by posterior pituitary directly into circulation:

ADH
Oxytocin

MB

OC

AL

PL

Anterior pituitary hormones:

GH, TSH, ACTH, LH/FSH, prolactin

Posterior pituitary hormones:

ADH, oxytocin

FIGURE 6.1. Secretion of hypothalamic and pituitary hormones. AL, anterior lobe; MB, mammillary bodies; OC, optic chiasm; PL, posterior lobe. (Adapted with permission from Gardner DG, Shoback D. *Greenspan's Basic & Clinical Endocrinology,* 8th ed. New York: McGraw-Hill, 2007: 106.)

TABLE 6.1.   Anterior Pituitary Hormones and Their Function

HORMONE	INCREASED BY	DECREASED BY	EXCESS	DEFICIENCY	TARGET ORGAN
ACTH	CRH, stress.	High cortisol.	Cushing's syndrome.	AI.	Adrenals.
TSH	TRH.	High T_4 and/or T_3.	Hyperthyroidism.	Hypothyroidism.	Thyroid.
LH/FSH	GnRH.	Gonadal sex steroids.		Hypogonadism.	Gonads.
GH	GHRH, hypoglycemia, dopamine.	Somatostatin.	Acromegaly.	Poor sense of well-being.	Multiple.
Prolactin	Pregnancy, nursing, TRH, stress.	Dopamine.	Galactorrhea, hypogonadism.	Inability to lactate.	Breasts.

- **Hormonal excess or deficiency:** See Tables 6.1 and 6.2.
- **Incidental discovery on imaging studies:** Up to 10% of the general population have pituitary incidentalomas.

DIFFERENTIAL

See Table 6.3.

DIAGNOSIS

- **Labs:** If the H&P or imaging is suggestive of tumor, check TSH, free T_4, prolactin, LH, FSH, IGF-1, and testosterone (in men) or estradiol (in women with amenorrhea) to assess for hormonal excess or deficiency. To check for AI, perform an early-morning cortisol or cosyntropin (Cortrosyn) stimulation test. To check for cortisol excess, perform a dexamethasone suppression test.
- **Pituitary imaging:** Order a **sellar-specific MRI** (see Figure 6.2). **A standard brain MRI may miss these small tumors!**
- **Formal visual field testing:** For macroadenomas or tumors compressing the optic chiasm.

TREATMENT

- **Medical:** Some tumors shrink with hormonal manipulation. Prolactinomas are treated primarily with dopamine agonists (eg, bromocriptine, cabergoline).
- **Surgical:** The **transsphenoidal** approach is successful in approximately 90% of patients with microadenomas.
- **Radiation:** Conventional radiotherapy or gamma-knife radiosurgery can be used as adjunctive treatment after surgery or in combination with medical treatment. Associated with a high risk of hypopituitarism.

> **KEY FACT**
>
> In acute 2° AI (eg, pituitary apoplexy), a cosyntropin stimulation test result is likely to be inappropriately "normal" because the adrenal glands have not had time to atrophy. So if suspicion for AI is high, treat with steroids!

TABLE 6.2.   Posterior Pituitary Hormones and Their Function

HORMONE	INCREASED BY	DECREASED BY	EXCESS	DEFICIENCY	TARGET ORGAN
ADH	↑ osmolality; hypovolemia.	↓ osmolality.	SIADH.	Diabetes insipidus (DI).	Kidneys, cardiovascular system.
Oxytocin	Distention of the uterus, cervix, and vagina; nipple stimulation. Estrogen enhances action.			Not required for parturition.	Uterus, breasts (causes contraction of smooth muscle).

TABLE 6.3.   **Differential Diagnosis of Sellar Lesions**

LESION	EXAMPLES
Pituitary adenoma	**Prolactinoma:** The most common pituitary microadenoma. **GH secreting:** Often very large. **Nonfunctioning:** One-third of all pituitary tumors; the most common macroadenoma. **ACTH secreting:** The most common cause of Cushing's syndrome. **TSH secreting:** Rare.
Physiologic enlargement of the pituitary gland	Hyperplasia due to pregnancy, 1° hypothyroidism, or 1° hypogonadism.
1° malignancies	Germ cell tumor, sarcoma, lymphoma, pituitary carcinoma.
Metastases	Breast cancer, lung cancer.
Cysts	Rathke's cleft, arachnoid, dermoid.
Infections in immunocompromised patients	Abscess, tuberculoma.
Other	Craniopharyngioma, meningioma, lymphocytic hypophysitis (autoimmune destruction of the pituitary, often postpartum).

KEY FACT

Sellar masses cause DI (by affecting posterior pituitary function) only when they are large and invade the suprasellar space. 1° pituitary tumors rarely cause DI.

COMPLICATIONS

- **Hypopituitarism:** See below.
- **Apoplexy:** Acute, spontaneous hemorrhagic pituitary infarction. A **neurosurgical emergency.** Treat with corticosteroids +/– transsphenoidal decompression.
- **DI or SIADH** (especially postoperatively; patients may recover).
- **Visual field defects.**

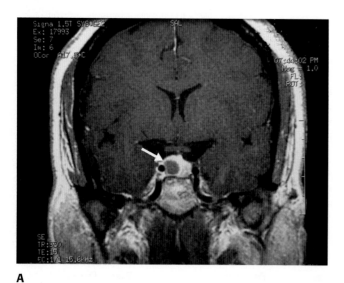
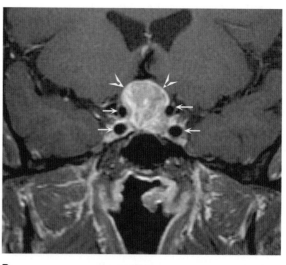

A   **B**

FIGURE 6.2.   **Pituitary adenomas.** Coronal gadolinium-enhanced MR images demonstrating **(A)** a microadenoma (arrow), which enhances less than the adjacent pituitary tissue, and **(B)** a pituitary macroadenoma (arrowheads) extending superiorly from the sella turcica to the suprasellar region. Arrows denote the internal carotid arteries. (Image A reproduced with permission from Schorge JO et al. *Williams Gynecology.* New York: McGraw-Hill, 2008, Fig. 15-8A. Image B reproduced with permission from Fauci AS et al. *Harrison's Principles of Internal Medicine,* 17th ed. New York: McGraw-Hill, 2008, Fig. 333-4.)

Prolactinoma

The **most common type of pituitary tumor.** The majority of lesions are microadenomas (< 1 cm).

SYMPTOMS/EXAM

- **Women:** Galactorrhea; amenorrhea; oligomenorrhea with **anovulation and infertility in 90% of cases.**
- **Men:** Impotence, ↓ libido, galactorrhea (very rare).
- **Both:** Headache, visual field cuts, hypopituitarism.

DIFFERENTIAL

See Table 6.4.

DIAGNOSIS

- **Labs:** ↑ prolactin with normal TFTs and a ⊖ **pregnancy test.**
- **Imaging:** Obtain an MRI if prolactin is ↑ in the absence of pregnancy or the medications listed in Table 6.4.

TREATMENT

- **Medical:** Dopamine agonists such as **bromocriptine or cabergoline.** Once prolactin is normalized, repeat pituitary MRI to ensure tumor shrinkage.
  - Cabergoline has fewer side effects but is associated with an ↑ risk of cardiac valvular disease.
  - Bromocriptine is preferred for ovulation induction and is likely **safe in pregnancy.**
- **Surgery:** Transsphenoidal resection is curative and is generally used if medical therapy is ineffective.
- **Radiation:** Conventional radiotherapy or gamma-knife radiosurgery may be used if the tumor is refractory to medical and surgical therapy.

KEY FACT

Women typically present with prolactinomas earlier than men because they develop amenorrhea and galactorrhea. Thus, women often have microprolactinomas (< 1 cm) at diagnosis, whereas men have macroprolactinomas.

KEY FACT

Always rule out pregnancy first in a woman presenting with amenorrhea and hyperprolactinemia.

KEY FACT

Prolactinoma is the most common functional pituitary tumor and can usually be treated medically with dopamine agonists (bromocriptine, cabergoline).

TABLE 6.4.   Etiologies of Hyperprolactinemia

| | PATHOLOGIC | | |
PHYSIOLOGIC	ADENOMA/HYPERPLASIA	DRUGS	OTHER DISORDERS
Pregnancy	**Lactotroph adenoma:** Micro- or macroprolactinoma.	Dopamine antagonists **(phenothiazines,** haloperidol, **risperidone,** metoclopramide, reserpine, methyldopa, cocaine).	**Hypothyroidism.** **CKD.**
Nipple stimulation			
Stress	**Lactotroph hyperplasia:** Usually due to disruption of normal dopamine inhibition of prolactin.	**Cimetidine.**	**Hypothalamic or pituitary stalk lesions** (craniopharyngioma of the hypothalamus, infiltrative diseases, other pituitary adenomas).
Exercise		**Verapamil.**	

(Adapted with permission from Gardner DG, Shoback D. *Greenspan's Basic & Clinical Endocrinology,* 8th ed. New York: McGraw-Hill, 2007: 119.)

GROWTH HORMONE (GH) EXCESS

A 60-year-old woman with DM presents for a routine checkup. On review of systems, she reports having headaches, arthralgias, a sensation of "generalized bone growth," and jaw and maxillary enlargement for > 10 years. Exam reveals an ↑ BP along with coarsened features with large hands and feet. What is the most likely diagnosis and management?

Acromegaly from a benign pituitary adenoma. IGF-1 should be ↑. Treatment consists of surgical resection.

Leads to acromegaly when it occurs in adulthood. Etiologies are as follows:

- **Benign pituitary adenoma:** GH-secreting pituitary adenomas are responsible for nearly all cases of acromegaly.
- **Iatrogenic:** Associated with treatment with human GH.
- **Ectopic GH or GHRH:** Extremely rare; seen with lung carcinoma, carcinoid tumors, and pancreatic islet cell tumors.

Symptoms/Exam

- **Almost all patients have soft tissue proliferation (hand/foot/jaw enlargement) and coarsening of facial features.** An ↑ in shoe, ring, or glove size is common.
- Headache and visual loss are direct effects of tumor.
- Additional symptoms are as follows:
    - **Cardiac:** Hypertension, cardiac hypertrophy.
    - **Endocrine:** ↑ insulin resistance with impaired glucose intolerance or overt DM; hypogonadism.
    - **Constitutional:** Heat intolerance, weight gain, fatigue.
    - **GI:** ↑ incidence of colonic polyps and colon cancer (**order a colonoscopy** after diagnosis).

Diagnosis

- **Labs:** Random GH is not helpful. ↑ **IGF-1 levels** are the hallmark.
- **Glucose tolerance test:** An ↑ GH level after a 100-g glucose load is diagnostic of excess GH secretion.
- **Radiology:** Pituitary MRI.

Treatment

- **Surgical:** Transsphenoidal resection is first-line therapy and is usually curative.
- **Medical:** If GH excess persists after surgery, long-acting somatostatin analogs (octreotide and lanreotide) may be added.
- **Radiotherapy:** For patients with inadequate responses to surgical and medical therapy.

Complications

Hypopituitarism, cardiovascular effects (hypertension, CHF, CAD), metabolic effects (type 2 DM), sleep apnea.

KEY FACT

In a patient with coarse facial features and new DM, check IGF-1 (not GH) to rule out acromegaly.

KEY FACT

Do an oral glucose load after the IGF-1 screening test. If GH levels do not drop after an oral glucose load, acromegaly is diagnosed.

KEY FACT

Treat GH-secreting pituitary adenomas with transsphenoidal surgery. If refractory, try medical therapy such as somatostatin analogs.

HYPOPITUITARISM

↓ or absent secretion of one or more pituitary hormones. Etiologies are outlined below.

SYMPTOMS/EXAM

Presentation depends on the particular hormone deficiency. In increasing order of importance, with **ACTH being preserved the longest,** pituitary hormones are lost in the following order:

- **GH deficiency:** May be asymptomatic in adults. Has been associated with ↑ fat mass, bone loss, and cardiovascular risk factors.
- **LH/FSH deficiency:** Hypogonadism. Manifested in men as lack of libido/impotence and in women as irregular menses/amenorrhea.
- **TSH deficiency:** Hypothyroidism.
- **ACTH deficiency:** AI (weakness, nausea, vomiting, anorexia, weight loss, fever, hypotension). Hyperkalemia is generally present only in 1° AI.
- **ADH deficiency (DI):** Seen only if the posterior pituitary is also involved.

KEY FACT

ACTH deficiency is the most life-threatening aspect of panhypopituitarism. However, ACTH function is generally preserved the longest.

DIFFERENTIAL

Remember the **"eight I's":** Invasive, Infiltrative, Infarction, Injury, Immunologic, Iatrogenic, Infectious, Idiopathic.

- **Invasive:** Pituitary adenomas, craniopharyngioma, 1° CNS tumors, metastatic tumors, anatomic malformations (eg, encephalocele and parasellar aneurysms).
- **Infiltrative:** Sarcoidosis, hemochromatosis, histiocytosis X.
- **Infarction:**
  - **Sheehan's syndrome:** Pituitary infarction associated with postpartum hemorrhage and vascular collapse. Typically presents with difficulty in lactation and failure to resume menses postpartum.
  - **Pituitary apoplexy:** Spontaneous hemorrhagic infarction of a preexisting pituitary tumor (see above).
- **Injury:** Severe head trauma can lead to anterior pituitary dysfunction and DI.
- **Immunologic: Lymphocytic hypophysitis**—destructive lymphocytic infiltration causing hypopituitarism during pregnancy or postpartum. May cause symptoms of mass lesion and ACTH insufficiency.
- **Iatrogenic:** Most likely after **pituitary surgery** or **radiation therapy.**
- **Infectious:** Rare; include TB, syphilis, and fungi.
- **Idiopathic: Empty sella syndrome**—an enlarged sella turcica that is not entirely filled with pituitary tissue; the pituitary gland may be flattened by CSF pressure. Most commonly congenital.

KEY FACT

In a man with hypopituitarism and skin bronzing, think hemochromatosis.

DIAGNOSIS

Specific hormonal testing includes the following:

- **ACTH/adrenal axis:** Abnormal ACTH and cortisol. See the discussion of AI below for details on the **cosyntropin test.** Note that the test may be normal in acute pituitary dysfunction; in this setting, the adrenals can still respond to a pharmacologic dose of ACTH.
- **Thyroid axis: Low free T$_4$** in 2° hypothyroidism (TSH levels are **not** reliable for this diagnosis, as levels may be low or normal).
- **Gonadotropins:** Low FSH/LH, testosterone, or estradiol.
- **GH:** Low IGF-1; abnormal GH stimulation testing.
- **ADH:** If DI is suspected, test as described in Table 6.5.

KEY FACT

Seventy-five percent or more of the pituitary must be destroyed before there is clinical evidence of hypopituitarism.

TABLE 6.5.   **Diagnosis of Central DI, Nephrogenic DI, and Psychogenic Polydipsia**

TEST	CENTRAL DI	NEPHROGENIC DI	PSYCHOGENIC POLYDIPSIA
Random plasma osmolality	↑	↑	↓
Random urine osmolality	↓	↓	↓
Urine osmolality during water deprivation	No change	No change	↑
Urine osmolality after IV DDAVP	↑	No change	↑
Plasma ADH	↓	Normal to ↑	↓

TREATMENT

Treat the underlying cause. Medical treatment consists of correcting hormone deficiencies:

- **ACTH:** Hydrocortisone 10–30 mg/day, two-thirds in the morning and one-third in the afternoon/evening.
- **TSH:** Replace with levothyroxine (adjust to a goal of normal free T_4).
- **GnRH:**
  - **Men:** Replace testosterone by injection, patch, or gel.
  - **Women:** If premenopausal, OCPs or HRT.
- **GH:** Human GH is available.
- **ADH:** Intranasal DDAVP 10 μg QD-BID.

DIABETES INSIPIDUS (DI)

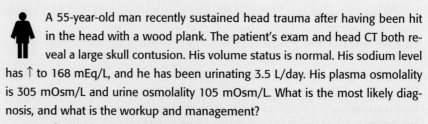

A 55-year-old man recently sustained head trauma after having been hit in the head with a wood plank. The patient's exam and head CT both reveal a large skull contusion. His volume status is normal. His sodium level has ↑ to 168 mEq/L, and he has been urinating 3.5 L/day. His plasma osmolality is 305 mOsm/L and urine osmolality 105 mOsm/L. What is the most likely diagnosis, and what is the workup and management?

Central DI occurs in patients with brain conditions such as cancer, infections, surgery, or trauma. Patients are usually euvolemic because they have the ability to retain sodium appropriately. Plasma osmolality exceeds urine osmolality because the kidneys are not retaining water appropriately for the level of hypernatremia. Treat with DDAVP.

Deficient ADH action resulting in copious amounts of extremely dilute urine and possibly hypernatremia. Subtypes are as follows:

- **Central DI:** Deficient ADH secretion by the posterior pituitary. Caused by hypothalamic masses, traumatic brain injury, infiltrative diseases (eg, Langerhans cell histiocytosis, sarcoidosis), and vascular conditions (eg, Sheehan's syndrome. May also be idiopathic.
- **Nephrogenic DI:** Normal ADH secretion, but impaired ability to act on the kidneys. Caused by congenital/inherited defects, CKD, hypercalcemia, hypokalemia, and **lithium.**

KEY FACT

The most common cause of acquired nephrogenic DI is lithium use.

Symptoms/Exam

- Characterized by **polyuria** and polydipsia.
- The hallmark is inappropriately **dilute urine** in the setting of ↑ **serum osmolality (urine osmolality < serum osmolality).**
- **Hypernatremia** occurs if the patient lacks access to free water or does not have an intact thirst mechanism.

Differential

Psychogenic polydipsia—polyuria due to ↑ drinking, usually > 5 L of water per day, leading to dilution of extracellular fluid and water diuresis.

Diagnosis

Diagnosed as follows (see also Table 6.5):

- **Plasma and urine osmolality.**
- **Water deprivation test to establish the diagnosis of DI:**
  - **Normal response:** Urine osmolality ↑ in response to water deprivation.
  - **DI:** Urine osmolality is low (≤ 300 mOsm/L) despite water restriction.
  - **Psychogenic polydipsia:** Urine osmolality ↑ more than plasma osmolality.
- **Desmopressin challenge test (DDAVP;** comparable to synthetic ADH) **to distinguish central or nephrogenic DI:** Urine osmolality ↑ in central DI but not in nephrogenic DI.
- If central DI is diagnosed, obtain a **pituitary MRI** to determine the etiology.

Treatment

- **Central DI:** DDAVP administration (IV, SQ, PO, or intranasally).
- **Nephrogenic DI:** Treat the underlying disorder if possible. A low-solute diet, thiazide diuretics, and amiloride may be helpful.

Thyroid Disorders

TESTS AND IMAGING

Thyroid Function Tests (TFTs)

Table 6.6 outlines the role of TFTs in diagnosing thyroid disorders. Figure 6.3 illustrates the hypothalamic-pituitary-thyroid axis.

- **Thyrotropin (TSH)** is the best screening test and the most sensitive indicator of thyroid dysfunction. If there is 2° (pituitary) thyroid dysfunction, TSH is unreliable, and FT_4 is used instead.
- If TSH is abnormal, then check FT_4.
- If TSH is low and FT_4 is normal, then check a **total or free T_3 (TT_3 or FT_3)** to rule out "T_3 thyrotoxicosis" (a predominance of T_3 production over T_4 production; usually seen in early hyperthyroidism). It is not necessary to check TT_3 or FT_3 in the evaluation of routine hypothyroidism.

Radionuclide Uptake and Scan of the Thyroid Gland

Most often used to determine the etiology of hyperthyroidism; not useful in the evaluation of hypothyroidism. ^{123}I is administered orally, and the percent of radioactive iodine (RAI) uptake is determined at 4–6 and 24 hours (see Table 6.7).

KEY FACT

Patients with DI have extremely dilute urine, with no change in urine output even if fluid intake is ↓. If urine osmolality is low in a hypernatremic patient, consider DI.

KEY FACT

To establish the diagnosis of DI, perform a water deprivation test. Water restriction should not influence urine output or osmolality in DI, since ADH production or action is impaired.

KEY FACT

If urine osmolality ↑ and urine output ↓ after DDAVP administration, you have diagnosed central DI. The next diagnostic test should be a pituitary MRI.

KEY FACT

Keeping up with fluid losses from massive polyuria is a key component of DI treatment.

KEY FACT

The single best screening test for evaluating thyroid function is TSH.

TABLE 6.6. **TFTs in Thyroid Disease**

	TSH	FREE T$_4$	T$_3$/FREE T$_3$
1° hypothyroidism	↑	↓	↓
2° (pituitary) hypothyroidism	↓/normal	↓	↓
3° (hypothalamic) hypothyroidism	↓	↓	↓
1° hyperthyroidism	↓	↑	↑
2° hyperthyroidism (rare; TSH-secreting adenoma)	↑	↑	↑
Exogenous hyperthyroidism	↓	↑	Mildly ↑
Euthyroid sick (acute)	↓/normal[a]	Rare ↑/normal/↓	↓
Euthyroid sick (recovery)	↑[b]	Normal	Normal

[a] ↓ (but not undetectable), especially if the patient has received dopamine, glucocorticoids, narcotics, or NSAIDs.
[b] Usually not > 20 mIU/L.

In iodine-sufficient areas such as the United States, amiodarone induces hypothyroidism more often than hyperthyroidism.

HYPOTHYROIDISM

Etiologies include the following:

- **Hashimoto's (autoimmune) thyroiditis:** The **most common cause in the United States.** Characterized by goiter in early disease and by a small, firm gland in late disease.
- **Late phase of subacute thyroiditis:** After the acute phase of hyperthyroidism, hypothyroidism may occur but is usually transient (see below).
- **Drugs:** Amiodarone, lithium, interferon, iodide (kelp, radiocontrast dyes).
- **Iatrogenic:** Postsurgical or post–RAI treatment.
- **Iodine deficiency:** Rare in the United States but common worldwide. Often associated with a grossly enlarged gland.

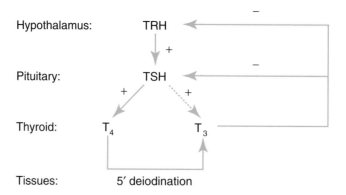

FIGURE 6.3. **The hypothalamic-pituitary-thyroid axis.** TSH is produced by the pituitary in response to TRH. TSH stimulates the thyroid gland to secrete T$_4$ and low levels of T$_3$. T$_4$ is converted in the periphery by 5′ deiodinase to T$_3$, the active form of the hormone. T$_3$ is also primarily responsible for feedback inhibition on the hypothalamus and pituitary. Most T$_4$ is bound to TBG and is not accessible to conversion; therefore, free T$_4$ provides a more accurate assessment of thyroid hormone level.

TABLE 6.7. Hyperthyroidism Differential Based on Radioiodine Uptake and Scan

DECREASED UPTAKE	DIFFUSELY INCREASED UPTAKE	UNEVEN UPTAKE
Thyroiditis Exogenous thyroid hormone ingestion Struma ovarii	Graves' disease	Toxic multinodular goiter (multiple hot and cold nodules). Solitary toxic nodule (one hot nodule; the remainder of the thyroid appears cold). Cancer (cold nodule).

- **Rare causes:** 2° hypothyroidism due to hypopituitarism; 3° hypothyroidism due to hypothalamic dysfunction; peripheral resistance to thyroid hormone.

SYMPTOMS/EXAM

- Presents with **fatigue, weight gain, cold intolerance, dry skin, menstrual irregularities, depression,** and **constipation.**
- Exam may reveal an enlarged thyroid gland, bradycardia, edema, dry/cold skin, hoarseness, coarse/brittle hair, and a delayed relaxation phase of DTRs.

DIAGNOSIS

- **Labs:** ↑ TSH (> 10 mIU/L) **and** ↓ FT$_4$. Hashimoto's thyroiditis is associated with ⊕ **antithyroperoxidase** (anti-TPO) and/or ⊕ **antithyroglobulin antibodies.**
- **Radiology:** RAI scan and thyroid ultrasound are generally not indicated.

TREATMENT

- **Thyroid hormone replacement:**
  - Levothyroxine (LT$_4$) is generally used. The replacement dose is usually 1.6 µg/kg/day.
  - In elderly patients or those with heart disease, **start low and go slow** (12.5–25.0 µg/day; then slowly ↑ the dose by 25-µg increments every month until euthyroid).
- **Subclinical hypothyroidism** (↑ TSH with normal FT$_4$; mild or no symptoms): Treatment is generally not indicated unless TSH is > 10 mIU/L or in the presence of thyroid antibodies, goiter, a ⊕ family history, or hyperlipidemia.

COMPLICATIONS

- **Myxedema coma:** Severe, life-threatening hypothyroidism characterized by weakness, **hypothermia, hypoventilation** with **hypercapnia,** hypoglycemia, hyponatremia, water intoxication, shock, and death. Treatment is supportive therapy with rewarming, intubation, and IV LT$_4$. Often precipitated by infection or other forms of stress. Consider glucocorticoids for AI, which can coexist with thyroid disease.
- **Other complications:** Anemia (normocytic), CHF, depression, hyperlipidemia.

KEY FACT

Autoimmune thyroid disease may be associated with other endocrine autoimmune disorders, most prominently pernicious anemia and AI.

HYPERTHYROIDISM

A 40-year-old woman presents with three months of palpitations and double vision. Her exam is notable for sinus tachycardia, exophthalmos (proptosis), a palpable goiter, and tremulousness. A thyroid panel reveals a TSH level of < 0.05 mIU/L with an ↑ T_4 and T_3 and thyroid-stimulating immunoglobulin (TSI). What are the best treatment options for this patient?

For hyperthyroidism of any cause, β-blockers will provide immediate relief of adrenergic symptoms such as palpitations. Both RAI and medications are treatment options. For medical treatment of Graves' disease or other non-thyroiditis-mediated hyperthyroidism, consider methimazole (MMI) or propylthiouracil (PTU). RAI ablation can worsen severe Graves' ophthalmopathy and thus may not be a good option for this patient; thyroidectomy is an option that may improve eye pathology.

The etiologies of hyperthyroidism include the following (see also Table 6.8):

- **Graves' disease (the most common cause):** Affects females more than males (by a ratio of 5:1). Peak incidence is at 20–40 years of age.
- **Solitary toxic nodule.**
- **Toxic multinodular goiter.**
- **Thyroiditis.**
- **Rare causes:** Exogenous thyroid hormone ingestion (thyrotoxicosis factitia), struma ovarii (ovarian tumor produces thyroid hormone), hydatidiform mole (hCG mimics TSH action), productive follicular thyroid carcinoma.

SYMPTOMS

Presents with weight loss, anxiety, **palpitations**, fatigue, hyperdefecation, **heat intolerance,** sweating, and amenorrhea.

EXAM

Findings include the following:

- **General:** Stare/lid lag, tachycardia, ↑ pulse pressure, hyperreflexia, restlessness, goiter (smooth and homogeneous in Graves' disease; irregular in multinodular goiter).
- **Graves' disease only:** Ophthalmopathy, infiltrative dermopathy (**pretibial myxedema: nonpitting**), thyroid bruit (due to ↑ vascularity), onycholysis (separation of the fingernails from the nail bed). Eye findings include **exophthalmos (bulging of the eye)** (see Figure 6.4), periorbital edema, and conjunctival inflammation.

DIAGNOSIS

Diagnostic methods include the following (see also Figure 6.5):

- **Labs:** TSH, FT_4, occasionally FT_3, thyroid antibodies (see above).
- **Radiology:** RAI uptake and scan can help determine the etiology of hyperthyroidism. Hyperthyroidism with **diffusely ↑ uptake** is associated with de novo hormone synthesis (**Graves' disease**); hyperthyroidism with **↓ uptake** suggests thyroid tissue destruction (**thyroiditis**) or an extrathyroidal source. Hold antithyroid medications at least seven days prior to testing.

KEY FACT

All patients with hyperthyroidism may have stare and lid lag. However, two physical findings are pathognomonic of Graves' disease: pretibial myxedema and exophthalmos.

KEY FACT

Elderly patients may present with apathetic hyperthyroidism, which is characterized by depression, slow AF, weight loss, and a small goiter.

TABLE 6.8. Causes and Treatment of Hyperthyroidism

Cause	Thyroid Exam	Unique Findings	Radioactive Iodine Uptake and Scan	Treatment
Graves' disease	Diffusely enlarged thyroid; bruit may be present.	**Exophthalmos**, periorbital edema, **pretibial myxedema.** TSI +/− TPO antibodies.	**Diffusely ↑ uptake.**	Meds (MMI, PTU), RAI; surgery for very large, obstructing goiters.
Solitary toxic nodule	Single palpable nodule.	Autoantibodies are usually absent. May have predominantly T_3 **toxicosis.**	Single focus of ↑ uptake.	**Definitive therapy is RAI** or surgery.
Multinodular goiter	**"Lumpy-bumpy," enlarged thyroid.**	Autoantibodies are usually absent. May have predominantly T_3 toxicosis.	Multiple hot and/or cold nodules.	Definitive therapy is RAI or surgery.
Thyroiditis (transient destruction of thyroid tissue)	**Tender**, enlarged thyroid.	Subacute thyroiditis occurs following a viral infection. Can also be postpartum or silent ("painless"); thought to have an autoimmune etiology. ↑ thyroglobulin. Classically followed by a hypothyroid phase and then by euthyroidism. Can be caused by meds (eg, **amiodarone**).	**Diffusely ↓ uptake.**	β-blockers, NSAIDs, steroids if indicated.
Exogenous hyperthyroidism	Normal or nonpalpable.	The patient may be taking weight loss medications or have psychiatric illness. Distinguish from thyroiditis by low thyroglobulin levels.	Diffusely ↓ uptake.	Discontinuation of thyroid hormone.

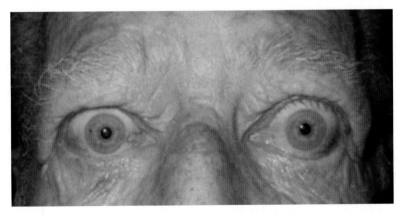

FIGURE 6.4. Graves' ophthalmopathy. Note the periorbital edema, injection of corneal blood vessels, and proptosis. (Reproduced with permission from USMLERx.com.)

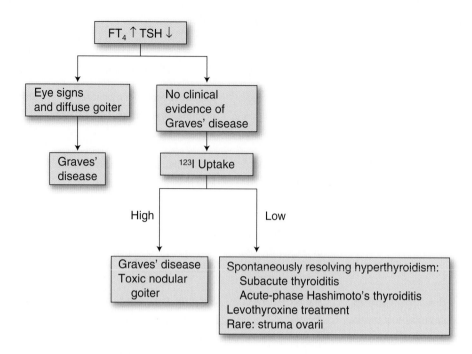

FIGURE 6.5.   **Algorithm for the diagnosis of hyperthyroidism.**

TREATMENT

- **Medications:** MMI and PTU can be used to ↓ thyroid hormone production. **In pregnancy, PTU is the first choice because MMI may be teratogenic. Liver toxicity can occur** (more so with PTU than with MMI).
    - In Graves' disease, treatment for 18 months can lead to complete remission in 50% of cases.
    - β-blockers can be used in the acute phase to control tachycardia and other symptoms.
- **RAI ablation therapy:**
    - The treatment of choice for solitary toxic nodules and toxic multinodular goiter, as these **conditions generally do not spontaneously remit with medical therapy. Contraindicated in pregnancy.**
    - A high cure rate is achieved after one dose, but treatment usually results in hypothyroidism, requiring subsequent thyroid hormone replacement therapy.
- **Surgery:**
    - Indicated for uncontrolled disease during pregnancy; for extremely large goiters causing obstruction; for amiodarone-induced thyroiditis that is refractory to medical management; or for patients who object to RAI therapy and cannot tolerate antithyroid drugs.
    - Risks include hypoparathyroidism and recurrent laryngeal nerve injury.

COMPLICATIONS

- **AF:** Particularly common in the elderly. Thyroid function should be checked in all cases of new AF. Associated with a higher risk of stroke than other causes of nonvalvular AF.
- **Ophthalmopathy:** Can lead to nerve or muscular entrapment (and thus to blindness or palsies). Can be precipitated or **worsened by RAI therapy, especially in smokers.** Treatment includes high-dose glucocorticoids and eye surgery.

- **Thyroid storm:**
  - Severe thyrotoxicosis, most commonly from Graves' disease. Frequently has an underlying precipitating factor (eg, infection, surgery, trauma, RAI therapy, ingestion). Characterized by exaggerated symptoms of hyperthyroidism such as **fever,** hypertension, severe tachycardia, delirium, agitation, diarrhea, vomiting, jaundice, and CHF.
  - Treatment involves high-dose propranolol, PTU (superior to MMI for thyroid storm), glucocorticoids (to inhibit conversion of T_4 to T_3), and iodide (to inhibit preformed thyroid hormone release).

THYROIDITIS

Can present with hyper-, hypo-, and/or euthyroid states (see Table 6.9).

SYMPTOMS/EXAM

- **Early stage:** Characterized by thyroid inflammation (high ESR) and release of preformed thyroid hormone, leading to clinical hyperthyroidism, suppressed TSH, and low RAI uptake.
- **Late stage:** Characterized by thyroid "burnout" and hypothyroidism.
- Most patients with acute thyroiditis eventually recover thyroid function.

TABLE 6.9. Clinical Features and Differential Diagnosis of Thyroiditis

TYPE	ETIOLOGY	CLINICAL FINDINGS	TESTS	TREATMENT
Subacute thyroiditis (de Quervain's)	Viral.	Hyperthyroid early; then hypothyroid. **Tender**, large thyroid; **fever.**	↑ **ESR**; no antithyroid antibodies; low RAI uptake.	β-blockers, NSAIDs, acetaminophen +/− steroids.
Hashimoto's thyroiditis	Autoimmune.	Usually hypothyroid; painless +/− goiter.	Ninety-five percent have ⊕ antibodies; anti-**TPO** is most sensitive.	Levothyroxine.
Suppurative thyroiditis	Bacteria > other infectious agents.	Fever, neck pain, tender thyroid.	TFTs are normal. No uptake on RAI scan; ⊕ **cultures.**	Antibiotics and drainage.
Amiodarone	Am**IOD**arone contains **IOD**ine.	Destructive thyroiditis is seen in the United States; iodine-induced hyperthyroidism is seen in iodine-deficient areas.	Three possible changes: 1. ↑ FT_4 and total T_4; then low T_3 and high TSH. 2. High TSH; low FT_4 and T_3. 3. Low TSH; high FT_4 and T_3.	1. No treatment is needed; will normalize eventually. 2. Gradual titration of levothyroxine. 3. As for other thyroiditis; stop amiodarone if possible.
Other medications	Lithium, α-interferon, interleukin-2.		Lithium typically causes hypothyroid profile.	Stop medication if possible.
Postpartum thyroiditis	Lymphocytic infiltration; seen after up to 10% of pregnancies.	Small, nontender thyroid.	May see hyper- or hypothyroidism. Antibodies are often ⊕; RAI uptake is low.	No treatment unless propranolol is needed for tachycardia. It is important to monitor TFTs in future pregnancies.

***T**REATMENT*

See Table 6.9.

THYROID DISEASE IN PREGNANCY

See the discussion in the Women's Health chapter.

NONTHYROIDAL ILLNESS (EUTHYROID SICK SYNDROME)

Seen in hospitalized or terminally ill patients, typically without symptoms. Results from impaired ability to convert T_4 to T_3 in peripheral tissues during acute illness. In mild illness, the **most common abnormality is a low T_3 level, with normal FT_4 and TSH levels.** During the course of the illness, FT_4 and T_3 may decline while TSH levels vary, often rising during the recovery phase; this should not be confused with hypothyroidism.

THYROID NODULES AND CANCER

Thyroid nodules are more common in women but are more likely to be malignant in men. Radiation exposure is a major risk factor. The "90%" mnemonic applies:

- **90% of nodules are benign.**
- **90% of nodules are cold** on RAI uptake scan; 15–20% of these are malignant (1% of hot nodules are malignant).
- **90% of thyroid malignancies present as a thyroid nodule.**
- **> 90%** of cancers are either papillary or follicular, which carry the best prognoses.

***S**YMPTOMS/**E**XAM*

- Present as a firm, palpable nodule.
- Cervical lymphadenopathy and hoarseness are concerning signs.
- Often found incidentally on radiologic studies that are ordered for other purposes.

***D**IFFERENTIAL*

May be benign or represent one of four main types of cancer:

- **1° thyroid cancer:**
  - **Papillary: Most common;** spreads lymphatically. Has an **excellent prognosis overall,** with more than a 95% five-year survival rate for all but metastatic disease.
  - **Follicular:** More aggressive; spreads locally and hematogenously. Can metastasize to the bone, lungs, and brain. Rarely produces thyroid hormone.
  - **Medullary:** A tumor of parafollicular C cells. May secrete calcitonin. Fifteen percent are familial or associated with multiple endocrine neoplasia (MEN) 2A or 2B.
  - **Anaplastic:** Undifferentiated. Has a **poor prognosis;** usually occurs in older patients.
- **Other:** Metastases to the thyroid (breast, kidney, melanoma, lung); lymphoma (1° or metastatic).

KEY FACT

Thyroid medications are not indicated in nonthyroidal illness; treat the underlying illness.

KEY FACT

Papillary and follicular thyroid cancers are the most common 1° thyroid cancers and also have the best prognosis.

KEY FACT

Medullary thyroid cancer can produce ↑ levels of calcitonin and is often associated with MEN 2A or 2B.

DIAGNOSIS

- Check TSH. If TSH level is normal, proceed to fine-needle aspiration (FNA) of the nodule (see Figure 6.6).
- Thyroid/neck ultrasound to determine nodule size, detect lymphadenopathy, and evaluate for other nodules. Size > 3 cm, high intravascular flow, irregular shapes/borders, and microcalcifications should raise concern for malignancy.
- If TSH level is low, proceed to RAI uptake and scan, as this indicates that there is an ↑ likelihood of a hot nodule. Do **not** biopsy a hot nodule.
- **All euthyroid and hypothyroid nodules should be biopsied with FNA.** If the nodule is not palpable, this may be done under ultrasound guidance. Four pathologic results are possible:
    - **Malignant:** Surgery.
    - **Benign:** Serial follow-up. The use of LT$_4$ to suppress the growth of benign nodules is no longer recommended, as it is often ineffective and may be associated with toxicity (especially in the elderly).
    - **Insufficient for diagnosis:** Repeat ultrasound-guided FNA after six weeks.
    - **Follicular neoplasm or "suspicious for malignancy":** Surgery.
- If a multinodular goiter is present, FNA of the most suspicious nodule (by radiologic features) or the dominant nodule (largest nodule > 1 cm) is acceptable, although it will not diagnose all cases of malignancy. Such patients should be followed, and nodules that ↑ in size should be considered for FNA.

KEY FACT

If a palpable nodule is associated with a normal TSH, proceed directly to FNA.

KEY FACT

Thyroglobulin is a good marker for the presence of thyroid tissue. If present after total thyroidectomy and RAI remnant ablation, it can indicate thyroid cancer recurrence.

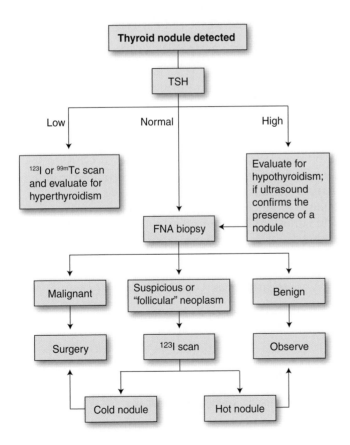

FIGURE 6.6.   Evaluation of a thyroid mass. (Adapted with permission from Gardner DG, Shoback D. *Greenspan's Basic & Clinical Endocrinology,* 8th ed. New York: McGraw-Hill, 2007: 270.)

TREATMENT

- Nodules: See Figure 6.6.
- Papillary/follicular thyroid cancer:
  - First: Surgical thyroidectomy.
  - Second: RAI remnant ablation.
  - Third: LT_4 to suppress TSH.
- Medullary or anaplastic thyroid cancer:
  - First: Surgical thyroidectomy with neck dissection.
  - Second: Chemotherapy if metastatic disease is present.

Adrenal Gland Disorders

A 56-year-old woman with rheumatoid arthritis and diabetes presents with persistent fatigue. She is usually on ASA, metformin, calcium, vitamin D, and prednisone (10 mg/day), but she stopped her prednisone two months ago because she was concerned that it was the cause of her osteopenia. Her exam is normal, including her skin color, except for a BP of 85/50 mm Hg and an HR of 70 bpm. Labs are as follows: Na^+ 133 mEq/L, K^+ 4 mEq/L, BUN 13 mg/dL, creatinine 0.7 mg/dL, glucose 87 mg/dL, and a normal WBC count with 8% eosinophils. What is the likely reason for her fatigue?

2° AI from chronic prednisone use that was unmasked by abrupt prednisone withdrawal. The patient is euvolemic and has mild hyponatremia from SIADH, normal potassium, hypoglycemia, and eosinophilia.

The adrenal gland is under control of the hypothalamus and pituitary (see Figure 6.7):

- **Medulla:** Produces catecholamines (epinephrine, norepinephrine, dopamine).
- **Cortex:** Composed of three zones—remember as **GFR:**
  - Glomerulosa: Produces mineralocorticoids (**aldosterone**).
  - Fasciculata: Produces **cortisol** and androgens.
  - Reticularis: Produces androgens and cortisol.
- ACTH and cortisol follow a circadian rhythm; levels are highest at around 6:00 A.M.

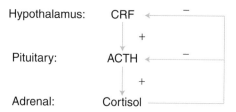

FIGURE 6.7.   The hypothalamic-pituitary-adrenal axis.

ADRENAL INSUFFICIENCY (AI)

2° AI (due to ACTH deficiency from pituitary disease) is much more common than 1° AI (adrenal failure). Etiologies are as follows (see also Table 6.10):

- **1° AI (Addison's disease):** Because of high adrenal reserve, > 90% of both adrenal cortices must fail to cause clinical AI.
  - **Autoimmune adrenalitis:** The **most common** etiology of 1° AI. Often accompanied by other autoimmune disorders (eg, Hashimoto's thyroiditis, type 1 DM).
  - **Metastatic malignancy** and **lymphoma.**
  - **Adrenal hemorrhage:** Seen in critically ill patients, pregnancy, anticoagulated patients, and **antiphospholipid antibody syndrome.**
  - **Infection:** TB, fungi (*Histoplasma*), CMV, HIV.
  - **Infiltrative disorders:** Amyloid, hemochromatosis.
  - Congenital adrenal hyperplasia.
  - Adrenal leukodystrophy.
  - **Drugs:** Ketoconazole, etomidate, metyrapone.
- **2° AI:**
  - **Iatrogenic:** Glucocorticoids (**most common**); anabolic steroids (eg, megestrol).
  - **Pituitary or hypothalamic tumors.**

SYMPTOMS/EXAM

- Presents with weakness, fatigue, anorexia, weight loss, nausea, vomiting, diarrhea, unexplained abdominal pain, and postural lightheadedness. Salt craving and postural dizziness may be seen in 1° AI (but not in 2° AI, as mineralocorticoid function is not impaired).
- 1° AI presents with **hyperpigmentation** of the oral mucosa and palmar creases, dehydration, and **hypotension.**
- ↓ pubic/axillary hair is seen in women.

DIAGNOSIS

- **Labs: Hyponatremia,** hyperkalemia (only in 1° AI), eosinophilia, azotemia due to volume depletion, mild metabolic acidosis, hypoglycemia, hypercalcemia.

KEY FACT

The most common cause of AI is exogenous glucocorticoid use.

KEY FACT

Hyperpigmentation indicates 1° AI (most notable in the oral mucosa, palmar creases, and recent scars) due to compensatory high levels of ACTH that stimulate melanocytes to produce excess melanin.

KEY FACT

A poststimulation cortisol level of < 18 μg/dL suggests AI.

KEY FACT

If a patient presents with shock and you suspect acute AI, stabilize the patient with IV fluids and stress-dose steroids.

TABLE 6.10.   1° vs. 2° Adrenal Insufficiency

	1°	**2°**
ACTH	High	Low
Cortisol	Low	Low
Hyperkalemia	Common	No
Hyponatremia	May be present	May be present
Hyperpigmentation	May be present	No
Mineralocorticoid replacement needed	Yes	No

KEY FACT

For suspected shock due to AI, treat with dexamethasone + fludrocortisone if the cosyntropin stimulation test has not been done yet, as hydrocortisone will interfere with test results.

KEY FACT

Autoimmune diseases travel together. Think of polyglandular autoimmune syndrome type 2 (Schmidt syndrome) if you see the following three diseases together: type 1 DM, thyroiditis, and 1° AI.

KEY FACT

If a type 1 DM patient who had previously been well controlled on an insulin regimen presents with new-onset hypoglycemia, consider 1° AI (Addison's disease).

KEY FACT

If a patient with newly diagnosed 1° AI is also found to have hypothyroidism, treat the AI first or you may precipitate an adrenal crisis.

- An A.M. cortisol level of < 3 µg/dL suggests AI, but confirm with a cosyntropin stimulation test (see below). Any random cortisol level ≥ 18 µg/dL rules out AI except in critical illness. However, a low or normal value is not useful.
- **Cosyntropin stimulation test:** Obtain baseline ACTH and cortisol and then administer cosyntropin (synthetic ACTH) 250 µg IM or IV. After 30–60 minutes, poststimulation cortisol should be ≥ 18 µg/dL.
  - **High baseline ACTH + abnormal cosyntropin stimulation test:** 1° AI.
  - **Low baseline ACTH + abnormal cosyntropin stimulation test:** 2° AI.
  - **Further considerations** are as follows:
    - **Critical illness:** The diagnosis of AI in critically ill patients is controversial. Some authors suggest using a higher cutoff value for the poststimulation cortisol (20–30 µg/dL), a random cortisol level of < 15 µg/dL, or a poststimulation change in cortisol level ≤ 9 µg/dL.
    - **Imaging:** If the cause of 1° AI is not known, adrenal imaging is warranted. If the cause of 2° AI is not known (eg, there is no exogenous corticosteroid exposure), order a pituitary MRI.

TREATMENT

- **1° AI:** Requires both mineralocorticoid and glucocorticoid replacement. Use fludrocortisone 0.05–0.10 mg/day to replace the mineralocorticoid component.
- **2° AI:** Requires glucocorticoid replacement only.
- **Glucocorticoid replacement:** Use hydrocortisone 10–30 mg/day, two-thirds in the morning and one-third in the afternoon/evening. Dexamethasone or prednisone can also be used. When patients are under stress due to illness or surgery, they require temporarily higher doses of glucocorticoids ("stress doses").

COMPLICATIONS

Adrenal crisis—acute deficiency of cortisol, usually due to major stress in a patient with preexisting AI. Characterized by shock, headache, nausea, vomiting, confusion, and fever. **Fatal if not treated with immediate steroid therapy.**

CUSHING'S SYNDROME

A 28-year-old woman presents with severe fatigue and weight gain for several months. On exam, she has ↑ facial hair, purple abdominal striae, central obesity, and thin skin that bruises easily. Her 24-hour urinary cortisol is ↑; cortisol is suppressed with high-dose but not low-dose dexamethasone. Her plasma ACTH level is high. What is the most likely diagnosis?

An ACTH-secreting pituitary adenoma. A high ACTH level indicates an ACTH-dependent etiology for this patient's Cushing's syndrome. High-dose dexamethasone suppresses pituitary ACTH but not ectopic ACTH. The next step in the workup is a pituitary MRI.

A syndrome due to excess cortisol. Etiologies are as follows:

- **Exogenous corticosteroids: The most common cause overall.**
- **Endogenous causes:**
  - **Cushing's disease** (70% of endogenous cases): Due to ACTH hypersecretion from a **pituitary** adenoma (most are microadenomas). More common in women.
  - **Ectopic ACTH** (15%): From nonpituitary neoplasms producing ACTH (eg, small cell lung carcinoma, bronchial carcinoids). Rapid increases in ACTH levels lead to marked hyperpigmentation, metabolic alkalosis, and hypokalemia, sometimes without other cushingoid features. More common in men.
  - **Adrenal** (15%): Adenoma, carcinoma, or nodular adrenal hyperplasia.

SYMPTOMS/EXAM

Table 6.11 lists the clinical characteristics of Cushing's syndrome.

DIAGNOSIS

- **Lab abnormalities:** Metabolic alkalosis, hypokalemia, hypercalciuria, leukocytosis with relative lymphopenia, hyperglycemia, glucose intolerance.
- Principles of evaluation are as follows (see also Figure 6.8):
  - **Step 1:** Confirm excess cortisol production. Do either (1) a low-dose (1-mg) dexamethasone suppression test or (2) a 24-hour urine free cortisol level. If either test is abnormal, confirm with the other test.
  - **Step 2:** Check ACTH level. High cortisol normally inhibits ACTH production completely. Thus, **high** or "normal" ACTH indicates **ACTH-dependent** Cushing's syndrome (**pituitary** or **ectopic** production of ACTH, which leads to high cortisol), whereas **low** ACTH indicates ACTH-independent Cushing's syndrome (**adrenal** disease that directly produces cortisol).
- **ACTH dependent:** Obtain a pituitary MRI. If the pituitary MRI is ⊖ or equivocal, consider inferior petrosal sinus sampling (IPSS).
- **ACTH independent:** Obtain a CT/MRI of the abdomen/pelvis to evaluate for adrenal adenoma vs. carcinoma.

TREATMENT

- **Cushing's disease:** Transsphenoidal pituitary adenoma resection.
- **Ectopic ACTH:**
  - Treat the underlying neoplasm.
  - If the neoplasm is not identifiable or treatable, options are as follows:
    - Pharmacologic blockade of steroid synthesis (ketoconazole, metyrapone, aminoglutethimide).

TABLE 6.11. Clinical Features of Cushing's Syndrome

GENERAL	DERMATOLOGIC	MUSCULOSKELETAL	NEUROPSYCHIATRIC	GONADAL DYSFUNCTION	METABOLIC
Truncal obesity	Plethora	Osteopenia	Emotional lability	Menstrual disorders	Glucose intolerance/diabetes
Hypertension	Striae		Depression	Impotence, ↓ libido	Hyperlipidemia
Moon facies	Acne		Psychosis		Polyuria
Dorsocervical fat pad	Bruising				Kidney stones
("buffalo hump")					

(Adapted with permission from Gardner DG, Shoback D. *Greenspan's Basic & Clinical Endocrinology*, 8th ed. New York: McGraw-Hill, 2007, Table 10-12.)

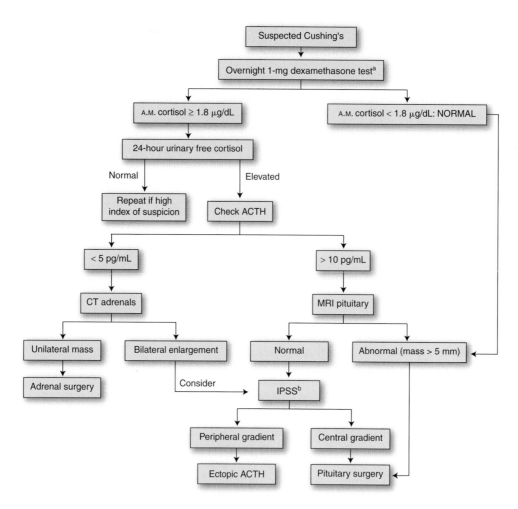

FIGURE 6.8. **Evaluation and diagnosis of Cushing's syndrome.**
[a]Overnight 1-mg dexamethasone test: Give the patient 1 mg of dexamethasone PO to be taken at 11:00 P.M. The following morning, check cortisol between 7:00 and 9:00. Normal cortisol is < 1.8 μg/dL.
[b]IPSS = inferior petrosal sinus sampling. Catheters are used to measure levels of ACTH draining from the pituitary and periphery before and after CRH stimulation. If the gradient is greater from the pituitary, it suggests a central source. If greater from the periphery, the source is peripheral.

- Potassium replacement (consider spironolactone to aid potassium maintenance, as these patients require industrial doses of potassium replacement).
- Bilateral adrenalectomy if all else fails.
  - **Adrenal tumors:** Unilateral adrenalectomy.

COMPLICATIONS

Complications are associated with long-term glucocorticoid therapy and include DM, hypertension, CAD, obesity, osteoporosis, and susceptibility to infections such as *Nocardia*, PCP, and other opportunistic pathogens.

HYPERALDOSTERONISM

May account for 0.5–10% of patients with hypertension. Etiologies are as follows:

- **Aldosterone-producing adenoma (Conn's disease):** Accounts for 60% of cases of 1° aldosteronism.

- **Idiopathic hyperaldosteronism:** One-third of 1° aldosteronism cases; CT shows normal-appearing adrenals or bilateral hyperplasia.
- **2° hyperaldosteronism:** Refers to extra-adrenal disorders such as renin-secreting tumors, renovascular disease (renal artery stenosis, malignant hypertension), and edematous states with ↓ effective arterial volume (CHF, cirrhosis, renal disease).

SYMPTOMS/EXAM

- **Hypertension and hypokalemia** are classic features, although low K⁺ is not necessary for diagnosis. Metabolic alkalosis, mild hypernatremia, and hypomagnesemia may also be seen.
- Most patients are asymptomatic, and there are no characteristic physical findings.

DIAGNOSIS

- **Measure plasma aldosterone concentration (PAC) and plasma renin activity (PRA):**
  - **1° hyperaldosteronism:** PAC is ↑, PRA is suppressed, and the **PAC/PRA ratio is elevated** (the cutoff is laboratory dependent and is usually > 25).
  - **2° hyperaldosteronism:** Both PAC and PRA are ↑, and the PAC/PRA ratio is < 10 (see Figure 6.9).
- **Confirmatory testing:**
  - **IV saline loading** (2 L of saline infused over 2–4 hours) will fail to suppress PAC into the normal range in patients with 1° aldosteronism (as opposed to low-renin essential hypertension).
  - After three days of salt loading (U_{Na} > 200 mEq), **24-hour urine collection for aldosterone** will not suppress PAC to < 14 μg in patients with 1° aldosteronism.
  - If 1° aldosteronism is diagnosed, obtain an **adrenal CT** to distinguish between Conn's and idiopathic hyperaldosteronism (see Figure 6.10).
  - If CT findings are equivocal and in older patients (in whom adrenal incidentaloma is more common), consider **adrenal vein sampling** to localize the plasma aldosterone source.

KEY FACT

A high PAC/PRA ratio and an absolute PAC ≥ 15 are characteristic of 1° aldosteronism.

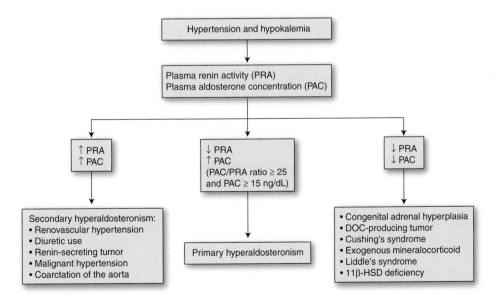

FIGURE 6.9. **Evaluation of hypertension with hypokalemia.**

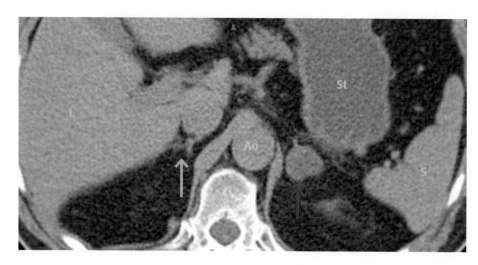

FIGURE 6.10. **Adrenal adenoma.** Cropped transaxial image from a noncontrast CT scan shows a small, low-density mass in the left adrenal gland (red arrow). Blue arrow = normal right adrenal gland, L = liver, Ao = aorta, St = stomach, S = spleen. (Reproduced with permission from USMLERx.com.)

TREATMENT

- **Spironolactone** (in high doses up to 400 mg/day) or **eplerenone** blocks the mineralocorticoid receptor and usually normalizes K$^+$. In men, the most common side effect of spironolactone is **gynecomastia,** but other side effects may occur (eg, rash, impotence, epigastric discomfort).
- **Unilateral adrenalectomy** is recommended for patients with a single adenoma.

PHEOCHROMOCYTOMA

Rare tumors that **produce epinephrine and/or norepinephrine.** Subtypes are as follows:

- Adrenal tumor (90% of pheochromocytomas).
- Extra-adrenal locations (paragangliomas).

SYMPTOMS/EXAM

- Presents with **episodic attacks** of throbbing in the chest, trunk, and head, often precipitated by movements that compress the tumor.
- **Headaches, diaphoresis, palpitations,** tremor and anxiety, nausea, vomiting, fatigue, abdominal or chest pain, weight loss, cold hands and feet, and constipation may also be seen.
- Most patients are hypertensive, but hypertension is episodic in 25% of cases. Orthostasis is usually present.

DIAGNOSIS

- **Step 1:** Make a biochemical diagnosis. Screen with **24-hour urinary catecholamines and fractionated metanephrines.** A less specific screening test is **plasma fractionated metanephrines.** Levels are usually 2–3 times above normal.
- **Step 2:** Localize the tumor. Obtain a **CT or MRI of the abdomen/pelvis** to localize pheochromocytoma (see Figure 6.11).
- If imaging is normal, a ^{123}**I-MIBG** scintiscan (an imaging study that injects radioactive tracer) can localize extra-adrenal lesions (paragangliomas) and metastases.

MNEMONIC

Pheochromocytoma rule of 10s:

10% normotensive
10% occur in children
10% familial
10% bilateral
10% malignant
10% extra-adrenal (called paragangliomas)

KEY FACT

Suspect pheochromocytoma in patients with a family history of MEN 2, neurofibromatosis, or von Hippel–Lindau disease.

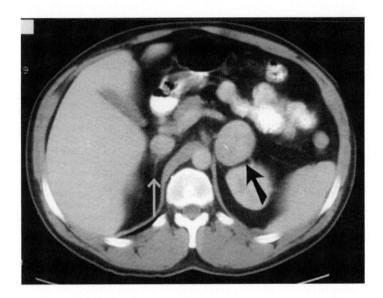

FIGURE 6.11.   Left adrenal pheochromocytoma. Note the large heterogeneously enhancing mass with a thin area of calcification in the left adrenal gland (black arrow) on a transaxial image from a contrast-enhanced CT scan. Blue arrow = normal right adrenal gland, L = liver, S = spleen. (Reproduced with permission from Brunicardi FC et al. *Schwartz's Principles of Surgery*, 9th ed. New York: McGraw-Hill, 2010, Fig. 38-46A.)

TREATMENT

- **Pharmacologic preparation for surgery:**
  - **Phenoxybenzamine:** An α-adrenergic blocker; a key first step.
  - **β-blockers:** Used to control heart rate, but only **after** BP is controlled and good α-blockade has been achieved.
- **Hydration:** It is essential that patients be well hydrated before surgery.
- **Surgery: Surgical resection** by an experienced surgeon is the definitive treatment for these tumors. Associated with a **90% cure rate.**
- **Postoperative complications include hypotension and hypoglycemia.** Always hang dextrose-containing IV fluids in the recovery room!
- **Follow-up:** Should include 24-hour urine for metanephrines and normetanephrines two weeks postoperatively. If levels are normal, surgical resection can be considered complete. Patients should then undergo yearly biochemical evaluation for at least 10 years.

COMPLICATIONS

Hypertensive crises, MI, cerebrovascular accidents, arrhythmias, renal failure, dissecting aortic aneurysm, cardiomyopathy.

ADRENAL INCIDENTALOMAS

Adrenal lesions are found incidentally in approximately 2% of patients undergoing abdominal CT for unrelated reasons.

EXAM

Exam findings depend on whether the lesion is functioning or nonfunctioning (see above).

KEY FACT

Always achieve α-blockade (with phenoxybenzamine) before using β-blockers in patients with pheochromocytoma, because unopposed β-blockade can lead to paroxysmal worsening of the hypertension.

KEY FACT

Always rule out pheochromocytoma (which can be life-threatening) and Cushing's syndrome (because subclinical disease is relatively common) in a patient found to have an adrenal incidentaloma.

DIFFERENTIAL

- **Functional adenoma:** Cushing's syndrome, pheochromocytoma, aldosteronoma.
- **Nonfunctional adenoma.**
- **Adrenal carcinoma:** Often large (> 4 cm) and high density on CT scan. Sixty percent are functional, usually secreting androgens or cortisol (or both hormones). **Virilization** in the presence of an adrenal mass suggests malignancy.
- **Metastases:** Most commonly arise from the lung, GI tract, kidney, or breast.
- **Other:** Myelolipoma (look for the presence of fat on CT scan), cysts, hemorrhage (usually bilateral).

DIAGNOSIS/TREATMENT

- **Evaluate function:**
  - Obtain a 24-hour urine collection for catecholamines and fractionated metanephrines or plasma fractionated metanephrines to rule out pheochromocytoma.
  - Order a 1-mg dexamethasone suppression test to rule out Cushing's.
  - Determine PRA and aldosterone level to screen for aldosteronoma in patients with hypertension or hypokalemia.
- **Treatment is based on the size and functional status of the mass.** Resect the mass if it is > 6 cm (4- to 6-cm tumors can be observed or resected). If the tumor is < 4 cm, observe and repeat imaging at 6–12 months.

Disorders of Lipid and Carbohydrate Metabolism

DIABETES MELLITUS (DM)

 A 53-year-old healthy man with a family history of type 2 DM presents for follow-up for a high HbA_{1c}. Three months ago, his HbA_{1c} was 8.7% on routine screening. Today, after adjusting his diet and exercise regimen, it is 8.2%. What is the best management strategy?

Start metformin, which is the first-line treatment for mild persistent hyperglycemia. According to American Diabetes Association (ADA) guidelines, if HbA_{1c} remains ≥ 7% for three months, one should continue metformin and exercise one of two options: (1) add a sulfonylurea or basal insulin (preferred), or (2) add pioglitazone (a thiazolidinedione) or a GLP-1 agonist (eg, exenatide injection).

Per the ADA, the presence of any one of the following is diagnostic for DM (see Table 6.12 for screening criteria):

- Symptoms of diabetes (polyuria, polydipsia, unexplained weight loss) plus a random glucose concentration ≥ 200 mg/dL (11.1 mmol/L).
- A fasting (≥ 8 hours) plasma glucose level ≥ 126 mg/dL (7 mmol/L).
- A two-hour plasma glucose level ≥ 200 mg/dL (11.1 mmol/L) during an oral glucose tolerance test with a 75-g glucose load.
- An HbA_{1c} ≥ 6.5%.

The diagnosis of DM should be confirmed on a subsequent day unless there are obvious signs of hyperglycemia.

TABLE 6.12.   Diabetes Screening Criteria

CONSIDER SCREENING EVERY THREE YEARS	CONSIDER SCREENING SOONER AND MORE FREQUENTLY

All individuals ≥ 45 years of age.	If the patient is overweight (BMI ≥ 25 kg/m²) and:
	  ▪ Is physically inactive.
	  ▪ Has a first-degree relative with diabetes.
	  ▪ Is a member of a high-risk ethnic group (African American, Hispanic, Native American, Asian American, Pacific Islander).
	  ▪ Has delivered a baby weighing ≥ 9 lbs or has been diagnosed with gestational DM.
	  ▪ Is hypertensive.
	  ▪ Has low HDL (< 35 mg/dL) or high TG levels (> 250 mg/dL).
	  ▪ Has a clinical condition associated with insulin resistance (eg, PCOS, acanthosis nigricans).
	  ▪ Has vascular disease.

SYMPTOMS/EXAM

- Presents with the **three "polys": polyuria, polydipsia,** and **polyphagia.**
- Rapid weight loss, dehydration, blurry vision, neuropathy, altered consciousness, acanthosis nigricans (indicates insulin resistance), and candidal vulvovaginitis may also be seen
- **Signs of DKA** include **Kussmaul respirations** (rapid, deep breaths) and a **fruity breath odor** from acetone.

DIFFERENTIAL

- **Type 1 DM:** Autoimmune destruction of the pancreatic islet cells leading to absolute insulin deficiency; associated with a genetic predisposition. The classic patient is young and thin and requires insulin **at all times.** Three **autoantibodies** are commonly found in patients with type 1 DM:
  - Anti–glutamic acid decarboxylase (GAD) antibody.
  - Anti–ICA 512 antibody.
  - Anti-insulin antibody (useful only in the first 1–2 weeks after insulin therapy is initiated).
- **Type 2 DM:** Associated with obesity, insulin resistance, and relative insulin deficiency; accounts for roughly 90% of DM cases in the United States. Has a strong polygenic predisposition.
- **2° causes of DM:** Insulin deficiency or resistance from many causes, such as CF, pancreatitis, Cushing's syndrome, and medications (glucocorticoids, thiazides, pentamidine). May also be due to genetic defects in β-cell function (eg, mature-onset diabetes of the young).
- **Latent autoimmune diabetes in adults:** Generally considered a form of type 1 DM seen in adults. Patients have autoantibodies, but the course is less severe than that in children.

TREATMENT

- **Routine diabetic care:** See Table 6.13.
- **Glycemic control:** Lowering HbA_{1c} is associated with fewer microvascular and neuropathic complications and possibly macrovascular disease. The UK Prospective Diabetes Study (UKPDS) trial defined the goal HbA_{1c} to be < 7%. For therapeutic goals, see Table 6.14.
- **Oral medications for type 2 DM:** See Table 6.15.
  - Metformin is first-line therapy in type 2 DM (in the absence of contraindications such as Cr > 1.5 mg/dL). Often a second or third oral agent or basal insulin is needed to keep HbA_{1c} at the goal as the disease progresses.

KEY FACT

Age does not necessarily determine the type of DM; more children are being diagnosed with type 2 DM and more adults with type 1 DM.

KEY FACT

First-line treatment of type 2 DM in an obese patient with normal renal function (Cr < 1.4–1.5) is metformin.

KEY FACT

Hold metformin immediately before and after radiologic studies with IV contrast because of the risk of lactic acidosis. Do not use in CHF or liver failure.

KEY FACT

Initiate medical therapy and lifestyle changes at the time of diagnosis. Check HbA_{1c} every three months until the goal of < 7% has been attained.

TABLE 6.13.   Routine Diabetic Care

Test	Frequency	Comments
GLYCEMIC CONTROL		
HbA$_{1c}$	Every three months when titrating meds.	Goal < 7%. Check every six months when stable.
MICRO- AND MACROVASCULAR COMPLICATIONS		
BP	Each visit.	Goal < 130/80 mm Hg. First-line therapy is usually ACEIs or ARBs, but calcium channel blockers, β-blockers, and diuretics may also be used.
Lipid control	Annually.	Goal LDL < 70–100 mg/dL. TG < 150, HDL > 40 mg/dL.
ASA	Each visit.	**1° prevention:** For patients > 40 years of age or those with cardiovascular risk factors. **2° prevention:** For all diabetics.
Dilated eye exam	Annually.	**Type 1 DM:** Within 3–5 years of diagnosis. **Type 2 DM:** At the time of diagnosis. Refer more often in the setting of significant retinopathy. Laser therapy can ↓ the risk of vision loss.
Foot exam	Annually.	**Comprehensive exam:** Note pulses, loss of peripheral sensation with monofilament, ulcers, fungal infections, calluses, or any foot deformities. Refer to podiatry for any abnormality. Perform visual inspection at each visit.
Microalbuminuria and creatinine	Annually.	Microalbuminuria = spot urine albumin/creatinine > 30–300 mg/g. ACEIs/ARBs can slow progression to overt nephropathy.
OTHER HEALTH CARE MAINTENANCE		
Influenza vaccine	Annually.	
Pneumococcal vaccine	Once.	Repeat × 1 if the first vaccine was given before age 65 and > 5 years ago.

TABLE 6.14.   Treatment Goals for Nonpregnant DM Patients (both type 1 and type 2)

	Normal	Goal	Additional Action Suggested
Preprandial capillary plasma glucose	< 100 mg/dL	70–130 mg/dL	< 90 mg/dL or > 150 mg/dL
Peak postprandial capillary plasma glucose	< 140 mg/dL	< 180 mg/dL	Target only if preprandial glucose is at target and HbA$_{1c}$ is still elevated
HbA$_{1c}$	< 6%	< 7%	> 8%

TABLE 6.15. **Non-Insulin Medication Options in Type 2 DM**

MEDICATION	ACTION/USE	CLINICAL APPLICATION	COMMENTS
Biguanides (metformin)	↓ glucose production and insulin resistance.	First-line drug. **Hold two days before elective surgery and before contrast studies.**	**GI side effects, lactic acidosis (rare), no weight gain. Contraindications: Renal insufficiency** (Cr > 1.4 mg/dL); LFTs more than three times normal.
Sulfonylureas (glyburide, glipizide, glimepiride)	**Stimulate insulin release.**	Second-line drug. Exercise caution in the elderly because of hypoglycemia.	Act like insulin (**hypoglycemia, weight gain**). **Contraindication:** Severe sulfa allergy. Only glipizide is safe in renal failure.
Thiazolidinediones (TZDs) (pioglitazone, rosiglitazone)	↓ peripheral insulin resistance.	Do not use in CHF or liver disease.	**"Fat and fluid" retention;** fracture risk. **Contraindications:** CHF, active liver disease. **Caution: Rosiglitazone carries a potential risk of MI.**
Meglitinides (repaglinide, nateglinide)	Stimulate insulin release from the pancreas.	Effects are similar to an oral form of ultra-short-acting insulins. Good for postprandial glucose. Acceptable in renal failure.	Hypoglycemia, weight gain.
α-glucosidase inhibitors (acarbose, miglitol)	Prevent glucose adsorption from the gut.	Not commonly used because of GI side effects. Good for postprandial glucose.	GI effects, especially flatulence and bloating.
GLP-1 receptor agonists (exenatide, liraglutide)	Incretin mimetics; potentiate insulin actions. Early satiety; slow gastric absorption. Incretin hormones are secreted by the gut.	Approved for combination use with metformin, sulfonylureas, and TZDs.	Nausea, weight loss. Given as an SQ injection.
DPP-4 inhibitors (sitagliptin, saxagliptin)	Prevent breakdown of GLP-1, thus increasing GLP-1.	Approved for monotherapy or in combination with metformin or a TZD.	Hypersensitivity, weight neutral.
Amylin analog (pramlitide)	Hormone secreted by pancreatic β cells to slow gastric emptying and ↓ postprandial hyperglycemia.	Treat ↑ fasting glucose using combination therapy with insulin.	Nausea, weight loss. Cuts insulin dose by 50%. Administered as an SQ injection before meals.

TABLE 6.16. **Summary of Insulin Characteristics**

	INSULIN TYPE	ONSET	PEAK ACTION	DURATION
Ultra–short acting (SQ)	Lispro, aspart, glulisine	5–15 minutes	60–90 minutes	3–4 hours
Short acting (SQ)	Regular	15–30 minutes	1–3 hours	5–7 hours
Intermediate acting (SQ)	NPH	2–4 hours	8–10 hours	18–24 hours
Long acting (SQ)	Glargine, detemir	3–4 hours	Glargine has virtually no peak; detemir peaks at 6–8 hours	Up to 24 hours

KEY FACT

Rosiglitazone, a TZD, is associated with ↑ rates of MI, although this is still controversial. The ADA recommends against routine use of rosiglitazone given the safety profile and availability of alternative medications.

KEY FACT

If you need to use a TZD, use pioglitazone, which is not associated with MIs. Like rosiglitazone, however, it is associated with CHF—so use with caution.

KEY FACT

The DPP-4 inhibitors (sitagliptin and saxagliptin) can be used in renal failure.

- The goal is to minimize micro- and macrovascular risk factors, with special priority given to cardiovascular risk reduction.
- **Insulin:** For all type 1 DM and many type 2 DM patients (see Table 6.16). Potential insulin regimens include "**basal-bolus**" (basal coverage with intermediate- to long-acting insulin plus a short-acting **bolus** before meals) and **continuous SQ insulin infusion** delivered via an SQ catheter ("insulin pump"). See Figures 6.12 through 6.14 for recommendations on the initiation and titration of insulin.
- **Pancreatic/islet cell transplant:** Experimental.

COMPLICATIONS—ACUTE

Acute complications of DM include the following (see also Table 6.17):

- **DKA:** Can be the initial manifestation of type 1 DM, but may also occur in patients with type 1 or type 2 DM when a stressor is present (eg, infection, infarction, surgery, medical noncompliance). Often presents with abdominal pain, vomiting, Kussmaul respirations, a fruity breath odor, and

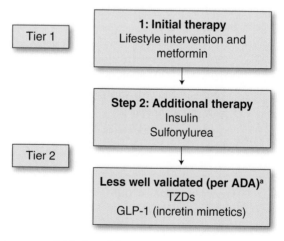

FIGURE 6.12. **Initiation of therapy for type 2 diabetes.**
ªAlthough not listed in ADA guidelines, other medication options for specific settings include α-glucosidase inhibitors, meglitinides, amylin analogs, and DPP-4 inhibitors.

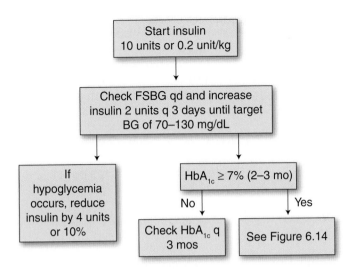

FIGURE 6.13.   Initiation of insulin therapy.

anion-gap metabolic acidosis. Mortality is < 5%. Look for and treat the precipitating event when possible.

- Close the anion gap with an IV **insulin drip;** the glucose will ↓ as the gap closes. Once the glucose level is < 250 mg/dL, add dextrose to IV fluids. When the anion gap has closed, insulin may be switched to SQ. Start SQ insulin **before** discontinuing the insulin drip to prevent "rebound" hyperglycemia.
- **Fluids:** Start with NS. If the patient is not in shock, sodium is normal or ↑, and/or potassium must be repleted concurrently, switch to 1/2 NS or $D_5$1/2 NS.

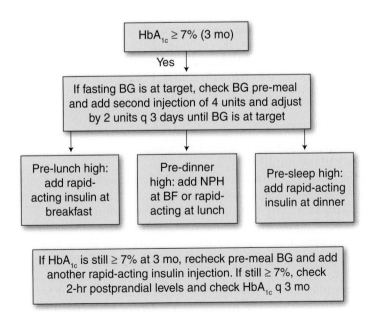

FIGURE 6.14.   Titration of insulin for intensive treatment of diabetes.

TABLE 6.17. DKA vs. Hyperosmolar Coma

	DKA	HYPEROSMOLAR COMA
Serum HCO$_3$	Low (< 15 mEq/L)	Normal or slightly low
pH	< 7.3	> 7.3
Blood glucose	< 800 mg/dL; can be normal	Often > 800 mg/dL
Serum ketones	> 5 mmol/L	< 5 mmol/L
Urine ketones	Large	Small

> **KEY FACT**
>
> For DKA, continue an insulin drip until the anion gap closes **even after glucose has normalized.** For both DKA and hyperosmotic coma, continue the insulin drip until two hours after the first SQ injection when switching to SQ insulin; otherwise you may risk rebound hyperglycemia.

- **Potassium:** Usually falsely elevated due to acidosis. Start K$^+$ replacement at 4.0–4.5 mEq/L, as levels will fall with treatment.
- Bicarbonate, magnesium, and phosphate are usually not needed.
- Hyperosmolar nonketotic coma:
  - Seen in type 2 DM. Significant hyperglycemia (often > 600 mg/dL), hyperosmolality, and dehydration without ketosis are characteristic. Mortality is 40–50%; frequently occurs in elderly patients with multiple comorbidities. There is often a precipitating event (infection, infarction, intoxication, medical noncompliance).
  - Presents with "polys," weakness, lethargy, and confusion (when osmolarity is > 310 mOsm/L) or with coma (> 330 mOsm/L). Treatment is similar to that for DKA; treat the underlying stressor and give fluids, an insulin drip, and electrolyte replacement.
    - **Fluids:** Often need 6–10 L. Start with NS and then follow with 1/2 NS; add D5 when glucose levels are < 250 mg/dL. Watch for pulmonary edema and volume overload in elderly patients.
    - **Insulin drip:** See the DKA section above.
    - **Potassium:** See the DKA section above.
    - **Sodium:** In both DKA and hyperosmotic coma, sodium is often **falsely low due to hyperglycemia.** For each 100 mg/dL that glucose exceeds 100 mg/dL, Na ↓ by 2.4 mEq/L.

> **KEY FACT**
>
> Two landmark trials show that lowering HbA$_{1c}$ prevents **microvascular** complications: the Diabetes Control and Complications Trial for type 1 DM and the UK Prospective Diabetes Study for type 2 DM. There is conflicting evidence on whether lowering HbA$_{1c}$ prevents macrovascular complications.

COMPLICATIONS—CHRONIC

Chronic complications include the following:
- Microvascular complications:
  - **Retinopathy:** Occurs after DM has been present for 3–5 years. Prevent with a yearly eye exam and laser therapy for retinal neovascularization.
  - **Nephropathy:** The first sign is usually microalbuminuria. Prevent with BP control, glucose control, and ACEIs or ARBs.
  - **Neuropathy:** Often progressive, involving the distal feet and hands. Prevent ulcers with foot care, careful inspection, and podiatry as needed.
- **Macrovascular complications:** Associated with an ↑ risk of MI and stroke. Prevent with ASA therapy in high-risk patients; maintain a low threshold for cardiac stress testing; and keep LDL < 100 mg/dL (or < 70 mg/dL in high-risk patients with known CAD).
- **Infections:** DM patients are at ↑ risk of unusual infections such as necrotizing fasciitis or myositis, mucormycosis, emphysematous cholecystitis, and malignant otitis externa.
- **Tight glycemic control** can ↓ the incidence of chronic complications, especially microvascular disease.

> **KEY FACT**
>
> Autonomic symptoms from hypoglycemia can be blunted in patients on β-blockers or in those whose repeated hypoglycemic episodes have rendered them unaware of hypoglycemia.

GESTATIONAL DIABETES

See the Women's Health chapter.

HYPOGLYCEMIA

A 42-year-old woman with type 2 DM and depression presents with recurrent episodes of lightheadedness, diaphoresis, and tremulousness. She has been on stable doses of glargine, mealtime insulin lispro (Humalog), benazepril, and citalopram. She undergoes a supervised fast in the hospital with the following lab results when she develops similar symptoms: ↑ insulin levels, ↓ C-peptide, and ↓ glucose. What is the diagnosis?

Possible insulin abuse. Patients with surreptitious use of insulin or sulfonylureas will have ↑ insulin levels. Insulin administration is associated with ↑ insulin levels and ↓ C-peptide levels.

Although most hypoglycemic reactions occur in patients being treated with insulin, they may also be seen in those on sulfonylureas, meglitinides, and, rarely, other medications (usually when used in combination with sulfonylureas or insulin).

SYMPTOMS/EXAM

- **Neuroglycopenic symptoms** (low glucose delivery to the brain): Mental confusion, stupor, coma, focal neurologic findings mimicking stroke, death.
- **Autonomic symptoms:** Tachycardia, palpitations, sweating, tremulousness, nausea, hunger.

DIFFERENTIAL

- **Insulin reaction:** Too much insulin, too little food, or too much exercise can cause hypoglycemia in patients on insulin.
- **Sulfonylurea overdose:** Especially problematic in elderly patients or in those with renal failure causing ↓ medication clearance.
- **Factitious hypoglycemia:** A surreptitious or inadvertent hypoglycemic agent used in a nondiabetic patient (eg, incorrect medication dispensed).
- **Insulinomas:** Rare tumors of the pancreatic islets cells that secrete insulin. Usually single, benign tumors that can be surgically resected.
- **Reactive hypoglycemia:** Hypoglycemia after a meal may be seen in patients with "dumping syndrome" following bariatric surgery; otherwise rare.
- **Autoimmune hypoglycemia:** A rare condition with anti-insulin antibodies that cause hypoglycemia.

DIAGNOSIS

- Check glucose level when symptoms arise to confirm hypoglycemia.
- Conduct a supervised fast for up to 72 hours. When glucose levels are < 45 mg/dL and the patient experiences the characteristic symptoms of hypoglycemia, measure simultaneous glucose, insulin, C-peptide, proinsulin, and sulfonylurea levels (see Table 6.18).

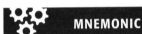

MNEMONIC

Causes of hypoglycemia—

REEXPLAIN

Renal failure
EXogenous (eg, sulfonylurea)
Pituitary failure
Liver failure
Alcohol
Insulinoma, **I**nfection
Neoplasm

KEY FACT

Hypertriglyceridemia can cause milky-appearing serum when the TG level is > 350 mg/dL.

TABLE 6.18. Diagnosis of Hypoglycemic Disorders[a]

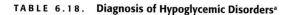

	INSULIN	C-PEPTIDE	SULFONYLUREA SCREEN
Insulinoma	High	High	–
Factitious insulin ingestion	High	Low	–
Sulfonylureas	High	High	+

[a]A 72-hour fast is necessary to rule out insulinoma. Insulin and C-peptide levels should be measured when glucose level is < 45 mg/dL and is accompanied by characteristic symptoms of hypoglycemia.

TREATMENT

- **Conscious patients:** Glucose tablets; orange juice or other sugar-containing beverages.
- **Unconscious patients:** Give 1 mg glucagon IM or 50% glucose solution IV. If these are not available, honey, syrup, or glucose gel may be rubbed into the buccal mucosa.

KEY FACT

For familial hyperlipidemia syndromes, treatment is similar to that of nonhereditary hyperlipidemias:

- ↑ TG = diet and anti-TG medications.
- ↑ LDL = statins +/– ezetimibe or niacin.

FAMILIAL LIPID ABNORMALITIES

Table 6.19 outlines the presentation of various familial lipid abnormalities. See the Ambulatory Care chapter for routine hyperlipidemia treatment guidelines and management.

TABLE 6.19. Common Familial Lipid Abnormalities

DISEASE	MAIN CHOLESTEROL FINDINGS	CLINICAL PRESENTATION
Lipoprotein lipase deficiency (AR)	↑↑ TG (1000s).	Childhood diagnosis. Eruptive cutaneous **xanthomas**, lipemia retinalis, acute pancreatitis, hepatosplenomegaly.
Apo C-II deficiency (AR)—required cofactor for lipoprotein lipase	↑↑ TG (1000s).	Childhood diagnosis. Eruptive cutaneous **xanthomas**, lipemia retinalis, acute pancreatitis, hepatosplenomegaly.
Familial hypertriglyceridemia (AD)	Mildly ↑ TG (200–500).	Eruptive cutaneous **xanthomas**, lipemia retinalis, acute pancreatitis.
Familial hypercholesterolemia—deficiency or malfunction of LDL receptor (AD)	TC > 500 in homozygotes (275–500 in heterozygotes); ↑↑ LDL, ↑ TG.	Premature CAD, **tendon xanthomas.** Homozygous: **CAD in the first decade.**
Familial defective ApoB100—impaired LDL binding	TC > 500 in homozygotes (275–500 in heterozygotes); ↑↑ LDL, ↑ TG.	Premature CAD, **tendon xanthomas.**
Familial combined hyperlipidemia (AD)—can be isolated ↑ TG, ↑ LDL, or both	↑ TC, ↑ TG, ↑ LDL, or both.	Premature CAD. Associated with insulin resistance.
Familial dysbetalipoproteinemia—ApoE2 isoform (AR)	Mildly ↑ TC and ↑ TG (both 250–500).	**Palmar and tubular xanthomas.**

AR = autosomal recessive; AD = autosomal dominant; TG = triglycerides; TC = total cholesterol.

Mineral Metabolism and Metabolic Bone Disease

CALCIUM METABOLISM

Figure 6.15 delineates the hormonal control of calcium metabolism. Figure 6.16 graphically depicts the mechanisms of vitamin D metabolism. The **25-hydroxyvitamin D** (25-HD) level indicates body vitamin D stores, and **1,25-dihydroxyvitamin D** (1,25-DHD) is the biologically active hormone.

HYPERCALCEMIA

An asymptomatic 35-year-old woman presents to her primary care physician for an annual exam. On routine laboratory testing, she is found to have a serum calcium level of 10.8 mg/dL. Her father also has mild hypercalcemia. Follow-up testing reveals a mildly ↑ PTH level of 65 pg/mL. What is the most likely diagnosis?

Benign familial hypocalciuric hypercalcemia. Urinary calcium excretion is low in this disorder but high in 1° hyperparathyroidism. No treatment is necessary, but always evaluate first-degree relatives.

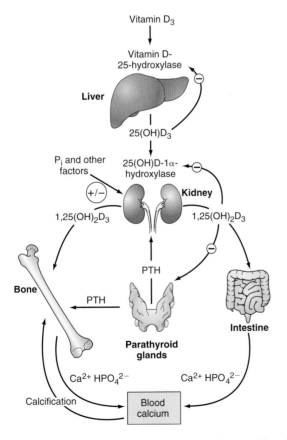

FIGURE 6.15. Hormonal control loop for calcium metabolism and function. Low serum calcium levels prompt a proportional increase in PTH concentration, which mobilizes calcium from the bone. PTH also increases the synthesis of $1,25(OH)_2$ vitamin D in the kidney, which in turn stimulates the mobilization of calcium from bone, increases absorption of calcium in the intestine, and downregulates PTH synthesis. (Reproduced with permission from Kasper DL et al. *Harrison's Principles of Internal Medicine,* 16th ed. New York: McGraw-Hill, 2005: 2246.)

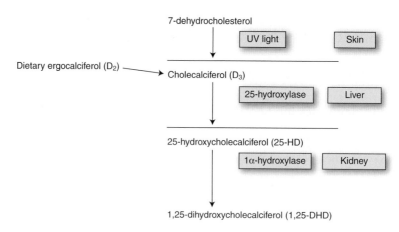

FIGURE 6.16. Vitamin D metabolism. Vitamin D is derived when UV light from the sun hits the skin, converting 7-dehydrocholesterol into cholecalciferol (D₃), or when ergocalciferol (D₂) is ingested and then converted to D₃. D₃ is 25-hydroxylated to 25-hydroxycholecalciferol (25-HD) in the liver. 25-HD is the primary storage form. 25-HD is converted to 1,25-dihydroxy-cholecalciferol (1,25-DHD) in the kidney under PTH regulation. 1,25-DHD is the active form of the hormone.

Most commonly presents as an incidentally discovered laboratory abnormality in an asymptomatic patient. Can be classified as PTH-mediated hypercalcemia (1° hyperparathyroidism) or as conditions in which PTH is suppressed.

SYMPTOMS/EXAM

Best remembered by the mnemonic "**psychic moans, abdominal groans, stones, and bones**" (see Table 6.20).

DIFFERENTIAL

- **1° hyperparathyroidism:** See the section below.
- **Malignancy-associated hypercalcemia:** Occurs in 10–15% of malignancies and portends a poor prognosis. Has three mechanisms:
    - **Tumor release of PTHrP (most common):** Homologous to PTH, but **not** detected by intact PTH serum assay, and does not ↑ 1,25-DHD production. Seen with solid tumors (eg, breast, lung, renal cell, ovarian, and bladder carcinoma).
    - **1,25-DHD production by tumor:** Due to 1α-hydroxylase activity; associated with lymphomas.
    - **Local osteolysis from metastases or adjacent tumor mass:** Typically multiple myeloma, breast cancer, or lymphoma.

TABLE 6.20. Signs and Symptoms of Hypercalcemia

PSYCHIC MOANS	ABDOMINAL GROANS	STONES	BONES	OTHER
Lethargy	Nausea	Nephrolithiasis	Osteitis fibrosa	Weakness
Depression	Vomiting	Nephrocalcinosis	Arthritis	Hypertonia
Psychosis	Constipation	Nephrogenic DI (polyuria,	Fractures (depending on	Bradycardia
Ataxia	Anorexia	polydipsia)	the cause)	Shortened QT
Stupor		Uremia		Band keratopathy[a]
Coma				

[a]A mottled-looking band stretching horizontally across the cornea.

- **Granulomatous disorders:** Sarcoidosis and TB result in ↑ 1,25-DHD production. Can be treated with glucocorticoids to suppress 1α-hydroxylase enzyme.
- **Endocrinopathies:**
  - **Thyrotoxicity:** Ten percent of thyrotoxic patients have mild hypercalcemia.
  - **Adrenal insufficiency:** Pheochromocytoma, VIPoma (rare).
- **Hypervitaminosis A and D:**
  - Vitamin A excess leads to bone resorption and associated hypercalcemia.
  - Vitamin D intoxication leads to ↑ 25-HD levels, which stimulate ↑ intestinal absorption of calcium and ↓ renal excretion.
- **Drug induced:** Thiazides, lithium, calcium-based antacids, estrogens, androgens, teriparatide (PTH 1-84).
- **Immobilization:** Usually seen in adolescents or others with high bone turnover states (Paget's, hyperthyroidism) due to marked increases in bone resorption. Associated with hypercalciuria.
- **Milk-alkali syndrome:** Occurs when large quantities of calcium are ingested with absorbable antacids and cause hypercalcemia, alkalosis, nephrocalcinosis, and kidney dysfunction.
- **Familial: Benign familial hypocalciuric hypercalcemia.** An autosomal dominant disorder characterized by hypercalcemia and hypocalciuria with normal to ↑ PTH levels.

DIAGNOSIS

- Check ionized calcium or correct for albumin level:

  Corrected Ca⁺⁺ = serum Ca (mg/dL) + [0.8 × (4.0 − albumin (g/dL)]

  ie, for each 1.0-mg/dL ↓ in albumin, add 0.8 mg/dL to measured total serum calcium.
- Determine PTH. If ↑, the differential should include PTH-mediated causes of hypercalcemia; if suppressed, check PTHrP, 25-HD, and 1,25-DHD (see Table 6.21).

TREATMENT

- **Hydration with NS is the essential element in treating acute hypercalcemia.** Often requires 2.5–4.0 L of NS per day; use caution in the setting of CHF.
- **Loop diuretics** are indicated **only after complete rehydration.**
- **IV bisphosphonates** (pamidronate or zoledronic acid):
  - The treatment of choice in suspected hypercalcemia of malignancy to ↓ bone resorption.

KEY FACT

Eighty percent of hospitalized hypercalcemia cases are due to malignancy. Eighty percent of outpatient hypercalcemia cases are due to 1° hyperparathyroidism.

KEY FACT

Lithium can lead to hypercalcemia by increasing PTH.

MNEMONIC

Causes of hypercalcemia—

CHIMPANZEES

Calcium supplementation
Hyperparathyroidism
Iatrogenic/**I**mmobility
Milk-alkali syndrome
Paget's disease
Adrenal insufficiency
Neoplasm
Zollinger-Ellison syndrome
Excess vitamin A
Excess vitamin D
Sarcoidosis

KEY FACT

Think of 1° hyperparathyroidism in a patient with ↑ PTH and ↑ calcium. Phosphorus is usually low-normal.

TABLE 6.21. Laboratory Findings Associated with Hypercalcemia

	CALCIUM	PHOSPHORUS	PTH	PTHRP	OTHER
PTH mediated	↑	↓	↑	↓	
PTHrP mediated	↑	↓	↓	↑	
1,25-DHD mediated	↑	↑	↓	↓	↑ 1,25-DHD
Vitamin D intoxication	↑	↑	↓	↓	↑ 25-HD

KEY FACT

First-line treatment for hypercalcemia is normal saline infusion to counteract volume depletion. If hypercalcemia is persistent and the patient has severe symptoms, add calcitonin. For patients with known cancer, add an IV bisphosphonate instead of calcitonin (eg, pamidronate, zolendronate).

- Their effect on serum calcium will be **delayed at least 24 hours,** and the calcium nadir will occur approximately 3–5 days after injection. Hypocalcemic effects will last 4–6 weeks.
  - Side effects include a mild ↑ in serum creatinine, transient fever and myalgias, and hypophosphatemia. **Also associated with osteonecrosis of the jaw.**
- **Calcitonin (SQ):**
  - Use only in the presence of severe symptomatic hypercalcemia.
  - Works faster than bisphosphonates, but efficacy is lost after three days owing to tachyphylaxis.
- **Glucocorticoids:** First-line treatment in patients with vitamin D– or vitamin A–mediated hypercalcemia, including ↑ 1,25-DHD production from lymphoma or granulomatous disease.

1° HYPERPARATHYROIDISM

Eighty percent of cases are due to a single parathyroid adenoma; the rest are due to multigland hyperplasia and cancer. Can be part of **MEN 1 or MEN 2A syndrome.**

SYMPTOMS/EXAM

- Like hypercalcemia, it presents with **"psychic moans, abdominal groans, stones, and bones."**
- **Eighty-five percent of patients are asymptomatic and are diagnosed on screening labs.**
- **Musculoskeletal:** Osteoporosis, weakness, and fatigue.
- **Renal: Nephrolithiasis;** gradual onset of **renal insufficiency** from nephrocalcinosis and nephrogenic DI.
- **Osteitis fibrosa cystica:** ↑ bone turnover causing bone pain and pathologic fractures. Also characterized by ↑ alkaline phosphatase. Radiographs of the phalanges and skull reveal subperiosteal resorption of cortical bone (see Figure 6.17). Osteolytic lesions due to brown tumors (cystic bone lesions containing fibrous tissue) may also be apparent.

KEY FACT

Hyperparathyroidism causes the greatest bone loss at the forearm, followed by the hip (sites of cortical bone). The spine (trabecular bone) is least affected.

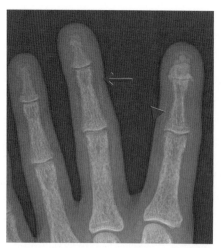
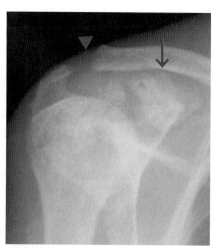

A   **B**

FIGURE 6.17. **Skeletal changes of hyperparathyroidism. (A)** Subperiosteal resorption of the phalanges (arrow) and digital artery calcifications (arrowhead). **(B)** Resorption of the distal clavicle (arrowhead) and soft tissue calcifications (arrow). (Reproduced with permission from Imboden JB et al. *Current Rheumatology Diagnosis & Treatment,* 2nd ed. New York: McGraw-Hill, 2007, Fig. 54-5.)

DIFFERENTIAL

- **Familial benign hypocalciuric hypercalcemia:** Distinguished from 1° hyperparathyroidism by normal or mildly ↑ PTH and marked **hypocalciuria. Requires no therapy.**
- **MEN syndromes:** See the section on MEN below.
- **Lithium therapy:** Lithium shifts the set point for PTH secretion, resulting in hypercalcemia.

DIAGNOSIS

Made by laboratory tests showing ↑ **PTH,** ↑ **Ca⁺⁺, and** ↓ or normal **phosphorus.** Further evaluation should include the following:

- Measurement of 24-hour urinary calcium and creatinine.
- Evaluation of renal function with creatinine.
- Bone mineral density (BMD) evaluation by dual-energy x-ray absorptiometry (DEXA).
- Measurement of 25-HD level. Low levels can cause 2° hyperparathyroidism and can predispose to hungry bone syndrome (see below).
- Imaging studies of the parathyroid glands (neck ultrasound and parathyroid sestamibi scan) are **not useful for diagnosis** but may be helpful in preoperative planning.

TREATMENT

- **Parathyroidectomy** is the treatment of choice. The **cure rate is 95%,** and the complication rate (hypoparathyroidism, recurrent laryngeal nerve injury) is < 1%. **Surgery is recommended under the following conditions:**
    - Age < 50 years.
    - Serum calcium 1.0 mg/dL above the upper normal level.
    - Creatinine clearance < 60 mL/min.
    - BMD with a T-score < −2.5 at any site.
    - Patient preference or inability to follow up.
- **Medical therapy:** Usually reserved for symptomatic patients who either refuse or are unsuitable candidates for surgery. Bisphosphonates can prevent bone loss. Cinacalcet, which ↓ PTH secretion, can ↓ serum calcium, but it is currently approved by the FDA only for 2° hyperparathyroidism from CKD or hypercalcemia from parathyroid carcinoma.

COMPLICATIONS

- Hypercalcemia, nephrolithiasis, nephrocalcinosis with renal insufficiency, osteoporosis.
- **Hungry bone syndrome:** Severe hypocalcemia occurring after parathyroidectomy, usually as a result of chronic bone disease.

HYPOCALCEMIA

A 65-year-old man undergoes a thyroidectomy for papillary thyroid carcinoma. On postoperative day 2, he complains of perioral numbness and bilateral hand cramping and muscle spasms. What is the most likely explanation for his symptoms, and how should he be treated?

Acquired hypocalcemia from hypoparathyroidism as a complication of thyroidectomy. Treat acutely with an IV calcium drip and correct any hypomagnesemia. Also initiate therapy with oral calcium, and add calcitriol if his symptoms persist.

Chronic hypocalcemia results from deficiency or failure to respond to either PTH or vitamin D. Acute hypocalcemia can occur even when PTH is high if adaptive mechanisms are overwhelmed. Etiologies are outlined in Table 6.22.

SYMPTOMS/EXAM

- **Neuromuscular excitability:** Paresthesias, seizures, organic brain syndrome, or **tetany** (a state of spontaneous tonic muscular contraction). Often heralded by numbness and tingling of the fingertips and perioral zone, its classic component is carpopedal spasm.
- **Chvostek's sign:** Contraction of facial muscles in response to tapping of the facial nerve.
- **Trousseau's sign:** Elicited by inflating a BP cuff to 20 mm Hg above systolic BP for three minutes. A ⊕ response is carpal spasm.
- **Soft tissue calcium deposition:** Cataracts; calcification of basal ganglia.
- **Cardiac:** Prolonged QT interval.
- **Dermatologic:** Dry, flaky skin with brittle nails.

DIAGNOSIS

First check calcium and correct for albumin or check ionized calcium; then check phosphorus, magnesium, and PTH (see Table 6.23). If PTH is ↑ or normal, check 25-HD and renal function.

TREATMENT

- **Acute:** In the setting of tetany, initiate a continuous IV calcium drip while starting oral calcium; give calcitriol if needed.
- **Chronic:** Oral calcium and calcitriol if needed.

TABLE 6.22.   Etiologies of Hypocalcemia

PATHOLOGY	MECHANISM/NOTES
Hypoparathyroidism	Most often postsurgical.
	Also autoimmune, congenital, or infiltrative (hemochromatosis, Wilson's disease, sarcoidosis).
Pseudohypoparathyroidism (PTH resistance)	A rare, heritable disorder of **target organ resistance to PTH.** Usually presents in childhood.
Vitamin D deficiency	Deficiency can result from lack of sunlight, malabsorption, or liver/renal disease. Diagnosed by low 25-HD level; treat with high-dose PO ergocalciferol.
	Long-standing deficiency leads to osteomalacia in adults (myopathy, poor bone mineralization with pseudofractures) or to rickets in children.
Extravascular deposition	Pancreatitis, rhabdomyolysis, tumor lysis, osteoblastic metastases, hungry bone syndrome.
Sepsis or severe illness	
Hypomagnesemia	Malabsorption, chronic alcoholism, cisplatin therapy.
	Diuretics, aminoglycosides.
Drugs	Calcium chelators **(citrated blood products).**
	Bisphosphonates, cinacalcet, **cisplatin.**

TABLE 6.23. Laboratory Findings Associated with Hypocalcemia

	CALCIUM	PHOSPHORUS	PTH	OTHER
Hypoparathyroidism	↓	↑	↓	
PTH resistance	↓	↑	↑	
Vitamin D deficiency	↓	↓	↑	↓ 25-HD
1,25-DHD resistance	↓	↓	↑	↑ 1,25-DHD

MEN AND 2° OSTEOPOROSIS

2° osteoporosis is defined as osteoporosis due to an identifiable underlying disease. See the Women's Health chapter for information regarding postmenopausal osteoporosis.

SYMPTOMS/EXAM

Typical osteoporotic fractures are hip, vertebral compression, and Colles' fractures (a type of distal radius fracture).

DIAGNOSIS

- See the Women's Health chapter for a discussion of DEXA scores and osteoporosis diagnosis.
- Further evaluation should include a search for 2° causes of osteoporosis based on clinical suspicion (see also Table 6.24):
  - 25-HD level.
  - Serum calcium, phosphorus, and PTH.
  - 24-hour urinary calcium and creatinine.
  - SPEP/UPEP.
  - **Testosterone level.**
  - TSH, especially in those with a history of hyperthyroidism or on levothyroxine replacement.

TREATMENT

See the Women's Health chapter for a discussion of treatment.

KEY FACT

2° osteoporosis should also be considered in women, especially those with Z-scores < −2. Z-score indicates a 2° cause of osteoporosis (think **"Z"** for "**Z**ebra" causes).

KEY FACT

As with female osteoporosis, first-line therapy for male osteoporosis centers on bisphosphonates.

TABLE 6.24. 2° Causes of Osteoporosis

ENDOCRINE CAUSES	GI DISORDERS	MARROW/HEMATOLOGIC DISORDERS	OTHER
Cushing's syndrome	Liver disease (1° biliary cirrhosis)	**Multiple myeloma**	Immobilization
Hypogonadism (male or female)	**Malabsorptive conditions** (mediated primarily	Leukemias/lymphomas	**Alcohol abuse**
Hyperprolactinemia (by inducing	via vitamin D deficiency):	Systemic mastocytosis	Tobacco use
hypogonadism)	▪ **Celiac disease**	Hemophilia	Osteogenesis imperfecta
Hyperthyroidism	▪ Gastrectomy	Thalassemia	RA
Hyperparathyroidism	▪ Inflammatory bowel disorders	Polycythemia vera	Ankylosing spondylitis
Vitamin D deficiency	▪ **Gastric bypass**		Eating disorders
Acromegaly	▪ Pancreatic insufficiency		Corticosteroid use
Osteomalacia			

COMPLICATIONS

Fractures. Hip fractures are associated with 30% mortality in men (higher mortality rate than for women). Vertebral fractures are associated with chronic pain and disability.

PAGET'S DISEASE

Accelerated bone turnover and remodeling, resulting in impaired bone integrity and overgrowth.

SYMPTOMS

Presents with pain, fractures, and skeletal deformity, most commonly in the **sacrum, spine, femur, skull, and pelvis.** Two-thirds of patients are asymptomatic.

EXAM

Depends on which bones are involved. Exam may reveal skull enlargement, frontal bossing, bowed legs, and cutaneous erythema, warmth, and tenderness over the affected site.

DIFFERENTIAL

Includes any localized bony tumor or cancer.

DIAGNOSIS

- **Labs:** ↑ **alkaline phosphatase** and bone turnover markers (eg, osteocalcin, urinary hydroxyproline, N-telopeptide). Ca^{++} and phosphorus are normal.
- **Imaging:**
  - **Plain radiography:** Involved bones are expanded and denser than normal (see Figure 6.18). Erosions are seen in the skull (osteoporosis circumscripta). Affected weight-bearing bones may be bowed.
  - **Bone scan:** ↑ uptake is seen in affected areas but can be nonspecific.

The most common fractures in Paget's disease are vertebral crush fractures.

Paget's is one of the rare causes of high-output CHF due to hypervascularity of bony lesions.

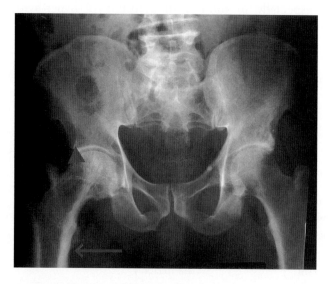

FIGURE 6.18. Paget's disease, right femur. Note the thickened cortex (arrow), thickened trabeculae (arrowhead), and expansion of the right femoral head and neck in comparison to the left femur. (Reproduced with permission from Fauci AS et al. *Harrison's Principles of Internal Medicine,* 17th ed. New York: McGraw-Hill, 2008, Fig. 349-3.)

TABLE 6.25.   **Complications of Paget's Disease**

RHEUMATOLOGIC	NEUROLOGIC	CARDIAC	NEOPLASTIC[a]	METABOLIC
Osteoarthritis Gout	Deafness (from involvement of cranial nerves, with bony entrapment) Spinal cord compression leading to paraplegia Peripheral nerve entrapment (carpal and tarsal tunnel syndromes)	High-output CHF	**Osteosarcoma or chondrosarcoma** Giant cell tumor	Immobilization-induced hypercalcemia/ hypercalciuria Nephrolithiasis

[a]Occur in 1% of Paget's cases.

TREATMENT

Bisphosphonates are the treatment of choice and lead to remission in most patients. Choices include IV pamidronate or zoledronic acid, oral alendronate, risedronate, and IV/PO ibandronate.

COMPLICATIONS

The complications of Paget's disease are outlined in Table 6.25.

Male Hypogonadism

The testes are composed of seminiferous tubules, where sperm are produced (80–90% of testicular mass), and Leydig cells, which produce androgens.

SYMPTOMS/EXAM

Postpubertal androgen deficiency: ↓ libido, erectile dysfunction, low energy. If prolonged, a ↓ in facial and body hair may be seen.

DIFFERENTIAL

- **Hypothalamic/pituitary disorders:** Low testosterone with normal or ↓ LH and FSH.
  - **Panhypopituitarism.**
  - **LH and FSH deficiency** associated with **anosmia: Kallmann's** syndrome.
- **Testicular disorders (primary hypogonadism):** Usually characterized by ↓ testosterone and ↑ LH and FSH.
  - **Klinefelter's syndrome: The most common genetic cause of male hypogonadism.** XXY karyotype. Can be associated with intellectual impairment.
  - **Adult seminiferous tubule failure:** Characterized by infertility, normal virilization, and **normal testosterone** levels (because the Leydig cells are unaffected). May be due to orchitis, leprosy, irradiation, alcoholism, uremia, cryptorchidism, lead poisoning, and chemotherapeutic agents (eg, cyclophosphamide, methotrexate).
  - **Adult Leydig cell failure (andropause):** A gradual ↓ in testicular function after age 50, with declining testosterone levels.
- Defects in androgen action:
  - **Complete androgen insensitivity:** Also known as **testicular feminization**—XY, with female phenotype, absence of uterus, absence of sexual hair, and infertility. Patients are usually raised as girls.
  - **Incomplete androgen insensitivity:** Phenotype varies with degree of insensitivity.

KEY FACT

Hypogonadism is suggested with a low serum testosterone. If LH and FSH are ↑, the cause is testicular damage (1° hypogonadism). If LH and FSH are ↓, the cause is the pituitary or hypothalamus.

KEY FACT

If LH and FSH are ↓ and a patient has delayed puberty and anosmia along with male relatives with similar symptoms, consider Kallmann's syndrome.

KEY FACT

If LH and FSH are ↑, consider Klinefelter's syndrome (XXY), the most common cause of male hypogonadism. The patient may be lanky and youthful-looking and may have gynecomastia, small testicles, executive functioning impairment, and fertility problems.

TABLE 6.26. Diagnosis of Male Hypogonadism Based on Lab Tests

ETIOLOGY	TESTOSTERONE	LH/FSH	PROLACTIN	NEXT STEPS
Testicular failure	↓	↑	Normal	Testosterone supplementation.
Age-related decline	↓	Normal	Normal	Testosterone supplementation.
Pituitary disease	↓	↓	↑	Pituitary MRI, lab tests.

DIAGNOSIS

Check testosterone first. If low, repeat testosterone with LH and FSH (see Table 6.26). Diagnosis requires low testosterone measured with a reliable assay in the morning (due to normal diurnal variation) on several occasions.

TREATMENT

- **Androgen replacement:** IM testosterone injections, patches, or gel.
- If an underlying disorder is diagnosed (eg, pituitary tumor), treat appropriately.
- Treatment with testosterone requires monitoring for adverse effects such as prostatic enlargement or unmasking of clinically silent prostate cancer (PSA), erythrocytosis (CBC), low HDL (lipid panel), and obstructive sleep apnea.

COMPLICATIONS

Infertility; osteoporosis can develop in the absence of androgens but can usually be prevented with appropriate testosterone replacement.

Endocrine Tumors

MULTIPLE ENDOCRINE NEOPLASIA (MEN)

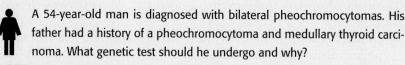

A 54-year-old man is diagnosed with bilateral pheochromocytomas. His father had a history of a pheochromocytoma and medullary thyroid carcinoma. What genetic test should he undergo and why?
RET proto-oncogene mutation testing, which is responsible for most cases of MEN 2. When inherited, MEN 2 is transmitted in an autosomal dominant pattern.

A group of **autosomal dominant** syndromes characterized by multiple endocrine tumors due to defective tumor suppressor genes.

- **MEN 1:** Parathyroid, pancreatic, and pituitary tumors. If there is a ⊕ family history, screen with serum calcium/PTH, serum gastrin, and serum prolactin.
- **MEN 2:** Medullary thyroid cancer and pheochromocytoma +/– 1° hyperparathyroidism. Screen for the RET proto-oncogene mutation if there is a ⊕ family history of MEN 2 or in any patient with medullary thyroid can-

KEY FACT

If LH is low in the setting of a low testosterone level, check a prolactin level to rule out hyperprolactinemia.

KEY FACT

Androgen therapy in hypogonadal men can lead to gynecomastia.

KEY FACT

MEN 1 can be remembered as the **"3 P's"**—**P**arathyroid, **P**ancreas, and **P**ituitary.

KEY FACT

MEN 2 can be remembered as the **"2 C's"**—**C**arcinoma of the **thyroid** and **C**atecholamines (pheochromocytoma) plus parathyroid (MEN 2A) or mucocutaneous neuromas (MEN 2B).

cer or bilateral pheochromocytomas. Prophylactic thyroidectomy is recommended in the setting of a ⊕ RET mutation, as 95% of patients will develop thyroid cancer.

CARCINOID TUMORS/CARCINOID SYNDROME

GI neuroendocrine tumors that are most commonly located in the small bowel. Most are hormonally inert, but some can secrete excessive **serotonin**, prostaglandins, and kinins.

SYMPTOMS/EXAM

- Classic carcinoid syndrome consists of episodic **flushing**, watery **diarrhea**, and **hypotension** with or without asthma.
- **Valvular heart disease** is a common complication.
- Emotional stress, certain foods (eg, tryptophan-containing foods), and straining with defecation can provoke symptoms.
- Carcinoid crisis can occur spontaneously or after tumor palpation, chemotherapy, or hepatic arterial embolization. Symptoms include labile blood pressure, bronchoconstriction, and arrhythmias.

DIAGNOSIS

- Order a **24-hour urine for 5-HIAA** (5-hydroxyindoleacetic acid, a serotonin metabolite).
- An indium-labeled octreotide scan can detect occult lesions (see Figure 6.19).
- Stage with CXR and a chest/abdominal CT.

TREATMENT

- Surgical resection is first-line treatment.
- Symptomatic relief may be obtained with octreotide.

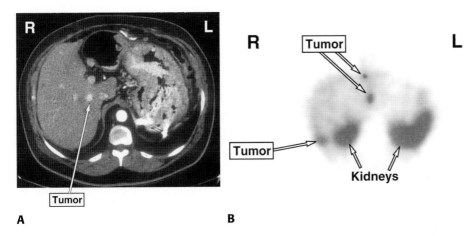

A   **B**

FIGURE 6.19. **Metastatic carcinoid tumor.** (**A**) Transaxial image from a contrast-enhancing staging CT showing a hypervascular liver metastasis. (**B**) Transaxial image from a SPECT indium-labeled octreotide scan showing other hepatic metastases. Uptake of radiotracer in the kidneys is a normal finding related to renal excretion. (Reproduced with permission from Fauci AS et al. *Harrison's Principles of Internal Medicine*, 17th ed. New York: McGraw-Hill, 2008, Fig. 344-3.)

ZOLLINGER-ELLISON SYNDROME (GASTRINOMA)

Hypersecretion of **gastrin** by tumors of the pancreas or duodenum.

Symptoms/Exam

Usually presents as refractory PUD despite *H pylori* treatment or multiple ulcers in the duodenum and jejunum.

Differential

Other causes of ↑ gastrin should be considered, including **therapy with PPIs or H$_2$ blockers,** pernicious anemia, chronic atrophic gastritis, and gastric carcinoma.

Diagnosis

- ↑ **fasting serum gastrin levels** are seen in the presence of gastric acid (pH < 5) and **refractory PUD.**
- If the patient is taking an H$_2$ blocker or a PPI, it must be stopped for at least one week before diagnostic testing.
- Localize by abdominal imaging or octreotide scan.

Treatment

Surgical resection is recommended.

CHAPTER 7

Gastroenterology and Hepatology

Anuj Gaggar, MD, PhD
Ma Somsouk, MD, MAS
Scott W. Biggins, MD, MAS

Upper GI Tract

INFECTIOUS ESOPHAGITIS

> A 37-year-old man presents to his primary care physician with pain and difficulty swallowing. His mouth has some small superficial and painful ulcerations, along with white exudate that can be scraped off with a tongue depressor. While an HIV test is pending, what would be the appropriate treatment for this patient?
>
> Fluconazole. This patient is demonstrating oral thrush and likely has *Candida* esophagitis. Although his oral ulcerations could be due to HSV, CMV, or *Histoplasma* infection, it would still be reasonable to empirically treat for *Candida* to assess for a response, as this is the most likely diagnosis.

Most common in immunosuppressed patients (eg, those with AIDS or malignancies, posttransplant patients, and patients undergoing chemotherapy) and in the setting of chronic steroid or recent antibiotic use. Common pathogens include *Candida albicans*, HSV, and CMV.

SYMPTOMS/EXAM

- Presents with odynophagia (pain as food passes through the esophagus), dysphagia (inability to swallow), and chest pain.
- *C albicans* is the etiologic agent in 75% of cases and CMV or HSV in < 50%.

DIFFERENTIAL

- **Noninfectious esophagitis:** Reflux, pill, caustic ingestion, radiation, eosinophilic, autoimmune (eg, Crohn's, Behçet's).
- **Other:** Functional dyspepsia, esophageal stricture, mass lesion, motility disorders, graft-versus-host disease.

DIAGNOSIS

- In immunocompromised patients, attempt a trial of empiric antifungal therapy (eg, fluconazole). In immunocompetent hosts, odynophagia and dysphagia are alarm symptoms; proceed with endoscopy.
- Upper endoscopy with biopsy is the diagnostic test of choice if the empiric trial yields no response. Findings are as follows:
  - *C albicans:* Linear, adherent plaques that may be yellow or white.
  - **CMV:** Few large, superficial ulcerations.
  - **HSV:** Numerous small, deep ulcerations.
  - **Idiopathic AIDS ulcers:** Low CD4 count; large ulcerations.

TREATMENT

- Treat or adjust underlying immunosuppression.
- *C albicans:* Treatment depends on host immune status.
  - **Immunocompetent patients:** Topical therapy; nystatin swish and swallow five times a day × 7–14 days. Test for HIV.
  - **Immunocompromised patients:** Oral therapy, initially with fluconazole 100–200 mg/day. If the patient is unresponsive, try increasing fluconazole or giving itraconazole, other azoles, caspofungin, or amphotericin.

KEY FACT

Oral thrush with odynophagia likely reflects underlying *Candida* esophagitis.

- **CMV:** Ganciclovir IV × 3–6 weeks.
- **HSV:** Acyclovir 200 mg PO five times a day or valacyclovir 1000 g PO BID.
- **Idiopathic ulcers:** Trial of prednisone.

COMPLICATIONS

Stricture, malnutrition, hemorrhage.

PILL ESOPHAGITIS

Variables include contact time, drug type, and pill characteristics. Most cases arise without preexisting swallowing problems. Pills can remain in a normal esophagus for > 5 minutes or for much longer in the presence of stricture or dysmotility. The risk is higher if pills are large, round, lightweight, or extended-release formulations.

SYMPTOMS/EXAM

Presents with odynophagia, dysphagia, and chest pain.

DIFFERENTIAL

Infectious and other noninfectious esophagitis, GERD, functional dyspepsia, esophageal stricture or mass lesion, esophageal motility disorders.

DIAGNOSIS

- **Review medications.** Common causative agents include the following:
    - **NSAIDs:** ASA, naproxen, ibuprofen, indomethacin.
    - **Antibiotics:** Tetracyclines (especially doxycycline), clindamycin (look for a young patient with acne presenting with odynophagia).
    - **Antivirals:** Foscarnet, AZT, ddC.
    - **Supplements:** Iron and potassium.
    - **Cardiac medications:** Quinidine, nifedipine, captopril, verapamil.
    - **Bisphosphonates:** Alendronate, pamidronate.
    - **Antiepileptics:** Phenytoin.
    - **Asthma/COPD medications:** Theophylline.
- **Upper endoscopy:** Evaluate for stricture or mass lesion (if no response is elicited to stopping the potentially offending agent).

TREATMENT

- Discontinue the suspected drug. Expect symptom relief within 1–6 weeks.
- Patients should drink eight ounces of water with each pill and remain upright at least 30 minutes afterward.
- Proton pump inhibitors (PPIs) may facilitate healing in the setting of concurrent GERD.

ACHALASIA

An idiopathic esophageal motility disorder with loss of peristalsis, high lower esophageal sphincter (LES) resting pressure, and failure of LES relaxation when swallowing. Age at onset is 25–60; incidence ↑ with age. Indistinguishable from esophageal dysmotility caused by **Chagas' disease**.

SYMPTOMS/EXAM

- Presents with progressive dysphagia to solids and then to liquids as well as with slow eating (**"last person at the table to finish meal"**).
- Regurgitation of undigested food, weight loss, and chest pain are also characteristic. Heartburn may result from the fermentation of retained food.

KEY FACT

You can diagnose pill esophagitis by history alone. There is no need for endoscopy.

KEY FACT

Patients with achalasia often lift their arms over their heads or extend their necks to aid in swallowing.

TABLE 7.1.   Differential Diagnosis of Dysphagia

	ACHALASIA	DIFFUSE ESOPHAGEAL SPASM	SCLERODERMA
Peristalsis	Absent	Simultaneous contractions	Absent
LES tone	Normal to ↑ with incomplete relaxation	Normal to ↑	↓
Esophageal body tone (amplitude)	Low	Normal to high	Low
Predominant symptom	Progressive dysphagia	Chest pain	Heartburn and dysphagia

DIFFERENTIAL

Chagas' disease (*Trypanosoma cruzi*), esophageal tumors, pseudoachalasia (a process mimicking achalasia that is typically 2° to tumor invasion into the esophageal neural plexus), webs, strictures, Zenker's diverticulum, oropharyngeal dysphagia (muscular dystrophies, myasthenia gravis, Parkinson's disease), spastic dysmotility disorders (diffuse esophageal spasm, nutcracker esophagus; see Table 7.1), esophageal hypomotility (scleroderma).

DIAGNOSIS

- **CXR:** Demonstrates an air-fluid level in a dilated esophagus.
- **Barium esophagography:** May reveal a dilated esophagus with loss of peristalsis and poor emptying or a smooth, symmetrically tapered distal esophagus with a **"bird's beak"** appearance (see Figure 7.1A).
- **Endoscopy:** Required to exclude esophageal strictures and tumor.
- **Endoscopic ultrasound:** Occasionally used to exclude pseudoachalasia.

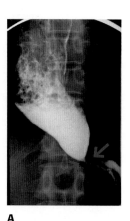

A

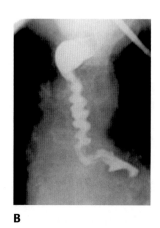

B

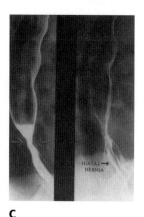

C

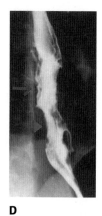

D

FIGURE 7.1.   Esophageal disease on barium esophagram. (A) Achalasia. Note the dilated esophagus tapering to a "bird's-beak" narrowing (arrows) at the lower esophageal sphincter. **(B) Esophageal spasm. (C) Peptic stricture** (arrow) secondary to GERD above a hiatal hernia (right). **(D) Barrett's esophagus** with adenocarcinoma. Note the nodular mucosa of Barrett's esophagus (arrow) and the raised filling defect (arrowhead) representing adenocarcinoma in this patient. (Image A reproduced with permission from Doherty GM. *Current Diagnosis & Treatment: Surgery,* 13th ed. New York: McGraw-Hill, 2010, Fig. 20-5. Image B reproduced with permission from USMLERx.com. Images C and D reproduced with permission from Chen MY et al. *Basic Radiology.* New York: McGraw-Hill, 2004, Figs. 10-14 and 10-19.)

TREATMENT

- **Nitrates and calcium channel antagonists:** Relax LES tone, but have only modest efficacy.
- **Botulinum toxin injection:** Injected into the LES. Performed endoscopically and associated with an 85% initial response, but > 50% of patients require repeated injection within six months. Ideal if the patient is a poor candidate for more invasive treatment.
- **Pneumatic dilation:** Of those treated, > 75% have a durable response. The perforation rate is 3–5%. Does not compromise surgical therapy.
- **Surgery:** Laparoscopic Heller myotomy with partial fundoplication (preventing severe reflux that can occur with myotomy). Of all cases, > 85% have a durable response.

DIFFUSE ESOPHAGEAL SPASM

Diffuse esophageal spasm is marked by uncoordinated contractions. There is a female predominance; onset is usually after age 40.

SYMPTOMS/EXAM

- Substernal chest pain is seen in 80% of patients; pain is nonexertional and worsens with meals.
- A globus ("lump in the throat") sensation is also characteristic.
- Associated with dysphagia to both solids and liquids.
- Regurgitation is less common than in achalasia. Weight loss is rare.

DIFFERENTIAL

Cardiac chest pain, GERD, achalasia, Chagas' disease, esophageal tumors, esophageal dysmotility, peptic stricture, esophagitis, diverticula.

DIAGNOSIS

Diagnose as follows (see also Table 7.1):

- **Barium esophagography:** Peristalsis is present but with delayed transit; esophageal spasms occur at multiple sites and have a **"corkscrew"** or **"rosary bead"** appearance (see Figure 7.1B).
- **Endoscopy:** Not useful in diagnosis, but excludes other differential diagnoses, such as stricture, tumor, and esophagitis.
- **Esophageal manometry:** Shows simultaneous contractions.
- **Ambulatory esophageal pH:** Used to evaluate for gastroesophageal reflux.

TREATMENT

- **Nitrates and calcium channel antagonists:** Relax LES tone, but have only modest efficacy.
- PPIs.
- No clear benefit is derived from botulinum toxin injection, esophageal dilation, or surgical myotomy.

KEY FACT

Unlike achalasia, diffuse esophageal spasm often presents with chest pain rather than with dysphagia.

ESOPHAGEAL RINGS, WEBS, AND STRICTURES

 A 60-year-old man with a history of hypertension and tobacco use presents with four months of increasing difficulty swallowing solids. He is still able to drink liquids but has difficulty with solid foods such as meats. What is the most appropriate diagnostic test for this patient?

Upper endoscopy. This patient has a high risk for esophageal cancer given his age, tobacco use, and description of slowly progressive dysphagia for solids more than liquids. With a high suspicion for cancer, endoscopy will allow for definitive diagnosis with biopsy.

Esophageal rings, webs, and strictures are distinguished as follows (see also Tables 7.2 and 7.3):

- **Lower esophageal (Schatzki) rings:** Common (found in 6–14% of upper GI exams); located in the distal esophagus. Often associated with hiatal hernia, congenital defects, or GERD.
- **Webs:** Less common; located in the proximal esophagus. Congenital.
- **Strictures:** Result from injury (eg, reflux, caustic, anastomosis).

SYMPTOMS/EXAM

Dysphagia with solids is more severe than that with liquids.

DIFFERENTIAL

Cardiac chest pain, GERD, achalasia, Chagas' disease, esophageal tumors, esophageal hypomotility (scleroderma), peptic stricture.

DIAGNOSIS

- **Barium esophagography:** May be diagnostic. Normal peristalsis; luminal abnormality is seen (see Figure 7.1C).
- **Endoscopy:** Required to exclude esophageal stricture or tumor.

TREATMENT

Esophageal dilation; PPIs to ↓ the recurrence of peptic stricture.

KEY FACT

Schatzki rings cause intermittent large-bolus solid-food dysphagia ("steakhouse syndrome").

KEY FACT

Plummer-Vinson syndrome includes esophageal webs, dysphagia, and iron deficiency anemia.

TABLE 7.2. Differential of Esophageal Rings, Webs, and Strictures

	RING	**WEB**	**STRICTURE**
Etiology	Congenital or peptic injury.	Congenital.	Peptic injury, caustic injury.
Esophageal location	Distal.	Proximal.	Mid-distal.
Treatment	Dilation.	Dilation.	Dilation.

TABLE 7.3.   Causes of Esophageal Dysphagia

CAUSE	CLUES TO DIAGNOSIS
Mechanical obstruction:	**Solids more than liquids:**
Schatzki ring	Intermittent dysphagia; not progressive
Peptic stricture	Chronic heartburn; progressive dysphagia
Esophageal cancer	Progressive dysphagia; age over 50
Motility disorders:	**Solid and liquids:**
Achalasia	Progressive dysphagia
Diffuse esophageal spasm	Intermittent, not progressive; may be accompanied by chest pain
Scleroderma	Chronic heartburn; Raynaud's phenomenon

(Adapted with permission from McPhee SJ et al. *Current Medical Diagnosis & Treatment 2010.* New York: McGraw-Hill, 2010, Table 15-8.)

BARRETT'S ESOPHAGUS

Intestinal metaplasia of the distal esophagus 2° to chronic GERD. Normal esophageal squamous epithelium is replaced by columnar epithelium and goblet cells ("specialized epithelium"). Found in 5–10% of patients with chronic GERD, and incidence ↑ with GERD duration. Most common in Caucasian men > 55 years of age; overall incidence is greater in males than in females. The risk of adenocarcinoma is 0.5% per year. Risk factors include male gender, Caucasian ethnicity, and smoking.

DIAGNOSIS

- **Upper endoscopy:** Suggestive but not diagnostic, as it is a histologic diagnosis. **Salmon-colored islands or "tongues"** are seen extending upward from the distal esophagus (see Figure 7.2).
- **Biopsy:** Diagnostic.
  - Shows metaplastic **columnar epithelium** and **goblet cells.**
  - Specialized intestinal metaplasia on biopsy is associated with an ↑ risk of **adenocarcinoma** (not squamous cell carcinoma).

TREATMENT

- Indefinite PPI therapy (GERD should be treated prior to surveillance, as inflammation may confound the interpretation of dysplasia).
- Adenocarcinoma surveillance is necessary only if patients are candidates for esophagectomy.
- Upper endoscopy with four-quadrant biopsies every 2 cm of endoscopic lesions.
- Screening (based on criteria from the American Society of Gastrointestinal Endoscopy) is as follows:
  - After initial diagnosis, repeat EGD in one year for surveillance with biopsies.
  - Proceed according to EGD findings:
    - **No dysplasia:** Repeat EGD every three years.
    - **Low-grade dysplasia:** Repeat EGD within six months. If findings are unchanged, extend surveillance to yearly intervals.

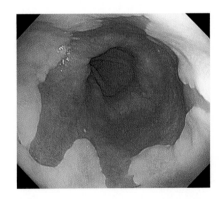

FIGURE 7.2.   Barrett's esophagus on endoscopy. Note the pink tongues characteristic of Barrett's. (Reproduced with permission from Fauci AS et al. *Harrison's Principles of Internal Medicine,* 17th ed. New York: McGraw-Hill, 2008, Fig. 285-3A.)

■ **High-grade dysplasia:** Management is controversial but includes early esophagectomy or intensive endoscopic surveillance every three months until cancer is diagnosed, followed by esophagectomy. Verify with an expert pathologist. Ablative therapies may be attempted (eg, photodynamic therapy, argon plasma coagulation, endoscopic mucosal resection).

DYSPEPSIA

Typically defined as one or more of the following: postprandial fullness, early satiation, and epigastric burning or pain. Distinct from but can present with GERD (retrosternal burning). In the United States, the prevalence of dyspepsia is 25%, but only 25% of those affected seek care. Of these, > 60% have **nonulcerative dyspepsia and < 1% have gastric cancer.**

SYMPTOMS/EXAM

May present with upper abdominal pain or discomfort, fullness, bloating, early satiety, belching, nausea, and retching or vomiting.

DIFFERENTIAL

Nonulcerative dyspepsia (> 60%), food intolerance (overeating, high-fat foods, alcohol, lactose intolerance), drug intolerance (NSAIDs, iron, narcotics, alendronate, theophylline, antibiotics), PUD (10–25%), GERD (15–20%), gastric cancer (< 1%), chronic pancreatitis, pancreatic cancer, biliary colic, IBS.

DIAGNOSIS/TREATMENT

■ **Look for alarm features:** May include new-onset dyspepsia in patients **> 50 years** of age, unintended **weight loss, melena, iron deficiency anemia, persistent vomiting, hematemesis, dysphagia, odynophagia,** abdominal mass, a history of PUD, previous gastric **surgery,** and a family history of **gastric cancer.**
  ■ **If alarm features are present:** Perform prompt endoscopy.
  ■ **If no alarm features are present:** Assess diet and provide education; discontinue suspect medications. Consider a trial of empiric acid suppression; consider testing for and treating *H pylori* (see below).
■ **Determine the local prevalence of *H pylori*.**
  ■ **If > 10%:** Test for *H pylori* by serology, stool antigen, or breath test. If ⊕, institute *H pylori* eradication therapy. If ⊖, initiate a trial of acid suppression × 4–8 weeks.
  ■ **If < 10%:** Institute a trial of acid suppression × 4–8 weeks.
■ **For persistent symptoms:**
  ■ If the patient received *H pylori* therapy, test for eradication with a stool antigen or breath test, **not with serology.** If disease is not eradicated, attempt a different regimen. If eradicated, refer to endoscopy.
  ■ If the patient received a trial of PPIs, refer to endoscopy.
■ **Endoscopy:**
  ■ **If unrevealing:** Diagnose with nonulcerative dyspepsia and provide reassurance; consider a trial of low-dose TCAs (desipramine 10–25 mg QHS) and possible cognitive-behavioral therapy.
  ■ **If revealing:** Manage as indicated.
■ Table 7.4 summarizes treatment options for PUD.

TABLE 7.4. **Treatment Options for PUD**

FINDINGS	TREATMENT OPTIONS[a]

Active *H pylori*–associated ulcer	1. Treat with an anti–*H pylori* regimen × 10–14 days. Possible treatment options include the following:
	  ▪ PPIs BID, clarithromycin 500 mg BID, amoxicillin 1 g BID (or metronidazole 500 mg BID if penicillin allergic).
	  ▪ PPIs BID, bismuth subsalicylate two tablets QID, tetracycline 500 mg QID, metronidazole 250 mg QID.
	2. After completion of a 10- to 14-day course of *H pylori* eradication therapy, continue treatment with PPIs QD or H_2 receptor antagonists (as below) × 4–8 weeks to promote healing. Inasmuch as there is a 20% *H pylori* treatment failure rate, check for *H pylori* eradication with a stool antigen or urea breath test, **not with serology.**

Active ulcer not attributable to *H pylori*	**Consider other causes**—eg, NSAIDs, Zollinger-Ellison syndrome, gastric malignancy. Treatment options are as follows:
	1. **PPIs:**
	  ▪ **Uncomplicated duodenal ulcers:** Treat for four weeks.
	  ▪ **Uncomplicated gastric ulcers:** Treat for eight weeks.
	2. **H_2 receptor antagonists:**
	  ▪ **Uncomplicated duodenal ulcers:** Cimetidine 800 mg, ranitidine or nizatidine 300 mg, famotidine 40 mg QD at bedtime × 6 weeks.
	  ▪ **Uncomplicated gastric ulcers:** Cimetidine 400 mg, ranitidine or nizatidine 150 mg, famotidine 20 mg BID × 8 weeks.
	  ▪ **Complicated ulcers:** PPIs are the preferred drugs.

Prevention of ulcer relapse	1. **NSAID-induced ulcers:** Prophylactic therapy for high-risk patients (patients with prior ulcer disease or ulcer complications; those on corticosteroids or anticoagulants; those > 70 years of age with serious comorbid illnesses). Treatment options include the following:
	  ▪ PPIs QD.
	  ▪ COX-2-selective NSAIDs (celecoxib).
	  ▪ In special circumstances, misoprostol 200 μg TID-QID.
	2. **Chronic "maintenance" therapy:** Indicated in patients with recurrent ulcers who are *H pylori* ⊖ or have failed attempts at eradication therapy. Give once-daily PPIs or H_2 receptor antagonists at bedtime (cimetidine 400–800 mg, nizatidine or ranitidine 150–300 mg, famotidine 20–40 mg).

[a]PPIs are administered before meals. Avoid metronidazole regimens in areas of known high resistance or in patients who have failed a course of treatment that included metronidazole.

(Adapted with permission from McPhee SJ et al. *Current Medical Diagnosis & Treatment 2010.* New York: McGraw-Hill, 2010, Table 15-10.)

GASTROESOPHAGEAL REFLUX DISEASE (GERD)

Caused by transient relaxation of the LES. In the United States, 40% of adults report having GERD symptoms at least once per month, and 7% report having daily symptoms. Although most patients have mild GERD, 40–50% develop esophagitis, 5% ulcerative esophagitis, 4–20% esophageal strictures, and 5–10% Barrett's esophagus. Risk factors include pregnancy and hiatal hernia.

SYMPTOMS

▪ Typical presentation:
  ▪ A retrosternal burning sensation (heartburn) accompanied by regurgitation that begins in the epigastrium and radiates upward (typically occurring within one hour of a meal, during exercise, or when lying recumbent) and is at least partially relieved by antacids.

- **Water brash** (excess salivation), **bitter taste,** globus sensation (throat fullness), odynophagia, dysphagia, halitosis, and otalgia are also commonly seen.
- **"Atypical" symptoms (up to 50%):** Nocturnal cough, asthma, hoarseness, noncardiac chest pain.

EXAM

Exam is often normal, or patients may present with **poor dentition** and wheezing.

DIFFERENTIAL

Infectious esophagitis (CMV, HSV, *Candida*), pill esophagitis (alendronate, tetracycline), PUD, dyspepsia, biliary colic, angina, esophageal dysmotility.

DIAGNOSIS

- For **typical symptoms,** treat with an empiric trial of PPIs × 4–6 weeks. Response to PPIs is diagnostic.
- If the patient is **unresponsive** to therapy or has **alarm symptoms** (dysphagia, odynophagia, weight loss, anemia, long-standing symptoms, blood in stool, age > 50), proceed as follows:
  - **Barium esophagography:** Has a limited role, but can identify strictures (see Figure 7.1C).
  - **Upper endoscopy with biopsy:** The standard exam in the presence of **alarm symptoms** (dysphagia, odynophagia, weight loss, bleeding, anemia). Normal in > 50% of patients with GERD (most have nonerosive reflux disease), or may reveal endoscopic esophagitis grades 1 (mild) to 4 (severe erosions, strictures, Barrett's esophagus). Strictures can be dilated.
  - **Ambulatory esophageal pH monitoring:** The gold standard, but often unnecessary. Indicated for correlating symptoms with pH parameters when endoscopy is normal and (1) symptoms are unresponsive to medical therapy, (2) antireflux surgery is being considered, or (3) there are atypical symptoms (eg, chest pain, cough, wheezing).

TREATMENT

- **Behavioral modification:** Elevate the head of the bed six inches; stop tobacco and alcohol use. Advise patients to eat smaller meals, reduce fat intake, lose weight, avoid recumbency after eating, and avoid certain foods (eg, mint, chocolate, coffee, tea, carbonated drinks, citrus and tomato juice). Effective in 25% of cases.
- **Antacids (calcium carbonate, aluminum hydroxide):** For mild GERD. Fast, but afford only short-term relief.
- **H$_2$ receptor antagonists (cimetidine, ranitidine, famotidine, nizatidine):** For mild GERD or as an adjunct for nocturnal GERD while the patient is on PPIs. Effective in 50–60% of cases.
- **PPIs (omeprazole, lansoprazole, rabeprazole, pantoprazole, esomeprazole):** The mainstay of therapy for mild to severe GERD. Daily dosage is effective in 80–90% of patients. **Fewer than 5%** of patients are **refractory** to twice-daily dosage. Long-term use of PPIs has been associated with an ↑ risk of osteoporosis. Acid suppression from PPIs or H$_2$ receptor antagonists may ↑ the risk of *C difficile* and pneumonia.
- **Surgical fundoplication (Nissen or Belsey wrap):**
  - Often performed laparoscopically. Indicated for patients who cannot tolerate medical therapy or who have persistent regurgitation. **Contraindicated** in patients with an esophageal motility disorder.

- **Outcome:** More than 50% of patients require continued acid-suppressive medication, and > 20% develop new symptoms (dysphagia, bloating, dyspepsia).
- **Endoscopic antireflux procedures:** Remain investigational.

COMPLICATIONS

- **Peptic strictures:** Affect 8–20% of GERD patients; present with dysphagia. Malignancies must be excluded via endoscopy and biopsy; can then be treated with endoscopic dilation followed by indefinite PPI therapy.
- **Upper GI bleeding:** Hematemesis, melena, anemia 2° to ulcerative esophagitis.
- **Posterior laryngitis:** Chronic hoarseness from vocal cord ulceration and granulomas.
- **Asthma:** Typically has an adult onset; nonatopic and unresponsive to traditional asthma interventions.
- **Cough:** Affects 10–40% of GERD patients, most without typical GERD symptoms.
- **Noncardiac chest pain:** After a full cardiac evaluation, consider an empiric trial of PPIs or ambulatory esophageal pH monitoring.
- **Other:** Barrett's esophagus, adenocarcinoma.

GASTROPARESIS

Delayed gastric emptying in the absence of obstruction. Most commonly related to diabetes, viral infection, neuropsychiatric disease, or postsurgical complications.

SYMPTOMS/EXAM

- Presents with postprandial fullness, bloating, abdominal distention, early satiety, nausea, and vomiting of digested food.
- Exam is normal. Mild to moderate upper abdominal tenderness may be seen during episodes. Occasionally, a **succussion splash** is heard.

DIFFERENTIAL

- Poor glycemic control, postsurgical complications (**postvagotomy or Roux-en-Y**), nonulcer dyspepsia, medications (anticholinergics, opiates).
- Hypothyroidism, scleroderma, muscular dystrophies, paraneoplastic syndrome (small cell lung cancer), amyloidosis.

DIAGNOSIS

- **Solid-phase nuclear medicine gastric emptying scan:** Following the administration of a radiolabeled meal, normal gastric retention is < 90%, < 60%, and < 10% at 60, 120, and 240 minutes, respectively.
- **Labs:** Electrolytes, hemoglobin A_{1c} (HbA_{1c}), ANA, TSH.
- **Endoscopy:** To rule out structural lesions and ulcers causing obstruction.
- **Gastroduodenal manometry:** Not widely available, but can often distinguish myopathic from neuropathic patterns.

TREATMENT

- **Dietary:** Small, frequent meals; low-fat, low-fiber diet.
- Tight glycemic control in diabetics.
- ↓ or discontinue opiates and anticholinergics.

KEY FACT

For true GERD, PPIs are highly effective, with < 5% of patients unresponsive to twice-daily doses.

KEY FACT

After surgical fundoplication for GERD, > 50% of patients still require continued acid-suppressive medication, and > 20% develop new symptoms (dysphagia, bloating, dyspepsia).

KEY FACT

Gastroparesis can be a sign of undiagnosed diabetes.

KEY FACT

"Idiopathic" gastroparesis can result from viral infections in young, healthy patients and is often self-limited, remitting within a few months.

- **Medications:**
    - **Cisapride:** Most effective, but its use is restricted owing to **QT-interval prolongation.**
    - **Metoclopramide:** A dopamine antagonist used as an antiemetic. ↓ effectiveness and adverse effects (extrapyramidal symptoms) are seen with long-term use.
    - **Domperidone:** A dopamine antagonist that is not approved for use in the United States.
    - **Erythromycin:** IV use has short-term efficacy; PO use is less effective chronically.
- **Jejunostomy tube:** For intractable, severe gastroparesis without small bowel dysmotility.
- **Total parenteral nutrition (TPN):** For intractable, severe gastroparesis with small bowel dysmotility.
- **Gastric pacing:** Investigational.

Lower GI Tract

ACUTE DIARRHEA

 A 21-year-old woman presents with diarrhea, cramps, and fever 10 days after she returned from a trip to India. She did not eat any raw meat but did stay with her family while there. She is febrile and mildly hypotensive. While stool samples are being ordered, should she receive antibiotics?

Yes. In this case, given her travel history to India visiting relatives, this patient's risk for typhoid fever is high. Although she could have traveler's diarrhea, the relative delay from her arrival makes typhoid more likely. She should start on empiric quinolones or a cephalosporin while stool and blood cultures are pending.

Defined as diarrhea of < **14 days'** duration. Usually toxin mediated or infectious, mild, and self-limited; cases are managed on an outpatient basis. Diarrhea accounts for 1.5% of all hospitalizations in the United States. ↑ morbidity is seen in children, the elderly, and the immunosuppressed. Etiologies include the following:

- **Bacterial:** *E coli, Campylobacter* (associated with Guillain-Barré syndrome), *Salmonella, Shigella, C difficile, Yersinia, Aeromonas.*
- **Viral:** Adenovirus, rotavirus, norovirus.
- **Parasites:** *Entamoeba histolytica* (associated with liver abscesses); *Giardia lamblia; Cryptosporidium, Microsporidium,* and *Mycobacterium avium* complex (MAC) in those with AIDS.
- **Drugs:** Antibiotics, NSAIDs, quinidine, β-blockers, magnesium-base antacids, PPIs, colchicine, theophylline, acarbose.
- **Other:** Food allergies; initial presentation of chronic diarrhea.

SYMPTOMS/EXAM

- Diarrhea accompanied by urgency, tenesmus, abdominal bloating, and pain.
- Exam may reveal tachycardia, orthostasis, ↓ skin turgor with dehydration, abdominal pain, and distention.

DIFFERENTIAL

Causes of chronic diarrhea (food intolerance, pancreatic insufficiency, medications, IBD, laxatives, malignancy).

DIAGNOSIS

- **Alarm features:** Evaluation is indicated in the presence of alarm features—eg, a fever of > 38.5°C (101.3°F), severe abdominal pain, bloody diarrhea, immune compromise, age > 70 years, or severe dehydration (see Table 7.5).
- **No alarm features** (short duration, nonbloody diarrhea, nontoxic exam): Treat with oral rehydration and symptomatic therapy. If no improvement is seen, evaluation is indicated.
- Evaluation includes the following:
  - **Blood tests:** CBC, electrolytes, BUN, creatinine, ESR, ameba serology.
  - **Stool tests:** Stool culture and sensitivity, O&P, *Giardia* antigen, *C difficile* toxin, leukocytes.
  - **Endoscopy:** Flexible sigmoidoscopy or colonoscopy with biopsy.

KEY FACT

Acute diarrhea (diarrhea of < 4 weeks' duration) is usually infectious and self-limited.

TREATMENT

- **Mild diarrhea:**
  - Oral rehydration (Pedialyte, Gatorade).
  - BRAT diet (bananas, rice, applesauce, toast).
  - **Antidiarrheals:** Loperamide 4 mg initially and then 2 mg after each stool (maximum 8 mg/day).
- **Severe diarrhea:** Oral or IV rehydration.
- **Empiric antibiotics:**
  - Indicated only in the presence of a fever of > 38.5°C (101.3°F), tenesmus, bloody stools, and fecal leukocytes (awaiting culture).
  - Ciprofloxacin × 3–5 days.
  - Antibiotics are **not** recommended for nontyphoidal *Salmonella*, *Campylobacter*, *Aeromonas*, *Yersinia*, or *E coli* O157:H7.
  - Antibiotics are recommended for shigellosis, cholera, extraintestinal salmonellosis, traveler's diarrhea, and amebiasis.
  - Giardiasis and *C difficile* are treated with metronidazole.

TABLE 7.5. Causes of Acute Infectious Diarrhea

| | **PATHOGEN** | | |
SUBTYPE	**VIRAL**	**PROTOZOAL**	**BACTERIAL**
Noninflammatory diarrhea	Norovirus, rotavirus.	*Giardia lamblia*, *Cryptosporidium*.	**Preformed endotoxin production:** *S aureus, Bacillus cereus, Clostridium perfringens.* **Enterotoxin production:** Enterotoxigenic *E coli* (ETEC), *Vibrio cholerae.*
Inflammatory diarrhea	CMV.	*E histolytica.*	**Cytotoxin production:** Enterohemorrhagic *E coli* (EHEC), *Vibrio parahaemolyticus, C difficile.* **Mucosal invasion:** *Shigella, Campylobacter jejuni, Salmonella,* enteroinvasive *E coli* (EIEC), *Aeromonas, Plesiomonas, Yersinia enterocolitica, Chlamydia, Neisseria gonorrhoeae, Listeria monocytogenes.*

(Reproduced with permission from Tierney LM et al. *Current Medical Diagnosis & Treatment,* 44th ed. New York: McGraw-Hill, 2005: 527.)

CHRONIC DIARRHEA

Diarrhea of > **4 weeks'** duration. Table 7.6 lists the etiologies of chronic diarrhea.

SYMPTOMS/EXAM

- Presents with diarrhea accompanied by abdominal bloating and pain.
- Exam reveals tachycardia, orthostasis, ↓ skin turgor with dehydration, abdominal pain, and distention.

TABLE 7.6. Causes of Chronic Diarrhea

TYPE	CLUES	CAUSES
Osmotic diarrhea	↓ stool volume with fasting; ↑ stool osmotic gap.	**Medications:** Antacids, lactulose, sorbitol. **Disaccharidase deficiency:** Lactose intolerance. **Factitious diarrhea:** Magnesium (antacids, laxatives).
Secretory diarrhea	Large volume (> 1 L/day): Little change with fasting; normal stool osmotic gap.	**Hormonally mediated:** VIPoma, carcinoid, medullary carcinoma of the thyroid (calcitonin), Zollinger-Ellison syndrome (gastrin). Factitious diarrhea (laxative abuse); senna. Villous adenoma. Bile salt malabsorption (ileal resection, Crohn's ileitis, postcholecystectomy). Medications.
Inflammatory conditions	Fever, hematochezia, abdominal pain.	**IBD:** Ulcerative colitis, Crohn's disease. **Malignancy:** Lymphoma, adenocarcinoma (with obstruction and pseudodiarrhea). **Other:** Microscopic colitis, radiation enteritis.
Malabsorption syndromes	Weight loss, abnormal lab values, fecal fat > 10 g/24 hrs.	**Small bowel mucosal disorders:** Celiac sprue, tropical sprue, Whipple's disease, small bowel resection (short bowel syndrome), Crohn's disease. **Lymphatic obstruction:** Lymphoma, carcinoid, infectious (TB, *Mycobacterium avium–intracellulare*), Kaposi's sarcoma, sarcoidosis. **Pancreatic disease:** Chronic pancreatitis, pancreatic carcinoma. **Bacterial overgrowth:** Motility disorders (diabetes, vagotomy), scleroderma, fistulas, small intestinal diverticula.
Motility disorders	Systemic disease or prior abdominal surgery.	**Postsurgical:** Vagotomy, partial gastrectomy, blind loop with bacterial overgrowth. **Systemic disorders:** Scleroderma, DM, hyperthyroidism. **IBS.**
Chronic infections		**Parasites:** *G lamblia, E histolytica.* **AIDS related:** ■ **Viral:** CMV. ■ **Bacterial:** *C difficile*, MAC. ■ **Protozoal:** Microsporidia (*Enterocytozoon bieneusi, Cryptosporidium, Isospora belli*)

(Adapted with permission from McPhee SJ et al. *Current Medical Diagnosis & Treatment 2010.* New York: McGraw-Hill, 2010, Table 15-5.)

DIAGNOSIS

Diagnose as follows (see also Table 7.7):

- Rule out acute diarrhea, lactose intolerance, parasitic infection, ileal resection, medications, and systemic disease.
- **Characterize the diarrhea:** Watery, inflammatory, fatty/malabsorption.
- **Conduct a focused initial evaluation:**
  - **Blood tests:** CBC, electrolytes, ESR, albumin, HbA_{1c}. Clues are as follows:
    - **ESR:** ↑ if diarrhea is inflammatory.
    - **Iron deficiency anemia:** Divalent cations such as iron absorbed through the duodenum. The presence of iron deficiency anemia may point to celiac sprue.
  - **Antigliadin or antiendomysial antibodies:** Associated with celiac sprue.
  - **Neuroendocrine tumors:** VIP (VIPoma), calcitonin (medullary thyroid carcinoma), gastrin (Zollinger-Ellison syndrome), glucagon.
  - **Stool tests:** Electrolytes (calculate osmotic gap), 24-hour collection for weight and quantitative fat, standard cultures plus tests for *Aeromonas* and *Plesiomonas*, O&P, and AIDS-related infection (MAC, *Cryptosporidium, Microsporidium*, CMV).
- **Stool test clues:**
  - **Weight:** If the 24-hour stool weight is > 1000 g, suspect secretory diarrhea; if < 250 g, suspect factitious diarrhea or IBS.
  - **Osmotic gap:** Calculated as 290 − 2 × (stool Na + stool K). A gap of < 50 mOsm/kg suggests secretory diarrhea; > 125 mOsm/kg suggests osmotic diarrhea.
  - **pH:** A pH < 5.6 implies carbohydrate malabsorption.
  - **Fecal occult blood test (FOBT):** Suggests inflammatory diarrhea, but often ⊕ with other types.

TABLE 7.7. Differential Diagnosis of Chronic Diarrhea

	SUBTYPE			
VARIABLE	**OSMOTIC**	**SECRETORY**	**INFLAMMATORY**	**FATTY/ MALABSORPTION**
History	Stool volume ↓ with fasting.	Large stool volume (> 1 L/day); no change with fasting.	Fever, abdominal pain, hematochezia.	Weight loss, greasy stools.
Exam		Severe dehydration.	Abdominal tenderness.	Glossitis.
Blood tests		Neuroendocrine peptides.	Leukocytosis, ↑ ESR.	Anemia, hypoalbuminemia.
Stool tests	Osm gap > 125, Mg > 45, pH < 5.6.	24-hour stool weight > 1000 g, osm < 50.	Leukocytes, fecal blood.	7–10 g fat/24 hrs.
Differential	Laxative use, carbohydrate malabsorption.	Bacterial, viral, bile acid malabsorption, collagenous colitis, vasculitis, neuroendocrine, nonosmotic laxatives.	IBD, *C difficile* colitis, invasive bacterial, viral, parasitic, ischemic, radiation, lymphoma, colon cancer.	Pancreatic exocrine insufficiency, celiac sprue, Whipple's disease, small bowel bacterial overgrowth, mesenteric ischemia.

(Adapted with permission from McPhee SJ et al. *Current Medical Diagnosis & Treatment 2010.* New York: McGraw-Hill, 2010, Table 15-6.)

- **Leukocytes:** Presence suggests inflammatory diarrhea.
- **Fat:** Spot testing is not specific; a 24-hour fat > 7–10 g implies malabsorption.
- **Laxative screen:** ↑ magnesium (> 45 mmol/L), phosphate, sulfate levels.
- **Urine test clues:** Neuroendocrine tumors: 5-HIAA (carcinoid), VMA, metanephrines, histamine.
- **Endoscopy:** Flexible sigmoidoscopy or colonoscopy with biopsy; consider upper endoscopy.
- **Other:** A ⊕ H_2 breath test after a glucose/lactulose load suggests bacterial overgrowth or lactose intolerance.

TREATMENT

- **Mild diarrhea:** See the previous section.
- **Osmotic diarrhea:**
    - **Carbohydrate malabsorption (lactose, fructose, sorbitol):** Dietary modification, lactase supplements.
    - **Celiac sprue:** Gluten restriction.
    - **Whipple's disease/tropical sprue:** Antibiotics.
    - **Bacterial overgrowth:** Antibiotics; ↑ glycemic control in diabetics.
- **Secretory diarrhea:**
    - Clonidine PO TID.
    - Octreotide SQ TID.
    - Cholestyramine PO QD to QID.
- **Inflammatory diarrhea: IBD**—sulfasalazine, 5-ASA (mesalamine), corticosteroids, azathioprine, 6-mercaptopurine (6-MP).
- **Fatty diarrhea: Pancreatic exocrine insufficiency**—pancreatic enzyme supplements.
- **AIDS diarrhea:** Rule out CMV. Eighty-seven percent of cases resolve following immune reconstitution inflammatory syndrome with HAART when CD4 levels are > 50/μL.

> **KEY FACT**
>
> In the United States, surreptitious laxative use accounts for 15% of referrals for chronic diarrhea and 25% of documented cases of secretory diarrhea.

CELIAC SPRUE

 A 34-year-old woman presents with chronic diarrhea and steatorrhea, iron deficiency anemia, and pruritic vesicles over her elbows and knees. Her primary care physician sends tests to rule out celiac sprue, and anti–tissue transglutaminase (anti-TTG) and antiendomysial antibodies are ⊖. What should the next test be?

Quantitative IgA level. A high percentage of patients with celiac sprue will also have IgA deficiency, and as the antibodies tested are IgA in nature, they may be falsely ⊖ in this patient population. This patient presents with features highly suggestive of celiac sprue (including dermatitis herpetiformis), so the possibility of a false-⊖ result should be considered. If she were to have IgA deficiency, endoscopy with biopsy might be appropriate for making the diagnosis.

A **gluten-sensitive enteropathy** interfering with the digestion and absorption of food nutrients. Often presents with diarrhea and failure to thrive, although it may be asymptomatic. Its prevalence is estimated at 1 in 300 to 1 in 500 and is highest among those of western **European** descent. Shows a bimodal presentation in the first 8–12 months of life and between 20 and 40 years of age. It also has a strong hereditary component (10% prevalence among first-degree relatives). The mechanism is a cross-reaction of T cells to gluten peptides, leading to duodenal **villous atrophy, intraepithelial lymphocytes,** and **crypt hyperplasia.** The disease course may be complicated by intestinal **lymphomas and adenocarcinomas.**

SYMPTOMS/EXAM

- Presents with **chronic diarrhea,** steatorrhea, bloating, abdominal pain, flatulence, and weight loss.
- Fatigue, anemia, bleeding diathesis, osteopenia, and stunted growth are also seen.
- **Dermatitis herpetiformis** (pruritic papulovesicles over the extensor surfaces; see Figure 7.3) is a common feature, as are cheilosis and glossitis.
- Associated conditions include diabetes, Down syndrome, abnormal AST/ALT, hypothyroidism, and hyposplenism.

DIFFERENTIAL

Bacterial overgrowth, collagenous colitis, IBD, IBS, pancreatic insufficiency, lactose intolerance, infectious gastroenteritis.

DIAGNOSIS

- **Serology: Anti-TTG** and **antiendomysial antibodies** have high sensitivity and specificity. Levels may fluctuate with disease activity and may be absent in IgA deficiency. Antigliadin antibody is less sensitive and specific.
- **Labs:** Reveal anemia (iron deficiency from iron malabsorption, folate), hypocalcemia, hypokalemia, and hypomagnesemia.
- **Endoscopy:** Shows **blunted duodenal villi.**
- Definitive diagnosis is made with the triad of a ⊕ serology, histology, and clinical/serologic response to the withdrawal of gluten from the diet.

TREATMENT

- Treatment is dietary but may include steroids for refractory disease.
- **Diet:** Removal of gluten is essential but may be difficult given the ubiquity of wheat flour.
- **Steroids:** Consider in the small percentage of patients who are refractory to a gluten-free diet. Consider malignancy in patients who are unresponsive to corticosteroids.
- **Calcium and vitamin D** for osteopenia; **pneumococcal vaccine** for hyposplenism.

KEY FACT

Iron deficiency anemia may be present in celiac sprue as a result of iron malabsorption.

KEY FACT

Consider celiac sprue whenever you are considering a diagnosis of IBS in a young woman. Like IBS, celiac sprue may manifest as abdominal bloating and cramping. Celiac sprue may also present with iron deficiency anemia, which may be incorrectly attributed to menses.

KEY FACT

Celiac sprue improves with the removal of gluten from the diet. Consider steroid therapy or rule out malignancy in those failing to respond to dietary changes.

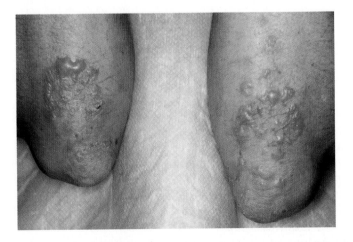

FIGURE 7.3. **Dermatitis herpetiformis.** Note the grouped papulovesicles. (Reproduced with permission from Fauci AS et al. *Harrison's Principles of Internal Medicine,* 17th ed. New York: McGraw-Hill, 2008, Fig. 52-8.)

COMPLICATIONS

- The risk of **malignancy** (enteropathy-associated T-cell and non-Hodgkin's **lymphoma, adenocarcinoma**) is ↑.
- Compliance in pregnant women is important because of the ↑ risk of miscarriage and congenital malformation.
- Noncompliance during childhood leads to failure to thrive or stunted growth.

IRRITABLE BOWEL SYNDROME (IBS)

Abdominal **discomfort or pain** during the **prior three months** that is relieved by defecation and associated with a change in stool frequency or form. Forty percent of patients have impaired ability to work, avoid social functions, cancel appointments, or stop travel because of the severity of their symptoms. Onset is typically in the late teens to 20s and/or **after infectious gastroenteritis.** In the developed world, women are more commonly affected than men, but in India the opposite is the case. Some 30–40% of patients have a **history of physical or sexual abuse.**

SYMPTOMS/EXAM

- Intermittent or chronic abdominal discomfort or pain; bloating, belching, excess flatus, early satiety, nausea, vomiting, diarrhea, constipation.
- Exam is often normal, or patients present with mild to moderate abdominal tenderness.

DIFFERENTIAL

IBD, colon cancer, chronic constipation (low-fiber/low-fluid intake, drugs, hypothyroidism), chronic diarrhea (**celiac sprue,** parasitic infections, bacterial overgrowth, lactase deficiency), chronic pancreatitis, endometriosis.

DIAGNOSIS

- Exclude organic disease.
- **Labs:** CBC, TFTs, serum albumin, ESR, FOBT.
- **If diarrhea:**
  - Stool for O&P and *C difficile* toxin.
  - Celiac sprue serology (antiendomysial and antigliadin antibodies; anti-TTG antibodies).
  - **24-hour stool collection:** A value > 300 g is atypical for IBS.
  - **Severe upper abdominal pain/dyspepsia:** Consider endoscopy (flexible sigmoidoscopy for those < 40 years of age; colonoscopy for those > 40 years).

KEY FACT

New-onset IBS often follows a diagnosis of infectious gastroenteritis.

TREATMENT

- Provide reassurance.
- Tactfully explain visceral hypersensitivity and validate symptoms.
- **Dietary trials:** Lactose-free, high-fiber diet.
- **Antispasmodics:** Dicyclomine, hyoscyamine, peppermint oil.
- **Antidepressants:** Desipramine, amitriptyline, fluoxetine, paroxetine.
- **Constipation-predominant type:**
  - ↑ fluid intake.
  - Provide bowel habit training.
  - Osmotic laxatives.
  - Lubiprostone (if symptoms are severe and other approaches prove unsuccessful).
- **Diarrhea-predominant type:** Loperamide, cholestyramine.

CONSTIPATION

Normal bowel movement frequency is 3–12 per week. Constipation is defined as < 3 bowel movements per week or excessive difficulty and straining at defecation. Prevalence is high in the Western world and is **highest among children and the elderly**. Etiologies are as follows:

- **Dietary:** Low fiber, inadequate fluids.
- **Behavioral:** Short-term stress, travel, disrupted routine.
- **Structural:** Colonic mass or stricture, rectal prolapse, Hirschsprung's disease, solitary rectal ulcer syndrome.
- **Systemic:** Diabetes, **hypothyroidism, hypokalemia, hypercalcemia,** autonomic dysfunction.
- **Medications:** Narcotics, diuretics, calcium channel blockers, anticholinergics, psychotropic drugs, clonidine.
- **Dysmotility:** Pelvic floor dysfunction, slow transit (pseudo-obstruction, psychogenic), IBS.

SYMPTOMS/EXAM

- Presents with abdominal bloating or pain as well as with nausea and anorexia.
- Exam is often normal but may present with abdominal distention, tenderness, and/or mass; external hemorrhoids, anal fissures, and fecal impaction; or rectal prolapse with straining.

DIAGNOSIS/TREATMENT

- Look for a history of the following:
    - Fewer than three bowel movements per week.
    - Excessive difficulty and straining at defecation.
    - Fecal incontinence, rectal prolapse, anal pain.
- **Initial evaluation:**
    - **Labs:** CBC, serum electrolytes **(especially potassium and calcium),** TSH, FOBT.
    - **Age < 50 years and normal labs:** Initiate a trial of ↑ fiber (20–30 g/day); fluid intake.
    - **Age ≥ 50 or < 50 with a failed fiber/fluid trial or fecal occult blood or anemia:** Barium enema; flexible sigmoidoscopy or colonoscopy.
- **Patients with no obstructive or medical disease:** ↓ or discontinue suspect drugs, followed by stepwise addition of (1) stool softeners (docusate), (2) osmotic laxatives (magnesium hydroxide, lactulose, sorbitol, polyethylene glycol), (3) enemas (tap water, mineral oil, soap suds, phosphate), and (4) colonic stimulants (bisacodyl, senna).
- **Refractory constipation:**
    - **Pelvic floor dysfunction:** Anorectal manometry and balloon expulsion studies and defecography. Treat with biofeedback.
    - **Slow-transit constipation:** Radiopaque marker studies and scintigraphy with serial examination of marker transit using radiographs.

DIVERTICULOSIS

Results from weakening of the colonic wall. In industrialized nations, has a 30–50% prevalence in patients > 50 years of age. Rates ↑ with low dietary fiber and advancing age. In the United States, the predominant location is the left colon.

KEY FACT

The first step in the evaluation of constipation is to understand the patient's true complaint.

KEY FACT

Normal bowel movement frequency ranges from 3 to 12 times per week.

SYMPTOMS

Approximately 70% of patients with diverticula remain asymptomatic; 20% will develop diverticulitis, and 10% will develop diverticular bleeding. In asymptomatic patients, the disorder is associated with excessive flatulence and pellet-like stools.

EXAM

Exam may be normal, or patients may present with mild abdominal distention and pellet-like stools.

DIFFERENTIAL

Colorectal cancer, IBS.

DIAGNOSIS

- No diagnosis is needed in patients who are asymptomatic.
- **Barium enema:** Accurate for diverticulosis, but insufficient to rule out colorectal cancer.
- **Colonoscopy:** Recommended for routine colorectal cancer screening in patients > 50 years of age.

TREATMENT

Dietary fiber 20–30 g/day; coarse bran or supplements (psyllium) to ↑ stool bulk and ↓ colonic pressure. May also prevent the formation of new diverticula.

COMPLICATIONS

- **Diverticular bleeding** affects 10–20% of patients with diverticulosis.
- Presents with painless rectal bleeding, usually from a single diverticulum (more frequently in the right colon).
- Spontaneous cessation is common (80%), but approximately one-third of patients have recurrent bleeding.
- Treat with colonoscopy and angiography with embolization; consider elective colonic resection after the second recurrence.

DIVERTICULITIS

Microperforation of the diverticula with associated inflammation. Occurs in 10–25% of those with diverticulosis and commonly affects the sigmoid colon; frequency ↑ with advancing age.

SYMPTOMS

LLQ pain (93–100%); fever, nausea, vomiting, constipation, diarrhea, urinary frequency ("sympathetic cystitis").

EXAM

Exam may reveal LLQ tenderness, localized involuntary guarding, percussion tenderness, and tender LLQ fullness or mass.

DIFFERENTIAL

Appendicitis, IBD, perforated colon cancer, UTI, ischemic colitis, infectious colitis, sigmoid volvulus.

DIAGNOSIS

- **Labs:** Reveal leukocytosis with PMN predominance.
- **UA:** Evaluate for UTI; consider colovesical fistula with pyuria and bacteriuria.
- **Flat and upright AXR:** A thickened colonic (sigmoid) wall is suggestive; free air suggests bowel perforation.
- **CT with IV contrast:** The test of choice; has high accuracy. Look for a thickened bowel wall, diverticula, and pericolonic fat stranding (see Figure 7.4). Evaluate for complications (bowel perforation, abscess, fistula).
- **Colonoscopy:** Exclude malignancy eight weeks after resolution.

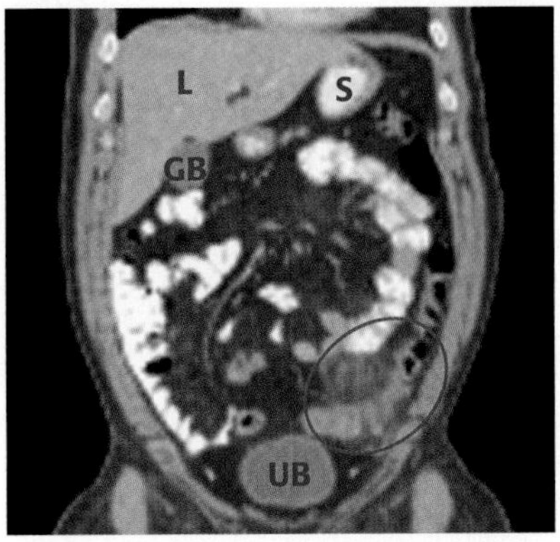

TREATMENT

- Outpatient treatment is sufficient if there are no significant comorbidities, minimal symptoms, and no peritoneal signs. Often requires hospitalization.
- Treat with IV fluids, bowel rest, and NG suction for ileus or obstruction.
- **Broad-spectrum antibiotics:** Cover anaerobes, gram-$\ominus$ bacilli, and gram-$\oplus$ coliforms. Administer a 7- to 10-day course. IV ampicillin/sulbactam (Unasyn) or piperacillin/tazobactam (Zosyn); PO quinolones; amoxicillin/clavulanate (Augmentin).
- **Surgery:** For perforation, abscess, fistula, obstruction, or recurrent diverticulitis (> 2 episodes).

COMPLICATIONS

- **Peritonitis:** Not excluded by the absence of free air. Associated with high mortality (6–35%); **necessitates urgent surgical intervention.**
- **Abscess:** Pelvic abscess is most common. Percutaneous CT-guided drainage is often possible.
- **Fistula:** Colovesical fistulas (to the bladder) are found in men more often than in women. Other fistulas are to the vagina, small bowel, and uterus. Surgical intervention is often postponed until the infection is treated.

FIGURE 7.4. **Acute diverticulitis.** Coronal reconstruction from a contrast-enhanced CT demonstrates sigmoid diverticula with perisigmoid inflammatory "fat stranding." The area of abnormality is circled in red. L= liver; S = stomach; GB = gallbladder; UB = urinary bladder. (Reproduced with permission from USMLERx.com.)

KEY FACT

Consider elective "prophylactic" resection after the second attack of diverticulitis or diverticular bleeding.

GI Bleeding

LOWER GASTROINTESTINAL BLEEDING (LGIB)

Defined as bleeding from a source distal to the ligament of Treitz, which divides the third and fourth portions of the duodenum. Of all cases, > 95% are from a colonic source and > 85% are self-limited. The hospitalization rate is 20 in 100,000 adults per year; risk $\uparrow$ 200-fold from the third to the ninth decade. Mortality is 3–5%. Etiologies include the following:

- Diverticulosis (40%).
- Vascular ectasia.
- Neoplasm, IBD, ischemic colitis, hemorrhoids, infectious, postpolypectomy.
- NSAID ulcers, radiation colitis, rectal varices, solitary rectal ulcer syndrome. Consider an upper GI source.

SYMPTOMS

Usually asymptomatic, but may present with abdominal cramps and, to a lesser extent, pain. Orthostasis is seen in severe cases.

EXAM

Hematochezia (bright red blood, maroon stools) or melena; pallor; abdominal distention with mild tenderness; hypotension; tachycardia.

DIAGNOSIS

- **Demographics and history:**
  - **Age group:** Distinguish elderly, asymptomatic patients (diverticular/vascular ectasias) from young patients who present with pain (infectious, inflammatory).
  - **Description of first blood seen by patient:** Bright red blood indicates a distal or rapid proximal source; black or maroon blood points to a more proximal source.
- Anoscopy to exclude an anal source; stool cultures if infection is suspected.
- **Mild to moderate LGIB:** Consider nasogastric lavage because 10% of upper GI bleeding (UGIB), especially if brisk, can present as hematochezia. Urgent colonic purge (over 4–6 hours); then colonoscopy.
- **Massive LGIB:**
  - **EGD:** UGIB must be excluded with EGD. **Ten percent of UGIB cases present with hematochezia.**
  - **Technetium-labeled RBC scan, CT angiography, and/or mesenteric angiography:** If > 6 units of blood are transfused, consider surgical intervention.
  - **Minimum bleeding rates:** Tagged RBC scan, 0.1–0.5 mL/min; mesenteric angiogram, 1.0 mL/min.
  - **Diagnostic colonoscopy:** Typically performed 12–48 hours after presentation and stabilization.

TREATMENT

- **Stabilization:**
  - NPO; consider an NG tube and place two large-bore IVs.
  - If the patient is in shock, treat with aggressive IV fluids and cross-matched blood with a **hematocrit goal of 25–30%.**
  - In the presence of active LGIB and a platelet count of < 50,000/μL or if there is known impaired function (uremia, ASA), transfuse platelets or desmopressin. With active LGIB and an INR of > 1.5, transfuse FFP.
- **Medical therapy:** H_2 receptor antagonists and PPIs have no role in the treatment of LGIB. Discontinue ASA and NSAIDs.
- **Urgent therapeutic colonoscopy:** Large-volume purge > 6 L; cautery or injection of epinephrine or clipping. Colonoscopy is technically challenging with brisk LGIB (urgent colonic purge requires sedation; visualization is often poor).
- **Mesenteric angiography/embolization:** The intervention of choice for brisk LGIB. Associated with 80–90% cessation rates for those with a diverticular or vascular ectasia etiology, although 50% experience rebleeding.
- **Surgery:** Indicated with active LGIB involving > 4–6 units of blood in 24 hours or > 10 units total. If the site is well localized, consider hemicolectomy; otherwise perform total abdominal colectomy.

TABLE 7.8.   **Risk Assessment in Patients with UGIB**

VARIABLE	RISK		
	LOW	MODERATE	HIGH
History	Age < 60.	Age < 60.	Age > 60, comorbidities, onset while in hospital.
Exam	SBP > 100, HR < 100.	SBP > 100, HR > 100.	SBP < 100, HR > 100.
EGD	Small, clean-based ulcer; erosions; no lesion found.	Ulcer with pigmented spot or adherent clot.	Active bleeding, varices, ulcer > 2 cm, visible vessel.
Rebleed risk	< 5%.	10–30%.	40–50%.
Triage	Ward/home.	Ward.	ICU.

ACUTE UPPER GASTROINTESTINAL BLEEDING (UGIB)

Incidence is 100 in 100,000 adults per year and ↑ with advancing age. Mortality is 10% and usually results from complications of underlying disease rather than from exsanguination. The risk of rebleeding is low if bleeding occurred > 48 hours before presentation (see Table 7.8). Etiologies include the following:

- PUD (55%) (see Figures 7.5 and 7.6).
- Gastroesophageal varices, vascular ectasia, Mallory-Weiss tear, erosive gastritis/esophagitis, Cameron's ulcer.
- **Other:** Dieulafoy's lesion, aortoenteric fistula, hemobilia.

SYMPTOMS/EXAM

- Patients present with nausea, retching, hematemesis (bright red blood or "coffee ground" emesis), dyspepsia, abdominal pain, melena or hematochezia, and orthostasis.
- Exam may reveal melena or hematochezia, pallor, hypotension, and tachycardia. Stigmata of chronic liver disease (spider angioma, ascites, jaundice) or a history of alcohol use is usually found among those with variceal hemorrhage.

DIAGNOSIS

- **History:** Assess NSAID use (peptic ulcer), retching prior to hematemesis (Mallory-Weiss tear), alcohol abuse (esophagitis, Mallory-Weiss tear, varices), prior abdominal aortic graft (aortoenteric fistula), chronic GERD (esophagitis), and weight loss/iron deficiency (malignancy).
- **NG tube lavage:** Useful if ⊕ (red blood, coffee grounds); if ⊖ (clear or bilious), does not exclude UGIB. **Ten percent** of UGIB cases have a ⊖ lavage.
- **EGD:** Perform after stabilization and resuscitation; often done > 12 hours from admission. Diagnostic, **prognostic**, and therapeutic.
- **H pylori testing:** Perform on all patients with peptic ulcers.

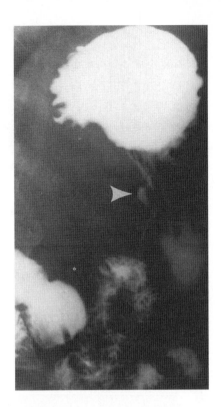

FIGURE 7.5.   **Gastric ulcer on barium upper GI.** A benign gastric ulcer can be seen as pooling of contrast (arrowhead) extending beyond the adjacent gastric wall. (Reproduced with permission from Chen MY et al. *Basic Radiology.* New York: McGraw-Hill, 2004, Fig. 10-21.)

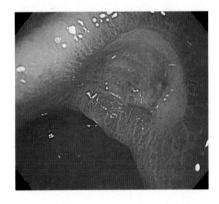

FIGURE 7.6.   **Benign gastric ulcer on endoscopy.** (Reproduced with permission from Fauci AS et al. *Harrison's Principles of Internal Medicine,* 17th ed. New York: McGraw-Hill, 2008, Fig. 285-2A.)

 KEY FACT

Ten percent of UGIB patients present with hematochezia.

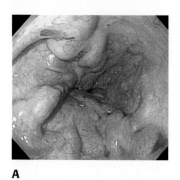 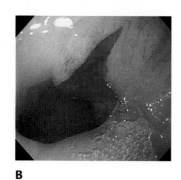 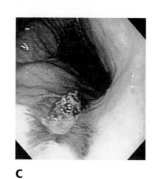 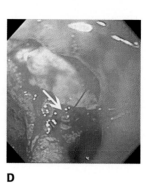

A   B   C   D

FIGURE 7.7.   Causes of upper GI bleed at endoscopy. (A) Esophageal varices. (B) Mallory-Weiss tear. (C) Gastric ulcer with protuberant vessel. (D) Duodenal ulcer with active bleeding (arrow). (Reproduced with permission from Fauci AS et al. *Harrison's Principles of Internal Medicine,* 17th ed. New York: McGraw-Hill, 2008, Figs. 285-16, 285-18, and 285-15D and E.)

KEY FACT

Hematocrit is a poor early indicator of the amount of blood loss in UGIB.

KEY FACT

As little as 50 mL of blood in the GI tract can cause melena.

KEY FACT

Ten percent of documented UGIB cases have a ⊖ NG tube lavage.

TREATMENT

- **Stabilization:** As with LGIB (see above).
- **Medical therapy:** H₂ receptor antagonists do not alter the outcome. Give high-dose oral PPIs twice daily on presentation. Initiate an IV PPI drip if EGD suggests a high risk of rebleeding (ie, active bleeding, visible vessel, adherent clot). Reduces the relative risk of bleeding by 50%. IV octreotide for suspected variceal hemorrhage; continue for three days if verified by EGD.
- **Endoscopy:** Of all patients with active UGIB at EGD (see Figure 7.7), > 90% can be effectively treated with banding, sclerosant, epinephrine, and/or electrocautery. Predictors of rebleeding include significant comorbidities, lesion size, and high-risk stigmata (visible vessel, adherent clot).
- **Refractory or recurrent UGIB:**
    - Esophageal balloon tamponade (Minnesota or Sengstaken-Blakemore tubes) for varices as a bridge to **TIPS.**
    - Angiogram with intra-arterial **embolization or surgery** for refractory nonvariceal bleeding.
- **H pylori eradication:** For all peptic ulcers causing UGIB. Given the 20% treatment failure rate, eradication should be confirmed with a stool antigen or urea breath test.

Inflammatory Bowel Disease (IBD)

Crohn's disease and ulcerative colitis are the 1° chronic autoimmune inflammatory diseases of the bowel. Table 7.9 and Figure 7.8 summarize the distinguishing features of both.

CROHN'S DISEASE

A 20-year-old man with a history of diarrhea presents with flank pain and is noted to have kidney stones. He notes years of having RLQ pain and occasional low-grade fevers. He is of Ashkenazi Jewish descent, and he has a family history of Crohn's disease. As he is awaiting an outpatient colonoscopy, serum anti–neutrophilic cytoplasmic antibody (p-ANCA) and anti–*Saccharomyces cerevisiae* antibody (ASCA) are sent. What pattern are these tests likely to show?

TABLE 7.9.   **Distinguishing Features of IBD**

FEATURE	CROHN'S DISEASE	ULCERATIVE COLITIS
Genetic predisposition	NOD2, CARD15, ATG16L1, IL23R.	Presumed genetic component.
Worse with smoking	Yes.	Possible improvement.
Age at onset	Bimodal: 15–25, 55–65 years.	Bimodal: 20–40, 60–70 years.
Abdominal pain	Sharp, focal.	Crampy; associated with bowel movement.
Bowel obstruction	Common.	Rare.
Gross hematochezia	Occasionally.	Common.
GI involvement	Mouth to anus; typically terminal ileum/proximal colon.	Colon only; rectum with continuous progression proximally.
Pattern	Segmental, transmural, eccentric.	Continuous, mucosal, circumferential.
Ulceration	Superficial to deep, linear, serpiginous.	Superficial.
Histology	Noncaseating granulomas.	Crypt abscesses.
p-ANCA ⊕	20%.	70%.
ASCA ⊕	65%.	15%.
Fistula/stricture	Common.	Uncommon.
Extraintestinal manifestations	Uncommon.	Common.
Infliximab response	Often.	Occasionally.
Surgery curative	Never.	Often.

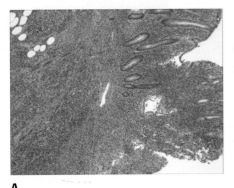

A

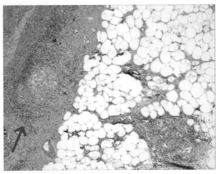

B

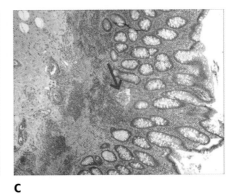

C

FIGURE 7.8.   Inflammatory bowel disease. (A)–(B) Crohn's disease. Transmural inflammation with noncaseating granulomas (arrow) is seen deep in the serosal fat on pathology. (C) Ulcerative colitis. Inflammation is confined to the mucosa and submucosa, with a crypt abscess (arrow). (Reproduced with permission from USMLERx.com.)

Labs will likely be p-ANCA ⊖ and ASCA ⊕. This patient's symptoms, family history, and risk factors (Ashkenazi Jewish ethnicity) are highly suggestive of Crohn's disease. p-ANCA and ASCA can be useful in distinguishing Crohn's disease from ulcerative colitis in that Crohn's is generally ASCA ⊕ (**A**lways **S**een in **C**rohn's), whereas ulcerative colitis is generally p-ANCA ⊕ (**A**lmost **N**ever in **C**rohn's).

A chronic, recurrent disease with patchy or **"skipped" transmural** inflammation of **any segment** of the GI tract from the mouth to the anus (see Figure 7.9). Demonstrates a propensity for the **ileum** and proximal colon, with 33% involving only the terminal ileum, 50% involving both the small bowel and colon, and 20% only the colon. Incidence is 4–8 in 100,000. More common among **Ashkenazi Jews,** those with a ⊕ family history, and smokers; **smoking** may exacerbate disease. Shows a **bimodal** age of onset at 15–25 and 55–65 years of age. The clinical course is characterized by the development of fistulas and strictures. **NOD2** mutations confer susceptibility.

SYMPTOMS

RLQ or periumbilical pain, **nonbloody diarrhea,** low-grade fever, malaise, weight loss, anal pain, oral aphthous ulcers, postprandial bloating, kidney stones (↑ oxalate absorption 2° to fat malabsorption).

EXAM

Fever, tachycardia, abdominal tenderness and/or mass, perianal fissures/fistulas/skin tags, extraintestinal manifestations (pyoderma gangrenosum, erythema nodosum, ankylosing spondylitis, sacroiliitis, uveitis).

DIFFERENTIAL

Ulcerative colitis, IBS, infectious enterocolitis (*Yersinia, E histolytica,* TB), mesenteric ischemia, intestinal lymphoma, celiac sprue.

KEY FACT

Of all IBD cases, > 10% cannot clearly be classified as ulcerative colitis or Crohn's disease.

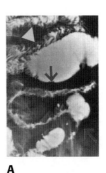 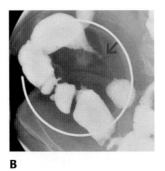 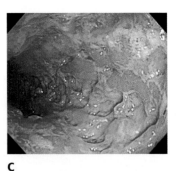

A   B   C

FIGURE 7.9. **Crohn's disease.** (**A**) Small bowel follow-through (SBFT) barium study shows skip areas of narrowed small bowel with nodular mucosa (arrows) and ulceration. Compare with normal bowel (arrowhead). (**B**) Spot compression image from SBFT shows "string sign" narrowing (arrow) due to stricture. (**C**) Deep ulcers in the colon of a patient with Crohn's disease, seen at colonoscopy. (Image A reproduced with permission from Chen MY et al. *Basic Radiology.* New York: McGraw-Hill, 2004, Fig. 10-30. Image B reproduced with permission from USMLERx.com. Image C reproduced with permission from Fauci AS et al. *Harrison's Principles of Internal Medicine,* 17th ed. New York: McGraw-Hill, 2008, Fig. 285-4B.)

DIAGNOSIS

- Labs:
  - Look for anemia (chronic disease, iron deficiency, vitamin B_{12} deficiency), leukocytosis, low serum albumin, ↑ CRP, and ↑ ESR.
  - There is a **poor correlation between lab results and disease severity.**
- **Stool studies:** Rule out infection with culture, O&P, and *C difficile* toxin.
- Colonoscopy:
  - Assess the extent and severity of disease. Key words are skipped lesions, cobblestone, stricture, fistula, and ulcerations (see Figure 7.9).
  - Biopsies demonstrate acute and chronic inflammation; **noncaseating granulomas** are seen < 25% of the time but are highly suggestive of Crohn's disease.
- **Small bowel follow-through:** Evaluate for small bowel involvement.
- **CT scan:** Consider if there is concern for abdominal abscess/fistula.
- **Immunologic markers:** Useful in indeterminate disease (Crohn's vs. ulcerative colitis, particularly if surgery is indicated). Markers used (see Table 7.10) include p-ANCA and ASCA.

TREATMENT

- 5-ASA agents:
  - **Sulfasalazine:** Released in the colon; **not active in the small bowel.** Used for induction and maintenance.
  - **Mesalamine (Pentasa, Asacol):** Asacol is released in the colon; Pentasa is **released in the small bowel.**
  - 5-ASA agents have limited effectiveness for small bowel disease.
- Antibiotics:
  - **Useful even with no obvious infection.**
  - Metronidazole or ciprofloxacin. Rifaximin (a nonabsorbable antibiotic) is also used.
- Corticosteroids:
  - Suppress acute flares; useful in small and large bowel disease.
  - Give prednisone 40–60 mg/day during acute flares with taper after response.
  - Significant long-term side effects include diabetes, hypertension, cataracts, metabolic bone disease, and psychosis.
  - Budesonide is an oral steroid with less systemic absorption; it is used for maintenance only.
- **Immunomodulatory drugs:**
  - Used for maintenance only, not for induction, as onset of action may take six weeks.
  - Used to minimize steroid exposure.
  - **Azathioprine (Imuran):** Therapeutic effects are delayed 6–8 weeks; significant bone marrow suppression requires frequent initial monitoring.

TABLE 7.10. Interpretation of p-ANCA and ASCA Values

TEST	RESULT	INTERPRETATION	CHARACTERISTICS
p-ANCA	−	Suggests Crohn's.	95% PPV, 92% specificity.
ASCA	+		
p-ANCA	+	Suggests ulcerative colitis.	88% PPV, 98% specificity.
ASCA	−		

KEY FACT

Smoking is associated with worsening Crohn's disease, while ulcerative colitis may **improve** with smoking.

KEY FACT

Crohn's colitis carries a risk of colon cancer similar to that of ulcerative colitis.

- **6-MP:** Similar to azathioprine. Thiopurine methyltransferase activity measurement may help with the titration of 6-MP.
- **Methotrexate:** Second- or third-line maintenance therapy.
- **Infliximab (Remicade):** Recombinant anti-TNF. IV infusion. For moderate to severe fistulizing disease; **contraindicated for disease with strictures.** Repeat IV infusions every 2–4 weeks for three doses; then consider maintenance doses every eight weeks. **TB must be ruled out** prior to use (PPD, CXR). Long-term treatment is associated with waning efficacy and ↑ allergic reactions. Certolizumab and adalimumab are other licensed options.
- **Natalizumab (Tysabri):** A humanized monoclonal antibody against cellular adhesion molecule α4-integrin. Blocks immune cells from extravasating out of the blood and into the intestinal tissue or through the blood-brain barrier (treatment of MS). Linked to rare cases of progressive multifocal leukoencephalopathy.
- **Surgery:** Some 50% of patients will require surgery for obstruction or abscess if the condition is refractory to medical therapy.

COMPLICATIONS

Strictures/obstruction, fistulas, abscess, colorectal cancer, malabsorption, nephrolithiasis, cholelithiasis.

ULCERATIVE COLITIS

A chronic, recurrent disease with diffuse **continuous** mucosal inflammation of the colon extending proximally from the rectum. Of all cases, > 50% are isolated to the rectum and sigmoid colon and < 20% involve the entire colon. Incidence is 3–15 in 100,000; age of onset is typically 20–40 years, but the disease also occurs in patients < 10 years of age and in the elderly. More common among Ashkenazi Jews, nonsmokers, and those with a family history; **smoking may attenuate disease.** Course is marked by repeated flares and remissions.

SYMPTOMS/EXAM

- Bloody diarrhea, crampy abdominal pain, fecal urgency, tenesmus, and weight loss are characteristic.
- Fever, tachycardia, and abdominal tenderness; red blood on DRE.
- Extraintestinal findings may include ankylosing spondylitis, sacroiliitis, erythema nodosum, pyoderma gangrenosum, and uveitis.

DIFFERENTIAL

Infectious colitis, ischemic colitis, Crohn's colitis.

DIAGNOSIS

- **Labs:**
  - Anemia (chronic disease, iron deficiency, hematochezia), leukocytosis, low serum albumin, ↑ CRP, ↑ ESR.
  - There is a **good correlation between labs (hematocrit, albumin, ESR) and disease severity.**
  - ↑ **alkaline phosphatase** is seen in the presence of coexisting primary sclerosing cholangitis.
- **Stool studies:** Rule out infection with culture, O&P, and C *difficile* toxin.
- **Imaging:** For moderate and severe activity. KUB reveals loss of haustrations, leading to a **"lead pipe"** appearance and colonic dilation (see Figure 7.10).

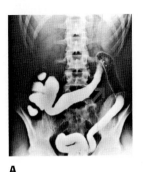 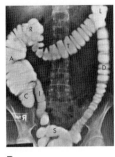 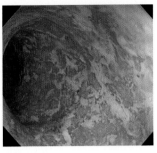

A   **B**   **C**

FIGURE 7.10. Ulcerative colitis. (A) Radiograph from a barium enema showing a feature-less ("lead pipe") colon with small mucosal ulcerations (arrow). Compare with normal haustral markings in **(B)**. **(C)** Diffuse mucosal ulcerations and exudates at colonoscopy in chronic ulcerative colitis. (Image A reproduced with permission from Doherty GM. *Current Diagnosis & Treatment: Surgery*, 13th ed. New York: McGraw-Hill, 2010, Fig. 30-17. Image B reproduced with permission from Chen MY et al. *Basic Radiology.* New York: McGraw-Hill, 2004, Fig. 10-10A. Image C reproduced with permission from Fauci AS et al. *Harrison's Principles of Internal Medicine,* 17th ed. New York: McGraw-Hill, 2008, Fig. 285-4A.)

- **Colonoscopy:**
    - Avoid if there is a severe flare. Evaluate the colon and terminal ileum. Look for rectal involvement (95–100%), **continuous circumferential ulcerations,** and **pseudopolyps.** The terminal ileum is occasionally inflamed from **"backwash ileitis."**
    - Biopsies demonstrate acute and chronic inflammation, **crypt abscesses,** and absence of granulomas.

TREATMENT

- Treatment depends on **severity** and on the **location** of active disease.
    - **Distal disease:** Mesalamine or hydrocortisone suppository (rectal involvement) or enema (up to the splenic flexure).
    - **Distal and proximal disease:** Oral or IV agents.
    - **Mild to moderate activity:**
        - Sulfasalazine PO.
        - Mesalamine PO.
        - Prednisone 40–60 mg PO QD if no response after 2–4 weeks.
    - **Severe activity:**
        - Methylprednisolone IV or hydrocortisone IV.
        - Roughly 50–75% of patients achieve remission in 7–10 days.
        - If no response is seen within 7–10 days, **colectomy** is usually indicated.
        - Consider a trial of cyclosporine or an anti-TNF agent prior to colectomy.
    - **Maintenance therapy:**
        - Sulfasalazine PO.
        - Mesalamine PO.
- **Surgery:**
    - Can be curative and can eliminate the risk of colon cancer.
    - Proctocolectomy with ileostomy is curative.
    - Proctocolectomy with ileoanal anastomosis is often curative, but 25% have "pouchitis," or inflammation of the neorectum.

COMPLICATIONS

Toxic megacolon (dilated colon, leukocytosis, fever, rebound tenderness), primary sclerosing cholangitis, colorectal cancer, extraintestinal manifestations (see Table 7.11).

KEY FACT

NSAID use can induce a flare of ulcerative colitis or Crohn's disease.

KEY FACT

The risk of colon cancer in those with ulcerative colitis for > 10 years is 0.5–1.0% per year; colonoscopy is recommended every 1–2 years beginning eight years after diagnosis.

TABLE 7.11. **Extraintestinal Manifestations of Ulcerative Colitis and Their Relationship to Disease Activity**

Related	Often Related	Unrelated
Arthritis	Pyoderma gangrenosum	Ankylosing spondylitis
Erythema nodosum	Uveitis	Primary sclerosing
Oral aphthous ulcers		cholangitis
Episcleritis		

Ischemic Bowel Disease

ACUTE MESENTERIC ISCHEMIA

Most common in the elderly and in those with valvular heart disease, atrial fibrillation (AF), or atherosclerotic disease. In young patients, it occurs with **AF, vasculitis, hypercoagulable** states (OCP use in young female smokers), and vasoconstrictor abuse. After infarction, mortality is 70–90%.

SYMPTOMS

Presents with acute-onset, severe abdominal pain (**"out of proportion to exam"**) as well as with sudden forceful bowel movements, often with maroon or bright red blood and nausea.

EXAM

- **Early:** Agitation, writhing, a soft abdomen with hyper- or hypoactive bowel sounds, ⊕ fecal blood.
- **Later:** Distention, progressive tenderness, peritoneal signs, hypotension, fever.

DIFFERENTIAL

Pancreatitis, diverticulitis, appendicitis, aortic dissection, perforated peptic ulcer, nephrolithiasis.

DIAGNOSIS

- Maintain a **high index of suspicion** for patients > 50 years of age with CHF, cardiac arrhythmias, recent MI, recent catheterization, or hypotension.
- **Labs:** Leukocytosis, metabolic acidemia (late finding only), ↑ serum **amylase** (with normal lipase) and lactate.
- **AXR:** Demonstrates air-fluid levels and **"thumbprinting"** in the small bowel wall.
- **CT:** Shows bowel wall thickening, luminal dilation, pneumatosis intestinalis and portal venous gas, a nonenhancing bowel wall, and vascular thrombosis.
- **Visceral angiogram:** Important diagnostically; may also be therapeutic (see Figure 7.11).

TREATMENT

- Correct hypotension, hypovolemia, and cardiac arrhythmias.
- Bowel rest; broad-spectrum IV antibiotics.
- Angiography followed by thrombolysis or immediate surgery.
- Anticoagulation should be postponed until > 48 hours after laparotomy.

KEY FACT

Early visceral angiography is critical in the diagnosis and management of acute mesenteric ischemia.

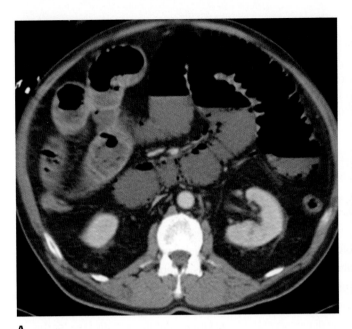

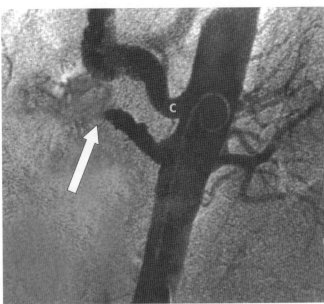

A   **B**

FIGURE 7.11.   Acute mesenteric ischemia. (A) Transaxial image from a contrast-enhanced CT in a patient with a history of atrial fibrillation and acute-onset, severe abdominal pain. Note the dilated loops of bowel in the midabdomen with pneumatosis intestinalis and a nonenhancing bowel wall. **(B)** Lateral midstream aortogram in a patient with a similar history and presentation shows acute occlusion of the superior mesenteric artery (arrow) by an embolus. C = celiac axis. (Image A reproduced with permission from USMLERx.com. Image B reproduced with permission from Brunicardi FC et al. *Schwartz's Principles of Surgery,* 9th ed. New York: McGraw-Hill, 2010, Fig. 23-38.)

ISCHEMIC COLITIS

Most common in the elderly and in patients with atherosclerotic or cardiovascular disease. Ranges from self-limited to life-threatening disease. **Watershed areas** (the splenic flexure and rectosigmoid junction of the colon) are the most common sites affected. Exsanguination and infarction are uncommon.

SYMPTOMS/EXAM

- Crampy left lower abdominal pain, hematochezia, nausea.
- Abdominal exam is benign or reveals mild LLQ tenderness.

DIFFERENTIAL

IBD, infectious colitis, diverticulitis.

DIAGNOSIS

- **Labs:** Leukocytosis, anemia.
- **AXR:** "Thumbprinting" is seen on the colon wall.
- **CT:** Shows bowel wall thickening, luminal dilation, and pericolonic fat stranding in watershed areas with the rectum spared (because of dual blood supply in the rectum). Vascular occlusion (eg, mesenteric venous thrombosis) is uncommon.
- **Flexible sigmoidoscopy:** Contraindicated if peritoneal signs are present. Performed with minimal insufflation. Look for **segmental changes sparing the rectum** (due to preserved collateral circulation from hemorrhoidal plexus) and hemorrhagic nodules. Pale, dusky, ulcerative mucosa.

> **KEY FACT**
>
> Ischemic colitis typically affects the colonic "watershed" areas of the splenic flexure and rectosigmoid junction but spares the rectum.

TREATMENT

- Correct hypotension, hypovolemia, and cardiac arrhythmias.
- Minimize vasopressors; give broad-spectrum IV antibiotics.
- Monitor for progression with serial exams and radiographs.
- If there are signs of infarction (guarding, rebound tenderness, fever), laparotomy, revascularization, or bowel resection may be needed.

Pancreatic Disorders

ACUTE PANCREATITIS

 A 43-year-old woman with a history of diabetes presents with severe abdominal pain of acute onset. Her exam is notable for a fever, tachycardia and hypotension, and tenderness to palpation in the epigastric region and the RUQ. Her labs reveal an ↑ WBC count, ↑ amylase and lipase, and ↑ total bilirubin. What is the likely diagnosis and the next important therapeutic step for this patient?

Gallstone pancreatitis and ERCP. This patient appears to have gallstone pancreatitis with evidence of biliary sepsis. While the patient is resuscitated and given empiric antibiotics, it will be important to remove the offending gallstone, preferably within the first 48 hours of presentation.

In the United States, > 80% of acute pancreatitis cases result from binge drinking or biliary stones; only 5% of heavy drinkers develop pancreatitis. Twenty percent of cases are complicated by necrotizing pancreatitis. Etiologies are as follows:

- **EtOH** and **gallstones** and, to a lesser extent, trauma.
- **Drugs:** Azathioprine, pentamidine, sulfonamides, thiazide diuretics, 6-MP, valproic acid, didanosine.
- **Metabolic:** Hyperlipidemia or hypercalcemia.
- **Mechanical:** Pancreas divisum, sphincter of Oddi dysfunction, masses.
- **Infectious:** Viruses (eg, mumps) and, to a lesser extent, bacteria and parasites (eg, *Ascaris lumbricoides*).
- **Other:** Scorpion bites, hereditary pancreatitis (an autosomal dominant mutation of the trypsinogen gene), CF, pregnancy.

SYMPTOMS

- Presents with sudden-onset, persistent, deep epigastric pain, often with radiation to the back, that **worsens when patients are supine and improves when they sit or lean forward.**
- Severe nausea, vomiting, and fever are also seen.

EXAM

- Exam reveals upper abdominal tenderness with guarding and rebound.
- Other findings include the following:
  - **Severe cases:** Distention, ileus, hypotension, tachycardia.
  - **Rare:** Umbilical (**Cullen's sign**) or flank (**Grey Turner's sign**) ecchymosis.
  - **Other:** Mild jaundice with stones or xanthomata with hyperlipidemia.

> **KEY FACT**
>
> *Ascaris lumbricoides* causes up to 20% of cases of acute pancreatitis in Asia.

> **KEY FACT**
>
> Gallstones and alcohol are the main causes of pancreatitis in the United States.

DIFFERENTIAL

Biliary colic, cholecystitis, mesenteric ischemia, intestinal obstruction/ileus, perforated hollow viscus, inferior MI, dissecting aortic aneurysm, ectopic pregnancy.

DIAGNOSIS

- **Labs** (see also Table 7.12):
  - Leukocytosis (10,000–30,000/µL); ↑ amylase (more sensitive) and lipase (more specific).
  - There is no clinical use for serial amylase or lipase.
  - High serum glucose.
  - An **ALT > 3 times normal suggests biliary stones over EtOH; an AST/ALT ratio of > 2 favors EtOH.** CRP ↓ with improvement.
- **Differential for ↑ amylase:** Pancreatitis, pancreatic tumors, cholecystitis, perforation (esophagus, bowel), intestinal ischemia or infarction, appendicitis, ruptured ectopic pregnancy, mumps, ovarian cysts, lung cancer, macroamylasemia, renal insufficiency, HIV, DKA, head trauma. **Lipase is usually normal in nonpancreatic amylase elevations.**
- **AXR:** May show gallstones, **"sentinel loop"** (an air-filled small bowel in the RUQ), and **"colon cutoff sign"** (abrupt ending of the transverse colon).
- **RUQ ultrasound:** May reveal cholelithiasis without cholecystitis. Choledocholithiasis (common duct stones) are often missed or have passed. However, biliary dilation may still be seen.
- **CT:** Performed initially to exclude abdominal catastrophes (see Figure 7.12). At 48–72 hours, exclude necrotizing pancreatitis. There is an ↑ risk of **renal failure** from contrast dye.

KEY FACT

CT is prognostic in severe pancreatitis and is used to evaluate for necrotizing pancreatitis. Necrotizing pancreatitis warrants empiric antibiotics (imipenem).

TREATMENT

- NPO with nasojejunal tube feeds or TPN with severe disease and anticipated NPO status for > 3–5 days.
- Aggressive IV hydration.
- Pain control with narcotics. Avoid morphine, as it ↑ sphincter of Oddi tone.
- Broad-spectrum IV antibiotics (imipenem) for severe necrotizing pancreatitis.
- For **gallstone pancreatitis** (↑ serum bilirubin, signs of biliary sepsis), perform ERCP for stone removal and cholecystectomy following recovery **but prior to discharge.**

KEY FACT

For persistent pancreatitis, no improvement on antibiotics (> 1 week), or suspicion of infected necrosis, consider CT with FNA to rule out infected necrosis, which requires surgical debridement.

TABLE 7.12. **Assessment of Pancreatitis Severity by Ranson's Criteria**[a]

24 HOURS: "GA LAW"	48 HOURS: "C HOBBS"
Glucose > 200 mg/dL	**C**a < 8 mg/dL
Age > 55	**H**ematocrit drop < 10%
LDH > 350 U/L	**O**2, arterial Po2 < 60 mm Hg
AST > 250 U/L	**B**ase deficit > 4 mEq/L
WBC > 16,000/µL	**B**UN rise > 5 mg/dL
	Sequestered fluid > 6 L

[a] Mortality risk: 1% with 0–2 criteria; 16% with 3–4 criteria; 40% with 5–6 criteria; 100% with 7–8 criteria.

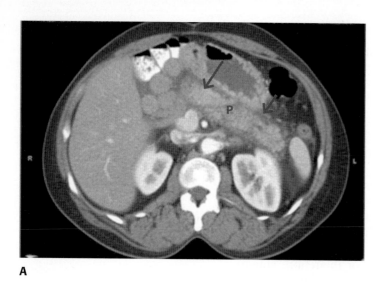
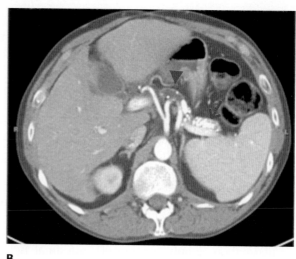

A   **B**

FIGURE 7.12.   Pancreatitis. Transaxial contrast-enhanced CT images. **(A) Uncomplicated acute pancreatitis.** Peripancreatic fluid and fat stranding can be seen (arrows). P = pancreas. **(B) Chronic pancreatitis.** Note the dilated pancreatic duct (arrowhead) and pancreatic calcifications (arrow). (Reproduced with permission from USMLERx.com.)

COMPLICATIONS

- **Necrotizing pancreatitis:**
  - Suspected in the setting of a persistently ↑ WBC count (7–10 days), high fever, and shock (organ failure).
  - Has a poor prognosis (up to 30% mortality and 70% risk of complications).
  - If infected necrosis is suspected, perform percutaneous aspiration. If organisms are present on smear, surgical debridement is indicated.
- **Pancreatic pseudocyst:** A collection of pancreatic fluid walled off by granulation tissue. Occurs in approximately 30% of cases but resolves spontaneously in about 50%. Drainage is not required unless the pseudocyst is present for > 6–8 weeks and is enlarging and symptomatic.
- **Other:** Pseudoaneurysm, renal failure, ARDS, splenic vein thrombosis (which can lead to isolated gastric varices).

CHRONIC PANCREATITIS

Persistent inflammation of the pancreas with irreversible histologic changes, recurrent abdominal pain, and loss of exocrine/endocrine function. Marked by atrophic gland, dilated ducts, and calcifications, although all are late findings. Characterized by the size of pancreatic ducts injured; "big duct" injury is from EtOH. Risk factors include EtOH and smoking. Associated with an ↑ risk of pancreatic cancer; 10- and 20-year survival rates are 70% and 45%, with death usually resulting from nonpancreatic causes. Etiologies are as follows:

- **EtOH (80%)** and, to a lesser extent, hereditary pancreatitis (CF, trypsinogen mutation).
- **Autoimmune:** Rare and associated with diffuse enlargement of the pancreas, ↑ IgG4, and autoantibodies; associated with other autoimmune disorders (eg, Sjögren's syndrome, SLE, primary sclerosing cholangitis).
- **Obstructive:** Pancreas divisum, sphincter of Oddi dysfunction, mass.
- **Metabolic:** Malnutrition, hyperlipidemia, hyperparathyroid-associated hypercalcemia.

Symptoms

- Presents with recurrent, deep epigastric pain, often radiating to the back, that worsens with food intake and when patients lie supine and **improves when they sit or lean forward.** Episodes may last anywhere from hours to 2–3 weeks.
- Also presents with anorexia, fear of eating (**sitophobia**), nausea/vomiting, and, later, weight loss and steatorrhea.

Exam

- Exam is normal. Mild to moderate upper abdominal tenderness may be found during episodes.
- Rarely, there may be a palpable epigastric mass (pseudocyst) or spleen (from splenic vein thrombosis).

Differential

Biliary colic, mesenteric ischemia, PUD, nonulcer dyspepsia, inferior MI, perforation, IBS, drug-seeking behavior.

Diagnosis

Diagnosis is as follows (see also Table 7.13):

- No single test is adequate; routine labs are normal. Amylase and lipase are not always ↑ during episodes.
- **Functional tests:**
  - Often normal in "small duct" chronic pancreatitis; not ⊕ until 30–50% of the gland is destroyed.
  - **Seventy-two-hour fecal fat test on 100-g/day fat diet:** ⊕ in the presence of > 7 g of fat in stool.
  - **Stool chymotrypsin and elastase:** Absent or low levels.
  - **Secretin test:** Most sensitive, but impractical. Give IV secretin and then measure pancreatic secretion via a nasobiliary tube.
  - **Structural tests:** Except for endoscopic ultrasound (**EUS**), imaging studies are insensitive, as architectural changes do not occur until late in the disease course; diagnosis is improved with EUS +/− FNA. Pancreatic calcifications are visualized on plain AXRs (30%); calcifications and a dilated pancreatic duct may be seen on CT.
- **Histology:** The gold standard, but impractical; obtained by EUS FNA. Reveals fibrosis, mixed lymphocyte and monocyte infiltrate, and architectural changes.

KEY FACT

Chronic pancreatitis of the "small duct" type may exhibit very subtle structural changes and is often associated with normal functional tests but marked symptoms.

TABLE 7.13. Diagnosis of Chronic Pancreatitis

CRITERION	"BIG DUCT"	"SMALL DUCT"
Seen on ultrasound or CT	Yes	No
Seen on ERCP	Yes	Maybe
Etiology	EtOH	Non-EtOH >> EtOH
Loss of function (exocrine/endocrine)	Common	Less common
Responsive to decompression (stenting, surgery)	Often	Rarely

TREATMENT

- Alcohol abstinence.
- Fat-soluble vitamins (vitamins A, D, E, and K); pancreatic enzymes.
- Pain control with narcotics (avoid morphine) and celiac plexus injection.
- ERCP with short-term pancreatic duct stenting and stone removal.
- **Surgical therapy** is appropriate for intractable pain and failure of medical therapy; modalities include pancreatectomy, pancreaticojejunostomy (Puestow), and pseudocyst drainage.

COMPLICATIONS

- **Malabsorption:** Fat-soluble vitamins (A, D, E, and K); pancreatic enzymes.
- **Metabolic bone disease:** Osteopenia (33%) and osteoporosis (10%). Manage with calcium, vitamin D, and bisphosphonates.
- **Other:** Brittle DM, pancreatic pseudocyst, pseudoaneurysm, hemosuccus pancreaticus (bleeding from the pancreatic duct into the GI tract), splenic vein thrombosis, pancreatic cancer.

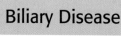

Biliary Disease

Tables 7.14 and 7.15 classify diseases with jaundice and biliary tract disease.

TABLE 7.14. Classification of Jaundice

TYPE OF HYPERBILIRUBINEMIA	LOCATION AND CAUSE
Unconjugated hyperbilirubinemia (predominant indirect-acting bilirubin)	↑ bilirubin production (eg, hemolytic anemias, hemolytic reactions, hematoma, pulmonary infarction). Impaired bilirubin uptake and storage (eg, posthepatitis hyperbilirubinemia, Gilbert's syndrome, Crigler-Najjar syndrome, drug reactions).
Conjugated hyperbilirubinemia (predominant direct-acting bilirubin)	**Hereditary cholestatic syndromes:** Faulty excretion of bilirubin conjugates (eg, Dubin-Johnson syndrome). **Hepatocellular dysfunction:** <ul><li>Biliary epithelial damage (eg, hepatitis, hepatic cirrhosis).</li><li>Intrahepatic cholestasis (eg, certain drugs, biliary cirrhosis, sepsis, postoperative jaundice).</li><li>Hepatocellular damage or intrahepatic cholestasis resulting from miscellaneous causes (eg, spirochetal infections, infectious mononucleosis, cholangitis, sarcoidosis, lymphomas, industrial toxins).</li></ul> **Biliary obstruction:** Choledocholithiasis, biliary atresia, carcinoma of the biliary duct, sclerosing cholangitis, choledochal cyst, external pressure on the common duct, pancreatitis, pancreatic neoplasms.

(Adapted with permission from McPhee SJ et al. *Current Medical Diagnosis & Treatment 2010.* New York: McGraw-Hill, 2010, Table 16-1.)

TABLE 7.15. Diseases of the Biliary Tract

Pathology	Clinical Features	Laboratory Features	Diagnosis	Treatment
Asymptomatic gallstones	None.	Normal.	Ultrasound.	None.
Symptomatic gallstones	Biliary colic.	Normal.	Ultrasound.	Laparoscopic cholecystectomy.
Porcelain gallbladder	Usually asymptomatic; high risk of gallbladder cancer.	Normal.	X-ray or CT.	Laparoscopic cholecystectomy.
Acute cholecystitis	Epigastric or RUQ pain, nausea, vomiting, fever, Murphy's sign.	Leukocytosis.	Ultrasound, HIDA scan, or CT.	Antibiotics, laparoscopic cholecystectomy.
Chronic cholecystitis	Biliary colic, constant epigastric or RUQ pain, nausea.	Normal.	Oral cholecystography, ultrasound (stones), cholecystectomy (nonfunctioning gallbladder).	Laparoscopic cholecystectomy.
Choledocholithiasis	Asymptomatic or biliary colic, jaundice, fever; gallstone pancreatitis.	Cholestatic LFTs; leukocytosis and blood cultures in cholangitis; ↑ amylase and lipase in pancreatitis.	Ultrasound (dilated ducts), ERCP.	Endoscopic sphincterotomy and stone extraction; antibiotics for cholangitis.

(Adapted with permission from McPhee SJ et al. *Current Medical Diagnosis & Treatment 2010.* New York: McGraw-Hill, 2010, Table 16-7.)

CHOLELITHIASIS (GALLSTONES) AND ACUTE CHOLECYSTITIS

A 50-year-old woman presents with abdominal pain after having suffered recurrent bouts of abdominal pain for years. A KUB shows a normal bowel gas pattern but a heavily calcified gallbladder. What is the next most appropriate step for this patient?

Cholecystectomy. This patient is demonstrating evidence of a porcelain gallbladder, which carries a risk of gallbladder cancer. For this reason, prophylactic cholecystectomy may improve symptoms and may also prevent the development of malignancy.

More common in women; incidence ↑ with age. In the United States, 10% of men and 20% of women > 65 years of age are affected; > 70% are cholesterol stones (see Table 7.16). Among patients with incidental asymptomatic gallstones, only 15% have biliary colic at 10 years, and 2–3% have cholecystitis/cholangitis.

■ **Cholecystitis:** The most common complication of cholelithiasis. More than 90% of cases are due to cholelithiasis with stone impacted in the

TABLE 7.16.   **Types of Gallstones**

	SUBTYPE		
VARIABLE	**CHOLESTEROL**	**BLACK PIGMENTED**	**BROWN PIGMENTED**
Regional/ethnic predictors	Western countries, Pima Indians, Caucasians >> blacks.	Africa, Asia.	Africa, Asia.
Risk factors	Age, female gender, pregnancy, estrogens, DM, obesity, rapid weight loss, ↑ triglycerides, prolonged fasting, ileal disease **(Crohn's)**, ileal resection, CF.	Chronic hemolysis **(sickle cell),** cirrhosis, high-protein diet.	Biliary infections, foreign bodies (stents, sutures), low-protein diet.

cystic duct. Spontaneous resolution occurs in > 50% of cases within 7–10 days.

- **Acalculous cholecystitis (without gallstones):** Usually seen in critically ill patients with no oral intake or following major surgical procedures; occurs after ischemia-related chronic gallbladder distention.

SYMPTOMS

- **Cholelithiasis:** Often asymptomatic or may present as follows:
  - **Common:** Biliary colic (crampy, wavelike RUQ pain), abdominal bloating, dyspepsia.
  - **Uncommon:** Nausea/vomiting (except in small bowel obstruction from **gallstone ileus**).
- **Cholecystitis:** Sudden-onset, severe RUQ or epigastric pain that may radiate to the right shoulder, accompanied by nausea/vomiting and fever. Jaundice suggests common bile duct stones (choledocholithiasis) or compression of the common bile duct by an inflamed, impacted cystic duct **(Mirizzi's syndrome).**

EXAM

- **Cholelithiasis:** RUQ tenderness is commonly seen, but exam may be normal.
- **Cholecystitis:** RUQ tenderness and voluntary guarding; ⊕ **Murphy's sign** (inspiratory arrest with palpation of the RUQ); fever; jaundice in < 25% of cases.

DIFFERENTIAL

- Choledocholithiasis, cholangitis, perforated peptic ulcer, acute pancreatitis.
- Diverticulitis (hepatic flexure, transverse colon), right-sided pneumonia.

DIAGNOSIS

- **Cholelithiasis:** Often an incidental finding on abdominal ultrasound or CT.
- **Cholecystitis:**
  - **Labs:** Leukocytosis with neutrophil predominance; ↑ total bilirubin (1–4 mg/dL) and transaminases (2–4 times normal) even without choledocholithiasis. ↑ alkaline phosphatase and amylase.

KEY FACT

Acalculous cholecystitis is generally seen in the critically ill with no oral intake or after major surgical procedures.

- **RUQ ultrasound:** Less sensitive than HIDA scan but more readily available. Shows gallbladder wall **thickening, pericholecystic fluid,** and localization of stones (see Figure 7.13). A sonographic **Murphy's sign** (focal gallbladder tenderness under a transducer) has a 90% positive predictive value. Low sensitivity (50%) for choledocholithiasis.
- **HIDA scan:** High sensitivity (95%) and specificity (90%). Assesses cystic duct patency; ⊕ in the setting of a ⊖ gallbladder uptake with preserved excretion into the small bowel. **CCK** stimulation assesses gallbladder contractility and aids in the diagnosis of acalculous cholecystitis.

TREATMENT

- **Asymptomatic cholelithiasis:** No specific treatment is indicated (even in DM).
- **Symptomatic cholelithiasis:**
  - Consider prophylactic cholecystectomy.
  - Cholecystectomy can be postponed until recurrent symptoms are seen.
  - The risk of **recurrent symptoms is 30–50% per year;** the risk of **complications is 1–2% per year.**
- Cholecystitis:
  - **Antibiotics can be withheld** in the setting of **mild and uncomplicated disease.**
  - **IV antibiotics:** Provide coverage of gram-⊖ enteric bacteria and enterococcus with antibiotics such as ampicillin and gentamicin (or ampicillin/sulbactam if the patient is ill).
  - Bowel rest.
  - Cholecystectomy should be performed after symptom resolution but prior to discharge.

COMPLICATIONS

- **Gangrenous cholecystitis:** The most common complication of cholecystitis (affects up to 20%), particularly in diabetics and the elderly. Patients appear septic.
- **Emphysematous cholecystitis:** 2° infection of the gallbladder with gas-forming organisms. More common in diabetics and the elderly; associated with high mortality. Gangrene and perforation may follow.

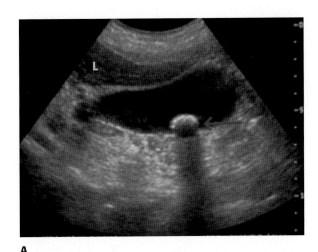

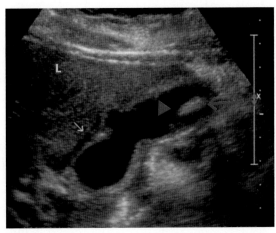

A   B

FIGURE 7.13.   Gallstone disease. (A) Cholelithiasis. Ultrasound image of the gallbladder shows a gallstone (arrow) with posterior shadowing. **(B) Acute cholecystitis.** Ultrasound image shows a gallstone (red arrow), a thickened gallbladder wall (arrowheads), and pericholecystic fluid (white arrow). L = liver. (Reproduced with permission from USMLERx.com.)

- **Cholecystenteric fistula:** Uncommon. Stone erodes through the gallbladder into the duodenum. Large stones (> 2.5 cm) can cause small bowel obstruction (**gallstone ileus**).
- **Mirizzi's syndrome:** Common bile duct obstruction by an inflamed impacted cystic duct. Uncommon.
- **Gallbladder hydrops:** Gallbladder mucocele with massive enlargement of the gallbladder due to cystic duct obstruction.
- **Porcelain gallbladder:** Intramural calcification. Associated with an ↑ risk of gallbladder cancer; cholecystectomy is indicated.

CHOLEDOCHOLITHIASIS AND CHOLANGITIS

Choledocholithiasis is defined as stones in the common bile duct. Cholangitis can be defined as biliary tree obstruction and subsequent suppurative infection.

SYMPTOMS

- **Choledocholithiasis:** Similar to cholelithiasis, except **jaundice is more common in choledocholithiasis.** Other symptoms include biliary colic (crampy, wavelike RUQ pain), abdominal bloating, and dyspepsia. May be asymptomatic.
- **Cholangitis:** Similar to cholecystitis but frequently more severe, presenting with fever, jaundice, and RUQ pain (Charcot's triad). May also include mental status changes and hypotension (Reynolds' pentad).

EXAM

- **Choledocholithiasis:** Exam is normal or reveals mild RUQ tenderness along with jaundice.
- **Cholangitis:**
  - Fever and RUQ tenderness with peritoneal signs (90%), jaundice (> 80%), hypotension, and altered mental status (15%).
  - **Charcot's triad (RUQ pain, jaundice, fever):** Present in only 70% of patients.
  - **Reynolds' pentad (Charcot's triad plus hypotension and altered mental status):** Points to impending septic shock.

DIFFERENTIAL

- **Choledocholithiasis:** Mass lesions (eg, pancreatic and ampullary carcinoma, cholangiocarcinoma, bulky lymphadenopathy), parasitic infection (eg, ascariasis), AIDS cholangiopathy, primary sclerosing cholangitis, recurrent pyogenic cholangitis.
- **Cholangitis:** Perforated peptic ulcer, hepatitis, acute pancreatitis, appendicitis, hepatic abscess, diverticulitis, right-sided pneumonia.

DIAGNOSIS

- **Choledocholithiasis:**
  - **Labs:** No leukocytosis; ↑ total bilirubin (> 2 mg/dL), transaminases (2–4 times normal), and alkaline phosphatase.
  - **RUQ ultrasound:** Has low sensitivity (< 50%).
  - **CT:** Has higher sensitivity than RUQ ultrasound.
- **Cholangitis:**
  - **Labs:** Leukocytosis with neutrophil predominance; ↑ total bilirubin (> 2 mg/dL), transaminases (> 2–4 times normal), alkaline phosphatase, and amylase; bacteremia.

KEY FACT

Charcot's triad = RUQ pain, jaundice, and fever/chills. Reynolds' pentad = Charcot's triad plus hypotension and altered mental status.

- **RUQ ultrasound:** Shows dilation of the common bile duct and chole-lithiasis. Less likely to visualize choledocholithiasis.
- **ERCP:** Perform < 48 hours after presentation, ideally after IV antibiotics and fluids. Requires sedation. Both diagnostic and therapeutic.
- **MRCP:** Noninvasive and sensitive for diagnosis.
- **EUS:** The most sensitive diagnostic study.
- **Percutaneous transhepatic cholangiography (PTHC):** An alternative if ERCP is unavailable, unsafe, or unsuccessful. Does not require sedation.

TREATMENT

- **Choledocholithiasis:**
  - **High suspicion** (total bilirubin > 2, alkaline phosphatase > 150, ↑ AST/ALT): ERCP with sphincterotomy/stone removal prior to surgery followed by laparoscopic cholecystectomy.
  - **Intermediate suspicion:** Intraoperative cholangiography, MRCP, or EUS. If MRCP or EUS is ⊕ for choledocholithiasis, proceed to ERCP.
- **Cholangitis:**
  - **Broad-spectrum IV antibiotics:** IV ampicillin/sulbactam (Unasyn) or ticarcillin/clavulanate (Timentin). If the patient is responsive to antibiotics, biliary decompression can be elective; otherwise, it is indicated emergently.
  - **ERCP:** Biliary decompression and drainage (sphincterotomy, stone removal, biliary stenting).
  - **PTHC:** A temporary alternative to ERCP that allows for biliary decompression (stenting and drainage).
  - Cholecystectomy after recovery for cholangitis due to gallstones.
- **Recurrent pyogenic cholangitis:** Affects Southeast Asians between 20 and 40 years of age; characterized by pigmented intrahepatic bile duct stones, biliary strictures, and repeated cholangitis. Treatment includes stenting and drainage. Often isolated to the left lobe of the liver; resection may be considered.

COMPLICATIONS

Gallstone pancreatitis, gram-⊖ sepsis, intrahepatic abscesses.

AIDS CHOLANGIOPATHY

An opportunistic biliary infection caused by CMV, *Cryptosporidium*, or *Microsporidium*. CD4 count is usually < 200/mL.

SYMPTOMS/EXAM

Presents with RUQ pain/tenderness, fever, hepatomegaly, and diarrhea. Jaundice is uncommon.

DIFFERENTIAL

Biliary stones, cholecystitis, primary sclerosing cholangitis.

DIAGNOSIS

- **Labs:** Markedly ↑ alkaline phosphatase.
- **ERCP or MRCP:** Intra- and/or extrahepatic biliary stricturing; papillary stenosis.
- **Aspiration and culture of bile are key to diagnosis.**

TREATMENT

- ERCP with sphincterotomy and biliary stenting.
- IV antibiotics based on bile cultures.
- Treat underlying immunosuppression/HIV.

PRIMARY SCLEROSING CHOLANGITIS

 A 46-year-old man with a recent diagnosis of ulcerative colitis presents with fatigue and pruritus that have been worsening over several months. His exam is largely normal, and his labs are notable for ↑ alkaline phosphatase and total bilirubin levels. An RUQ ultrasound shows hepatomegaly with mild dilation of the intrahepatic ducts with a normal gallbladder and common bile duct. What test will best establish this patient's diagnosis?

Cholangiography. This patient has primary sclerosing cholangitis. This will best be seen on cholangiogram, which would show the classic "beads on a string" appearance of the biliary tree. Although serology could be used to aid in the diagnosis, p-ANCA and ANA are not specific or sensitive enough to confirm the diagnosis.

A chronic cholestatic disease characterized by fibrosing inflammation of the intrahepatic and extrahepatic biliary system **without an identifiable cause.** Most common among middle-aged males; median survival from the time of diagnosis is 12 years. Commonly associated with **IBD** (more frequently ulcerative colitis than Crohn's) and, to a lesser extent, with other autoimmune disorders (sarcoidosis, Sjögren's syndrome, SLE, autoimmune hepatitis). Also associated with an ↑ risk of **cholangiocarcinoma.**

SYMPTOMS/EXAM

- Presents with gradual onset of fatigue and severe pruritus followed by jaundice and weight loss. Fever occurs with recurrent cholangitis.
- Exam reveals jaundice, hepatosplenomegaly, hyperpigmentation, xanthomas, excoriations, and stigmata of fat-soluble vitamin deficiency.

DIFFERENTIAL

Secondary sclerosing cholangitis—biliary stones, congenital anomalies, infections, AIDS cholangiopathy, recurrent pyogenic cholangitis.

DIAGNOSIS

- Maintain a high clinical suspicion in patients with IBD, as the **diagnosis of IBD typically precedes that of primary sclerosing cholangitis.** Diagnosis can be confirmed only by ERCP (see Figure 7.14). Magnetic resonance cholangiography is less sensitive and less specific.
- **Labs:** Look for a **cholestatic pattern** consisting of alkaline phosphatase > 1.5 times normal for six months plus a modest ↑ in bilirubin and transaminases.
- **Autoantibodies:** The sensitivity of **p-ANCA** is 70%; that of ANA is 25%.
- **Liver biopsy:** Look for pericholangitis and the classic "**onion skin**" periductal fibrosis, focal proliferation and obliteration of bile ducts, cholestasis, and copper deposition.
- **ERCP:** Shows irregularity of the intra- and extrahepatic biliary tree, classically with a "**beads on a string**" appearance. 2° causes of sclerosing cho-

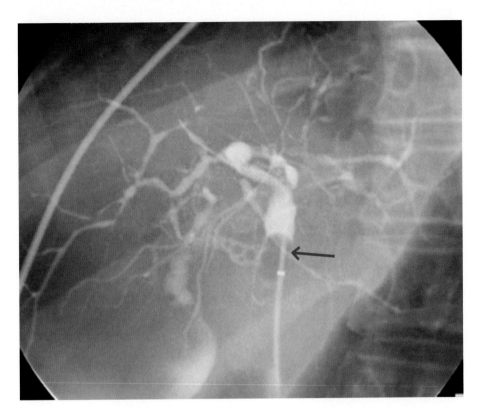

FIGURE 7.14. **Primary sclerosing cholangitis.** Images from ERCP after contrast injection through a catheter in the common bile duct with the balloon (blue arrow) inflated. Multifocal stricturing and dilation of the intrahepatic bile ducts is present. (Reproduced with permission from USMLERx.com.)

langitis usually have **only** extrahepatic bile duct involvement except with recurrent pyogenic cholangitis (intrahepatic biliary dilation and stones).

TREATMENT

- Focus on symptom control and on the prevention and management of complications. Medical therapy to prevent or delay disease progression is largely ineffective.
- **Symptom control:** Treat pruritus (cholestyramine, ursodiol, phenobarbital, rifampin).
- **Medical therapy: The natural history of primary sclerosing cholangitis is not significantly changed by current medical therapy.**
- **Liver transplantation:** The treatment of choice for end-stage liver failure; five-year survival is 75%.

COMPLICATIONS

- **Steatorrhea/fat-soluble vitamin deficiency:** Treat with bile acids, digestive enzymes, and vitamins A, D, E, and K.
- **Metabolic bone disease:** Treat with Ca++ and bisphosphonates.
- **Recurrent bacterial cholangitis and dominant strictures:** Treat with antibiotics and biliary stent and drainage.
- **Other:** Biliary stones, **cholangiocarcinoma,** portal hypertension, end-stage liver disease.

KEY FACT

Primary sclerosing cholangitis is diagnosed by ERCP and shows a "beads on a string" appearance involving both intra- and extrahepatic bile ducts.

KEY FACT

Unlike primary biliary cirrhosis, the natural history of primary sclerosing cholangitis is not improved by ursodeoxycholic acid.

PRIMARY BILIARY CIRRHOSIS

A chronic cholestatic disease that primarily affects **middle-aged women of all races.** Prevalence is 19–240 cases in one million; 90–95% are women. Age of onset is 30–70; often associated with **autoimmune** disorders such as Sjögren's syndrome, RA, thyroid disease, celiac sprue, and CREST syndrome.

SYMPTOMS

May be asymptomatic (50–60% at the time of diagnosis) or present with fatigue, **severe and intractable pruritus prior to jaundice,** and malabsorptive diarrhea.

EXAM

- Exam reveals hepatomegaly, splenomegaly, skin pigmentation, excoriations (from pruritus), xanthelasma, and xanthomas. Kayser-Fleischer rings are rare (result from copper retention, as in Wilson's disease).
- Late findings include jaundice and the stigmata of cirrhosis.

DIFFERENTIAL

Biliary obstruction (stones, benign or malignant masses), autoimmune hepatitis, primary and secondary sclerosing cholangitis, drug-induced cholestasis (phenothiazines, steroids, TMP-SMX, tolbutamide), infiltrative diseases (sarcoidosis, lymphoma, TB).

DIAGNOSIS

- Suspect in the setting of unexplained cholestasis or ↑ serum alkaline phosphatase.
- **Labs:**
  - **Cholestatic pattern:** Look for an alkaline phosphatase level > 3–4 times normal, an ↑ GGT, and a slight ↑ in transaminases. Serum bilirubin is normal early in disease but is ↑ later in the disease course.
  - **Serum autoantibodies: Antimitochondrial antibodies (AMA)** are detected in **95% of cases.** ANA (70%), SMA (66%), RF (70%), and antithyroid antibodies (40%) are also seen.
  - **Other:** ↑ **serum IgM,** total cholesterol, HDL, ceruloplasmin, and urinary copper.
- **Imaging:** Ultrasound is initially useful for excluding biliary tract obstruction; MRI/CT can show nonprogressive periportal adenopathy. Signs of portal hypertension are usually absent at the time of diagnosis.
- **Liver biopsy:** Important for diagnosis, staging, and prognosis. The pathognomonic finding is the **"florid" duct lesion** (duct degeneration with periductular granulomatous inflammation), which is uncommon.
- **ERCP:** Needed only to exclude primary and secondary sclerosing cholangitis.

TREATMENT

- Disease-modifying therapy has limited efficacy. Symptom control and the prevention and treatment of complications are most important in management.
- **Ursodeoxycholic acid:** The only FDA-approved disease-modifying agent; promotes endogenous bile acid secretion and may also have immunologic effects. Give 13–15 mg/kg/day. Colchicine and methotrexate are less commonly used.

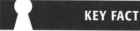

KEY FACT

Antimitochondrial antibody (present in 95% of patients) and ↑ serum IgM are the best laboratory diagnostic tools for primary biliary cirrhosis.

- **Liver transplantation:** The most effective treatment for decompensated primary biliary cirrhosis. Five-year survival is 85%; rates of recurrent primary biliary cirrhosis at 3 and 10 years are 15% and 30%, respectively. The need for liver transplantation can be predicted by the Mayo Clinic model (based on patient age, total bilirubin, PT, and serum albumin).

COMPLICATIONS

- **Malabsorption:** Treat with fat-soluble vitamins (A, D, E, and K) and pancreatic enzymes.
- **Metabolic bone disease:** Osteopenia (affects 33%) and osteoporosis (affects 10%). Manage with calcium, vitamin D, and bisphosphonates.
- **Cirrhosis:** Late ascites, encephalopathy, portal hypertension.

Hepatitis

HEPATITIS A (HAV) AND HEPATITIS E (HEV)

Spread by fecal-oral transmission; cause acute (**not chronic**) hepatitis. More common in developing countries. The annual incidence of HAV in the United States is 70,000, whereas **HEV is rare and limited to travelers of endemic regions** (Southeast and Central Asia, the Middle East, Northern Africa, and, to a lesser extent, Mexico). HAV is typically asymptomatic, benign, and self-limited in children but can range from mild to severe acute hepatitis in adults. The rate of fatal acute liver failure from HAV is < 4% in patients < 49 years of age but can be as high as 17% in those > 49 years of age. **HEV is more severe** than HAV, **particularly in pregnancy,** a setting in which **mortality is approximately 20%.**

SYMPTOMS

- Presents with flulike illness, malaise, anorexia, weakness, fever, RUQ pain, jaundice, and pruritus. Children are typically asymptomatic.
- Atypical presentations include acute liver failure, cholestasis (prolonged, deep jaundice), and relapsing disease (2–18 weeks after initial presentation).
- Figure 7.15 illustrates the typical course of HAV.

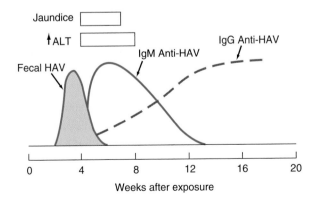

FIGURE 7.15. **Typical course of acute HAV.** (Reproduced with permission from Fauci AS et al. *Harrison's Principles of Internal Medicine*, 17th ed. New York: McGraw-Hill, 2008, Fig. 298-2.)

EXAM

Jaundice, RUQ tenderness.

DIFFERENTIAL

Acute HBV or, less frequently, HCV; mononucleosis, CMV, HSV, drug-induced hepatitis, acute alcoholic hepatitis, autoimmune hepatitis.

DIAGNOSIS

- **History:** Inquire about ill contacts, substandard water supply, travel (HEV), and contaminated food (**shellfish and green onions**).
- **Labs:**
    - **HAV:** Anti-HAV IgM (acute infection); anti-HAV IgG (prior exposure, vaccination); anti-HAV total measures IgM and IgG (acute infection, prior exposure, vaccination).
    - **HEV:** Anti-HEV IgM (acute infection); anti-HEV (prior exposure).

TREATMENT

- No specific drug treatment is available for HAV or HEV.
- Supportive care.
- Consider early delivery for pregnant women with HEV (no proven benefit).

PREVENTION

- **Vaccination:** The HAV vaccine is safe and effective, but no vaccine for HEV is currently available.
- **Indications for HAV vaccine:** Travelers to endemic regions, men who have sex with men, IV drug users, Native Americans, those with chronic liver disease (**all HCV ⊕**), food handlers, day care center workers.
- **HAV immunoglobulin:** Effective for postexposure prophylaxis. For those traveling immediately to endemic areas, supplement with the first HAV vaccine shot.

> **KEY FACT**
>
> HAV and HEV cause variably severe acute hepatitis but do not cause chronic hepatitis.

> **KEY FACT**
>
> Hepatocellular carcinoma can occur before cirrhosis from HBV, but this is not true of HCV.

HEPATITIS B (HBV) AND HEPATITIS D (HDV)

A 50-year-old man from China presents to his new physician with a history of hepatitis B. His labs reveal that he is HBsAg ⊕, anti-HBs ⊖, HBeAg ⊕, and anti-HBc ⊕ and has an HBV DNA level of 2000 IU/mL. He has no stigmata of liver disease, and his INR, albumin, and transaminase levels are all normal. In addition to ensuring that sexual and household contacts are vaccinated, what measures would constitute appropriate surveillance for hepatocellular carcinoma (HCC) in this patient?

Abdominal CT or ultrasound every six months. Hepatitis B does not need to progress to cirrhosis before HCC can arise; therefore, this patient with active HBV needs active surveillance. AFP can also be measured but is not required, and by itself it is insufficient as a screening test for HCC.

Some 400 million people worldwide have chronic HBV, including > 1 million in the United States. Transmission can be perinatal (the most common cause worldwide), sexual, or percutaneous. Age at infection is **inversely related** to the risk of chronic infection. Of all patients with chronic HBV, 15–20% develop cirrhosis and 10–15% develop HCC. **HDV infection re-**

quires **HBV coinfection.** In the United States, HDV is found primarily among IV drug users and hemophiliacs.

SYMPTOMS

- **Acute HBV:** Presents with flulike illness, malaise, weakness, low-grade fever, serum sickness–like symptoms (arthritis, urticaria, angioedema), and RUQ pain followed by jaundice (see Figure 7.16).
- **Chronic HBV:** Can be asymptomatic.
- **Extrahepatic manifestations:** Serum sickness, polyarteritis nodosa, glomerulonephritis.

EXAM

- **Acute:** Icteric sclera, arthritis, RUQ tenderness.
- **Chronic:** Stigmata of cirrhosis (spider angiomata, palmar erythema, gynecomastia).

DIFFERENTIAL

- **Other acute viral diseases:** HAV, HCV, mononucleosis, CMV, HSV.
- Spirochetal (**leptospirosis,** syphilis) and rickettsial disease (**Q fever**).
- **Other chronic liver diseases:** Autoimmune disease, hemochromatosis, α_1-antitrypsin deficiency, Wilson's disease, alcoholic/nonalcoholic steatohepatitis.

DIAGNOSIS

- **HBsAg:** Surface antigen indicates **active** infection (see Table 7.17).
- **Anti-HBs:** Antibody to HBsAg indicates past viral infection or immunization.
- **Anti-HBc:** IgM is an early marker of infection; IgG is the best marker for prior HBV exposure. IgM may also become detectable in reactivation of HBV.

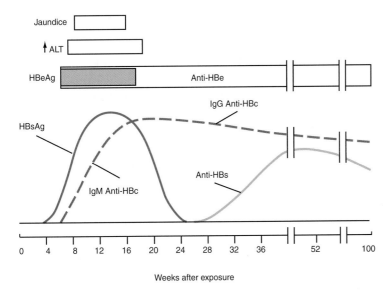

FIGURE 7.16. **Typical course of acute HBV.** (Reproduced with permission from Fauci AS et al. *Harrison's Principles of Internal Medicine,* 17th ed. New York: McGraw-Hill, 2008, Fig. 298-4.)

TABLE 7.17. Serologic Patterns in HBV Infection and Their Interpretation

HBsAg	Anti-HBs	Anti-HBc	HBeAg	Anti-HBe	INTERPRETATION
+	−	IgM	+	−	Acute hepatitis B.
+	−	IgG[a]	+	−	Chronic hepatitis B with active viral replication.
+	−	IgG	−	+	Chronic hepatitis B with low viral replication.
+	+	IgG	+ or −	+ or −	Chronic hepatitis B with heterotypic anti-HBs (about 10% of cases).
−	−	IgM	+ or −	−	Acute hepatitis B.
−	+	−	−	−	Vaccination (immunity).
−	−	IgG	−	−	False ⊕; less commonly, infection in remote past.

[a]Low levels of IgM anti-HBc may also be detected.

(Reproduced with permission from McPhee SJ et al. *Current Medical Diagnosis & Treatment 2010*. New York: McGraw-Hill, 2010, Table 16-5.)

- **HBeAg:** Proportional to the quantity of intact virus and therefore infectivity. Some HBV variants (called **precore mutants**) cannot make HBeAg. Precore mutants have lower spontaneous remission, are less responsive to treatment, and are associated with a higher risk of cirrhosis and HCC. Precore mutants are diagnosed by their high HBV DNA and ⊖ HBeAg.
- **Anti-HDV:** Indicates past or present HDV infection. **Does not indicate immunity.**
- **HBV DNA:** Indicates active replication. A level of $> 10^5$ copies/mL is considered active; $> 10^2$ copies/mL are detectable by new assays.
- **Liver biopsy:** Not routinely needed prior to treatment. Indicated if the diagnosis is in question or to determine the degree of inflammation or fibrosis/cirrhosis.

TREATMENT

- **Acute exposure/needlestick prophylaxis:** The CDC recommends that hepatitis B immune globulin (HBIG) be given **within 24 hours along with vaccine** if the patient was not previously immunized.
- **Chronic hepatitis B:** The decision to treat depends on HBeAg status, ALT level, HBV DNA level, and the presence of cirrhosis.
  - In general, treatment is reserved for patients with evidence of active hepatic inflammation (ALT > 2 times the upper limit of normal or at least moderate inflammation on liver biopsy) with moderate levels of detectable HBV virus.
  - If there is evidence of cirrhosis (radiographically or histologically), treatment with oral agents is generally recommended in the setting of any detectable HBV virus regardless of the degree of hepatic inflammation. Interferon is contraindicated in patients with cirrhosis and HBV infection.
- **Nucleoside analogs:** Given PO; generally well tolerated. Several agents are currently available, and the treatment of choice is dependent on resistance profile, cost, and potency. **Tenofovir** and **entecavir** are first-line therapy; other agents include **lamivudine, adefovir,** and **telbivudine.**
- **Pegylated interferon-α_{2a}:** Given SQ; associated with many side effects (eg, constitutional, psychiatric, bone marrow toxicity, flare of autoimmune disease, hepatic decompensation). Contraindicated in cirrhosis. The best re-

sponses to treatment are obtained with active hepatic inflammation (high ALT) and low HBV DNA levels.

- Treat HDV by treating HBV.
- **HBV cirrhosis:** Treat indefinitely with an antiviral agent if HBV DNA is detectable.
- **Liver transplantation:** The treatment of choice for decompensated cirrhosis.

HEPATITIS C (HCV)

Transmitted by percutaneous or mucosal blood exposure. Risk factors include blood transfusions before 1992, IV drug use, and occupational exposure (needlesticks). Spontaneous resolution occurs in 15–45% of patients, with the highest rates of resolution in children and young women. Chronic infection occurs in the remainder of patients. Cirrhosis occurs in 20% within 20–30 years. The risk of carcinoma is 1–4% per year after cirrhosis.

SYMPTOMS

- **Acute HCV:** Presents with flulike illness, malaise, weakness, low-grade fever, myalgias, and RUQ pain followed by jaundice. Only 30% of patients are symptomatic in acute disease.
- **Chronic HCV:** Often asymptomatic, or may present with cryoglobulinemia associated with a vasculitic skin rash (**leukocytoclastic vasculitis**), **arthralgias**, sicca syndrome, and **glomerulonephritis**. In the setting of cirrhosis, presents with fatigue, muscle wasting, dependent edema, and easy bruising.

EXAM

- **Acute:** Icterus; RUQ tenderness.
- **Chronic:** Stigmata of cirrhosis (spider angiomata, palmar erythema, gynecomastia, ascites).

DIFFERENTIAL

- **Other acute viral diseases:** HAV, HBV, mononucleosis, CMV, HSV.
- Spirochetal (**leptospirosis, syphilis**) and rickettsial disease (**Q fever**).
- **Other chronic liver diseases:** HBV, hemochromatosis, α_1-antitrypsin deficiency, Wilson's disease, nonalcoholic steatohepatitis, autoimmune hepatitis.

DIAGNOSIS

- **Screening:** HCV antibody ($\oplus$ 4–6 weeks after infection); qualitative PCR (in acute infection; can be $\oplus$ 1–2 weeks after infection). Screen patients with risk factors or persistently ↑ transaminases.
- **Confirmatory:** Qualitative PCR or recombinant immunoblot assay (RIBA).
- **Prognostic:** Liver biopsy.

TREATMENT

- **Regimen:** Treat with SQ interferon (pegylated or standard) and PO ribavirin × 24 weeks (non–genotype 1) or × 48 weeks (genotype 1). Check quantitative RNA at 12 weeks; if there is less than a 2-log drop, consider stopping treatment.
  - **Predictive:** Quantitative PCR (a low viral load indicates a better treatment response). Genotypes 2 and 3 are associated with a better treatment response than genotype 1.

- **Indications for treatment:** Age 18–60, HCV viremia, ↑ aminotransferase levels.
- **Contraindications:** Psychosis, severe depression, symptomatic coronary or cerebrovascular disease, **decompensated cirrhosis,** uncontrolled seizures, severe bone marrow insufficiency, pregnancy or inability to use birth control, retinopathy, autoimmune disease.

- **Acute infection/needlestick prophylaxis:** After known exposure, serial testing for HCV antibody, HCV PCR, AST, and ALT is recommended both immediately and at 4, 8, and 12 weeks.
  - Consider treatment with high-dose standard interferon or **pegylated interferon** (83–100% sustained virologic response) if no spontaneous clearance is seen at 12 weeks. The benefit of ribavirin combination therapy is unclear.
  - A treatment delay of 8–12 weeks to document lack of spontaneous clearance does not affect the probability of treatment response.
- **Chronic HCV:** Treatment is curative in up to 80% of genotype 2/3 cases but is < 50% for genotype 1.
  - Combination treatment with **ribavirin** daily and **pegylated interferon** weekly is the current standard of care. Treatment duration is dependent on genotype and generally consists of 24 weeks for genotype 2 or 3 and 48 weeks for genotype 1. Baseline viral load also predicts the likelihood of successful treatment.
  - Side effects are common and include hemolytic anemia and cough (ribavirin), bone marrow suppression (leukopenia, anemia, thrombocytopenia), flulike symptoms, and exacerbations or occurrence of autoimmune disorders (thyroid disease, sarcoidosis, psoriasis, type 1 DM), related to interferon. Ribavirin has teratogenic effects. Patients who may be pregnant should have pregnancy testing prior to treatment and use two methods of birth control during treatment.
  - New HCV agents such as **telaprevir** and **boceprevir,** used in combination with ribavirin and pegylated interferon, may ↑ cure rates for HCV genotype 1 by 20–30%.
- **Cryoglobulinemia:** Treatment of acute flares includes plasmapheresis +/– steroids. Long-term effectiveness is seen with interferon plus ribavirin, and data on rituximab appear promising.

AUTOIMMUNE HEPATITIS

Characterized by hypergammaglobulinemia, periportal hepatitis, and autoimmune markers. Typically chronic, but 25% of cases are characterized by acute onset and rare fulminant hepatic failure. Prevalence depends on gender and ethnicity; women are affected three times more often than men. Incidence among Northern American and European Caucasians is 1 in 100,000. Less common in non-Caucasians; in Japan, incidence is 0.01 in 100,000. The risk of cirrhosis is 17–82% at five years. The main prognostic factors are severity of inflammation/fibrosis on liver biopsy and HLA type. Associated with other autoimmune diseases.

SYMPTOMS

Fatigue (85%), jaundice, RUQ pain. **Pruritus suggests an alternate diagnosis.**

EXAM

- Hepatomegaly, jaundice, splenomegaly (with or without cirrhosis).
- **Acute:** Icteric sclera, arthritis, RUQ tenderness.
- **Chronic:** Stigmata of cirrhosis (spider angiomata, palmar erythema, gynecomastia, ascites).

KEY FACT

Advanced liver disease is a poor prognostic sign for treatment response but not a contraindication to the treatment of autoimmune hepatitis.

DIFFERENTIAL

Wilson's disease, viral hepatitis (HBV, HCV), α_1-antitrypsin deficiency, hemochromatosis, drug-induced hepatitis, alcoholic and nonalcoholic steatohepatitis.

DIAGNOSIS

- **International Autoimmune Hepatitis Group (IAHG) criteria:** A definite or probable diagnosis of autoimmune hepatitis is made according to the following criteria: (1) magnitude of hypergammaglobulinemia, (2) autoantibody expression, and (3) certainty of exclusion of other diagnoses (see Table 7.18).
- **Extrahepatic associations:** Present in 10–50% of cases.
- **Frequent:** Autoimmune thyroid disease, ulcerative colitis, synovitis.
- **Uncommon:** RA, DM, CREST syndrome, vitiligo, alopecia.

TREATMENT

- **Treatment indications:** Active symptoms, biochemical markers (↑ ALT, AST, or gamma globulin), histologic markers (periportal hepatitis, bridging necrosis). The best treatment responses are obtained in the setting of active hepatic inflammation (high ALT).
- **Relative contraindications:** Asymptomatic patients with mild biochemical inflammation (AST < 3 times normal); cirrhosis without histologic necroinflammation.
- **Prednisone monotherapy:** Give 60 mg QD; tapering schedule varies and is controversial.
- **Steroid-sparing therapy:** Lower-dose prednisone (30 mg QD); then taper over 4–6 weeks in combination with azathioprine.
- **Treatment end points:** Defined at the end of steroid taper.
- **Remission:** No symptoms; AST < 2 times normal; normalization of bilirubin and gamma globulin; biopsy with minimal inflammation.
- **Treatment failure:** Progressive symptoms; AST or bilirubin > 67% of pretreatment values.
- **Liver transplantation:** Should be considered in the presence of decompensated liver disease, severe inflammation, and necrosis on liver biopsy with treatment failure or no biochemical improvement during the first two weeks of therapy.

KEY FACT

The decision to treat autoimmune hepatitis depends on the severity of hepatic inflammation, not hepatic dysfunction.

KEY FACT

Autoimmune hepatitis is associated with a high rate of anti-HCV false ⊕s, so the diagnosis must be confirmed by checking a PCR assay for HCV viremia.

TABLE 7.18. Differential Diagnosis of Immunologic Disease of the Liver

DISEASE	GENDER	LFTS	OTHER LABS	DIAGNOSIS	ASSOCIATION	TREATMENT
Primary sclerosing cholangitis	M > F	AP > 1.5 times ULN.	p-ANCA.	ERCP or MRCP reveals "beads on a string."	Ulcerative colitis in 70%.	Liver transplant.
Primary biliary cirrhosis	F >> M	AP > 3–4 times ULN; total bilirubin ↑.	AMA (95%), IgM.	Biopsy reveals paucity of bile ducts and granulomatous cholangitis.	Autoimmune (thyroiditis, CREST, sicca in 50%).	Ursodeoxycholic acid → liver transplant.
Autoimmune hepatitis	F > M	↑ AST/ALT.	ANA, ASMA, anti-LKM antibody, ↑ IgG.	Biopsy reveals interface hepatitis and plasma cell infiltrate.		Prednisone, azathioprine.

ULN = upper limit of normal; AP = alkaline phosphatase; ASMA = anti–smooth muscle antibody; anti-LKM antibody = anti–liver/kidney microsome antibody.

DRUG-INDUCED HEPATITIS

Ranges from subclinical disease with abnormal LFTs to fulminant hepatic failure. Accounts for 40% of acute hepatitis cases in U.S. adults > 50 years of age; for 25% of cases of fulminant hepatic failure; and for 5% of jaundice cases in hospitalized patients. Drug-induced hepatitis can be characterized as intrinsic (direct toxic effect) or idiosyncratic (immunologically mediated injury) and as necroinflammatory (hepatocellular), cholestatic, or mixed. Risk factors include advanced age, female gender, use of an increasing number of prescription drugs, underlying liver disease, renal insufficiency, and poor nutrition.

SYMPTOMS/EXAM

May present with constitutional symptoms, jaundice, RUQ pain, and pruritus. Often asymptomatic.

DIFFERENTIAL

Viral hepatitis, ischemic hepatitis, Wilson's disease, α_1-antitrypsin deficiency, hemochromatosis, nonalcoholic steatohepatitis.

DIAGNOSIS

Diagnose as follows (see also Table 7.19):

- **Exclude other causes:** Obtain a liver ultrasound with duplex (to evaluate for acute hepatic vasculature thrombosis) and hepatitis serologies.
- **History:** Take a detailed drug history that includes dosage, duration, and use of concurrent OTC, alternative, and recreational drugs.
- **Labs:** ↑ serum LDH; transaminases typically range from 2–4 times normal (subclinical) to 10–100 times normal.
- **Drug withdrawal:** Most drug-induced hepatitis will improve with discontinuation of the toxic agent.
- **Liver biopsy:** Most useful for **excluding** other etiologies. Eosinophilic inflammatory infiltrate suggests drug-induced hepatitis; histologic patterns can implicate drug classes.

T A B L E 7 . 1 9 .   Characterization of Drug-Induced Hepatitis

	INTRINSIC	**IDIOSYNCRATIC**
Relation to dosage	Dose dependent.	Dose independent.
Frequency	More common.	Less common.
Onset	Hours to days after starting drug.	Weeks to months after starting drug.
Toxicity	Direct toxic effect.	Immune-mediated toxicity.
Prognosis	Good.	Poor.
Implicated drugs	Acetaminophen, carbon tetrachloride, alcohol, *Amanita phalloides,* aflatoxins.	NSAIDs, INH, sulfonamides, valproic acid, phenytoin, ketoconazole.

TREATMENT

- Discontinue the implicated drug.
- Supportive care.
- **Liver transplantation:** Drug-induced fulminant hepatic failure has a low likelihood of spontaneous recovery.

ACETAMINOPHEN TOXICITY

- The most common cause of drug-induced hepatitis and drug-induced fulminant hepatic failure. The toxic dose is > 4 g in nonalcoholics and > 2 g in alcoholics, but much higher doses are frequently associated with fulminant hepatic failure.
- **Dx:**
    - Maintain a high clinical suspicion with marked elevation of transaminases.
    - **Acetaminophen level:** Predict toxicity with the Rumack-Matthew nomogram (assesses acetaminophen concentration, time after ingestion, and risk for toxicity). ↑ levels precede transaminitis.
    - **Prognostic factors predicting death or need for liver transplant:** Arterial blood pH < 7.3 **or** hepatic encephalopathy grade 3 **or** 4 with INR > 6.5 and serum creatinine > 3.4 mg/dL.
- **Tx:**
    - N-acetylcysteine PO or IV.
    - Liver transplantation.

KEY FACT

Acetaminophen in modest doses (eg, < 2 g/day) is much safer than NSAIDs for patients with cirrhosis.

ALCOHOLIC LIVER DISEASE

Alcohol accounts for 100,000 deaths per year in the United States, and 20% of these deaths are related to alcoholic liver disease, which carries a risk of progressive liver disease. Patients at risk include those exceeding the critical intake threshold (80 g/day in men and 20 g/day in women), females, African Americans, those with poor nutritional status, and those with HBV or HCV infection. The spectrum of disease includes fatty liver (steatosis), acute alcoholic hepatitis, and alcoholic (**Laënnec's**) cirrhosis.

KEY FACT

Alcoholic hepatitis is not a prerequisite to alcoholic cirrhosis.

SYMPTOMS

- **Steatosis:** Asymptomatic or mild RUQ pain.
- **Acute alcoholic hepatitis:** Fever, anorexia, RUQ pain, jaundice, nausea, vomiting.
- **Alcoholic cirrhosis:** Patients may be asymptomatic or may present with anorexia, fatigue, and ↓ libido. Associated with an ↑ risk of variceal hemorrhage.

EXAM

- Exam may reveal hepatomegaly, splenomegaly, cachexia, jaundice, spider telangiectasias, **Dupuytren's contractures**, parotid gland enlargement, gynecomastia, and testicular atrophy.
- There are no symptoms specific to alcoholic liver disease.

DIFFERENTIAL

Nonalcoholic steatohepatitis, nonalcoholic fatty liver disease, autoimmune hepatitis, hemochromatosis, α_1-antitrypsin deficiency, Wilson's disease, viral hepatitis, toxic or drug-induced hepatitis.

KEY FACT

Discriminant function (DF) measures the severity of alcoholic hepatitis. A DF > 32 predicts one-month mortality as high as 50%. DF = [4.6 × (patient's PT − control PT)] + serum bilirubin.

DIAGNOSIS

- **History of habitual alcohol consumption:** The **CAGE questionnaire** is sensitive for alcohol abuse.
- **Alcoholic steatosis:** Modest elevation of **AST > ALT in a 2:1 ratio**; liver biopsy shows small (microvesicular) and large (macrovesicular) fat droplets in the cytoplasm of hepatocytes.
- **Alcoholic hepatitis:** Marked leukocytosis, modest elevation of AST > ALT in a 2:1 ratio, and markedly ↑ serum bilirubin. Liver biopsy shows steatosis, hepatocellular necrosis, **Mallory bodies** (eosinophilic hyaline deposits), ballooned hepatocytes, and **lobular PMN inflammatory infiltrate.**
- **Alcoholic cirrhosis:** Liver biopsy shows micro- or macronodular cirrhosis and perivenular fibrosis that is not usually seen in other types of cirrhosis.

TREATMENT

- The mainstays of treatment are alcohol abstinence and improved nutrition. Social support (eg, AA) and medical therapy (eg, disulfiram, naltrexone) can assist with abstinence.
- **Alcoholic steatosis:** Can resolve with abstinence and improved nutrition.
- **Alcoholic hepatitis:**
  - **Corticosteroids: Improve survival** when DF is > 32 **and** there are no contraindications (active GI bleeding, active infection, serum creatinine > 2.3 mg/dL). DF is a function of PT/INR and total bilirubin.
  - **Other therapies under study: Medium-chain triglycerides** and **pentoxifylline.** Pentoxifylline has anti-TNF effects but is less effective than corticosteroids when DF is > 32.
  - **Long-term therapy:** Antioxidants, S-adenosylmethionine (SAMe), silymarin, vitamins A and E.
- **Alcoholic cirrhosis:** Hepatic function can significantly improve with abstinence and improved nutrition.
- **Liver transplantation:** Often precluded by active or recent alcohol abuse or use. Recidivism rates are high. Most transplant centers require at least six months of documented abstinence prior to listing for liver transplant.

KEY FACT

Alcoholic hepatitis can be treated with corticosteroids when DF is > 32 and there are no contraindications (active GI bleeding, active infection, serum creatinine > 2.3 mg/dL).

NONALCOHOLIC FATTY LIVER DISEASE

A 37-year-old man is being evaluated for ↑ AST/ALT over one year. He has hypertension and diabetes but denies using any acetaminophen, supplements, or other medications not prescribed for his known medical conditions. On exam, his body mass index (BMI) is 32, and labs show his ALT/AST at 200% of the upper limit of normal. Workup for hepatitis is ⊝, including serologies for hepatitis A, B, and C as well ANA, AMA, ceruloplasmin, ferritin, and transferrin. An ultrasound shows a diffusely hyperechoic liver with patent vessels. What interventions are likely to improve his symptoms?

Weight loss and good control of BP and diabetes. This man likely has nonalcoholic fatty liver disease given his metabolic profile and overall ⊝ workup. There is no established treatment for this condition aside from improving predisposing conditions such as weight, hypertension, triglyceridemia, and diabetes.

The spectrum of disease ranges from benign steatosis (fatty liver) to steatohepatitis (hepatic inflammation). Prevalence in the United States is 15–25%. Steatohepatitis is found in 8–20% of morbidly obese individuals independent of age. Disease is generally benign and indolent but can progress to cirrhosis in 15–20% of cases. Risk factors for severe disease include female gender, age > 45 years, BMI > 30, AST/ALT > 1, and type 2 DM.

SYMPTOMS

Presents with fatigue, malaise, and, to a lesser extent, RUQ fullness or pain. Asymptomatic in > 50% of patients.

EXAM

- Hepatomegaly is common, but examination may be limited in the obese.
- Stigmata of chronic liver disease.

DIFFERENTIAL

- Alcoholic liver disease.
- **Nutrition:** TPN, kwashiorkor, rapid weight loss.
- **Drugs:** Estrogens, corticosteroids, chloroquine.
- **Metabolic:** Wilson's disease, abetalipoproteinemia.
- **Iatrogenic:** Weight reduction surgery with jejunoileal bypass, gastroplasty, or small bowel resection.

DIAGNOSIS

- Exclude causes of liver disease, specifically alcoholic liver disease.
- **Aminotransaminases:**
  - Typically **ALT > AST (× 2–4) (vs. alcoholic liver disease, in which AST > ALT)**; poor correlation with the presence and extent of inflammation. **A normal AST and ALT cannot exclude nonalcoholic fatty liver disease.**
  - **The AST/ALT ratio ↑ with severity of liver disease,** which is typical of cirrhosis of all etiologies.
- BMI is an independent predictor of the degree of hepatocellular fatty infiltration.
- Ultrasound, CT scan, or MRI.
- Liver biopsy is the gold standard. The grade of inflammation and stage of fibrosis predict disease course and response to therapeutic intervention.

TREATMENT

- Gradual weight loss. Rapid weight loss may ↑ inflammation and fibrosis.
- Treat hyperlipidemia and diabetes.
- No FDA-approved therapy is available.
- Vitamin E and pioglitazone have shown benefit in histologically proven disease with reduction in hepatic steatosis and inflammation. Pioglitazone is associated with weight gain.

Metabolic Liver Disease

HEREDITARY HEMOCHROMATOSIS

An **autosomal recessive** disease. Homozygote prevalence is 1 in 300 persons. The most common genetic disease in Northern Europeans; the Caucasian carrier rate is 1 in 10. Associated with a major mutation in chromosome 6, the **HFE gene.** Patients have a normal life expectancy if there is no cirrhosis and the patient is adherent to treatment; survival is lower if the patient has **cirrhosis at the time of diagnosis.** Cirrhosis with hereditary hemochromatosis

KEY FACT

Nonalcoholic fatty liver disease can occur in the absence of obesity.

KEY FACT

Nonalcoholic fatty liver disease is the third most common cause of abnormal LFTs in adult outpatients after medication and alcohol.

KEY FACT

Normal LFTs do not exclude nonalcoholic fatty liver disease.

carries a high risk of hepatocellular carcinoma (200 times that of the control population).

SYMPTOMS

Arthritis (pseudogout), skin color change, RUQ pain, symptoms of chronic liver disease (fatigue, anorexia, muscle wasting), loss of libido, impotence and dysmenorrhea, heart failure, DM. Often asymptomatic (10–25%).

EXAM

Hepatomegaly, skin hyperpigmentation (bronze skin), stigmata of chronic liver disease, hypogonadism.

DIFFERENTIAL

- **Chronic liver diseases:** HBV, HCV, alcoholic liver disease, nonalcoholic fatty liver disease, Wilson's disease, α_1-antitrypsin deficiency, autoimmune hepatitis.
- **2° iron overload diseases:** Homozygous α-thalassemia; multiple previous blood transfusions.

DIAGNOSIS

- Suspect hereditary hemochromatosis with an unexplained **high serum ferritin or iron saturation even with normal LFTs.**
- **Fasting serum TS and ferritin:** If TS is > 45% and ferritin is ↑, hereditary hemochromatosis is suggested; check HFE genotype. A TS of < 45% and normal ferritin exclude hereditary hemochromatosis.
- **HFE genotyping:** Homozygote is diagnostic **only if** (1) the patient is < 40 years of age, (2) serum ferritin level is < 1000 µg/L, and (3) transaminases are normal. Otherwise, confirmation with liver biopsy is necessary.
- **Liver biopsy:** The best means of making a definitive diagnosis; a hepatic Prussian blue stain with **iron index of > 1.9** is diagnostic. Also used for disease staging (influences prognosis; hepatocellular carcinoma screening is needed if the patient is cirrhotic).

TREATMENT

- Alcohol abstinence.
- Avoid high-dose vitamin C.
- **Phlebotomy:** Weekly or biweekly until serum ferritin is < 50 ng/mL; then 3–4 times per year indefinitely.
- Screen first-degree family members.
- In the setting of cirrhosis, screen for hepatocellular carcinoma.
- Liver transplantation is appropriate for decompensated liver disease.

COMPLICATIONS

DM, restrictive cardiomyopathy, joint disease (chondrocalcinosis, degenerative arthritis, pseudogout), hepatocellular carcinoma, ↑ incidence of bacterial infections (especially *Vibrio*, *Yersinia*, and *Listeria* spp).

α_1-ANTITRYPSIN DEFICIENCY

α_1-antitrypsin protects tissues from protease-related degradation. The deficiency is encoded on chromosome 14 and has an **autosomal codominant** transmission. The Z allele is the most common deficiency, particularly in those of Northern European descent. α_1-antitrypsin deficiency is severe when homozygous (eg, PiZZ) and is intermediate when heterozygous (eg, PiMZ).

Liver disease can be seen in the neonatal period. The incidence of liver disease at ages 20, 50, and > 50 is 2%, 5%, and 15%, respectively, with males affected more often than females. There is a high incidence of HCC in those with cirrhosis. A high prevalence of HBV and HCV markers suggests synergistic liver injury.

SYMPTOMS/EXAM

- Neonatal cholestasis, occult cirrhosis, shortness of breath/dyspnea on exertion, panniculitis.
- Exam reveals signs of cirrhosis (spider angiomata, palmar erythema, gynecomastia) and emphysema (clubbing, barrel chest).

DIFFERENTIAL

- **Other metabolic liver diseases with childhood presentation:** Hereditary tyrosinemia, Gaucher's disease, glycogen storage disease, CF.
- **Chronic liver diseases:** HBV, HCV, hemochromatosis, Wilson's disease, autoimmune hepatitis, nonalcoholic fatty liver disease, alcohol.

DIAGNOSIS

- **Extrahepatic manifestations:** Basilar and panacinar emphysema, pancreatic fibrosis, panniculitis.
- **Serum α_1-antitrypsin concentration:** For screening; α_1-antitrypsin is an acute-phase reactant. False-$\oplus$ tests may be obtained with inflammation (even in PiZZ).
- **Serum α_1-antitrypsin phenotyping:** The screening and diagnostic test of choice.
- **Liver biopsy:** Characteristic eosinophilic α_1-antitrypsin globules are seen in the endoplasmic reticulum of periportal hepatocytes.

TREATMENT

- Avoid cigarette smoking and alcohol; weight loss if the patient is obese.
- Liver transplantation.

WILSON'S DISEASE

An 18-year-old woman with recent-onset depression and "bizarre" behavior (as described by her family) presents to the ER in an altered state. She is noted to have normal vital signs, but her labs reveal a low hematocrit, an ↑ total bilirubin level (with an ↑ unconjugated fraction), and an AST/ALT ratio five times the upper limit of normal. A toxicology screen is normal, and a blood smear shows active hemolysis. What tests would help make the diagnosis?

Ceruloplasmin, urinary copper excretion, a slit-lamp exam, and liver biopsy. This patient has many features of Wilson's disease, including hemolytic anemia, new psychiatric changes, and ↑ LFTs. Although there is no highly sensitive and specific test for Wilson's disease, the aforementioned tests can be useful in a setting where suspicion is high. If there are no neurologic symptoms, the slit-lamp exam may not be as useful.

An uncommon **autosomal recessive** disease. Usually presents between ages 3 and 40; associated with mutations in the WD gene on chromosome 13. ↓ biliary copper excretion results in toxic copper deposition in tissues.

MNEMONIC

Characteristics of Wilson's disease—

ABCD

Asterixis
Basal ganglia deterioration
Ceruloplasmin ↓
Cirrhosis
Copper ↑
Carcinoma (hepatocellular)
Choreiform movements
Dementia

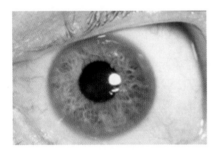

FIGURE 7.17. Kayser-Fleischer ring. (Reproduced with permission from USMLERx. com.)

SYMPTOMS

- Presents with abnormal behavior, personality change, psychosis, tremor, dyskinesia, arthropathy (pseudogout), and jaundice.
- **Clinical presentation:** Can be acute, subacute, or chronic.
- **Organ involvement** (in descending order of frequency): Hepatic, neurologic, psychiatric, hematologic, renal (Fanconi's syndrome), other (ophthalmologic, cardiac, skeletal, endocrinologic, dermatologic).
- The mean age at onset of hepatic symptoms is 8–12 years.

EXAM

- Exam reveals Kayser-Fleischer rings (see Figure 7.17), icterus, slowed mentation, hypophonia, and tremor.
- Clinical stigmata of cirrhosis are associated with **chronic** disease.

DIFFERENTIAL

- **Infiltrative diseases:** Hemochromatosis.
- **Chronic liver diseases:** HBV, HCV, hemochromatosis, α_1-antitrypsin deficiency, autoimmune hepatitis.
- **Copper overload diseases:** Hereditary aceruloplasminemia, idiopathic copper toxicosis, Indian childhood cirrhosis.

DIAGNOSIS

- Suspect Wilson's disease in patients **3–40 years of age** with unexplained LFTs or liver disease associated with **neurologic or psychiatric changes, Kayser-Fleischer rings, hemolytic anemia,** and a ⊕ family history.
- **Liver biochemistry tests:** Show characteristically low alkaline phosphatase, marked hyperbilirubinemia, and modest aminotransaminase elevations (AST > ALT).
- **Ceruloplasmin (CP):** Typically **low in Wilson's disease,** but a low CP is both insensitive (15% of cases have normal CP, since CP is an acute-phase reactant) and nonspecific (CP is also low in nephrotic syndrome, protein-losing enteropathy, and malabsorption).
- **Urinary copper excretion: High** if symptomatic (100–1000 µg/24 hrs; level may indicate disease severity). Normal excretion is < 40 µg/24 hrs.
- **Liver biopsy:** Shows high hepatic copper concentration (> 250 µg/g); may also be seen in primary biliary cirrhosis, primary sclerosing cholangitis, fibrosis, or cirrhosis.
- **Other:** Serum copper concentration, slit-lamp exam.

TREATMENT

- D-**penicillamine:** Improvement lags 6–12 months following treatment; maintenance is typically required.
- **Other:** Trientine, zinc, ammonium.
- **Liver transplantation:** For acute hepatic or medically refractory Wilson's disease; reverses metabolic defect and induces copper excretion.

Advanced Liver Disease

CIRRHOSIS

The final common pathway of many liver diseases that cause hepatocellular injury and lead to fibrosis and nodular regeneration. Reversal may occur with treatment of some chronic liver diseases (eg, HBV, HCV).

SYMPTOMS

- Fatigue, anorexia, muscle wasting, loss of libido, impotence, dysmenorrhea.
- Decompensation associated with GI bleeding, encephalopathy (sleep-wake reversal, ↓ concentration), ascites.
- **Platypnea** (dyspnea induced by sitting upright and relieved by recumbency) and **orthodeoxia** (low PaO_2 when sitting upright that is relieved by recumbency).

EXAM

- **Stigmata of chronic liver disease:** Palmar erythema, spider telangiectasia (see Figure 7.18).
- **Dupuytren's contractures,** gynecomastia, testicular atrophy, bilateral parotid enlargement, **Terry's nails** (white, obscure nails).
- **Portal hypertension: Caput medusae,** splenomegaly, ascites.
- **Hepatic encephalopathy: Fetor hepaticus,** asterixis, confusion.

DIFFERENTIAL

- HCV, HBV, alcohol.
- Hemochromatosis.
- Primary sclerosing cholangitis, primary biliary cirrhosis, Wilson's disease, α_1-antitrypsin deficiency, cryptogenic liver disease, nonalcoholic steatohepatitis, autoimmune hepatitis, vascular disease (Budd-Chiari syndrome, veno-occlusive disease, right heart failure).
- Drug toxicity (methotrexate, amiodarone, nitrofurantoin), other (sarcoidosis, schistosomiasis, hypervitaminosis A, CF, glycogen storage disease).

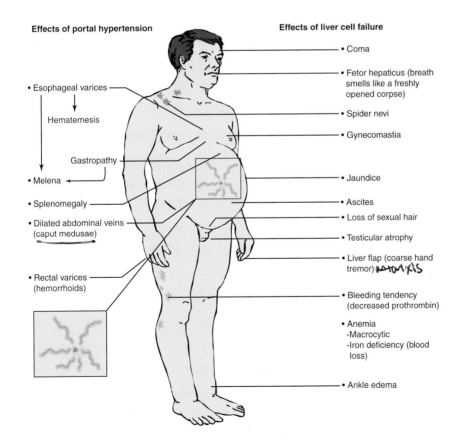

FIGURE 7.18. Clinical effects of cirrhosis. (Modified with permission from Chandrasoma P, Taylor CE. *Concise Pathology*, 3rd ed. Originally published by Appleton & Lange. Copyright © 1998 by The McGraw-Hill Companies, Inc.)

TABLE 7.20. Child-Turcotte-Pugh Scoring

	1 POINT	2 POINTS	3 POINTS
Ascites	Absent	Nontense	Tense
Encephalopathy	Absent	Grades 1–2	Grades 3–4
Bilirubin (mg/dL)	< 2.0	2–3	> 3.0
Albumin (mg/dL)	> 3.5	2.8–3.5	< 2.8
PT (seconds over normal)	1–3	4–6	> 6

KEY FACT

The Model for End-Stage Liver Disease (MELD) score is more accurate than the Child-Turcotte-Pugh score at predicting mortality with cirrhosis. MELD is based on three serum laboratory tests: INR, total bilirubin, and creatinine.

KEY FACT

Vaccination for HAV and HBV is indicated for all nonimmune patients with chronic liver disease, including cirrhotics.

DIAGNOSIS

Diagnose as follows (see also Tables 7.20 and 7.21):

- **Liver biopsy:** The gold standard; can be useful in assessing etiology.
- **Physical exam.**
- **Labs:** Thrombocytopenia (splenic sequestration); ↑ INR and low albumin (↓ hepatic synthetic function); ↑ alkaline phosphatase, serum bilirubin, and GGT (cholestasis); normal or ↑ transaminases.
- **Imaging:** Ultrasound with duplex (ascites, biliary dilation, hepatic masses, vascular patency), CT (more specific than ultrasound for cirrhosis and masses, portal hypertension), MRI (excellent specificity for hepatic masses; see Figure 7.19).

TREATMENT

- Avoid alcohol, iron supplements (except in iron deficiency), NSAIDs, and benzodiazepines; minimize narcotics; limit acetaminophen to < 2 g/day.
- Fluid restriction is unimportant (unless serum Na is < 125), and protein restriction should not be recommended.
- Administer pneumococcal and influenza vaccines.
- Prophylactic measures are as follows:
  - **1° prophylaxis:** HAV and HBV vaccination; nonselective β-blockers for documented esophageal varices.
  - **2° prophylaxis:** Antibiotics for spontaneous bacterial peritonitis (SBP); esophageal variceal banding or nonselective β-blockers +/– long-acting nitrates. Patients typically show low adherence/tolerance to β-blockers/nitrates.
- Treat underlying disease.
- Consider screening for hepatocellular carcinoma with ultrasound and serum AFP every six months.
- Treat complications (see below).

TABLE 7.21. Child-Turcotte-Pugh Classification

CTP SCORE	CHILD-PUGH CLASS	THREE-YEAR SURVIVAL (%)
5–6	A	> 90
7–9	B	50–60
10–15	C	30

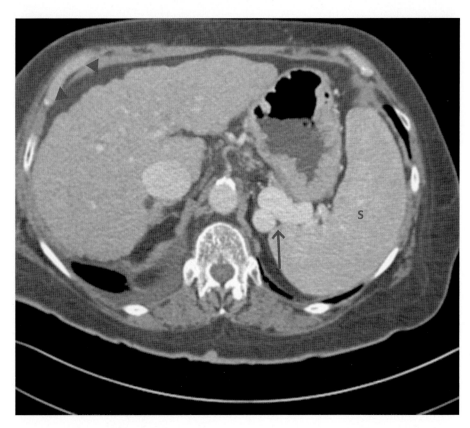

FIGURE 7.19. **Cirrhosis.** Transaxial image from contrast-enhanced CT shows a nodular liver contour (arrowheads) and the stigmata of portal hypertension, including splenomegaly (S) and perisplenic varices (arrow). (Reproduced with permission from USMLERx.com.)

- **Liver transplantation:** Refer to a transplant center when there is clinical evidence of decompensated liver disease (portal hypertensive bleeding, hepatic encephalopathy, ascites), evidence of hepatocellular carcinoma, a Child-Turcotte-Pugh score of > 6, or a MELD score of > 15.

COMPLICATIONS

Hepatic encephalopathy, varices, ascites/SBP, hepatorenal syndrome, hepatopulmonary syndrome, hepatocellular carcinoma; portopulmonary syndrome.

VARICES

- Esophageal variceal hemorrhage (EVH) accounts for one-third of all deaths in cirrhotics. **Mortality with each EVH episode is 30–50%.** Alcoholic cirrhotics are at highest risk.
- **Tx:**
  - **Acute variceal hemorrhage:** Large-bore IVs, resuscitation (goal hematocrit of 28%, platelets > 50, INR < 1.6), octreotide drip, empiric antibiotics, PPI, and early endoscopy. A hematocrit greater than 30% is associated with ↑ portal pressures.
  - **Esophageal variceal bleeding prophylaxis:**
    - 1°: Nonselective β-blockers (nadolol, propranolol).
    - 2°: Endoscopic ablation (banding or sclerotherapy); nonselective β-blockers +/– long-acting nitrates; portocaval shunt (TIPS or surgical).

- Gastric and rectal varices are not treatable endoscopically.
- **Portal hypertensive gastropathy:** A common source of bleeding. Treat with portocaval shunt (TIPS or surgical) or liver transplantation.

ASCITES AND SPONTANEOUS BACTERIAL PERITONITIS (SBP)

In the United States, > 80% of ascites cases are due to chronic liver disease (cirrhosis or alcoholic hepatitis). Some **10–30% of cirrhotics with ascites develop SBP every year.** Infection-related mortality is 10%, but the **overall in-hospital mortality rate is 30%.**

SYMPTOMS/EXAM

Characterized by shifting dullness, fluid wave, and bulging flanks (low sensitivity, moderate specificity). Imaging (ultrasound, CT) is superior to examination. **SBP is often asymptomatic,** but patients may have fever, abdominal pain, and sepsis.

DIFFERENTIAL

The serum-ascites albumin gradient (SAAG) is helpful (see Table 7.22).

DIAGNOSIS

- **Diagnostic paracentesis:** Indicated in the presence of new-onset ascites, ascites present at hospital admission, and ascites with symptoms or signs of infection.
- **Analysis:**
  - **Routine:** Cell count, culture, albumin, total protein.
  - **Optional:** Glucose, LDH, amylase, Gram stain, cytology.
  - **Not useful:** pH, lactate.
- **SBP diagnosis:** Ascites PMN > 250 cells/mL or a single organism on culture. **The presence of multiple organisms on ascites culture suggests 2° peritonitis.**

TREATMENT

- **Ascites:**
  - Dietary sodium restriction (< 2 g/day); furosemide and spironolactone (give doses in a 4:10 ratio—eg, 40 mg to 100 mg, 80 mg to 200 mg). Initiate fluid restriction only if serum Na < 125 mEq/dL.
  - Large-volume paracentesis, portocaval shunt (TIPS), liver transplantation.

KEY FACT

A SAAG ≥ 1.1 g/dL is 96% accurate in detecting portal hypertension.

KEY FACT

For SBP treatment, the addition of IV albumin to IV antibiotics significantly ↓ renal impairment and mortality.

KEY FACT

Ninety percent of cirrhotics presenting with ascites will respond to sodium restriction of < 2 g/day along with furosemide with spironolactone (at maximum doses of 160 mg and 400 mg, respectively).

TABLE 7.22.   Significance of SAAG Values

HIGH SAAG (≥ 1.1)	LOW SAAG (< 1.1)
Cirrhosis, hepatocellular carcinoma	Peritoneal carcinomatosis
Alcoholic hepatitis	Peritoneal TB, SBP
Heart failure	Nephrotic syndrome
Vascular (Budd-Chiari, portal vein thrombosis)	Bowel infarction
	Serositis
Myxedema	
Fulminant hepatitis	

- **SBP prophylaxis:** Fluoroquinolone or TMP-SMX. Indicated for cirrhotics hospitalized with GI bleed (three days), ascites with total protein < 1.5 g/dL (while hospitalized), or prior SBP (if the patient has ascites).
- **SBP treatment: Do not wait for culture results to begin treatment.** Give cefotaxime or ceftriaxone IV × 5 days and **IV albumin.**

HEPATIC ENCEPHALOPATHY

Neuropsychiatric changes in the setting of liver disease constitute hepatic encephalopathy until proven otherwise. Look for precipitating factors, including infection, GI bleeding, dehydration, hypokalemia, constipation/ileus, hepatocellular carcinoma, dietary protein overload, CNS-active drugs (narcotics, benzodiazepines, anticholinergics), uremia, hypoxia, hypoglycemia, and noncompliance with hepatic encephalopathy treatment.

SYMPTOMS/EXAM

Insomnia, sleep-wake reversal, personality change, confusion.

DIAGNOSIS

Diagnosis is clinical. **Blood ammonia levels are rarely helpful.**

TREATMENT

- Correct precipitating factors and anticipate treatment-related adverse effects.
- Oral/NG tube or rectally administered lactulose (adverse effects include dehydration and hypokalemia). For patients intolerant of or refractory to lactulose, add rifaximin.
- Zinc, short-term protein restriction, branched-chain amino acid–enriched diet.

HEPATORENAL SYNDROME

A 43-year-old man with HCV cirrhosis presents with malaise and fatigue. He is noted to have a distended abdomen with a total bilirubin of 3.5 mg/dL, an INR of 1.8, and an ↑ creatinine of 2.2 mg/dL. His ascites is tapped and does not show evidence of infection. His urine sodium level is < 10 mEq/L, and a small IV albumin challenge does not improve his creatinine level. What should be the next step for this patient?

Urgent referral to a liver transplant center. This patient is showing decompensated liver disease with evidence of hepatorenal syndrome as well. Given that his mortality within the next two weeks is quite high, referral to a transplant center would be appropriate, as his hepatorenal syndrome is unlikely to improve without transplantation.

The prognosis is grave; **median survival is 10–14 days.** Two-month mortality is 90%.

DIFFERENTIAL

Prerenal azotemia, acute tubular necrosis, drug-induced disorders (NSAIDs, antibiotics, radiographic contrast, diuretics), glomerulonephritis, vasculitis.

DIAGNOSIS

Exclude other cause of renal failure. Discontinue diuretics and then perform a plasma volume expansion trial with 1.5 L IV normal saline or 5% IV albumin. If serum creatinine ↓, suspect another diagnosis.

TREATMENT

Identify and treat precipitants. Restrict sodium to < 2 g/day if serum sodium is < 125 mEq/L; then restrict fluids to < 1.5 L/day. Treat infection; liver transplantation is often required. **Renal failure from hepatorenal syndrome reverses with liver transplantation.**

LIVER TRANSPLANTATION

Liver transplantation is a standard operation with excellent survival rates (80–90% at one year and 60–80% at seven years). The scarcity of available cadaveric donor livers is reflected in the high mortality rates (up to 20% per year) in those awaiting liver transplantation. Typical waiting times are **eight months to three years.** Living-donor liver transplants constitute a promising alternative but comprise < 5% of all liver transplants.

THE PROCESS

- Determine the presence of other viruses (HAV, HCV, mononucleosis/ EBV, CMV, HSV).
- Refer to a transplant center (often the rate-limiting step).
- There are no minimal listing criteria, yet an indication for transplant should be identified.
- Assess indications and contraindications (see below).
- Perform a psychosocial and financial evaluation.
- Present to a selection committee, where a decision is made on whether to place patient on wait list.
- Priority is determined by the MELD score, a function of INR, total bilirubin, and serum creatinine; the higher the score, the higher the priority. For hepatocarcinoma, a MELD score is assigned independent of the calculated MELD score.

INDICATIONS

- **Acute hepatic failure:** Acetaminophen overdose, idiosyncratic drug injury, toxins (*Amanita phalloides* ingestion), HAV, HBV flare, acute Budd-Chiari syndrome, Wilson's disease, acute fatty liver of pregnancy, others. As high as 17% have an indeterminate (nonidentifiable) cause.
- **Cirrhosis with decompensation** (in descending order): HCV, EtOH, cryptogenic, primary biliary cirrhosis, primary sclerosing cholangitis, HBV, autoimmune hepatitis.
- **Hepatocellular carcinoma:** Not exceeding stage 2 (≤ 3 lesions ≤ 3 cm in size or one lesion ≤ 5 cm with no extrahepatic metastasis). Liver biopsy is not required if two radiographic studies are supportive of the diagnosis.
- **Metabolic liver disease:** Hemochromatosis, α_1-antitrypsin deficiency, Wilson's disease, tyrosinemia, glycogen storage diseases.
- **Extrahepatic metabolic disease:** Urea cycle enzyme deficiency, hyperoxaluria.

KEY FACT

Liver graft allocation in the United States is a "sickest-first" system that is based on the MELD score (serum creatinine, total bilirubin, INR).

CONTRAINDICATIONS

- Compensated cirrhosis without complications (too early).
- Extrahepatic malignancy (excluding skin cancers).
- Hepatocellular carcinoma exceeding stage 2 (see above).
- Active substance abuse and alcohol abuse (generally defined as occurring within the last six months); some centers include active smoking.
- Active untreated sepsis.
- Advanced untreatable cardiopulmonary disease.
- Uncontrolled psychiatric disease.

COMPLICATIONS

- **Operative:** Biliary complications (25%), wound infections, death.
- **Immunosuppression:** Opportunistic infections (CMV, HSV, fungal, PCP, others), drug-related effects (hypertension, renal insufficiency, DM, cytopenias, tremor, headaches, nausea/vomiting, seizures, others), malignancies (lymphoma, others).
- **Recurrent disease** (in descending order): HCV (> 99% if viremic at transplantation), **alcoholism**, HBV, primary sclerosing cholangitis, primary biliary cirrhosis, autoimmune hepatitis.
- **Acute rejection:** Occurs in up to 30% within the first three months after transplant; usually treatable, and rarely results in graft loss.

KEY FACT

As many as 17% of patients with acute liver failure will have **no identifiable cause.**

NOTES

CHAPTER 8

Geriatrics

Christina A. Lee, MD
Stephanie Rennke, MD

Nutritional Recommendations

Nutritional guidelines for the elderly are similar to those for the general population. They include the following:

- Reduction of dietary fats.
- ↑ consumption of fruits, vegetables, and whole grains/fiber.

Patients > 75 years of age who are on restricted diets are at risk of protein-calorie malnutrition and inadequate intake of folate, vitamin B_{12}, calcium, and vitamin D.

VITAMIN D

- Older individuals are at higher risk for vitamin D deficiency because of:
  - ↓ ability of the skin to produce vitamin D.
  - ↓ sun exposure.
  - ↓ synthesis of 1,25-vitamin D due to a higher prevalence of renal dysfunction.
  - ↓ vitamin D intake.
- Vitamin D improves bone mineral density and may ↓ fracture risk by improving muscle function, thereby decreasing the risk of falls.
- Older adults should probably take 800–1000 IU daily to maintain adequate vitamin D levels. Treat vitamin D deficiency (< 20 ng/mL) with high-dose PO ergocalciferol.

VITAMIN E

There is no evidence that vitamin E is effective in cancer prevention, in the treatment of CAD, or in delaying the progression of dementia. **High-dose vitamin E (> 400 IU/day) may ↑ all-cause mortality.**

Weight Loss

Unintended weight loss is **not a normal part of aging.** Although the cause cannot be identified in 25% of cases, known etiologic factors include the following (see also the mnemonic **DETERMINE**):

- **Medical:** Chronic heart disease, chronic lung disease, dementia, poor dentition, changes in taste or smell, dysphagia, mesenteric ischemia, cancer, diabetes, hyper- or hypothyroidism.
- **Psychosocial:** Alcoholism, depression, social isolation, limited funds, difficulty shopping for or preparing food, need for assistance with feeding.
- **Pharmacologic:** NSAIDs, antiepileptics, digoxin, SSRIs.

DIAGNOSIS/TREATMENT

- Identify treatable medical, psychological, and social causes.
- Consider age-appropriate (and life expectancy–appropriate) cancer screening (eg, prostate, colon, breast).
- Discontinue any offending drugs.
- Appetite stimulants and dietary supplements may ↑ weight but do not improve mortality.
- Tube feeding has complications (aspiration, pneumonia, pain) and does **not** improve mortality in patients with dementia.

MNEMONIC

Causes of unintentional weight loss—

DETERMINE

Disease
Eating poorly
Tooth loss/mouth pain
Economic hardship
Reduced social contact
Multiple medicines
Involuntary weight loss/gain
Need for assistance in self-care
Elder years (> 85 years of age)

KEY FACT

Loss of lean body mass and ↑ % body fat are normal age-related changes; unintentional weight loss is not.

Complications

Associated with high morbidity within two years of onset, including falls, isolation, skin breakdown, and nursing home placement.

Immunizations

 A 69-year-old man with hypertension and osteoarthritis presents to his primary care physician for a routine office visit. His daughter would like to discuss vaccinations. What are your recommendations?

The CDC recommends that adults > 65 years of age receive the following vaccinations: influenza (yearly), pneumococcal polysaccharide (once), Td booster (every 10 years), varicella when the patient has no evidence of immunity by laboratory studies or history of varicella or zoster (two vaccinations during one's lifetime), and herpes zoster. MMR, hepatitis A, hepatitis B, and meningococcal vaccinations may be considered under certain circumstances (eg, for health care workers, outbreaks, travel, or chronic diseases). Immunocompromised patients should not receive live vaccines.

See the Ambulatory Medicine chapter for vaccination guidelines. In the elderly, give special consideration to the following:

- **Influenza vaccine:** Efficacy declines with age, but vaccination is still important in this high-risk group. Should be done yearly.
- **Pneumococcal vaccine:** ↓ the risk of pneumococcal **bacteremia** but has no significant effect on outpatient pneumonia or hospitalizations for pneumonia. Use if the patient is unvaccinated or if the patient's previous vaccination history is unknown. Administer a one-time revaccination five years or more after the first dose to patients ≥ 65 years of age if the first dose was given prior to age 65.
- **Tetanus vaccine:** Clinical tetanus is rare in the United States but commonly occurs in unvaccinated or underimmunized elderly patients or in those who have ulcers. Patients ≥ 65 years of age should receive a Td booster every 10 years.

Prophylaxis

ASPIRIN (ASA)

ASA prophylaxis is recommended for patients with a life expectancy of > 5 years, but its use must be weighed against the risk of GI and intracranial bleeding.

Cancer Screening

CERVICAL CANCER

- Most cervical cancer in the elderly results from inadequate screening at younger ages.
- Stop routine screening at age 65 in women who have had adequate recent screening with Pap smears and are not otherwise at high risk for cervical cancer (per the United States Preventive Services Task Force [USPSTF]).
- There is no evidence to support continued screening following total hysterectomy for benign disease.

BREAST CANCER

The USPSTF recommends stopping breast cancer screening after age 74, although older women may still benefit if they do not have significant comorbid disease.

COLON CANCER

- The incidence of colorectal cancer approximately doubles each decade from age 40 to 80.
- Unless there is a personal history of colorectal carcinoma or the patient has a particularly long life expectancy, it is reasonable to discontinue screening between ages 75 and 80.

PROSTATE CANCER

- There is insufficient evidence that prostate cancer screening at any age ↓ morbidity or mortality from prostate cancer.
- If a physician and a patient have decided to proceed with screening, it is reasonable to stop once that patient has less than a 10-year life expectancy.

Sensory Impairment

VISION LOSS IN THE ELDERLY

- Vision screening should be conducted by Snellen chart even on asymptomatic elderly patients.
- Arcus senilis (see Figure 8.1), defined as loss of pigment in the periphery of the iris, is a common nonpathologic finding in the elderly and does not interfere with vision.
- Common causes of vision loss in the elderly include age-related macular degeneration, glaucoma, cataracts, and diabetic retinopathy (see the section on chronic vision loss in the Ambulatory Medicine chapter).

KEY FACT

Stop screening for cervical cancer at age 65 or older if your patient has had normal recent Pap smears. Consider stopping breast and colon cancer screening if a patient has less than a 10-year life expectancy due to other comorbidities.

KEY FACT

Age-related macular degeneration, the most common cause of permanent vision loss in the elderly, is characterized by central vision loss and retinal drusen (yellow spots on the macula).

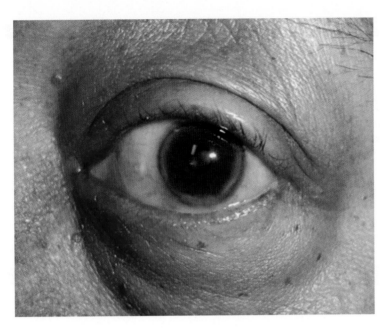

FIGURE 8.1. **Arcus senilis.** Note the opaque ring in the corneal margin. (Reproduced with permission from USMLERx.com.)

HEARING LOSS IN THE ELDERLY

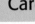 The prevalence of uncorrected hearing loss in the elderly is roughly 25%. Screening for hearing impairment should be conducted with otoscopic and audiometric testing for those who exhibit deficits.

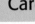 **Presbycusis,** a form of sensorineural hearing loss that is most often associated with aging, is felt to be due to loss of hair cells in the cochlea and neurons in CN VIII, leading to a **high-frequency, bilateral, symmetric** hearing loss.

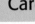 For further detail, refer to the discussion of hearing loss in the Ambulatory Medicine chapter.

 KEY FACT

Consider sensory impairment in the differential diagnosis of elderly patients with falls, depression, or increasing social isolation.

Cardiovascular Medicine

HYPERTENSION

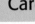 Patients between 60 and 80 years of age should be screened and treated for both systolic and diastolic hypertension.

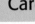 The Joint National Committee on Prevention, Detection, Evaluation, and Treatment of High Blood Pressure (JNC 7) recommends an upper limit of 140 mm Hg for systolic BP in the elderly. A target BP of < 140/90 mm Hg (< 130/80 mm Hg with hypertension and DM or renal disease) is associated with a ↓ in cardiovascular complications.

 KEY FACT

In patients > 85 years of age with multiple comorbidities, hypertension should be treated with caution to prevent orthostatic hypotension, which can contribute to falls.

HYPERLIPIDEMIA

- The USPSTF recommends continued screening according to life expectancy and overall risk factors.
- Evidence supports the treatment of hyperlipidemia in elderly patients for 2° prevention of cardiovascular outcomes. The goal for patients with CAD is an LDL of < 100 mg/dL.
- More controversial is the treatment of elders for the 1° prevention of cardiovascular disease.
- Dietary counseling should be based on the patient's overall nutritional status as well as the risk of malnutrition.
- Treatment is similar to that in younger patients. Statins are normally well tolerated. However, the side effect of rhabdomyolysis is more common in the elderly, most likely because of drug-drug interactions.

ATRIAL FIBRILLATION (AF)

- The incidence of AF ↑ with age and doubles with each decade over age 55.
- Age alone is not a risk factor for ↑ bleeding events on warfarin. However, older people tend to have more variability in their INR as a result of metabolic changes and the effects of polypharmacy.
- A meta-analysis showed that cost-effectiveness and improved quality of life resulted from the anticoagulation of older patients with AF plus stroke risk factors (eg, a history of CVA, hypertension, or DM).

Urinary Incontinence

 A 76-year-old woman presents to her primary care physician with worsening urinary incontinence over the past year. She experiences leakage of urine with coughing and laughing. She also has sudden onset of the urge to urinate and does not always make it to the bathroom in time. What is the most likely etiology of her incontinence?

Mixed stress and urge incontinence, the most common type of urinary incontinence in older women. Start with lifestyle modifications—eg, weight loss and avoidance of caffeinated products, pelvic muscle exercises (Kegel exercises), and treatment of exacerbating conditions such as cough and constipation. Antimuscarinics (eg, oxybutynin, trospium) should be used with caution in light of their anticholinergic side effects and may take several weeks to take effect.

A complaint of involuntary leakage of urine can result in physical, functional, and psychological morbidity as well as ↓ quality of life.

- Consider factors **outside the lower urinary tract,** including medical conditions, medications, and functional etiologies.
- **Lower urinary tract** causes include detrusor overactivity, impairment of urethral sphincter mechanisms, an underactive detrusor, and bladder outlet obstruction.
- Although a history, a physical exam, and a UA are often sufficient to provide a working diagnosis, a minority of patients require referral or specialized testing.

- See Table 8.1 and the mnemonic **DIAPPERS** for an overview of urinary incontinence.
- Bladder catheters may be considered in patients with incontinence but are associated with a high risk of infection. There are four indications for catheter placement:
  1. Inability to void. Usually due to outlet obstruction (eg, BPH), neurogenic bladder with retention, or medications.
  2. Incontinence **and** the following:
     - Open wounds needing protection (pressure ulcers).
     - Critical illness requiring close monitoring.
     - Palliative care and patient preference.
  3. After anesthesia (short term only).
  4. Severe cases of gross hematuria or pyuria with concerns for obstruction, monitoring, and/or irrigation.
- Incontinence alone is **not** an indication for catheter placement.

KEY FACT

Many of the medications used for urge incontinence/detrusor hyperactivity will actually worsen overflow incontinence as a result of their anticholinergic side effects. Make sure the cause of incontinence is correctly identified!

KEY FACT

Urinary incontinence alone is not an indication for catheter placement.

TABLE 8.1. Overview of Urinary Incontinence

Type of Incontinence	Mechanism	Characteristics	Treatment Options
Urge	Uninhibited bladder contraction/detrusor overactivity.	Most common in the elderly. Abrupt urgency with moderate to large leakage. Elevated postvoid residuals without outlet obstruction.	Behavioral therapy (frequent voiding, biofeedback). Goals include frequent voluntary voiding and training of CNS and pelvic mechanisms to inhibit detrusor contractions. If unsuccessful, add a bladder suppressant (eg, oxybutynin, tolterodine, trospium). Beware of anticholinergic side effects.
Stress	Intra-abdominal pressure overcomes sphincter closure mechanisms.	Primarily affects younger women. Involuntary leakage on exertion such as sneezing or coughing.	Pelvic floor exercises (Kegels), pessaries, bladder suspension surgery.
Overflow	Incomplete bladder emptying due to impaired detrusor activity and/or outlet obstruction.	Usually affects men with prostatic enlargement or patients with spinal cord injury. Can also be caused by urinary retention resulting from the use of anticholinergic medications. Leakage is small in volume but continuous. Elevated postvoid residuals; weak stream. Intermittency, hesitancy, and nocturia may also be seen.	α-adrenergic antagonists, 5α-reductase inhibitors, transurethral resection of prostate. For further treatment details, see the discussion of BPH in the Ambulatory Medicine chapter.
Functional	Inability to void in a commode owing to factors such as poor mobility, vision, or impaired cognition.	May be exacerbated by medical conditions (CHF, DM, low albumin) or by medications (especially diuretics).	Fluid management; pads/protective garments. Urinal/bedside commode. Regular toileting schedule. Catheters should be used only as a last resort.

Fecal Incontinence

Continuous or recurrent uncontrolled passage of fecal material (> 10 mL) for at least one month. A common **cause of nursing home placement.**

- Loss of continence can result from dysfunction of the anal sphincter, abnormal rectal compliance, ↓ rectal sensation, or a combination of any of these abnormalities.
- Dysfunction of the levator ani muscle appears to have a strong association with the severity of incontinence.
- Fecal incontinence is usually multifactorial, as these derangements often coexist (see Table 8.2).

DIAGNOSIS

- The rectal exam should assess for fecal impaction, anal tone, pelvic floor tone, and any masses.
- Inspection of the distal colon and anus with flexible sigmoidoscopy and anoscopy can exclude mucosal inflammation or masses.
- Complaints of diarrhea may be assessed with stool studies and a full colonoscopy.

TREATMENT

- **Medical therapy:** Antidiarrheal drugs, along with the elimination of medications that are known to cause diarrhea, may be of benefit.
  - The goal is to ↓ stool frequency and improve stool consistency.
  - Formed stool is easier to control than liquid stool.
  - Loperamide is more effective than diphenoxylate for reducing urgency.
  - Anticholinergic agents taken before meals may be helpful in patients who tend to have leakage of stools after eating.
- **Biofeedback therapy:** A painless, noninvasive means of cognitively retraining the pelvic floor and the abdominal wall musculature. However, insufficient evidence exists supporting its efficacy.

KEY FACT

Fecal incontinence affects 3–10% of community-dwelling elderly.

KEY FACT

Constipation is a common cause of fecal incontinence in the elderly.

TABLE 8.2. Etiologies of Fecal Incontinence

ETIOLOGY	CHARACTERISTICS
Vaginal delivery	Incontinence may occur either immediately or years after delivery. The most common injuries are anal sphincter tears and trauma to the pudendal nerve.
Surgical trauma	Surgery on the anal sphincter or surrounding structures.
DM	↓ internal anal sphincter resting pressure. Diarrhea is 2° to autonomic neuropathy.
↓ rectal compliance	Rectal filling fails to produce a sensation of rectal fullness and the urge to defecate.
Impaired rectal sensation	A number of conditions are associated, including DM, MS, dementia, meningomyelocele, and spinal cord injuries.
Fecal impaction	A common cause in the elderly. Produces constant inhibition of internal anal sphincter tone, permitting leakage of liquid stool around the impaction.

- **Surgery:**
    - A number of surgical approaches have been used for the treatment of fecal incontinence.
    - Colostomy should be reserved for those with intractable symptoms who are not candidates for other therapies.
- **Nerve stimulation:** Electrical stimulation of the sacral nerve roots can restore continence in patients with structurally intact muscles.
- **Supportive measures:** Can be instituted in most patients. May include avoiding foods or activities known to worsen symptoms, ritualizing bowel habits, and improving perianal skin hygiene. Stool impaction should be corrected and a bowel regimen instituted to prevent recurrence.

KEY FACT

Stool consistency can be improved by supplementing the diet with a bulking agent, but this may exacerbate incontinence in patients with ↓ rectal compliance (eg, those with radiation proctitis or a rectal stricture).

Sexual Dysfunction

Older men and women frequently remain interested in sex despite a ↓ in overall sexual activity. In men, ↓ activity may result from a variety of factors, including atherosclerosis, neurologic disorders, medications, psychological factors, endocrine problems, social issues, limited availability of partners, ↓ libido, and erectile dysfunction. In women, additional factors include vaginal dryness or burning and vaginal atrophy.

KEY FACT

Erectile dysfunction and loss of libido are not normal signs of aging.

SYMPTOMS

- **Men:** Symptoms in men include inadequate erections, ↓ libido, and orgasmic failure.
- **Women:** Symptoms in women include vaginal dryness or burning (atrophy), dyspareunia, slower time to orgasm, a need for prolonged clitoral stimulation, and ↓ libido.

DIFFERENTIAL

Medication effects (eg, SSRIs, β-blockers), psychosocial factors, anatomical problems, Peyronie's disease in men.

DIAGNOSIS

- Review the patient's medical problems and medication list.
- Ask about substance use (eg, alcohol, cigarettes, heroin, cocaine).
- Screen for depression.
- Assess time spent in foreplay or in stimulation.
- **Labs:**
    - For men, consider serum testosterone, although this is likely to be low yield if there are no other signs of hypogonadism.
    - If serum testosterone levels are low or low normal, consider a bioavailable testosterone level. LH and prolactin are not routinely necessary, as the hypothalamic-pituitary axis tends to become less responsive with aging.
    - Other lab tests should be dictated by the history and physical (eg, glycosylated hemoglobin, lipid panel).

KEY FACT

Screen for possible depression in older persons with sexual dysfunction.

TREATMENT

Counsel patients on lifestyle modifications (eg, ↓ alcohol intake, smoking cessation) and address any psychosocial issues. Discontinue offending medications if possible. Address underlying medical problems as appropriate. Specific treatments for sexual dysfunction include the following:

- **Men:**
  - **Pharmacologic:**
    - **Phosphodiesterase-5 (PDE-5) inhibitors (sildenafil, tadalafil, vardenafil):** Often effective, and the most acceptable option for patients. Contraindicated in patients who use nitrates, as hypotension may result.
    - **Testosterone:** Should be used only for true hypogonadism. Associated with multiple side effects and an ↑ risk of prostate disease. Contraindicated if the patient has a history of prostate cancer.
  - **Mechanical: Penile injections or vacuum devices** may be effective but are rarely acceptable to patients.
  - **Other options:** Constriction rings, counseling, surgery for Peyronie's disease, penile prostheses.
- **Women:** Topical estrogen creams or rings (if there is no hepatic or cardiac disease); ↑ stimulation time before intercourse. Consider counseling.

Falls

Falls are more common in inpatient settings and in the postdischarge period. It is important to differentiate between an accidental fall and syncope. Risk factors include the following:

- Gait instability
- ↓ positional sense and reflexes
- ↓ sensorium/vision
- Orthostatic hypotension
- Incontinence
- A history of a cerebrovascular event
- Parkinson's disease
- A history of syncope
- Alcohol use
- Medications (benzodiazepines, sedatives, neuroleptics, antihistamines, opiates)
- Environment (loose rugs, stairs)

PREVENTION

- Improved lighting and correction of visual deficits.
- Decreasing psychotropic or other known offending medications.
- Vitamin D replacement for those who are deficient (shown to ↓ falls and improve body sway).
- Exercise (particularly strength/flexibility/balance exercises such as tai chi).
- Environmental modifications such as installation of handrails, removal of rugs, use of shower rails and seats, use of ramps, and first-floor setup (placement of the bed, commode, and bath on the same floor, preferably on the main level of the residence).
- Use of assistive devices.
- Avoidance of pharmacologic and physical restraints.

KEY FACT

Physical restraints do not prevent falls and lead to ↑ mortality, ↑ hospital lengths of stay, pressure sores, nosocomial infection, and emotional distress.

COMPLICATIONS

- Roughly 50% of falls result in injury, and 10% require hospitalization.
- A prolonged amount of time spent on the floor can lead to rhabdomyolysis, dehydration, and hypothermia.
- Associated with nursing home placement and functional decline.

Hip Fractures

The one-year mortality rate for hip fracture is up to 25%; half of elderly patients are unable to continue to live independently after the fracture.

SYMPTOMS

Presents with hip or groin pain after a fall. Patients are often unable to bear weight.

EXAM

Leg shortening and external rotation when the patient is supine. Tenderness on palpation or internal/external rotation may be seen. Look for other fall-related trauma, such as head injury or rib fractures.

DIFFERENTIAL

Soft tissue injury, dislocation, avascular necrosis (AVN).

DIAGNOSIS

Radiographic studies generally establish the diagnosis, usually on AP pelvis or hip series. Rarely, an MRI is needed to diagnose a subtle fracture or to confirm AVN (see Figure 8.2).

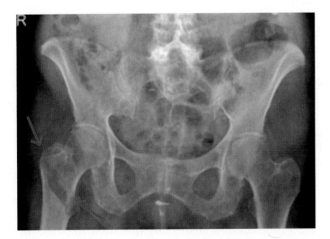

FIGURE 8.2. **Hip fracture.** Frontal radiograph of the pelvis shows an intertrochanteric fracture of the right femur (arrows). (Reproduced with permission from USMLERx.com.)

Treatment of hip fracture—

O-ROT

Orthopedic management (to include prophylactic anticoagulation until ↑ mobility)
Rehab
Osteoporosis treatment
Tertiary fall prevention

KEY FACT

Assess goals of care with the hip fracture patient and, if necessary, with the surrogate decision maker. Operative management may not always be consistent with a frail patient with preexisting immobility and a shortened life expectancy. However, unrepaired hip fractures are associated with extremely high morbidity.

TREATMENT

The major components of therapy are as follows (see also the mnemonic O-ROT):

- **Orthopedic management:** Usually required, with the exact procedure depending on the type of fracture. Most surgeons now recognize the importance of expediting operative repair (should occur within 24 hours of the fracture).
- **Postoperative rehabilitation:** Should begin immediately or as soon as allowed by surgical recommendations. Includes mobilization, DVT prophylaxis, pain management, prevention of complications, and functional adaptation.
- **Osteoporosis treatment:** Consider starting patients on a bisphosphonate if this has not been done already. Hip protectors may slightly ↓ fracture risk but do not prevent falls.
- **3° prevention of falls** (see above).

COMPLICATIONS

Immobility, venous thromboembolism, functional decline and death.

Pressure Ulcers

A higher incidence of pressure ulcers is found in hospitals and nursing homes than in homes with family caregivers. Causes may be extrinsic or intrinsic.

- **Extrinsic causes:**
    - Sustained pressure, primarily over bony prominences (eg, sacrum, ischium, heels, trochanters).
    - Shearing forces.
    - Infection, friction, or moisture.
- **Intrinsic causes:**
    - Immobility.
    - Cognitive dysfunction.
    - Impaired wound healing (may be 2° to diabetes, peripheral vascular disease, venous stasis, or poor nutritional status).
    - Changes in skin structure and integrity associated with aging.

DIAGNOSIS

- **Stage I:** Nonblanching erythema over intact skin.
- **Stage II:** Partial-thickness skin loss (epidermis +/– dermis).
- **Stage III:** Full skin loss down to but not through the fascia (see Figure 8.3A).
- **Stage IV:** Tissue loss down to the level of muscle, tendon, or bone. Any undermining/sinus tracts are also considered (see Figure 8.3B).
- **Unstageable:** Full-thickness tissue loss in which the base of the ulcer is covered by slough (yellow, tan, gray, green, or brown) and/or eschar (tan, brown, or black) in the wound bed. Slough and/or eschar can be removed to expose the base of the wound, and stage can be determined.
- **Suspected deep tissue injury:** A localized purple or maroon area of discolored intact skin or blood-filled blister due to damage of underlying soft tissue from pressure and/or shear.

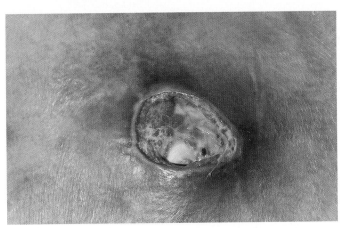
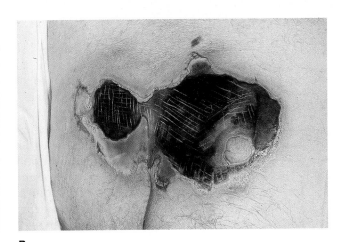

A   **B**

FIGURE 8.3. **Pressure (decubitus) ulcers.** (A) Stage III. (B) Stage IV. Note that the criss-cross marks in the necrotic area are from attempts to mechanically debride necrotic tissue. Surgical debridement of necrotic tissue under anesthesia revealed involvement of fascia and bone. (Reproduced with permission from Wolff K et al. *Fitzpatrick's Color Atlas & Synopsis of Clinical Dermatology,* 6th ed. New York: McGraw-Hill, 2009, Figs. 16-17 and 16-18.)

TREATMENT

- **Pressure relief:** Pressure-relieving mattresses and seat cushions; physical therapy; frequent repositioning (every two hours).
- **Debridement of dead or infected tissue:** Sharp, mechanical, or enzymatic debridement may be used.
- **Selection of topical dressing:** The goal is maintenance of a moist wound bed to promote healing.
- **Management of bacterial load: Not all wounds are infected!** There is no need for systemic antibiotics unless there are signs of cellulitis (erythema, pain, warmth, or increasing drainage/odor) or systemic infection.

PREVENTION

Preventive measures include competent nursing care, good hygiene and hydration, and adequate nutrition.

Sleep Disorders

Two sleep states have been identified: non–rapid eye movement (NREM) and rapid eye movement (REM). A typical night of sleep begins with NREM; REM occurs after 80 minutes. Both sleep states then alternate, with REM periods increasing as the night progresses. NREM includes four stages:

- **Stages 1 and 2:** Classified as light sleep. Stage 1 is a transition from wakefulness to sleep.
- **Stages 3 and 4:** Classified as deep, restorative sleep.

SYMPTOMS/EXAM

- Changes in sleep occur as a normal part of aging. Such changes may affect sleep pattern (the amount and timing of sleep), sleep structure (stages), or both. Specifically, stages 1 and 2 may ↑, while stages 3 and 4 ↓.
- Typical complaints from patients > 65 years of age include the following:
  - Difficulty falling asleep.
  - Midsleep awakening and ↑ arousal during the night.
  - Nonrestorative sleep (may be perceived as ↓ sleep time).
  - Earlier bedtime and earlier morning awakening.
  - Daytime napping or reversal of the sleep-wake cycle.

DIFFERENTIAL

- **1° sleep disorders:** Circadian rhythm disorders, sleep apnea, restless leg syndrome, REM behavior disorder.
- **Psychiatric:** Stress, depression, bereavement, anxiety.
- **Pain related:** Neuropathic pain, rheumatologic conditions, malignancy syndromes.
- **Physiologic:** Dyspnea resulting from cardiac and pulmonary conditions (COPD, CHF); nocturia due to DM, BPH, or medications; GERD.
- **Medication related (10–15%):**
  - **Respiratory medications:** Theophylline, β-agonists.
  - **Cardiovascular medications:** Furosemide, quinidine.
  - **Antidepressants:** Desipramine, nortriptyline, imipramine.
  - **Other:** Corticosteroids, caffeine, nicotine.

DIAGNOSIS/TREATMENT

There is limited evidence supporting specialized testing with polysomnography. However, the following issues should be addressed:

- **General measures:**
  - Diagnose and treat **sleep apnea.**
  - Identify any **stressors and psychiatric conditions.**
  - Encourage good **sleep hygiene:**
    - Adhere to a regular bedtime and morning rise time.
    - Limit daytime napping.
    - Exercise during the day but not at night.
    - Avoid caffeine, alcohol, and nicotine in the evening.
    - Limit nighttime fluid intake to diminish the urge to urinate during sleeping hours.
    - Control room noise, light, and temperature.
    - Avoid reading or watching television in bed.
- **Medications:** If all other measures fail and medications must be used, they should always be administered in the lowest effective dose and should be given as intermittent or short-term dosing only. Whereas no medications are recommended in the treatment of insomnia for the older patient, use of the following medications should be actively discouraged:
  - **Benzodiazepines:** ↑ the likelihood of falls, leading to hip fracture and motor vehicle accidents. Tolerance has been widely noted.
  - **Antihistamines (eg, diphenhydramine):** Anticholinergic effects.
  - **Melatonin:** Wide variability in dosage in different OTC formulations.

COMPLICATIONS

Untreated sleep disorders result in poor memory, impaired concentration, impaired function, ↑ numbers of accidents and falls, and chronic fatigue.

Depression

Greatly underdiagnosed and undertreated in older patients. Elderly patients may be more likely to present with somatic complaints or experience delusions and are less likely to report depressed mood. Risk factors include the following:

- A prior episode of depression
- A ⊕ family history
- Lack of social support
- Use of alcohol or other substances
- Parkinson's disease
- Recent MI
- A history of CVAs
- Cognitive impairment
- Loss of autonomy/functional impairment
- Multiple comorbid medical conditions
- Uncontrolled pain or insomnia

DIFFERENTIAL

- **Mild cognitive impairment:** Can precede dementia (patients are likely to have predominantly depressive symptoms).
- **Parkinson's disease:** The early presentation of Parkinson's may mimic depression. (However, a high percentage of Parkinson's patients also develop depression.)
- **Other:**
    - Fatigue and weight loss from DM, thyroid disease, malignancy, vitamin B_{12} deficiency, or anemia.
    - Sleep disturbance with daytime fatigue and depressed mood as a result of pain, nocturia, and sleep apnea.
    - Bereavement, delirium, substance abuse.

TREATMENT

The mainstay of treatment for major depression consists of medications +/– psychotherapy. The approach is similar to that taken for depression in younger patients.

- **Pharmacotherapy:** Medications for elderly patients are chosen largely on the basis of their side effect profiles (eg, anxiety, insomnia, pain, weight loss). **SSRIs** are generally first-line agents, usually initiated at half the typical starting dose. Side effects typically last < 4 weeks, but weight gain and sexual dysfunction may last longer. See Table 8.3.
- **Psychotherapy:** Cognitive-behavioral therapy, problem-solving therapy, and interpersonal psychotherapy are effective either alone or in combination with pharmacotherapy.
- **Electroconvulsive therapy (ECT):**
    - Associated with response rates of 60–70% in patients with refractory depression.
    - Side effects of confusion and anterograde memory impairment may persist for up to six months.
    - First-line therapy for patients who are severely depressed, for those who are at high risk for suicide, and in other situations when a rapid response is urgent (eg, when a medical condition is severely compromised by depression). Also an option for patients who are not eligible for pharmacotherapy as a result of hepatic, renal, or cardiac disease.

KEY FACT

Management of depression in elderly patients is similar to that of patients in other age groups. SSRIs are generally first line. Use caution with TCAs in light of their anticholinergic side effects.

KEY FACT

The side effects of mirtazapine (a norepinephrine antagonist and serotonin antagonist)—somnolence, ↑ appetite, and weight gain—may actually help elderly patients who have depression associated with sleep problems or unintentional weight loss.

TABLE 8.3. **Pharmacotherapy for Depression in the Elderly**

Class/Medication	Uses	Side Effects
SSRIs (sertraline, paroxetine, fluoxetine, citalopram)	First-line medications. Equally efficacious in elderly patients. **Usually initiated at half the listed starting dose in elderly patients.**	Nausea and sexual dysfunction are most common. Paroxetine and fluvoxamine also have anticholinergic side effects. Fluoxetine is rarely used because of its long half-life and inhibition of cytochrome P-450. If discontinued abruptly, patients can experience withdrawal (flulike symptoms, dizziness, headache). There is an ↑ risk of serotonin syndrome in patients taking SSRIs and/or MAOIs.
2° amine TCAs (nortriptyline)	May offer added benefit in patients with neuropathic pain, detrusor instability, or insomnia.	**Anticholinergic side effects** are common. Also associated with conduction abnormalities. Lethal in overdose, and should be avoided in patients with suicidal ideation.
MAOIs and 3° amine TCAs (phenelzine, amitriptyline, imipramine)	Rarely used because of side effect profiles and the likelihood of drug interactions.	Eating tyramine-containing foods while on MAOIs can cause serotonin syndrome. Both classes are lethal in overdose.
Mirtazapine	Beneficial for depression with sleep abnormalities and in patients with **unintentional weight loss** due to the side effect profile.	Somnolence, ↑ appetite, modest weight gain, dizziness.
Trazodone	Not as efficacious as other antidepressants. Used to treat insomnia.	Associated with **priapism.** Also causes somnolence.
Venlafaxine	In addition to antidepressant effects, also used to treat anxiety and neuropathic pain.	May ↑ diastolic BP.
Bupropion	Also reduces cravings in smoking cessation. Lowest risk of sexual side effects.	Seizure risk that is dose and titration related.
Psychostimulants (dextroamphetamine, methylphenidate)	Sometimes used in patients with predominantly vegetative symptoms.	Commonly associated with tachycardia, insomnia, and agitation.

Dementia

 An 85-year-old woman presents to her primary care provider's office after her family notices that she has exhibited strange behavior for the past year. She is emotionally labile with frequent outbursts of crying and laughing, and she has become fixated on hoarding magazines. Her short-term memory is intact on exam. What is the most likely diagnosis?

Frontotemporal dementia. Patients have progressive alterations in behavior and personality, including apathy, disinhibition, and stereotyped behaviors. Patients may also develop aphasia with changes in speech, comprehension, and motor impairment. In comparison to Alzheimer's disease, age of onset is earlier (50–70 years), and cognitive impairments appear later in the disease course. Brain imaging is required to exclude other diagnoses, such as tumor, CVA, subdural hematoma, or abscess.

An acquired syndrome involving a decline in memory plus at least one other cognitive domain—language (aphasia), motor function (apraxia), visuospatial capacity (agnosia), or executive function (abstract thinking, organization, problem solving)—that leads to impairments in occupation, social activities, or relationships and represents a change from a prior level of function. Risk factors are listed in Table 8.4.

Symptoms/Exam

Mild cognitive impairment may be seen in early dementia. Patients may have impairment in one or more domains (memory, language, visuospatial, executive) but have normal activities of daily living (ADLs) and general cognitive function. Examples include the following:

- Getting lost in familiar places.
- Personality changes such as poor impulse control or behavioral disturbance.
- Diminishment in simple problem-solving ability.
- Trouble with complex or routine tasks (eg, balancing the checkbook, making meals).
- Difficulty learning new things.
- Impaired or poor judgment.
- Language problems (eg, word finding).

See Table 8.5 for descriptions of specific types of dementia.

 KEY FACT

Alzheimer's disease is characterized by an insidious, progressive course without waxing and waning. Patients experience early loss of short-term memory.

 KEY FACT

Patients with Lewy body dementia classically have a dramatic worsening of extrapyramidal symptoms when given antipsychotic medications.

KEY FACT

Lewy body dementia can be distinguished from Alzheimer's by three characteristics not prominently seen in Alzheimer's: (1) fluctuations in attention and alertness (looks like delirium), (2) visual hallucinations (can be seen in late Alzheimer's), and (3) parkinsonism (gait/postural instability).

TABLE 8.4. **Risk Factors for Dementia**

Strong Risk Factors	Other Risk Factors
Age (particularly for Alzheimer's disease)	Head trauma with loss of consciousness
A family history in first-degree relatives	A history of depression
Apolipoprotein E ε4 genotype	Low educational achievement
DM	Female gender (for Alzheimer's disease)
Hypercholesterolemia	Gait impairment (for those without
Low and high BP	Alzheimer's disease)

TABLE 8.5. Subtypes of Dementia

Type of Dementia	Clinical Presentation	Treatment Considerations
Alzheimer's disease (the most common cause of dementia)	**Progressive loss of cognitive skills, eg, memory, language, judgment, and orientation.** **Early stage:** Starts with short-term memory loss; leads to progressive memory loss, personality changes, delusional thinking, and functional impairment. **Late stage:** Aphasia, agnosia, apraxia; assistance is needed for all ADLs. ↑ risk is associated with apolipoprotein E genotype ε4 allele, but testing is considered optional.	**Mild to moderate cognitive impairment: Acetylcholinesterase inhibitors** (donepezil, galantamine, rivastigmine). **Late stage: Memantine** (blocks NMDA glutamate receptors); small ⊕ effect. **Behavioral symptoms (delusions, hallucinations, agitation/sundowning):** Atypical antipsychotics are often used but are associated with ↑ mortality.
Vascular/multi-infarct dementia	Frequently characterized by **sudden** onset and **stepwise** decline due to multiple small strokes. Neurologic deficits on exam and imaging correlate with previous stroke location. Commonly coexists with Alzheimer's disease.	Treat any underlying causes of cerebral infarction. Physical and cognitive rehabilitation.
Lewy body dementia (the second most common cause of 1° degenerative dementia)	Presents with dementia, often followed by **parkinsonism** (gait instability and postural instability), **visuospatial impairment and hallucinations,** and REM sleep disorder. **Fluctuations in performance,** especially attention and alertness, are also seen. Intracytoplasmic Lewy body inclusions are found in the brainstem.	Patients have ↑ sensitivity to antipsychotic medications (vs. Alzheimer's patients). **Dopaminergic medications should be avoided** except in the presence of clinically significant parkinsonism, as these medications can worsen psychotic symptoms. Quetiapine is often used for hallucinations.
Frontotemporal dementia (Pick's disease)	Characterized by impaired executive function (initiating activity, planning), poor self-awareness of one's deficits, and **disinhibited behavior.** Pick's disease is one type (Pick bodies are found in the neocortex and the hippocampus). A family history in a first-degree relative is a major risk factor.	Monitor patients for the development of amyotrophic lateral sclerosis (ALS).
Other causes of dementia	**Medications:** Analgesics, anticholinergics, antipsychotics, sedatives. **Metabolic disorders:** Thyroid disease, vitamin B_{12} deficiency, hyponatremia, hypercalcemia, hepatic and renal insufficiency. **Other:** Alcohol, HIV, encephalitis, syphilis, Parkinson's disease, trauma, Huntington's disease.	
Pseudodementia	Depression presenting as dementia. Associated with an ↑ likelihood that the patient will develop dementia.	

(continues)

TABLE 8.5.   Subtypes of Dementia *(continued)*

TYPE OF DEMENTIA	CLINICAL PRESENTATION	TREATMENT CONSIDERATIONS
Creutzfeldt-Jakob disease	A rare, infectious, rapidly progressive dementia that is usually fatal within one year of onset. Presents with rapid cognitive impairment accompanied by motor deficits and seizures.	Diagnosis is made by autopsy; there is no treatment.
Normal pressure hydrocephalus	The classic presentation is "wet, wobbly, and wacky"—urinary incontinence, gait apraxia, and dementia. Gait is typically shuffling and unresponsive to antiparkinsonian medications.	Diagnosis is confirmed by ventriculomegaly on CT/MRI. CNS drainage (ventricular shunt) may improve symptoms.

DIAGNOSIS

- The Mini-Mental Status Exam (MMSE) is the best-studied instrument for screening dementia. Accuracy depends on age, language proficiency, and highest educational level completed.
- Workup includes CBC, electrolytes, creatinine, LFTs, calcium, TSH, vitamin B_{12}, RPR, and HIV.
- Neuroimaging is controversial, but patients can be screened with noncontrast CT or MRI. Neuroimaging may also be considered on the basis of risks for pathology—eg, for young patients (< 60 years of age), those with rapid onset of symptoms, or those with focal neurologic signs.
- Neuropsychiatric testing if diagnosis is uncertain or complicated by psychiatric illness (eg, depression).

TREATMENT

- Alzheimer's disease will progress despite treatment type.
- The following agents can be used to symptomatically treat memory (cognitive) decline:
  - **Cholinesterase inhibitors (donepezil, rivastigmine, galantamine, tacrine):** For **mild to moderate** Alzheimer's disease. Benefits include improvement or stabilization on neuropsychiatric scales, but benefits appear to be modest at two years. May also help treat behavioral symptoms of dementia.
  - **NMDA antagonists (memantine):** For **moderate to severe** Alzheimer's disease with or without concomitant acetylcholinesterase use.
- The following can be used to symptomatically treat behavior problems (depression, agitation, delusions, hallucinations):
  - **Typical antipsychotics** (eg, olanzapine, quetiapine): Use with caution in light of associated ↑ mortality in this population.
  - **Antidepressants** (eg, SSRIs).

COMPLICATIONS

Malnutrition, pressure ulcers, recurrent infections, depression, nursing home placement, caregiver burden.

KEY FACT

An MMSE score of > 26 is considered normal; 24–26 points to mild cognitive impairment; and < 24 is suggestive (but not diagnostic) of dementia. Note that attention may be preserved until the late stages of Alzheimer's disease, and MMSE may not pick up dementia in patients with high baseline IQ.

KEY FACT

For Alzheimer's disease, start a cholinesterase inhibitor for mild to moderate symptoms. As symptoms worsen, consider adding memantine or using memantine alone.

KEY FACT

No clear benefit has been shown for gingko biloba, selegiline, vitamin E, or estrogen in slowing the progression of dementia.

Delirium

Delirium is common in the elderly, especially among hospitalized patients. Although covered in detail in the Hospital Medicine chapter, it is mentioned here because it is a common mimicker of dementia and depression. Usually has a multifactorial etiology in elderly patients, with many risk factors:

- Preexisting cognitive impairment (especially dementia)
- Advanced age
- Severe underlying illness
- Number and severity of comorbid conditions
- Functional impairment
- Visual or hearing impairment
- Malnutrition and dehydration

Always consider drug-drug interactions due to polypharmacy and adverse drug reactions due to changes in medication distribution, metabolism, and clearance as a cause of delirium.

Iatrogenesis

- Elderly patients are at high risk for iatrogenic complications for many reasons:
  - More frequent admission to hospitals and nursing homes
  - Diminished reserves (cognitive, renal, hepatic)
  - Underdiagnosis or delayed diagnosis of medical conditions due to atypical presentations
  - Difficulty with adherence to complicated medical regimens
- Common iatrogenic complications include the following:
  - Nosocomial infections
  - Falls
  - Pressure ulcers
  - Delirium
  - Surgical/perioperative complications
  - Adverse drug reactions/drug-drug interactions
- Risk factors for the development of iatrogenesis are as follows:
  - Self-treatment
  - Lack of coordinated care
  - Recent hospital admission/discharge
  - Impaired cognition
  - Complicated medication regimens

KEY FACT

Comorbidities and functional status are more important than age alone when one is considering who is at risk for iatrogenic complications.

Polypharmacy

> A 92-year-old woman with hypertension, anxiety, and osteoporosis is admitted to the hospital with acute onset of severe low back pain for one week. She has been unable to get out of bed and is brought to the ER. Follow-up spinal radiographs reveal multiple compression fractures throughout the lumbar spine. Medications on admission include HCTZ, lorazepam, lisinopril, alendronate, cyclobenzaprine, and atenolol. She is started on IV morphine as needed for pain. On hospital day 1, she appears intermittently lethargic, apathetic, and incoherent. She refuses medication and food and has disturbed sleep. What is the most likely diagnosis?
>
> Delirium 2° to polypharmacy. Common offenders include benzodiazepines, opiates, and anticholinergics (eg, cyclobenzaprine). On admission, medications may be reinitiated or ↑ following a period of nonadherence as an outpatient, so obtain a medication history that includes compliance. A reasonable alternative therapy for this patient would be to add acetaminophen around the clock, physical therapy, and a low-dose opiate as needed.

Defined as the use of five or more medications. A significant cause of hospital admissions that **should be on the differential of any presentation in an older adult.** Changes in physiologic function and pharmacokinetics in the older patient promote ↑ sensitivity to medications and hence ↑ the possibility of complications and adverse drug events. Specific changes include the following:

- **Altered medication distribution:**
    - ↓ protein binding of some drugs (eg, warfarin, phenytoin) due to low serum albumin.
    - Water-soluble drugs become more concentrated, and fat-soluble drugs have longer half-lives (↑ volume of distribution).
- **Metabolism:** ↑ hepatic enzyme activity, affecting the metabolism of drugs with high first-pass metabolism (eg, propranolol).
- **Excretion:** Renal function ↓ by as much as 50% by age 85.
- **Absorption:** No clinically significant change in drug absorption occurs with normal aging. Chronic diseases and medications may ↑ gastric pH, motility, or gastric emptying time.

Symptoms/Exam

- **Delirium** can result from many drugs, including cold remedies, anticholinergics, and analgesics (common but often overlooked in the elderly).
- Other common symptoms/signs include nausea, anorexia, weight loss, parkinsonism, constipation, hypotension, balance disturbances, and acute renal failure.

Treatment

- Try **nonpharmacologic means** before drugs.
- Improve adherence by keeping the dosing schedule simple (once daily is best), the number of pills low, and medication changes infrequent.
- Continually review the drug list for potential discontinuations.
- Consider dose reduction or discontinuation of medications rather than treating an adverse drug effect with another medication.

KEY FACT

To prevent polypharmacy, "start low and go slow" (but conduct an adequate trial).

KEY FACT

Remember that OTC drugs, supplements, and herbals can cause adverse drug effects.

COMPLICATIONS

Adverse drug events, drug-drug interactions, duplication of drugs, ↓ quality of life, nonadherence, and financial burden of cost.

Palliative and End-of-Life Care

Generally accepted goals of end-of-life care include the following:

- To continue to treat potentially **reversible** disease.
- To help **alleviate suffering,** including physical, psychological, social, and spiritual distress.
- To help the patient **prepare for death.**

ETHICAL AND LEGAL ISSUES

Unique ethical considerations include the following:

- The concept of futile medical interventions, which may lead to conflicts between provider, patient, or family. Can often be resolved through discussions.
- The individual has the right to refuse or withdraw medical treatments. Ethically, there is no difference between *withdrawal* of life-sustaining treatment (eg, a mechanical ventilator) and *refusing to initiate* such an intervention.
- The potential to hasten death is permissible if the 1° intention is to provide comfort and dignity and to relieve suffering (ie, it is appropriate to prescribe as much morphine as needed to relieve suffering if congruent with patient goals of care). This is often termed the "ethical principle of **double effect.**"
- **Euthanasia** is defined as hastening a patient's death in response to their request, sometimes called "mercy killing." It is not legal in any state.
- **Physician-assisted suicide** involves a physician giving a patient the information or means to end his or her own life. This is currently legal, with multiple restrictions, only in the states of Oregon, Washington, and Montana.

MEDICAL DECISION MAKING

There are several ways patients can indicate their end-of-life wishes:

- **Advance directives:**
    - Defined as oral or written statements made by patients when they are competent with the purpose of guiding their care should they become incompetent.
    - Valid only for futile care or terminal illness.
    - Not legally binding in all states, but helps guide medical providers and family members in medical decision making based on the patient's previously recorded wishes.
- **Durable power of attorney for health care (DPOA-HC):**
    - The patient designates a surrogate decision maker.
    - The role of the surrogate is to offer "substituted judgment" such as that which would be offered if the patient could speak for himself/herself.
    - If a patient has not designated a health care agent, decisions default to the next of kin.

> **KEY FACT**
>
> The ethical principle of double effect allows for treatments that may hasten death if the **primary intention** is to relieve suffering.

- **"Do not resuscitate" (DNR) orders:**
    - Only 15% of all patients who undergo CPR in the hospital survive to hospital discharge. The survival rate for patients with metastatic cancer who undergo CPR is < 1%.
    - Patients should be informed about likely mortality outcomes as well as the potential adverse consequences of CPR and resuscitation attempts (eg, fractured ribs, neurologic disability, invasive procedures).
    - Requests for withdrawal of certain life-sustaining measures (eg, intubation, dialysis) must be respected when received from appropriately informed and competent patients or their surrogates.
    - Clinicians may recommend discontinuation of inappropriate interventions.

HOSPICE AND PALLIATIVE CARE

- Focuses on the patient and family rather than the disease; stresses the provision of comfort and pain relief rather than treating illness or prolonging life.
- Associated with ↑ patient satisfaction and ↓ family anxiety.
- Patients may be treated at home, in the hospital, or in an inpatient hospice care facility.
- Per Medicare guidelines, requires a physician's estimate of **< 6 months** of life remaining in order to be reimbursed. However, some patients remain in hospice care much longer, as life expectancy is notoriously difficult to estimate.

SYMPTOM MANAGEMENT

- **Pain:**
    - Very common, yet often undertreated.
    - Use a numeric or analog scale to assess.
    - Help the patient set pain management goals (strike a balance between sedation or "double effect" and total pain relief).
    - Treat chronic pain around the clock with long-acting drugs.
    - ↑ drugs as needed (there is no ceiling for pure opiates).
    - Use caution when combining analgesics (eg, acetaminophen and NSAIDs).
    - Sedation typically precedes significant respiratory depression.
    - Always add a bowel regimen to prevent constipation in patients receiving continuous opiates.
- **Dyspnea:**
    - Present in up to 50% of dying patients.
    - Identify and treat the underlying cause where possible.
    - Opiates are highly effective.
    - Nonpharmacologic measures include O_2, fresh air, and using fans to keep air moving.
    - Benzodiazepines treat the associated anxiety but not the dyspnea itself.
    - In patients with excessive secretions, a scopolamine patch may alleviate dyspnea and "choking" sensations.
- **Nausea and vomiting:**
    - If opiate related, consider a sustained-release formulation, a different agent at an equianalgesic dose, or the addition of a dopamine antagonist antiemetic.
    - If due to an intra-abdominal process (constipation, gastroparesis, gastric outlet obstruction), try small food portions, NG tube aspiration, laxa-

tive/bowel regimens, prokinetic agents, high-dose corticosteroids, or 5-HT$_3$ antagonists (eg, ondansetron).
- If related to ↑ ICP, use corticosteroids or palliative cranial irradiation as indicated.
- If due to vestibular disturbance, treat with anticholinergic or antihistaminic agents.
- Consider around-the-clock dosing of antiemetics.
- Benzodiazepines and dronabinol may also be effective.
- **Constipation:**
  - Often opiate related.
  - Behavioral treatments include increasing activity and fluid/fiber intake.
  - A bowel regimen is required for patients on opiates. Start stool softeners and bowel stimulants prophylactically, and add enemas and other treatments as needed.
- **Delirium and agitation:**
  - Many patients experience confusion before death.
  - Consider the usual reversible causes of delirium (see the previous section in this chapter), and treat if indicated.
  - Consider the psychoactive effects of current medications.
  - Haloperidol or risperidone may be used if reversible causes are not identified and behavioral management is unsuccessful. It may be acceptable to do nothing if the delirium does not bother the patient and family.

NUTRITION AND HYDRATION

- Dying patients who have stopped eating or drinking rarely experience hunger or thirst.
- Dry mouth can be managed with swabs and good oral care.
- Aggressive IV hydration can lead to dyspnea (pulmonary edema) and pain (lower extremity edema).

PSYCHOLOGICAL AND SOCIAL ISSUES

- Patients and families rank emotional support as one of the most important aspects of good end-of-life care.
- Clinicians can provide listening, assurance, and support as well as coordination with psychotherapy and group support.
- Depression must be treated and distinguished from normal anticipatory grief.

KEY FACT

The use of opiates for end-of-life care is **not** associated with the development of addiction or abuse.

KEY FACT

For patients with irreversible conditions, tube feeding has not been shown to improve mortality and comfort but has been shown to lead to complications.

Elder Abuse

- Elder abuse is widespread but often underreported. Adult children are the largest category of abusers in elderly patients.
- Patients should initially be interviewed alone. Ask about their perceived safety and dependency on family/caregivers.
- Table 8.6 details the subtypes and clinical characteristics of elder abuse.

MANAGEMENT

- The goal is to protect the safety of the elderly person while simultaneously respecting that person's autonomy.
- If the patient **does not have the capacity to accept or refuse intervention,** the physician should discuss with Adult Protective Services issues such as assistance with financial management, guardianship, and court proceedings.

REPORTING REQUIREMENTS

State laws and reporting requirements for elder abuse vary widely. In many states, the suspicion of abuse constitutes grounds for reporting, and physicians making reports in good faith are immune from legal liability. Often the reporter remains anonymous.

TABLE 8.6. Types and Characteristics of Elder Abuse

Type	Description
Domestic	Maltreatment of an older adult living at home or in a caregiver's home.
Institutional	Maltreatment of an older adult living in a residential facility.
Self-neglect	Behavior of an older adult who lives alone that threatens his or her own health or safety.
Physical abuse	Intentional infliction of physical pain or injury.
Financial abuse	Improper or illegal use of the resources of an older person without his/her consent, benefiting a person other than the older adult.
Psychological abuse	Infliction of mental anguish (eg, humiliating, intimidating, threatening).
Neglect	Failure to fulfill a caretaking obligation to provide goods or services (eg, abandonment; denial of food or health-related services).
Abandonment	Desertion of an elderly person by someone who has assumed responsibility for providing care to that person.
Sexual abuse	Nonconsensual sexual contact of any kind.

NOTES

CHAPTER 9

Hematology

Miten Vasa, MD
Thomas Chen, MD, PhD

Anemia

APPROACH TO ANEMIA

The best first steps in evaluation are measurement of the absolute reticulocyte count (see Figure 9.1) and review of the **peripheral smear**. The reticulocyte count can be used to categorize anemias as follows:

- **Hypoproliferative anemias:** Underproduction of RBCs with a low reticulocyte count. Classically subdivided by the MCV into **micro-, macro-,** and **normocytic** causes (see Table 9.1).
- **Hyperproliferative anemias:** ↑ destruction or loss of RBCs. **Reticulocyte count is ↑.**
    - The two most common causes are **bleeding** and **hemolysis** (covered in a subsequent section).
    - **MCV is not helpful in the evaluation of hyperproliferative anemias.**

IRON DEFICIENCY ANEMIA

Exacerbated by menstruation, pregnancy, and lactation.

Symptoms/Exam

- General findings of anemia are skin and conjunctival pallor.
- **Features associated with iron deficiency** include the following:
    - **Pica:** Craving for nonfood substances, especially clay.
    - **Pagophagia:** Craving for ice chips.
    - **Cheilosis:** Fissures at the corners of the mouth.
    - **Glossitis:** Smooth tongue.
    - **Koilonychia:** Spooning of the fingernails.
    - **Dysphagia:** Due to esophageal webs (**Plummer-Vinson syndrome**).

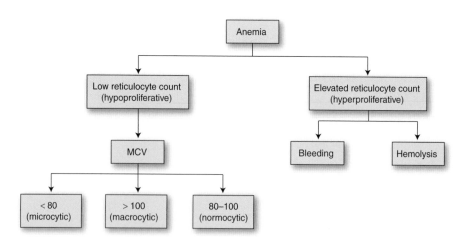

FIGURE 9.1. Algorithm for categorizing anemias.

TABLE 9.1.   Classification of Hypoproliferative Anemias

MICROCYTIC (MCV < 80)	MACROCYTIC (MCV > 100)	NORMOCYTIC (MCV 80–100)
"TAIL":	**Megaloblastic:**	ACD
Thalassemia trait	▪ B$_{12}$, folate deficiency	Aplastic anemia
Anemia of chronic disease	▪ Myelodysplasia	Myelodysplasia
(ACD)	▪ Myeloma	Renal insufficiency
Iron deficiency	▪ Aplastic anemia	Mixed disorder
Lead toxicity	▪ Pure red cell aplasia	Early disease process
	▪ Drug-induced bone	
	marrow suppression	
	▪ Alcohol	
	Nonmegaloblastic:	
	▪ Liver disease	
	▪ Hypothyroidism	

DIFFERENTIAL

- Causes of iron deficiency include blood loss from menstruation, GI bleed, and frequent phlebotomy. Inadequate iron ingestion or poor iron absorption is rare; the latter is sometimes associated with celiac disease.
- **Anemia of chronic disease (ACD):** Table 9.2 distinguishes ACD from iron deficiency.
- **Lead poisoning:** Presents with ↑ **RBC protoporphyrin, basophilic stippling,** and **lead lines** on the gums (the classic risk factor is occupation as a painter because of the lead in paint).

DIAGNOSIS

- Classic findings are **microcytic, hypochromic** RBCs on peripheral smear with marked **anisocytosis** (see Figure 9.2). However, these findings are present in only a minority of patients.
- **Serum ferritin** is the most useful screen for iron deficiency. Values of < 12 µg/L are diagnostic of iron deficiency. Although normal values do not rule it out, values of > 100 µg/L make iron deficiency unlikely. Other iron indices are listed in Table 9.2.
- **Bone marrow biopsy** is rarely indicated.
- A **therapeutic trial of iron may be diagnostic.** Reticulocytosis from iron typically begins 3–5 days after iron therapy. An ↑ in hemoglobin lags behind by several days.

KEY FACT

The most common presentation of celiac disease is iron deficiency anemia that is refractory to oral iron therapy.

KEY FACT

The total iron-binding capacity (TIBC) is often the simplest test to differentiate ACD from iron deficiency. TIBC is low in ACD and high in iron deficiency.

KEY FACT

A ferritin level of < 12 µg/L is diagnostic of iron deficiency.

TABLE 9.2.   ACD vs. Iron Deficiency Anemia

VARIABLE	ACD	IRON DEFICIENCY
MCV	Normal/low	Low
RDW	Normal	Normal or ↑
Ferritin	Normal/high	Low
TIBC	↓	↑
Soluble transferrin receptor	Normal	↑

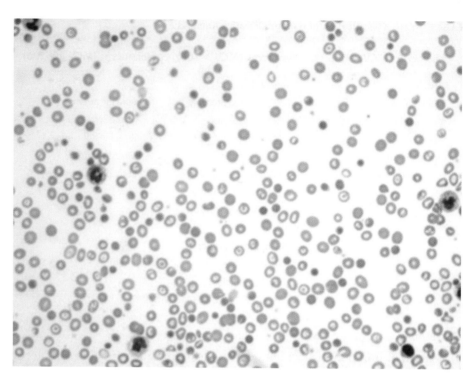

FIGURE 9.2. **Iron deficiency anemia.** Note the small RBCs with central pallor and targeting, indicative of a microcytic, hypochromic anemia from iron deficiency. (Reproduced with permission from USMLERx.)

TREATMENT

- **Oral iron replacement:** The goal is approximately 300 mg of elemental iron per day. The most common reason for treatment failure is noncompliance with or intolerance of iron (can cause constipation).
- **Parenteral iron:** Carries a risk of anaphylaxis; use only if the patient has a total inability to tolerate oral iron.
- Treat the underlying cause.

ANEMIA OF CHRONIC DISEASE (ACD)

Caused by sequestration of iron in the reticuloendothelial system as a result of an underlying inflammatory disorder. ACD is the **most common cause of anemia in the elderly population;** it often coexists with other causes.

SYMPTOMS/EXAM

Presents with symptoms of anemia and underlying disorders (eg, infectious diseases, rheumatologic disorders, cancer).

DIFFERENTIAL

Must often be differentiated from iron deficiency anemia (see Table 9.2).

DIAGNOSIS

A diagnosis of exclusion; peripheral smear is nonspecific.

TREATMENT

- Treat the underlying cause.
- High doses of erythropoietin (30,000–60,000 U/week) may be tried in patients with serum erythropoietin levels of < 100–500 IU/L.

ANEMIA ASSOCIATED WITH CHRONIC KIDNEY DISEASE (CKD)

Erythropoietin is produced by the kidneys, and patients with CKD often produce inadequate amounts. The anemia is usually normocytic and normochromic.

SYMPTOMS/EXAM

Presents with symptoms of anemia and of the underlying disorder (renal failure).

DIFFERENTIAL

Must be distinguished from hemolytic anemia, iron deficiency anemia, blood loss, and other causes of anemia.

DIAGNOSIS

- Evaluate hemoglobin, hematocrit, RBC indices, reticulocyte count, iron, TIBC, percent transferrin saturation, ferritin, and stool occult blood.
- If no other cause is identified and creatinine is ≥ 2 mg/dL, the anemia can be treated as anemia associated with CKD.
- Measurement of serum erythropoietin levels is generally not indicated.

TREATMENT

- Subcutaneous erythropoietin administration is recommended to target hemoglobin to 10–12 g/dL.
- Iron supplementation is usually required to maintain adequate iron stores.

VITAMIN B₁₂/FOLATE DEFICIENCY

The absorption of vitamin B_{12} requires many factors, including the secretion of intrinsic factor (IF) from the stomach and an intact terminal ileum. Vegans are at high risk for B_{12} deficiency, as B_{12} comes solely from animal products, whereas folate is derived from green, leafy vegetables. In developed countries, the 1° cause of B_{12} deficiency is **pernicious anemia (PA)** due to autoimmune destruction of parietal cells. PA is associated with other autoimmune disorders, including thyroiditis, vitiligo, and Addison's disease.

SYMPTOMS/EXAM

- Glossitis and atrophic gastritis (in PA).
- Mild icterus due to ineffective erythropoiesis, causing intramedullary hemolysis.
- Neurologic findings are present only in B_{12} deficiency and include the following:
  - **Peripheral sensory neuropathy:** Paresthesias in the distal extremities.
  - **Posterior column findings:** Loss of vibratory sensation and proprioception; gait instability.
  - Dementia or more subtle personality changes may occur at any time ("megaloblastic madness").
  - Neurologic changes are not always reversible with B_{12} replacement.

DIFFERENTIAL

The causes of B_{12} and folate deficiency are further outlined in Table 9.3.

KEY FACT

Anemia generally starts when creatinine clearance (CrCl) is < 45 mL/min and worsens with declining renal function.

KEY FACT

Use of erythropoietin-stimulating agents in kidney disease to boost hemoglobin levels above 10–12 g/dL may result in an ↑ in thromboembolic events.

KEY FACT

In developed countries, the most common cause of vitamin B_{12} deficiency is pernicious anemia.

KEY FACT

The neurologic changes associated with B_{12} deficiency are not always reversible with B_{12} replacement.

TABLE 9.3. Causes of B$_{12}$/Folate Deficiency

B$_{12}$ DEFICIENCY	FOLATE DEFICIENCY
Dietary deficiencies—very rare; typically found in strict vegans	**Inadequate intake:**
↓ IF—the most common cause; typically from PA (autoimmune destruction of parietal cells)	▪ Malnutrition
	▪ Alcoholism
Gastrectomy	▪ Malabsorption (eg, tropical sprue)
Ileal resection	↑ **demand:**
Crohn's disease	▪ Pregnancy
Tapeworm infestation (*Diphyllobothrium latum*)	▪ Hemodialysis (folate lost in dialysate)
Bacterial overgrowth of terminal ileum	▪ Chronic hemolytic anemia
	▪ Psoriasis

KEY FACT

MMA is a more sensitive test than B$_{12}$ level to evaluate for serum B$_{12}$ deficiency. In patients with borderline B$_{12}$ levels, an ↑ MMA is diagnostic of B$_{12}$ deficiency.

KEY FACT

In a patient with B$_{12}$ deficiency, anti-IF antibodies are virtually diagnostic for PA as the cause of B$_{12}$ deficiency.

DIAGNOSIS

▪ Labs:
   ▪ Low serum B$_{12}$ level or RBC folate level (RBC folate level is more reflective of long-term folate levels than serum folate level).
   ▪ Anemia with an **MCV > 100** (may see one without the other).
   ▪ Significant elevations in LDH and elevations in indirect bilirubin.
   ▪ Pancytopenia is seen in severe cases.
   ▪ ↑ levels of homocysteine or methylmalonic acid (**MMA**) may be seen. MMA is a more sensitive test than B$_{12}$ level and should be checked when B$_{12}$ is in the lower part of the normal range.
▪ **Smear:** Macro-ovalocytes and **hypersegmented neutrophils** (any neutrophil with ≥ 6 lobes or the majority with ≥ 4 lobes; see Figure 9.3).
▪ **Bone marrow:** Megaloblastic (hypercellular, ↓ myeloid/erythroid ratio, enlarged RBC precursors with relatively immature nuclei); **may mimic the blastic appearance of acute leukemia.**

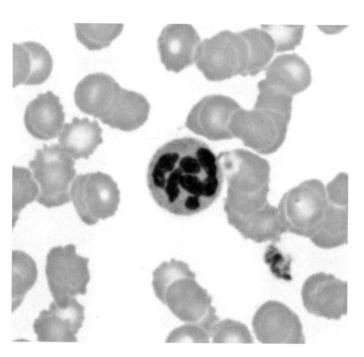

FIGURE 9.3. **Megaloblastic anemia.** Note the macro-ovalocytes and hypersegmented neutrophil. (Reproduced with permission from USMLERx.com.)

- **Schilling test:** Establishes the **cause** of B_{12} deficiency. Stages I and II may be combined by using different radioactive labels for each step (see Figure 9.4). This test is rarely done now.
- **Antibodies: Anti-IF antibodies are highly specific for PA** as the cause of B_{12} deficiency. **Anti–parietal cell antibodies** are less sensitive and specific.

TREATMENT

- **Parenteral B_{12}:** Recommended for the initial treatment of B_{12} deficiency in light of the possibility of generalized malabsorption.
- **Initial replacement:** Give 100 µg IM daily × 1 week, then every week × 1 month.
- **Maintenance:** Give 100 µg IM every month.
- **Oral B_{12}:** Equally effective for routine replacement, assuming that the patient is capable of absorbing. The recommended dose is 1–2 mg PO daily.
- **Oral folate:** A dose of 1 mg PO daily is adequate for folate deficiency.

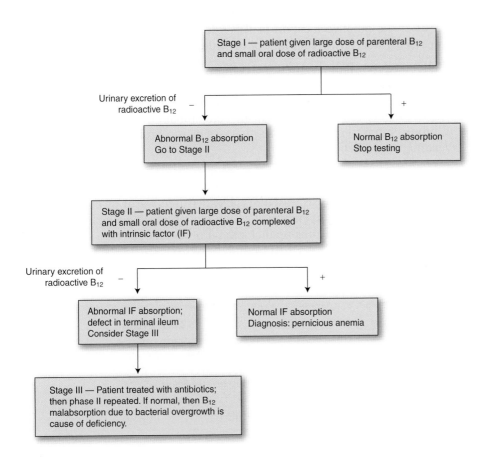

FIGURE 9.4.   Algorithm for the diagnosis of B_{12} deficiency.

HEMOLYTIC ANEMIA

 A 60-year-old woman with a history of chronic lymphocytic leukemia (CLL) complains of weakness and dark urine. Her CLL was last treated with chemotherapy three months ago. Exam reveals scleral icterus, cervical lymphadenopathy, and splenomegaly. Laboratory studies are as follows: hemoglobin 6.5 g/dL, platelet count 200,000/μL, reticulocyte count 13%, total bilirubin 6.0 mg/dL, LDH 357 U/L, and direct antiglobulin (Coombs') test ⊕ for IgG. What is the most likely diagnosis?

Warm antibody–mediated hemolytic anemia. Autoimmune hemolytic anemias may be idiopathic or result from drugs, lymphoproliferative disorders, collagen vascular diseases, or malignancies. CLL is a common cause. Treatment includes steroid therapy.

Hemolysis is classically categorized as either extravascular or intravascular on the basis of the putative location of RBC destruction and several associated features (see Table 9.4). **Other laboratory findings** include the following:

- **LDH** is often mildly ↑; striking elevations are characteristic of intravascular hemolysis.
- Indirect hyperbilirubinemia may be seen with bilirubin levels as high as 4 mg/dL; higher values usually indicate concomitant liver dysfunction.
- Chronic intravascular hemolysis may result in chronic hemoglobinuria, leading to iron deficiency.

DIFFERENTIAL

- **Immune hemolysis (extravascular):** Divided into **warm** or **cold** antibodies, referring to the temperature at which the responsible autoantibody will bind erythrocytes and thus predict several other characteristics (see Table 9.5).

> **KEY FACT**
>
> If a patient develops hemolytic anemia soon after starting a new medication—especially sulfas or dapsone—suspect G6PD deficiency and look for bite cells on peripheral blood smear or Heinz bodies on special stains.

TABLE 9.4. Extravascular vs. Intravascular Hemolytic Anemia

FEATURE	EXTRAVASCULAR	INTRAVASCULAR
Site of RBC destruction	Spleen	Bloodstream, liver
Peripheral smear findings	Spherocytes	Schistocytes (see Figure 9.5)
Serum haptoglobin	Normal or mildly ↓	Markedly ↓
Urine hemosiderin	Unchanged	↑
Examples	Warm antibody immune hemolysis Hypersplenism Delayed transfusion reaction	Cold antibody immune hemolysis Acute transfusion reaction Microangiopathic hemolysis Oxidative hemolytic anemia (eg, G6PD deficiency) Paroxysmal nocturnal hemoglobinuria Hemoglobinopathies (sickle cell anemia) Infection related (malaria, *Clostridium*, *Babesia*)

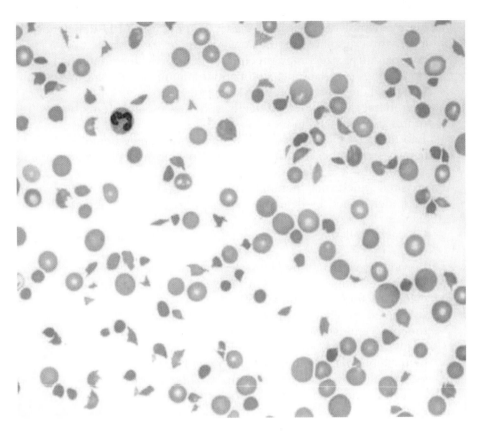

FIGURE 9.5. **Schistocytes.** A large number of fragmented RBCs is characteristic of microangiopathic or intravascular hemolysis. In this case, the patient had DIC. (Reproduced with permission from USMLERx.com.)

- **Microangiopathic hemolytic anemias (intravascular):** Characterized by **schistocytes** and a ⊖ **Coombs' test.** Usually caused by fibrin strands in damaged microvasculature, resulting in sheared RBCs. Almost all are associated with thrombocytopenia.

TABLE 9.5. Immune Hemolysis Categories

	WARM ANTIBODY	**COLD ANTIBODY**
Autoantibody	IgG	IgM
Direct antiglobulin test	⊕ for IgG	⊕ for IgM, complement
Peripheral smear	Spherocytes	Schistocytes
Site of RBC destruction	Spleen	Spleen
Associated conditions	Autoimmune diseases; CLL, lymphoma; α-methyldopa	*Mycoplasma* infection, EBV, CLL, lymphoma
Treatment	Steroids, splenectomy, immunosuppression	Warming extremities, plasmapheresis, alkylator medications, rituximab

- **Oxidative hemolytic anemia:** A classic example is **G6PD deficiency,** in which erythrocytes have ↓ ability to withstand oxidative stress.
  - **Any oxidative stress may precipitate hemolysis,** including viral infections, drugs (eg, dapsone, sulfonamides, antimalarials, and nitrofurantoin), and dietary factors (eg, fava beans).
  - **Peripheral smear** shows **bite cells, spherocytes,** and **Heinz bodies** (requires a special stain to see).
  - **Lab tests:** ↑ LDH, ↑ indirect bilirubin during acute hemolysis; G6PD activity (remember that measuring this during an acute hemolytic episode will result in a false-⊖ test).
- **Paroxysmal nocturnal hemoglobinuria (PNH):** A rare clonal stem cell disorder caused by defective expression of RBC membrane proteins (CD55 and CD59).
  - Characterized by episodic complement-mediated intravascular hemolysis.
  - Previously diagnosed by Ham's test (acidified serum hemolysis) or by the sucrose hemolysis test. Currently the **best test is to perform flow cytometry for CD55 and CD59.**
  - Associated with several hematologic complications, including **pancytopenia, venous thromboses** (especially Budd-Chiari), and progression to myelodysplasia, aplastic anemia, or AML. Can also cause massive hemoglobinuria, resulting in acute renal failure, as well as iron deposition, resulting in CKD and proximal tubule dysfunction.
- **Sickle cell anemia:** This subtype is covered in the hemoglobinopathy section below.

Microangiopathies

A 44-year-old woman presents with three days of increasing confusion and fevers. She has no medical problems, takes no medications, and is not sexually active. On exam, her temperature is 38.6°C (101.5°F), BP 136/72 mm Hg, HR 92, and RR 18. She appears confused but has an otherwise nonfocal neurologic exam. The remainder of her exam is normal except for petechiae at the sites of her blood pressure cuff. Labs reveal a WBC count of 12,000, a hemoglobin level of 8.5 g/dL, and a platelet count of 22,000/μL. Creatinine is 1.4 mg/dL, LDH is 1250 IU/L, and PT and PTT are normal, as are CXRs and UA. Peripheral smear demonstrates 2+ schistocytes. She is placed on empiric antibiotics for possible infection, and over the next two days her platelet count and hemoglobin continue to drop while her creatinine rises. Her blood and urine cultures remain ⊖ and LP results are normal, but she continues to spike intermittent fevers. On the third hospital day she has a seizure. Her brain MRI is normal. What is the most likely diagnosis, and what is the treatment for the suspected condition?

The combination of anemia and thrombocytopenia in this previously healthy woman raises suspicion for a microangiopathic hemolytic anemia (MAHA). The ↑ LDH lends further support to this diagnosis. Of the MAHAs, thrombotic thrombocytopenic purpura (TTP) is most likely based on the normal PT and PTT (ruling out DIC) and the presence of fever, neurologic findings, and acute renal failure. Treatment is plasma exchange with fresh frozen plasma (FFP).

Table 9.6 outlines the distinguishing features and treatment of microangiopathies.

TABLE 9.6.   **Differential and Treatment of Microangiopathies**

Causes of Microangiopathy	Distinguishing Features	Treatment
DIC	Associated with severe infection, sepsis, and intravascular thrombus. Consumptive coagulopathy. ↑ **PT and PTT;** low fibrinogen.	Treat the underlying condition; cryoprecipitate (FFP if indicated).
TTP	↑ LDH, neurologic symptoms, normal coagulation tests (unless concomitant DIC).	**Plasma exchange with FFP;** steroids; **no platelet transfusions.**
HUS	↑ LDH, renal insufficiency, normal coagulation tests (unless concomitant DIC).	Hemodialysis if necessary; may be self-limited.
Preeclampsia	Peripartum period; hypertension.	Early delivery; diuretics, antihypertensives.
HELLP syndrome	Peripartum period; ↑ liver enzymes; probably a variant of eclampsia.	Early delivery.
Malignant hypertension	Hypertension.	Antihypertensives.
Vasculitis	Features of specific vasculitis.	Treat the underlying condition.
Miscellaneous (metastatic cancer, mechanical heart valve, severe burns)		Treat the underlying condition.

THROMBOTIC THROMBOCYTOPENIC PURPURA (TTP)

A rare disorder of unknown etiology that is characterized by microangiopathy, ↑ **LDH,** and neurologic changes tempered by appropriate clinical suspicion. The **classic pentad—fever, microangiopathic hemolytic anemia, thrombocytopenia, neurologic changes, and renal failure**—is seen in < 10% of cases.

SYMPTOMS/EXAM

- Patients usually present with anemia, bleeding, or neurologic abnormalities.
- Neurologic changes can be subtle and may include personality changes, headache, confusion, lethargy, or coma.

DIFFERENTIAL

Associated conditions include the following:

- **Medications:** Cyclosporine, tacrolimus, quinine, ticlopidine, clopidogrel, mitomycin C, estrogens.
- **Pregnancy:** Overlaps with eclampsia and HELLP.
- **Autoimmune disorders:** SLE, antiphospholipid antibody syndrome, scleroderma, vasculitis.
- **HIV.**
- **Bone marrow transplantation:** Autologous or allogeneic.

KEY FACT

The classic pentad for TTP is fever, microangiopathic hemolytic anemia, thrombocytopenia, neurologic changes, and renal failure—but rarely are all five seen together.

KEY FACT

There is no one diagnostic test that is specific for TTP, but LDH is almost always ↑.

DIAGNOSIS

- Peripheral smear shows evidence of thrombocytopenia with microangiopathy (ie, **schistocytes**). **PT/PTT should be normal unless DIC is also present.**
- ADAMTS13, the von Willebrand factor–cleaving protease that is deficient in TTP, can be measured, but the test is not entirely reliable and is generally too slow to be clinically useful. No standardized lab test exists for TTP, but **LDH is almost always ↑**.
- **It is unusual for platelets to be < 50,000/µL** unless another disorder is also present.

TREATMENT

- **Plasmapheresis:** Plasma exchange using FFP has a high response rate but must be continued daily until neurologic symptoms resolve and LDH remains stable.
- If the patient is in a facility that lacks the capability for plasmapheresis, treatment can be temporized with FFP infusion.
- Splenectomy is also used for relapsing cases.
- Platelet transfusion is contraindicated unless serious bleeding is present.

HEMOLYTIC-UREMIC SYNDROME (HUS)

- Similar to TTP, but **without neurologic changes and with more prominent renal failure.**
- Sx/Exam:
  - Characterized by microangiopathy, ↑ LDH, and **renal failure.**
  - Primarily a self-limited disease in children that is **associated with diarrheal illnesses** (eg, *E coli* O157:H7, *Shigella*, *Campylobacter*) but may be associated with the same medications and conditions as TTP.
- Tx: Treat with supportive care and renal replacement therapy as needed for uremic symptoms. Plasma exchange is generally part of the treatment in adults unless the HUS is associated with diarrheal illness, in which case it has not been shown to be of benefit.

Hemoglobinopathies

THALASSEMIAS

- In normal patients, adult hemoglobin (HbA) is **primarily (97–99%) composed of two α chains plus two β chains** ($\alpha_2\beta_2$). In **thalassemia**, there is a ↓ amount of either α or β chain. As a result, HbA is ↓, while there is an ↑ in variant forms of hemoglobin such as HbA$_2$ and HbF. There are **two general types of thalassemias: α and β.**
  - **α-thalassemias:** Seen in patients from **Southeast Asia and China;** rarely seen in African Americans.
  - **β-thalassemias:** Seen in patients from the **Mediterranean;** rarely seen in Asians or African Americans.
- The severity of α-thalassemia depends on the number of α-globin genes functioning (see Table 9.7).
- β-thalassemia can be further subdivided into three types: β-thalassemia major, intermedia, and minor (see Table 9.8).
- Dx: Peripheral smear typically shows microcytosis, hypochromia, and basophilic stippling (β-thalassemia only). With increasing severity, ↑ nucleated RBCs and target cells are seen (see Figure 9.6).

TABLE 9.7. **Differential Diagnosis of α-Thalassemias**

	α-THALASSEMIA TRAIT	HEMOGLOBIN H DISEASE	HYDROPS FETALIS
α-globin chains	2–3	1	0
Hematocrit	28–40%	22–32%	N/A
Hemoglobin electrophoresis	**Normal**	10–40% HbH	N/A
Clinical course	Normal life span	Chronic hemolytic anemia, exacerbated by stress	Universally lethal as neonate

SICKLE CELL ANEMIA

A 30-year-old woman with sickle cell disease presents to the hospital with left-sided weakness. She has had many episodes of acute chest syndrome. Her medications include folic acid and hydroxyurea. MRI is consistent with an acute infarction in the right MCA territory. What is an appropriate means of preventing stroke in sickle cell disease patients?

Monthly erythrocyte transfusions of two units per month in adults ↓ stroke recurrence.

Characterized by a homozygous defect in the β-globin gene that produces HbS. Heterozygotes have the sickle cell trait and are clinically normal except under extreme stress. Sickling is ↑ by **dehydration, acidosis, or hypoxia.** Peripheral smear shows **target cells, Howell-Jolly bodies,** and classic **sickle cells** (see Figure 9.7).

TABLE 9.8. **Differential Diagnosis of β-Thalassemias**

	β-THALASSEMIA MAJOR (COOLEY'S ANEMIA)	β-THALASSEMIA INTERMEDIA	β-THALASSEMIA MINOR
β-globin synthesis	Almost complete absence	Moderately ↓	Near normal (heterozygous)
Hematocrit	< 10% without transfusions	Variably low	28–40%
HbA	0%	0–30%	80–95%
HbA$_2$	4–10%	0–10%	4–8%
HbF	90–96%	90–100%	1–5%
Life span	20–30 years	Adult	Normal
Transfusion dependent	Yes	Variable	No
Clinical notes	Bony anomalies, hepatosplenomegaly, jaundice, transfusional iron overload	Mild bony anomalies; mild hepatosplenomegaly	Asymptomatic; mild microcytic anemia

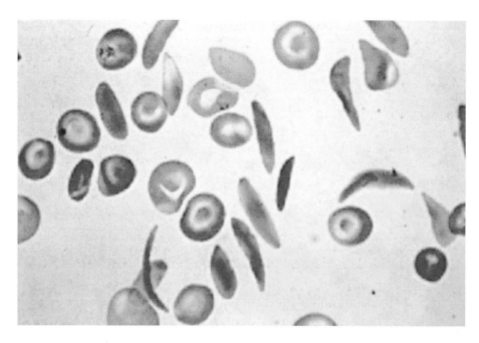

FIGURE 9.7. **Sickle cell anemia.** Multiple sickle forms are characteristic. (Reproduced with permission from USMLERx.com.)

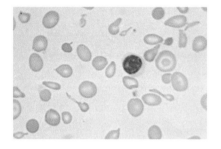

FIGURE 9.6. β-thalassemia intermedia. Note the microcytic and hypochromic RBCs. Many elliptical and teardrop-shaped red blood cells can also be seen. (Reproduced with permission from Fauci AS et al. *Harrison's Principles of Internal Medicine,* 17th ed. New York: McGraw-Hill, 2008, Fig. 99-5.)

SYMPTOMS/EXAM

The clinical manifestations of sickle cell anemia are due to unstable sickle cells that hemolyze and aggregate to cause vaso-occlusion.

- **Acute vaso-occlusion:** Manifests as pain crises, acute chest syndrome, priapism, stroke, and splenic sequestration.
- **Chronic vaso-occlusion:** Presents as renal papillary necrosis, avascular necrosis, autosplenectomy, and retinal hemorrhage (see Figure 9.8).
- **Chronic hemolytic anemia:** Presents as jaundice, pigment gallstones, and aplastic crisis.
- **Pain crises:**
  - Can result from vaso-occlusion in any organ or tissue, typically in bones.
  - Triggered by factors that promote sickling: hypoxia, dehydration, and infection.
  - Commonly manifest as pain in the back and long bones lasting for hours to days.
- **Acute chest syndrome:**
  - Results from vaso-occlusion in the pulmonary microvasculature; ↑ **mortality.**
  - Characterized by **chest pain, hypoxia, fever, pulmonary infarcts, or infiltrates on CXR.**
  - May be impossible to differentiate from pulmonary embolism (PE) and pneumonia.
  - Repeated episodes can lead to pulmonary hypertension and cor pulmonale.

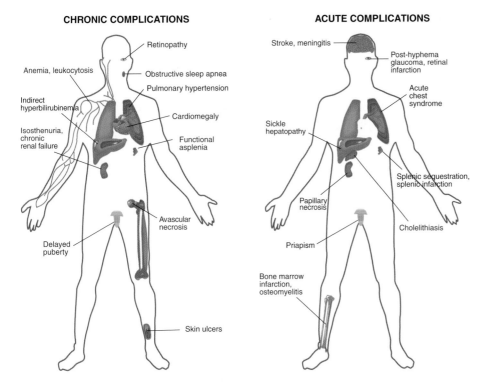

CHRONIC COMPLICATIONS

Retinopathy

Anemia, leukocytosis

Obstructive sleep apnea

Pulmonary hypertension

Indirect
hyperbilirubinemia

Cardiomegaly

Isosthenuria,
chronic
renal failure

Functional
asplenia

Avascular
necrosis

Delayed
puberty

Skin ulcers

ACUTE COMPLICATIONS

Stroke, meningitis

Post-hyphema
glaucoma, retinal
infarction

Acute
chest
syndrome

Sickle
hepatopathy

Splenic sequestration,
splenic infarction

Papillary
necrosis

Cholelithiasis

Priapism

Bone marrow
infarction,
osteomyelitis

FIGURE 9.8.   Chronic and acute complications of sickle cell disease.

TREATMENT

- **Maintenance:**
  - Although not universally accepted, folate supplementation may be required.
  - Pneumococcal vaccination.
  - Screen yearly for retinal disease and renal dysfunction.
  - Consider hydroxyurea in patients with > 3 pain crises per year requiring hospitalization or in those with repeated episodes of acute chest syndrome.
- **Acute episodes:**
  - Treat pain crises with aggressive hydration, analgesics, supplemental O_2, and incentive spirometry.
  - Transfusions should be avoided given the risk of alloimmunization and iron overload. However, transfusions are indicated for severe vaso-occlusive emergencies (acute chest syndrome, priapism, stroke). Transfuse until HbS is < 30%; initiate **exchange transfusion if necessary to keep hemoglobin ≤ 10 g/dL.**
- **Acute chest syndrome:** In addition to hydration, analgesics, O_2, and transfusion, acute chest syndrome should be treated with **antibiotics covering for *Streptococcus pneumoniae*, *Haemophilus influenzae*, *Mycoplasma pneumoniae*, and *Chlamydia pneumoniae*.** May require ICU admission.

KEY FACT

Acute chest syndrome should be treated with careful hydration, adequate analgesics, O_2, and either transfusion to a hemoglobin of 10 g/dL or exchange transfusion if the hemoglobin is already ≥ 10 g/dL. In addition, antibiotics to cover for *S pneumoniae*, *H influenzae*, *M pneumoniae*, and *C pneumoniae* should be administered.

TABLE 9.9. Causes of 2° Erythrocytosis

TYPE	ETIOLOGY
Congenital	High-affinity hemoglobin, congenitally low 2,3-DPG, autonomous high erythropoietin.
Arterial hypoxemia	High altitude, cyanotic heart disease, COPD, sleep apnea.
Renal lesions	Renal tumors, renal cysts, hydronephrosis, renal artery stenosis.
Liver lesions	Hepatoma, hepatitis.
Tumors	Adrenal adenoma, carcinoid, uterine fibroids, cerebellar hemangioblastoma.
Medications	Androgens.

Other CBC Abnormalities

ERYTHROCYTOSIS

Categorized mainly as 1° (polycythemia rubra vera) or 2° (reactive). The causes of **2° erythrocytosis** are listed in Table 9.9.

DIAGNOSIS

- If hematocrit is > 60% in males or > 56% in females, it is by definition an ↑ RBC mass, and measurement of RBC mass is not necessary.
- Exclude obvious causes of 2° erythrocytosis (see Table 9.9).
- See Table 9.10 for additional tests to consider.
- In smokers, pulse oximetry is sufficient to measure arterial O_2 saturation. An O_2 saturation of < 92% is low enough to cause erythrocytosis.
- In nonsmokers, an ABG with carboxyhemoglobin level is necessary.
- Low erythropoietin levels are suggestive of polycythemia vera but are not perfectly sensitive or specific.
- Low ferritin and high B_{12}/folate levels are associated with polycythemia vera and not with 2° erythrocytosis.

TREATMENT

No specific management of 2° erythrocytosis is necessary. The treatment of polycythemia vera is covered in a separate section.

KEY FACT

In a patient with an ↑ hematocrit who is not dehydrated or hypoxic, a low erythropoietin level is suggestive, but not diagnostic, of polycythemia vera.

TABLE 9.10. Evaluation of Erythrocytosis

LABS	IMAGING
Arterial O_2 saturation	RBC mass
Ferritin, B_{12}, folate, creatinine, LFTs, uric acid	Abdominal ultrasound or CT scan
Serum erythropoietin	
JAK2 mutation	

THROMBOCYTOPENIA

A 65-year-old woman presents to the hospital with a new diagnosis of right lower extremity DVT. Her past medical history is notable for a recent hospitalization in which she was given low-molecular-weight heparin (LMWH). Her CBC shows a platelet count of 100,000/μL. The patient is given IV unfractionated heparin, and 10 hours later her platelet count drops to 20,000/μL. What is the most appropriate next step in management?

Stop the unfractionated heparin and initiate argatroban. Heparin-induced thrombocytopenia (HIT) classically occurs 5–10 days after initial heparin exposure but may be delayed up to three months. As in this case, reexposure to heparin can result in a more rapid ↓ in platelet count. Management of suspected HIT requires stopping heparin and starting a direct thrombin inhibitor.

Defined as a platelet count of $< 150 \times 10^9$/L. Causes are outlined in Table 9.11.

DIAGNOSIS

- Examine a peripheral smear.
    - Rule out platelet clumping. Ask for a count/smear done in citrate, as EDTA (the anticoagulant most often employed in tubes used to collect a CBC) can cause clumping of platelets not seen on smear.
    - Look for evidence of microangiopathy (ie, schistocytes), marrow suppression (megaloblastic changes, dysplastic changes), and immature platelets (giant platelets) suggesting ↑ platelet turnover.

TABLE 9.11.   Causes of Thrombocytopenia

CAUSE	EXAMPLES
↑ destruction	**Immune thrombocytopenia:**
	▪ **1°:** Autoimmune (ITP).
	▪ **2°:** Lymphoid malignancies, HIV, SLE, alloimmunization from prior platelet transfusions.
	▪ **Drug induced:** Gold, abciximab, ticlopidine, quinine, heparin.
	▪ **Posttransfusion purpura.**
	Microangiopathies:
	▪ TTP, HUS, eclampsia.
	▪ DIC, sepsis.
	▪ Severe hypertension.
	Mechanical:
	▪ Artificial heart valves.
	▪ Hemangiomas.
	▪ Central venous catheters.
	Hypersplenism.
↓ production	Essentially any cause of marrow suppression can produce thrombocytopenia in isolation. See the pancytopenia discussion below.
	Probably the most important is drug-induced thrombocytopenia.
Other	**Dilutional:** From massive blood transfusions and fluid resuscitation.
	Pseudothrombocytopenia: From platelet clumping.

- Take a careful drug history.
  - Acetaminophen, H₂ blockers, sulfa drugs, furosemide, captopril, digoxin, and β-lactam antibiotics are all associated with thrombocytopenia.
  - Never forget **HIT** (see the discussion of clotting disorders below).
- Consider bone marrow biopsy if other findings suggest marrow dysfunction.
- Platelet-associated antibody tests are **not** useful.
- ITP is a diagnosis of exclusion.

TREATMENT

- Treat the underlying cause.
- Platelet transfusions in the absence of bleeding are usually unnecessary. Specific guidelines are given in the discussion of transfusion medicine. Platelet transfusions are **contraindicated** in TTP/HUS and HIT.

THROMBOCYTOSIS

Defined as a platelet count of $> 450 \times 10^9$/L. The main distinction is **reactive thrombocytosis** vs. **myeloproliferative disorder.** The steps involved in the evaluation of thrombocytosis are outlined in Table 9.12.

NEUTROPHILIA

- Defined as an absolute neutrophil count (ANC) of $> 10 \times 10^9$/L. The main distinction to be made is between myeloproliferative disorders (**typically CML**) and reactive neutrophilia.
- Reactive neutrophilia is readily apparent from the history (inflammation, infection, severe burns, glucocorticoids, epinephrine) and from examination of a peripheral smear (Döhle bodies, toxic granulations).

TABLE 9.12. Evaluation of Thrombocytosis

STEPS IN EVALUATION	COMMENTS
Repeat CBC and examine peripheral smear	An ↑ platelet count may be spurious or transient. Clues to reactive thrombocytosis may be present.
Stratify by degree of thrombocytosis	A platelet count of < 600k is unlikely to be essential thrombocythemia. A platelet count of > 1000k is less likely to be reactive thrombocytosis, but many "platelet millionaires" still have reactive thrombocytosis.
Identify causes of reactive thrombocytosis	Iron deficiency anemia, RA, IBD, infection or inflammatory states, postsplenectomy, active malignancy, myelodysplasia with 5q–, sideroblastic anemia.
Rule out other myeloproliferative syndromes	Consider testing for the JAK2 mutation for essential thrombocythemia. BCR-ABL by PCR in CML. Elevated RBC mass in polycythemia. Characteristic peripheral smear and splenomegaly in myelofibrosis.
Consider a bone marrow biopsy	Megakaryocyte morphology can suggest essential thrombocythemia. Examination for myelodysplasia, sideroblasts.

EOSINOPHILIA

- Defined as an absolute eosinophil count of $> 0.5 \times 10^9$/L. May be 1° (idiopathic) or 2°.
- **Idiopathic hypereosinophilia syndrome:**
  - Extremely rare and heterogeneous.
  - A prolonged eosinophilia of unknown cause with the potential to affect multiple organs by eosinophil infiltration.
  - Almost all cases have bone marrow infiltration, but heart, lung, and CNS involvement predicts a worse outcome.
  - Some cases are treatable with imatinib mesylate (Gleevec).
- **2° eosinophilia:** Remember the mnemonic **NAACP.**

MNEMONIC

Causes of 2° eosinophilia–

NAACP

Neoplastic
Asthma/**A**llergic
Addison's
Collagen vascular disease
Parasites

NEUTROPENIA

A 60-year-old woman who recently underwent a bone marrow transplant is rehospitalized with neutropenic fever. Empiric ceftazidime and vancomycin are begun, but her fever persists for > 72 hours despite ⊖ blood cultures. What is the next step in management?

Fungal and viral infections must be considered in patients with prolonged neutropenia. Consider adding caspofungin for the empiric treatment of possible invasive fungal infection.

- Defined as an ANC of $< 1.5 \times 10^9$/L (< 1.2 in African Americans). Causes are outlined in Table 9.13.
- **Gram-⊕ organisms** account for **60–70% of cases of neutropenic fever.**
- For further details, see the discussion of neutropenic fever in the Oncology chapter.

TABLE 9.13. Causes of Neutropenia

IMPAIRED PRODUCTION	↑ DESTRUCTION
Cytotoxic chemotherapy and other drugs	Autoimmune neutropenia
Aplastic anemia and other causes of marrow failure	Felty's syndrome
	Sepsis
Congenital	HIV
Cyclic neutropenia	Acute viral illness

TABLE 9.14. Summary of Peripheral Smear Morphology—RBCs

RBC Form	Associated Conditions
Schistocytes	Microangiopathy, intravascular hemolysis.
Spherocytes	Extravascular hemolysis, hereditary spherocytosis.
Target cell	Liver disease, hemoglobinopathy.
Teardrop cell	Myelofibrosis, thalassemia.
Burr cell (echinocyte)	Uremia.
Spur cell (acanthocyte)	Liver disease.
Howell-Jolly body	Postsplenectomy, functional asplenia.

PANCYTOPENIA

- Almost always represents ↓ or ineffective bone marrow activity. Differentiated as follows:
  - **Intrinsic bone marrow failure:** Aplastic anemia, myelodysplasia, acute leukemia, myeloma, drugs (chemotherapy, chloramphenicol, sulfonamides, antibiotics).
  - **Infectious:** HIV, post-hepatitis, parvovirus B19.
  - **Marrow infiltration:** TB, disseminated fungal infection (especially coccidioidomycosis and histoplasmosis), metastatic malignancy.
- **Dx:** Peripheral smear morphology is often helpful in diagnosis (see Tables 9.14 and 9.15).

TABLE 9.15. Summary of Peripheral Smear Morphology—WBCs

WBC Form	Associated Conditions
Atypical lymphocyte	Mononucleosis, toxoplasmosis, CMV, HIV.
Döhle body, toxic granulations	Infections, sepsis.
Hypersegmented neutrophil	B_{12} deficiency.
Auer rods	AML.
Pelger-Huët anomaly	Myelodysplasia, congenital.

Bone Marrow Failure Syndromes

APLASTIC ANEMIA

Marrow failure with hypocellular bone marrow and no dysplasia. Typically seen in young adults or the elderly. Subtypes are as follows:

- **Autoimmune (1°) aplastic anemia:** The **most common type.** Assumed when 2° causes have been ruled out.
- **2° aplastic anemia:** Can be caused by multiple factors.
  - **Toxins:** Benzene, toluene, insecticides.
  - **Drugs:**
    - Gold, chloramphenicol, clozapine, sulfonamides, tolbutamide, phenytoin, carbamazepine, allopurinol, and many others.
    - Post-chemotherapy or -radiation.
  - **Viral:** Post-hepatitis, parvovirus B19, HIV, CMV, EBV.
  - **Other:** PNH, pregnancy.

SYMPTOMS/EXAM

- Presents with symptoms of pancytopenia (fatigue, bleeding, infections).
- **Adenopathy and splenomegaly are generally not seen.**

DIAGNOSIS

- **Labs: Pancytopenia and markedly ↓ reticulocytes** are classically seen.
- **Peripheral smear:** Pancytopenia without dysplastic changes.
- **Bone marrow:** Hypocellular without dysplasia.

TREATMENT

- Supportive care as necessary (transfusions, antibiotics).
- **1° aplastic anemia:**
  - Definitive treatment is allogeneic bone marrow transplantation.
  - Remissions can sometimes be induced with antithymocyte globulin and cyclosporine.
- **2° aplastic anemia:** Treat by correcting the underlying disorder.

PURE RED CELL APLASIA (PRCA)

Marrow failure in erythroid lineage only.

SYMPTOMS/EXAM

Symptoms are related to anemia.

DIFFERENTIAL

After other causes of isolated anemia have been excluded, distinguish autoimmune PRCA from that stemming from abnormal erythropoiesis.

- **Autoimmune: Thymoma,** lymphoma/CLL, HIV, SLE, **parvovirus B19.**
- **Abnormal erythropoiesis:** Hereditary spherocytosis, sickle cell anemia, drugs (phenytoin, chloramphenicol).

KEY FACT

Suspect aplastic anemia in an otherwise healthy young adult with pancytopenia, no blasts on peripheral smear, and a hypocellular bone marrow. Take a careful history for meds and exposures, and send tests for viruses. For idiopathic aplastic anemia, consider antithymocyte globulin and cyclosporine or allogeneic bone marrow transplant.

KEY FACT

Immunosuppressive therapy with antithymocyte globulin and cyclosporine is effective in reducing transfusion requirements in > 70% of patients with aplastic anemia.

DIAGNOSIS

- **CBC:** Presents with anemia that is often profound, but WBC and platelet counts are normal. Reticulocytes are markedly ↓.
- **Peripheral smear:** No dysplastic changes.
- **Bone marrow biopsy:** Abnormal erythroid maturation and characteristic giant pronormoblasts are seen in parvovirus B19 infection.
- Obtain parvovirus B19 serology or PCR.

TREATMENT

- IVIG may be helpful in cases due to parvovirus.
- Remove thymoma if present.
- Immunosuppression with antithymocyte globulin and cyclosporine.

MYELODYSPLASTIC SYNDROME (MDS)

A 70-year-old man presents to his primary care physician with fatigue. CBC reveals a normal WBC and platelet count, but his hemoglobin level is 8.5 mg/dL with an MCV of 102 fL. He takes no medications or alcohol, and his B_{12} and folate levels are normal. What is the most likely diagnosis? Myelodysplasia, which commonly presents as isolated macrocytic anemia in older adults.

A clonal stem cell disorder that results in ineffective hematopoiesis and cytopenias and exists on a continuum with acute leukemia. **Eighty percent of patients are > 60 years of age.** MDS is associated with myelotoxic drugs and ionizing radiation. The prognosis is related to the percentage of blasts, cytogenetics, and the number of cytopenias.

SYMPTOMS/EXAM

Symptoms are related to those of cytopenias.

DIFFERENTIAL

Dysplasia can occur with vitamin B_{12} deficiency, viral infections (including HIV), and exposure to marrow toxins, so these factors must be ruled out before a diagnosis of MDS can be made.

DIAGNOSIS

Peripheral smear shows dysplasia.

- **RBCs:** Macrocytosis, macro-ovalocytes.
- **WBCs:** Hypogranularity; hypolobulation (pseudo–Pelger-Huët).
- **Platelets:** Giant or hypogranular.
- **Bone marrow:** Dysplasia; typically hypercellular. Cytogenetics can be normal or abnormal.

TREATMENT

- Supportive care with transfusions and growth factors.
- Chemotherapy with demethylating agents (eg, azacytidine or decitabine) or lenalidomide.
- Bone marrow transplantation is occasionally performed in younger patients.

Myeloproliferative Syndromes

A group of syndromes characterized by **clonal ↑ of bone marrow RBCs, WBCs, platelets, or fibroblasts.** Each is defined by the cell lineages predominantly affected. Syndromes have **considerable clinical overlap,** and it is often difficult to distinguish them (see Table 9.16).

POLYCYTHEMIA VERA

Defined as an abnormal ↑ in all blood cells, predominantly RBCs. The most common of the myeloproliferative disorders, it shows no clear age predominance.

Symptoms/Exam

- **Splenomegaly** is common.
- Symptoms are related to **higher blood viscosity** and expanded blood volume and include dizziness, headache, tinnitus, blurred vision, and plethora.
- **Erythromelalgia** is frequently associated with polycythemia vera and is characterized by erythema, warmth, and pain in the distal extremities. May progress to digital ischemia.
- Rarer findings include generalized **pruritus,** epistaxis, hyperuricemia, and iron deficiency from chronic GI bleeding.

Diagnosis

- Exclude 2° erythrocytosis.
- Bone marrow aspirate and biopsy with cytogenetics.
- A mutation of **JAK2,** a tyrosine kinase, is found in 65–95% of patients. Although not yet part of the diagnostic criteria, it can be used to help distinguish polycythemia vera from 2° erythrocytosis in unclear cases (but note that JAK2 is mutated in other myeloproliferative disorders and is not diagnostic for polycythemia vera).
- **Diagnostic criteria from the Polycythemia Vera Study Group** are outlined in Table 9.17.

KEY FACT

Erythromelalgia presents as erythema, warmth, and pain in the distal extremities, typically after a hot bath. It is often associated with polycythemia vera, and ASA relieves the symptoms.

KEY FACT

To diagnose polycythemia vera, you must have at a minimum an ↑ hemoglobin level (or RBC mass) **and** no other cause of 2° erythrocytosis. In polycythemia vera, JAK2 is often ⊕, and erythropoietin levels are low.

KEY FACT

The JAK2 mutation is seen in all myeloproliferative disorders but is most strongly associated with polycythemia vera.

TABLE 9.16.   Differentiation of Myeloproliferative Disorders

	WBC Count	**Hematocrit**	**Platelets**	**RBC Morphology**	**Comments**
Polycythemia vera	Normal or ↑	↑	Normal or ↑	Normal	JAK2 ⊕ in ~ 90% of cases.
CML	↑	Normal or ↓	Normal	Normal	Philadelphia chromosome or BCR-ABL ⊕ in > 95% of cases.
Myelofibrosis	Variable	**Usually** ↓	Variable	**Abnormal**	JAK2 ⊕ in 40–60% of cases.
Essential thrombocythemia	Normal or ↑	Normal	↑	Normal	JAK2 ⊕ in 50–60% of cases.

TABLE 9.17. Polycythemia Vera Study Group Criteria[a]

"A" Criteria	"B" Criteria
A1: Raised RBC mass or hematocrit ≥ 60% in males, 56% in females.	**B1:** Platelet count > 400,000.
A2: Absence of cause of 2° erythrocytosis.	**B2:** Neutrophil count > 10,000 (> 12,500 in smokers).
A3: Palpable splenomegaly.	**B3:** Splenomegaly by imaging.
A4: Abnormal marrow karyotype.	**B4:** Characteristic bone marrow colony growth (almost never used) or low serum erythropoietin.

[a]A1 + A2 + A3 or A4 = polycythemia vera; A1 + A2 + any two B = polycythemia vera.

TREATMENT

- No treatment clearly affects the natural history of the disease, so treatment should be aimed at controlling symptoms.
- Phlebotomy to keep hematocrit < 45% treats viscosity symptoms.
- Helpful medications include the following:
  - Hydroxyurea or anagrelide to keep the platelet count < 400,000/μL; both medications have been shown to prevent thromboses.
  - Allopurinol if uric acid is ↑.
  - The current standard is to recommend **low-dose ASA** in patients with erythromelalgia or other microvascular manifestations. **Avoid ASA in patients with a history of GI bleeding or a platelet count > 1 × 10^9/μL** (except in the setting of erythromelalgia or microvascular symptoms).

COMPLICATIONS

Predisposes to both clotting and bleeding; may progress to myelofibrosis or acute leukemia.

CHRONIC MYELOGENOUS LEUKEMIA (CML)

A 75-year-old man presents with headache and visual blurring of one week's duration. His neurologic exam is normal, including visual acuity, and the remainder of his physical exam is unremarkable except for mild splenomegaly. Labs show a WBC count of 322,000/μL, of which 85% are neutrophils, 7% are lymphocytes, 5% are basophils, and 3% are blasts. His hemoglobin level is 12 g/dL and platelet count 400,000/μL. The BCR-ABL fusion gene is detected by PCR. What treatment would you initiate to ↓ the patient's WBC count most quickly?

Hydroxyurea. This patient has CML complicated by leukostasis (as evidenced by headache and visual changes), and hydroxyurea will bring down his WBC count most quickly. However, this is just a temporizing measure, so therapy with imatinib should also be initiated to treat the underlying CML.

An excessive accumulation of neutrophils defined by chromosomal translocation t(9;22), the **Philadelphia chromosome**, producing the fusion protein **BCR-ABL**.

SYMPTOMS/EXAM

- Typically presents with an asymptomatic ↑ in WBC count or with nonspecific fatigue, night sweats, and hepatosplenomegaly.
- **Leukostasis syndrome** includes visual disturbances, headache, dyspnea, MI, TIA/CVA, and priapism, which are typically seen when the **WBC count is > 300,000/μL.**

DIAGNOSIS

- Markedly ↑ neutrophil count.
- Basophilia, eosinophilia, and thrombocytosis may also be seen (see Figure 9.9).
- The **Philadelphia chromosome is present in 90–95% of cases.** Detectable by **cytogenetics** or by **PCR** for the **BCR-ABL** fusion gene, performed on peripheral WBCs.
- Leukocyte alkaline phosphatase is low but rarely necessary.
- Bone marrow biopsy is not necessary for diagnosis but is often done to determine the prognosis.

TREATMENT

- **First line:** Major remissions can virtually always be achieved with **imatinib mesylate (Gleevec).** After five years, > 80% of patients remain in cytogenetic remission.
- The only curative therapy remains allogeneic bone marrow transplantation.
- Temporizing therapies to ↓ WBC counts include hydroxyurea, α-interferon, and low-dose cytarabine.

KEY FACT

CML is associated with the Philadelphia chromosome, t(9;22), in 90–95% of cases. First-line treatment is generally a tyrosine kinase inhibitor called imatinib that targets the unique gene product of the Philadelphia chromosome, BCR-ABL.

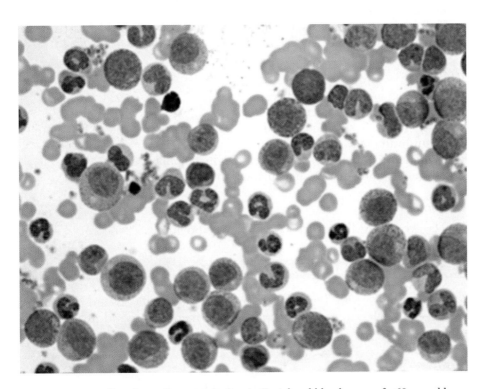

FIGURE 9.9. Chronic myelogenous leukemia. Peripheral blood smear of a 60-year-old man with a WBC count of 150,000/μL demonstrates markedly increased WBCs and large numbers of immature myeloid forms, including metamyelocytes, myelocytes, and promyelocytes, as well as a large number of eosinophils and basophils. (Reproduced with permission from USMLERx. com.)

COMPLICATIONS

- The disease has three phases based on the percentage of blasts in peripheral blood:
    - **Chronic phase:** Bone marrow and circulating blasts < 10%.
    - **Accelerated phase:** Bone marrow or circulating blasts 10–20%.
    - **Blast crisis:** Bone marrow or circulating blasts ≥ 20%.
- The natural history is progression from the chronic phase to the accelerated phase (median 3–4 years) and then to blast crisis.

MYELOFIBROSIS (AGNOGENIC MYELOID METAPLASIA)

Fibrosis of bone marrow leading to **extramedullary hematopoiesis** (marked splenomegaly; bizarre peripheral blood smear). Affects adults > 50 years of age and can be 2° to marrow insults, including other myeloproliferative disorders, radiation, toxins, and metastatic malignancies.

SYMPTOMS/EXAM

- Characterized by symptoms of cytopenia. Fatigue and bleeding are especially common.
- Abdominal fullness due to massive **splenomegaly and hepatomegaly.**

DIAGNOSIS

- CBC shows individual cytopenias or **pancytopenia.**
- Peripheral smear reveals **teardrops,** immature WBCs, nucleated RBCs, and giant degranulated platelets.
- The presence of the JAK2 mutation is not part of the diagnostic criteria but strongly supports the diagnosis.
- Bone marrow aspirate is frequently a **dry tap (no aspirate can be obtained);** biopsy shows marked fibrosis.

TREATMENT

- Treatment is mostly supportive.
- Give transfusions as necessary.
- Splenectomy or splenic irradiation is appropriate if the spleen is painful or if transfusion requirements are unacceptably high.
- α-interferon or thalidomide is occasionally helpful.
- Allogeneic bone marrow transplantation for selected patients.

COMPLICATIONS

May evolve into AML with an extremely poor prognosis.

ESSENTIAL THROMBOCYTHEMIA

A clonal disorder with ↑ platelet counts and a tendency toward thrombosis and bleeding. Has an indolent course with a **median survival of > 15 years** from diagnosis.

SYMPTOMS/EXAM

- Patients are usually asymptomatic at presentation.
- Occasionally presents with erythromelalgia, pruritus, and thrombosis (poses a risk for both arterial and venous clots).

DIAGNOSIS

- Primarily a **diagnosis of exclusion.** The first step is to rule out 2° causes of thrombocytosis (see separate section).
- Diagnosed by a persistent platelet count of > 600,000/µL with no other cause of thrombocytosis.
- As with polycythemia vera, it can be associated with mutation of the tyrosine kinase JAK2 (found in 50% of patients). This is not part of the diagnostic criteria but can be useful in distinguishing essential thrombocythemia from other causes of thrombocytosis.

TREATMENT

- No treatment is needed if there is no evidence of thrombotic phenomena and the platelet count is < 500,000/µL.
- Control platelet count with hydroxyurea, α-interferon, or anagrelide.
- Consider platelet pheresis for elevated platelets with severe bleeding or clotting.

COMPLICATIONS

The risk of conversion to acute leukemia is approximately 5% over a patient's lifetime.

Plasma Cell Dyscrasias

A group of disorders characterized by abnormal production of a paraprotein, often due to a monoclonal proliferation of plasma cells.

MULTIPLE MYELOMA

Symptoms are due to two aspects of myeloma:

- **Plasma cell infiltration:** Lytic bone lesions, hypercalcemia, anemia, plasmacytomas.
- **Paraprotein:** Depression of normal immunoglobulins leads to **infections;** excess protein may cause **renal tubular disease, amyloidosis,** or a **narrowed anion gap** (due to positively charged paraproteins).

DIAGNOSIS

The diagnostic criteria for multiple myeloma are delineated below and summarized in Table 9.18.

KEY FACT

The classic features of multiple myeloma are bone pain, anemia, hypercalcemia, and renal failure. However, don't forget subtle clues such as a narrowed anion gap and proteinuria that is dipstick ⊖ and detected only on specific urine protein testing (eg, 24-hour urine assay).

KEY FACT

Bone lesions in myeloma are purely osteolytic, so bone scans will be ⊖ and alkaline phosphatase will be normal. Order a plain film skeletal survey to evaluate for myeloma bone disease.

KEY FACT

The only potentially curative treatment for multiple myeloma is autologous stem cell transplantation, but this is feasible only in younger patients with good functional status.

TABLE 9.18.   Diagnostic Criteria for Multiple Myeloma[a]

MAJOR CRITERIA	MINOR CRITERIA
Bone marrow with > 30% plasma cells.	Bone marrow plasmacytosis 10–30%.
Monoclonal spike on SPEP > 3.5 g/dL for IgG or > 2 g/dL for IgA, or ≥ 1 g/24 hours of light chain on UPEP in the presence of amyloidosis.	Monoclonal globulin spike less than the levels in column 1.
	Lytic bone lesions.
Plasmacytoma on tissue biopsy.	Residual normal IgM < 50 mg/dL, IgA < 100 mg/dL, or IgG < 600 mg/dL.

[a]Diagnosis is established with one major and one minor criterion or with three minor criteria.

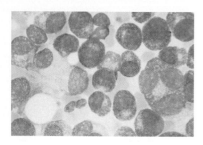

FIGURE 9.10. Multiple myeloma on bone marrow aspirate. Note the increased number of oval-shaped plasma cells with eccentric nuclei, dense nucleoli, and perinuclear clear space. (Reproduced with permission from Fauci AS et al. *Harrison's Principles of Internal Medicine,* 17th ed. New York: McGraw-Hill, 2008, Fig. 106-2.)

- **SPEP with immunofixation electrophoresis (IFE), UPEP with IFE:** To identify the M spike. Not all serum paraproteins are detectable in urine and vice versa.
- Bone marrow aspirate and biopsy (see Figure 9.10).
- **Skeletal bone plain film survey: Lytic lesions** are seen in 60–90% of patients (see Figure 9.11).
- Serum free light chains may be used to monitor response to therapy.

TREATMENT

Myeloma is rarely curable. The exception is a patient who can receive allogeneic stem cell transplantation. See Table 9.19 for treatment options.

COMPLICATIONS

Infection, renal failure, pathologic bony fractures, hypercalcemia, anemia.

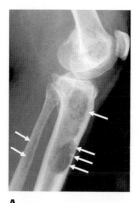

A

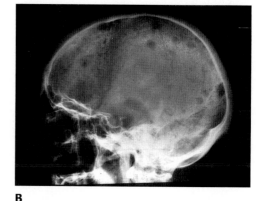

B

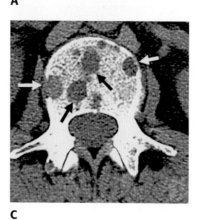

C

FIGURE 9.11. Multiple myeloma on plain film and CT. Characteristic lytic bony lesions of multiple myeloma involving the tibia and fibula (**A**) and the skull (**B**) as seen on plain films and the spine (**C**) as seen on CT. (Images A and C reproduced with permission from Lichtman MA et al. *Williams Hematology,* 8th ed. New York: McGraw-Hill, 2010, Fig. 109-13A. Image B reproduced with permission from Kantarjian HM. *MD Anderson Manual of Medical Oncology.* New York: McGraw-Hill, 2006, Fig. 8-1.)

TABLE 9.19.   **Treatment of Multiple Myeloma**

GOAL	TREATMENT
Reduce paraprotein	High-dose chemotherapy with autologous stem cell rescue (the standard of care, but limited to patients with good functional status). Steroid and alkylator combination chemotherapy. Biological molecules (thalidomide, lenalidomide, bortezomib).
Prevent skeletal complications	**IV bisphosphonate** if there is any evidence of skeletal compromise (bony lesions, osteopenia, hypercalcemia). No data exist for oral bisphosphonates. Radiation therapy and/or orthopedic surgery for impending pathologic fractures in weight-bearing bones.
Prevent infections	Pneumococcal and *Haemophilus* vaccines if not already immune.
Alleviate anemia	Reduce paraprotein. Consider erythropoietin or transfusion if severely symptomatic.
Prevent renal failure	Reduce paraprotein. Prevent hypercalcemia, dehydration.

AMYLOIDOSIS

A 54-year-old woman is evaluated for fatigue, weight loss, and dyspnea of two weeks' duration. Exam reveals a BP of 120/70 mm Hg reclining and 80/60 mm Hg while standing. She has bilateral lower extremity pitting edema and mild hepatomegaly. Laboratory studies are as follows: hemoglobin 12.8 g/dL, leukocyte count 8000/μL, platelet count 230,000/μL, INR 2.0, alkaline phosphatase 640 IU/L, and 4 g of protein in a 24-hour urine collection. Her ECG shows low voltage in all leads. What is the most likely diagnosis?

AL amyloidosis. Amyloidosis should be suspected in patients with multiorgan dysfunction and wasting. Common symptoms include weight loss, postural hypotension, hepatomegaly with ↑ alkaline phosphatase, a low-voltage ECG, and proteinuria. Macroglossia and cardiac involvement point to AL (light chain production) as the cause of amyloidosis.

A rare disorder characterized by the deposition of amyloid material throughout the body. Amyloid is composed of amyloid P protein and a fibrillar component. **The most common are AA and AL amyloid** (see Table 9.20).

SYMPTOMS/EXAM

The characteristics of amyloidosis are somewhat dependent on the type of amyloid and organs involved:

- **Renal:** Proteinuria, nephrotic syndrome, renal failure.
- **Cardiac:** Infiltrative cardiomyopathy, conduction block, arrhythmia, low-voltage ECG, hypertrophy, and a "speckled" pattern on echocardiography.
- **GI tract:** Dysmotility, obstruction, malabsorption.
- **Soft tissues: Macroglossia, carpal tunnel syndrome,** "shoulder pad" sign, "raccoon eyes."
- **Other:** Peripheral neuropathy, bleeding, factor X deficiency, lung nodules.

TABLE 9.20. Amyloid Types and Fibrillar Components

Type	Fibrillar Component	Association
AA	Acute-phase apolipoproteins	Chronic inflammation (TB, osteomyelitis, leprosy, familial Mediterranean fever)
AL	**Immunoglobulin light chain**	**Plasma cell dyscrasia (eg, multiple myeloma)**
ATTR	Transthyretin	Familial
AM	β_2-microglobulin	Hemodialysis

DIAGNOSIS

- **Tissue biopsy:** Amyloid yields the characteristic **apple-green birefringence** with Congo red stain.
- The choice of biopsy site depends on the clinical situation:
    - Biopsy of involved tissue has the highest yield.
    - Fat pad aspirate or rectal biopsies are generally low yield but minimally invasive.
- SPEP to screen for plasma cell dysplasias that cause AL amyloidosis.
- Once amyloid has been identified, investigate whether major organs are involved by ordering an ECG, echocardiography, and 24-hour urinary protein.

TREATMENT

Chemotherapy to ↓ the production of light chains is often recommended but is not very effective in AL amyloidosis.

KEY FACT

In chronic hemodialysis patients with carpal tunnel syndrome, consider AM amyloid from β_2-microglobulin accumulation in the wrists. This form of amyloid generally does not cause systemic disease.

OTHER DISEASES ASSOCIATED WITH A PARAPROTEIN

- **Monoclonal gammopathy of undetermined significance (MGUS):**
    - Presence of M spike without other criteria for myeloma.
    - One percent per year convert to myeloma, so monitor regularly for the development of myeloma.

TABLE 9.21. Distinguishing Features of Various Monoclonal Paraproteinemias

	Myeloma	MGUS	Waldenström's Macroglobulinemia	Amyloidosis
Abnormal cell	Plasma cell	Plasma cell	Lymphoplasmacytes	Plasma cell
Lytic bone lesions	**Present**	Absent	Absent	Absent
Paraprotein	> 3.5 g IgG or > 2 g IgA	Less than myeloma	Any **IgM**	Any
Bone marrow	> **10%** plasma cells	< **10%** plasma cells	Lymphoplasmacytes	Amyloid deposition
Tissue involvement	Plasmacytomas	None	None	Amyloid deposition
Splenomegaly or adenopathy	Absent	Absent	Present	Absent

- **Waldenström's macroglobulinemia** (see Table 9.21):
    - A low-grade indolent B-cell neoplasm characterized by **IgM** paraprotein.
    - Exam findings include lymphadenopathy, splenomegaly, hepatomegaly, and dilated, tortuous veins on retinal exam ("**sausage link**" veins). Treatment is the same as that for low-grade non-Hodgkin's lymphoma.
- **Hyperviscosity syndrome:** ↑ serum viscosity from IgM can occur, causing blurry vision, headaches, bleeding, and strokes. Emergent plasmapheresis can be used to ↓ serum viscosity by removing the IgM paraprotein.

> **KEY FACT**
>
> When you see splenomegaly and an IgM spike, think Waldenström's. Headache and visual changes are common symptoms of hyperviscosity, which is treated with emergent plasmapheresis.

Bleeding Disorders

APPROACH TO ABNORMAL BLEEDING

Excessive bleeding due to a defect in one of three variables: **blood vessels, coagulation factors,** or **platelets.**

Blood Vessel Disorders

- A rare cause of petechiae or purpura.
- Weakness of the vessel wall may be **hereditary** (eg, Ehlers-Danlos, Marfan's syndromes) or **acquired** (eg, vitamin C deficiency ["scurvy"], trauma, vasculitis).

> **KEY FACT**
>
> In a malnourished patient with gum bleeding and purple lesions located around the hair follicles of the legs, think scurvy and replace vitamin C.

Coagulation Factor Disorders

- Pose a significant bleeding risk only when clotting factor activity falls below 10%.
- **Hemarthroses** or deep tissue bleeds are most likely.
- Clotting factor disorders are either inherited or acquired (see also Tables 9.22 and 9.23).
- **Inherited disorders** include the following (see separate sections):
    - **Hemophilia A:** Deficiency in factor **VIII.**
    - **Hemophilia B:** Deficiency in factor **IX.**
    - **von Willebrand's disease (vWD).**

TABLE 9.22.   Diagnosis of Clotting Factor Disorders

CONDITION	PT	PTT	MIXING STUDY
Factor VII deficiency, warfarin use, vitamin K deficiency	Elevated	Normal	Corrects
Hemophilia	Normal	Elevated	Corrects
Heparin	Normal	Elevated	No correction unless heparin adsorbed
Factor VIII inhibitor	Normal	Elevated	No correction
Lupus anticoagulant	Normal	Elevated	No correction (test with Russell viper venom)
DIC	Elevated	Elevated	Minimal correction
Liver disease	Elevated	Elevated	Corrects
Dysfibrinogenemia	Elevated	Elevated	Variable correction (test with reptilase time)

TABLE 9.23. Comparison of Special Coagulation Tests

Test	Objective
Mixing study	To distinguish factor deficiency from inhibitor.
Reptilase time	To test for dysfibrinogenemia.
Russell viper venom test	To test for lupus anticoagulant.
Ristocetin cofactor assay	To test for vWF activity.

> **KEY FACT**
>
> Bleeding symptoms and hematologic abnormalities in patients with autoimmune disorders, in those with malignancy, or in the postpartum setting may be suggestive of an acquired factor VIII inhibitor. Mixing studies will not correct coagulation parameters.

- **Acquired disorders** are as follows:
  - **Factor inhibitors:** Elderly patients or patients with autoimmune diseases may acquire inhibitor, usually against factor VII or factor VIII.
  - **Anticoagulants:** Warfarin or heparin.
  - **Amyloid:** Associated with absorption of factor X in amyloid protein.
  - **Dysfibrinogenemia:** Seen in liver disease, HIV, lymphoma, and DIC.

Platelet Disorders

- Cause **petechiae**, mucosal bleeding, and menorrhagia; **exacerbated by ASA** and other medications.
- A prolonged bleeding time is seen but is not necessary for diagnosis.
- Defects may be **quantitative** (see the thrombocytopenia section) **or qualitative.**
- **Qualitative platelet disorders:**
  - The **most common inherited defect is von Willebrand's factor (vWF) deficiency** (see separate section).
  - **Others:** Medications (ASA, NSAIDs, IIB/IIIA inhibitors), uremia, and rare inherited defects (Glanzmann's thrombasthenia, Bernard-Soulier syndrome).

HEMOPHILIA

Hemophilias are **X-linked** deficiencies in clotting factors, so almost all patients are **male.**

- **Hemophilia A:** Factor VIII deficiency ("**A eight**").
- **Hemophilia B:** Factor IX deficiency ("**B nine**").

SYMPTOMS/EXAM

- Characterized by spontaneous bleeding in deep tissues, GI tract, and joints (hemarthroses).
- Variable in severity due to baseline percent factor activity.

DIAGNOSIS

- Labs reveal a normal PT and a prolonged PTT; a **mixing study corrects the defect (unless inhibitor is present).**
- Factor VIII or factor IX activity is low (0–10%).

TREATMENT

- There are two options for factor replacement:
  - **Recombinant factor:** Associated with less danger of HIV and HCV transmission than purified factor, but expensive.
  - **Purified factor concentrates:** Currently much safer than previous concentrates.
- Patients should be taught to self-administer factor in the event of spontaneous bleeding.
- Prophylaxis before procedures is as follows:
  - **Minor procedures:** For hemophilia A, DDAVP can be used if baseline factor VIII is 5–10%. Otherwise, replace with factor concentrates to 50–100% activity.
  - **Major procedures:** Replace with factor concentrate to 100% activity for the duration of the procedure with levels of at least 50% for 10–14 days (until the wound is healed).
- Acute bleeding:
  - **Minor bleeding:** Replace with factor concentrate to 25–50% activity.
  - **Major bleeding** (hemarthroses, deep tissue bleeding): Replace to 50% activity for 2–3 days.

VON WILLEBRAND'S DISEASE (vWD)

A 30-year-old woman presents with a 15-year history of heavy menses that last 10 days along with once-monthly episodes of epistaxis that have frequently required packing. Her mother and two sisters also have heavy menses, but gynecologic evaluation of the patient has identified no cause of menorrhagia. Her exam is normal. Labs are as follows: PT 11 sec, aPTT 40 sec, hemoglobin 9.6 g/dL, MCV 75 fL, platelet count 400,000/μL, and normal leukocyte count. What is the most likely cause of menorrhagia in this patient?

vWD with a history of mucosal bleeding and a mildly prolonged aPTT. Hemophilia is generally associated with marked prolongation of aPTT rather than with the mild prolongation seen here, and bleeding in patients with hemophilia most commonly occurs in the joints, not in the mucosa.

The **most common inherited bleeding disorder.** vWF complexes with factor VIII to induce platelet aggregation, and if there is dysfunction or deficiency of vWF, adequate platelet aggregation does not occur.

SYMPTOMS/EXAM

- Exhibits a bleeding pattern similar to that of a platelet disorder (**petechiae, mucosal bleeding/epistaxis, heavy menses, exacerbated by ASA**).
- Bleeding is generally provoked (eg, by ASA, trauma, surgery, circumcision, or dental work).

DIAGNOSIS

- There are three basic types; type I (↓ vWF) is the most common (see Table 9.24).
- Labs reveal a normal PT and a normal or prolonged PTT.
- If vWD is suspected, check ristocetin cofactor assay, von Willebrand antigen, and factor VIII activity level.

KEY FACT

Consider vWD in a patient with a normal platelet count in one of the following common clinical scenarios:
- Heavy menses.
- Bleeding after a minor dental procedure or arthroscopic surgery.
- A history of frequent epistaxis or epistaxis after starting ASA.
- A bleeding history that improves during pregnancy or on OCPs (estrogen ↑ vWF levels, so vWD often improves with the presence of additional hormones).

TABLE 9.24.   **Diagnosis of von Willebrand's Disease**

TYPE	FACTOR VIII ANTIGEN	vWF ACTIVITY (RISTOCETIN COFACTOR)	NOTES
I	Low/normal	Low	**The most common form.**
IIA	Low/normal	Absent	Abnormal vWF multimers.
IIB	Low/normal	Low/normal	Abnormal vWF multimers; **cannot use DDAVP.**
III	Low	Absent	

TREATMENT

- Avoid NSAIDs.
- Prophylaxis before procedures includes the following:
  - DDAVP is acceptable for minor procedures **except** in type IIB.
  - Purified factor VIII for major procedures.

DISSEMINATED INTRAVASCULAR COAGULATION (DIC)

- Consumptive coagulopathy characterized by **thrombocytopenia, ↑ PT and PTT,** and **schistocytes** on peripheral smear in association with serious illness.
- **Sx:** Acute DIC is often a catastrophic event and manifests as bleeding (eg, oozing from venipuncture sites) or clotting. In contrast, chronic DIC shows milder features and is associated with chronic illness (disseminated malignancy, intravascular thrombus).
- **Dx:** ↓ fibrinogen, ↓ platelets, prolonged PT/PTT, ↑ D-dimer, and **schistocytes.**
- **Tx:** Treat the underlying cause.
  - **Bleeding:** Cryoprecipitate can be given to achieve a fibrinogen level of > 100 mg/dL, and platelet transfusions can be administered to achieve a platelet count of $> 50 \times 10^9$ L.
  - **Clotting:** Low-dose IV heparin can be used to treat thrombotic complications. Given the risk of bleeding, a hematologist should be involved if a heparin drip is being used.

IMMUNE THROMBOCYTOPENIC PURPURA (ITP)

A disorder of reduced platelet survival, typically by immune destruction in the spleen. ITP commonly occurs in childhood with viral illnesses but may also affect young adults. Subtypes and their associated causes are as follows:

- 1°: No identifiable cause.
- 2°: Medications (gold, quinine, β-lactam antibiotics), CLL, SLE, HIV, HCV.

SYMPTOMS/EXAM

- Typically presents with **petechiae, purpura, mucosal bleeding, and menorrhagia.**
- Spleen size is normal.

KEY FACT

Isolated thrombocytopenia in an otherwise healthy young adult is most likely ITP. ITP is a clinical diagnosis, and bone marrow examination is not required. Bone marrow aspirate and biopsy are reserved for those who do not respond to prednisone therapy or who are > 60 years of age. 2° ITP may occur in SLE, HIV, CLL, and HCV.

TABLE 9.25. **Treatment of ITP**

TREATMENT	DOSE	EFFICACY	NOTES
Prednisone	1 mg/kg/day × 4–6 weeks	60% response rate	Time to remission is 1–3 weeks. **First-line treatment, but 90% of adults will relapse.**
IVIG	1 g/kg × 1 or 0.4 g/kg/day × 2	80–90% response rate	Rapid remission, but short-lived. Used for acute bleeding risk.
Splenectomy	N/A	70% remission rate	May require looking for accessory spleen.
Danazol	600 mg/day	10–80% response rate	Usually second line.
Anti-RhD	50 µg/kg × 1	80–90% response rate	Induces hemolytic anemia; works only with Rh-⊕ patients.
Rituximab	375 mg/m² q wk × 4 doses	30% response rate in chronic refractory ITP	Can cause allergic reactions.

DIAGNOSIS

- Diagnosis is made by excluding other causes of thrombocytopenia.
- Antiplatelet antibodies, platelet survival times, degree of ↑ in platelet count after platelet transfusion, and bone marrow biopsy are **not** needed for diagnosis. However, if the patient is > 60 years of age, a bone marrow biopsy is recommended to evaluate for myelodysplasia as the cause of thrombocytopenia.

TREATMENT

Consensus guidelines are that treatment is not necessary if platelet counts are > 30,000–50,000/µL and there is no bleeding. In the presence of acute bleeding, platelets can be transfused. Further treatment guidelines are given in Table 9.25.

Clotting Disorders

 A 70-year-old man is admitted to the ICU with severe sepsis from pneumonia. To facilitate early goal-directed therapy, a central venous catheter is inserted in his right internal jugular vein. Four days later, he develops right upper extremity swelling, and ultrasound reveals thrombosis of his right axillary vein. He has a normal creatinine level and weighs 187 pounds. He is started on LMWH and warfarin. Does his catheter need to be removed?

No, catheter-associated upper extremity DVTs do not require catheter removal. Remove the catheter as soon as it is no longer needed or it is not functioning properly.

Several days later the patient is transferred from the ICU to the ward, and discharge planning is begun. Assuming that the patient has no contraindications, what is the optimal duration of anticoagulation for upper extremity DVT, and does his catheter need to be removed?

Upper extremity DVTs carry same risk of PE as DVTs occurring at other sites and should thus be treated in the same manner. In this patient with a provoked DVT, three months of anticoagulation with warfarin adjusted to a goal INR of 2–3 is indicated.

KEY FACT

If a patient has ITP with a platelet count of > 30,000–50,000/µL and no bleeding, consideration should be given to surveillance with no active treatment.

KEY FACT

In ITP, avoid transfusing platelets unless the patient is actively bleeding.

KEY FACT

In an adult with ITP that is refractory to steroids, splenectomy is the most effective way to induce remission.

KEY FACT

In a patient with unprovoked DVT whose baseline PTT is prolonged, consider antiphospholipid antibody syndrome.

KEY FACT

Looking for very rare genetic conditions to explain a common problem is not cost-effective. Evaluation for rare causes of thrombophilia should be done only after common causes have been eliminated and in consultation with a hematologist.

KEY FACT

In a patient with active cancer who develops a DVT or PE, treatment with LMWH or fondaparinux for the first three months is superior to warfarin.

KEY FACT

In a patient with new DVT or PE, LMWH or fondaparinux is superior to unfractionated heparin for initial anticoagulation. Unfractionated heparin should be used only in the setting of renal failure, extreme obesity, or bleeding concerns.

APPROACH TO THROMBOPHILIA

Major risk factors for venous thromboembolism (VTE) include prior VTE, pregnancy, surgery, smoking, prolonged immobilization, hospitalization for any cause, and active malignancy. Suspect an **inherited thrombophilia** in the following conditions:

- An unprovoked clot occurring in a young person (< 50 years of age).
- A clot in an unusual location (eg, mesenteric vein, sagittal sinus).
- An unusually extensive clot.
- Arterial and venous clots.
- A strong family history.

DIFFERENTIAL

If arterial clots are present, the list of possible disorders shortens (see Table 9.26).

DIAGNOSIS

Diagnostic testing at time of diagnosis of VTE includes history and physical, CBC, PTT, and age-appropriate screening (see Table 9.26). Additional testing for hereditary thrombophilia is rarely indicated.

TABLE 9.26. **Differential Diagnosis of Clotting Disorders**

DIFFERENTIAL DIAGNOSIS	MODE OF EVALUATION
Arterial and venous:	
Malignancy	Age-appropriate cancer screening.
HIT syndrome	HIT antibody (antiplatelet factor 4).
Hyperhomocysteinemia	Homocysteine level.
PNH	**Flow cytometry** (to detect abnormal RBCs lacking CD55 and CD59).
Myeloproliferative disorders[a]	CBC.
Antiphospholipid antibody syndrome	Lupus anticoagulant, anticardiolipin antibody, anti-β_2 glycoprotein.
Venous only:	
Factor V Leiden	Check for factor V Leiden mutation.
Prothrombin 20210 mutation	Check for prothrombin 20210 mutation.
Protein C or S deficiency	Protein C and S levels.
Antithrombin III deficiency	Antithrombin III level.
Oral estrogens	N/A
Postsurgical, pregnancy, immobilization	N/A
Arterial only:	
Atherosclerosis	N/A
Vasculitis	N/A

[a]Essential thrombocythemia, polycythemia vera.

TREATMENT

Treatment is as follows (see also Table 9.27):

- **Provoked VTE** (eg, postop): Safe to treat for three months.
- **Unprovoked VTE:** Most patients are treated for 3–6 months at an INR of 2–3.
- **Exceptions** are as follows:
  - **Active cancer:** Treat with LMWH or fondaparinux for the first three months; continue treatment indefinitely as long the cancer is active.
  - **Antiphospholipid antibody syndrome:** Indefinite duration to ↓ the rate of recurrent VTE.
  - **Mechanical heart valves:** A higher INR (3–4) is indicated for lifelong treatment.
  - **Life-threatening VTE:** Many experts extend treatment to 12 months or indefinitely.

KEY FACT

If you see a patient with mesenteric vein thrombosis, pancytopenia, and dark urine (hemoglobinuria), think PNH and order flow cytometry to confirm.

TABLE 9.27.   Guide to Anticoagulant Medications

MEDICATIONS	PROS	CONS	TESTS USED TO MONITOR
Unfractionated heparin	Short half-life; can turn off quickly if the patient bleeds. Although falling out of favor, this is still appropriate for acute coronary syndromes, cardiopulmonary bypass, acute thrombotic events, mechanical heart valves, and anticoagulation in renal failure.	Requires continuous IV infusion. Long-term use is associated with osteoporosis. May cause HIT.	Need to monitor PTT and platelet count at least daily (for HIT). Reversible with **protamine**.
LMWH	No need to monitor PTT, as dosing is weight based.	Requires injection. Not reversible with protamine. Contraindicated in renal failure.	Will not prolong PTT; if monitoring is required, measure anti–factor Xa activity.
Warfarin	Oral.	Slow to reach therapeutic effect; requires the addition of unfractionated heparin or LMWH when starting for an acute clot. **Teratogenic;** many drug interactions. Warfarin skin necrosis (rare).	Monitor with INR; the usual goal range is an INR of 2–3. Duration varies with the clinical situation. Reversible with FFP or vitamin K.
Factor Xa inhibitors (fondaparinux)	No need for monitoring, as dosing is weight based. Once-daily dosing.	Requires injection. Contraindicated in renal failure. No reversing agent if the patient bleeds.	Will not prolong PTT.
Direct thrombin inhibitors (lepirudin or argatroban)	Used for anticoagulation in patients with HIT.	Irreversible thrombin inhibitors; require continuous IV infusion.	Monitor with PTT.

SPECIFIC THROMBOPHILIC DISORDERS

Factor V Leiden

- Associated with **venous** clots only. Gene frequency is highest (5%) in Caucasians, with a higher prevalence in those with VTE. Heterozygotes have a three- to eightfold ↑ in the risk of venous thrombosis; homozygotes have a 50- to 80-fold ↑ risk.
- **Dx:** Testing is generally not indicated, as it does not affect current treatment recommendations.

Prothrombin 20210 Mutation

- Similar to factor V Leiden; seen primarily in Caucasians, and associated with an ↑ risk of venous thrombosis.
- **Dx:** Testing is generally not indicated.

Protein C and S Deficiency/Antithrombin III Deficiency

- **Rarer but higher risk** than factor V Leiden or prothrombin mutations.
- **Dx:** Given the rarity of these deficiencies, **testing is extremely low yield** in the absence of strong evidence of familial thrombophilia.

Hyperhomocysteinemia

- Can be **genetic** (caused by a mutation in genes for cystathionine β-synthase or methylene tetrahydrofolate reductase) or **acquired** (due to a deficiency in B_6, B_{12}, or folate or to smoking, older age, or renal insufficiency). Carries an ↑ risk of **venous and arterial** thrombosis.
- **Dx/Tx:** Screening is generally not indicated because treatment has not been shown to ↓ the risk of future clots. Test with a fasting serum homocysteine level and treat with folate supplementation (often with vitamins B_6 and B_{12} as well).

Antiphospholipid Antibody Syndrome (APLA)

- A syndrome of **vascular thrombi** or **recurrent spontaneous abortions** associated with laboratory evidence of autoantibody against phospholipids. **Catastrophic APLA** is a rare severe form that is associated with multiorgan failure and high mortality.
- **Dx:** Diagnosis requires a **clinical event and** antiphospholipid antibody. Clinical characteristics are as follows:
  - Venous and/or arterial thrombi.
  - Thrombocytopenia.
  - Livedo reticularis.
  - Recurrent spontaneous abortions.
  - **Antiphospholipid antibody:** Can include a variety of autoantibodies, but only one need be present. However, the autoantibody needs to be present on repeated testing separated by about three months to exclude false-⊕ results.
    - **Lupus anticoagulant:** A clue to this may be prolonged PTT; confirm with a mixing study and a **Russell viper venom test.**
    - **Anticardiolipin antibody.**
    - Other: Anti-$β_2$ glycoprotein I, **false-⊕ VDRL.**

Heparin-Induced Thrombocytopenia (HIT)

There are two types of HIT, as outlined in Table 9.28. Type I is characterized by a mild fall in platelet count that occurs in the first two days after heparin is initiated and usually returns to normal with continued heparin use. It has

KEY FACT

Suspect antiphospholipid antibody syndrome in a young woman with recurrent spontaneous abortions and a prolonged PTT.

TABLE 9.28.   Types of Heparin-Induced Thrombocytopenia

TYPE	DOSE DEPENDENT	SEVERITY OF THROMBOCYTOPENIA	TIMING OF THROMBOCYTOPENIA	CLINICALLY SIGNIFICANT	ETIOLOGY
I	Yes	Mild	Immediate	No	Heparin-induced platelet clumping
II	No	Moderate/ severe	4–7 days after exposure	**Yes**	Antibody against heparin-platelet complex

no clinical consequences. Type II is the more serious type and is an immune-mediated disorder in which antibodies form against the heparin–platelet factor 4 (PF4) complex.

SYMPTOMS/EXAM

- Type II HIT presents as follows:
    - A ↓ in platelet count after 4–7 days of exposure to heparin.
    - May cause **arterial or venous clots**.
- Less common with LMWH than with unfractionated heparin.
- Exposure to any dose of heparin (heparin flushes, heparin-coated catheters, minidose SQ heparin) can cause this syndrome.

DIAGNOSIS

- Type II HIT requires a high degree of clinical suspicion.
- Lab testing includes the following:
    - **Antibody against PF4.**
    - **Functional assay:** Detects abnormal platelet activation in response to heparin (heparin-induced platelet activation, serotonin release).

TREATMENT

- If any suspicion exists, immediately stop all heparin; do not wait for lab tests, as catastrophic thrombosis and/or bleeding can occur.
- If the degree of suspicion is high, **treat with direct thrombin inhibitors** (lepirudin, argatroban) until platelet counts recover given the high risk of thrombosis.
- **Warfarin monotherapy is contraindicated in acute HIT** in view of the risk of skin necrosis.

> **KEY FACT**
>
> In a patient with a high suspicion of HIT II, stop heparin and LMWH immediately while waiting for HIT test results, and initiate treatment with a direct thrombin inhibitor (lepirudin or argatroban).

Transfusion Medicine

PRETRANSFUSION TESTING

Pretransfusion tests include the following:

- **Type and cross:** Use when transfusion is **probable** (eg, in an acutely bleeding patient). Test recipient plasma for reactivity against RBC from the donor—ie, perform an indirect Coombs' test on **donor** RBCs.
- **Type and screen** (aka "type and hold"): Use when transfusion is **possible** (eg, in preoperative evaluation). Screen recipient plasma for antibodies—ie, perform an indirect Coombs' test on **recipient** RBCs.
- Consider the risks of transfusions (see Table 9.29).

TABLE 9.29. Risks of Transfusion Therapy

	RISK	CLINICAL FEATURES	TREATMENT	CAUSE	COMMENTS
Febrile nonhemolytic reactions	1–4 in 1000	Chills, rigors within 12 hours of transfusion.	Acetaminophen, diphenhydramine.	WBC or bacterial contaminant, cytokines.	**Most common reaction.**
Allergic reaction	1–4 in 1000	**Urticaria or bronchospasm.**	As usual for urticaria or bronchospasm.	Allergic reaction to plasma contaminant.	**Seen in IgA deficiency;** prevented through use of washed RBCs.
Delayed hemolysis	1 in 1000	Extravascular **hemolysis 5–10 days after transfusion:** jaundice, ↓ in hematocrit, ⊕ Coombs' test, microspherocytes in peripheral smear.	Supportive care; send sample to blood bank to work up new alloantibody.	Low-titer antibodies against minor blood antigens.	Multiparous women or multiply transfused patients may be at ↑ risk.
Transfusion-related acute lung injury (TRALI)	1 in 5000	Noncardiogenic pulmonary edema, usually within six hours of transfusion.	Supportive care.	**Donor antibodies to recipient leukocytes** in pulmonary capillaries.	Most cases resolve after 96 hours.
Acute hemolytic transfusion reaction	1 in 12,000	Chills, fever, backache, headache, hypotension, tachypnea, tachycardia. DIC may occur in severe cases.	Vigorous hydration to prevent acute tubular necrosis. If hemolysis is severe, consider forced diuresis with mannitol and urinary alkalinization.	Severe intravascular hemolysis due to antibody against donor RBCs **(typically ABO incompatibility).**	Usually due to a clerical error.
HBV	1 in 66,000				
HCV	1 in 103,000				
HIV	1 in 676,000				

MANAGEMENT OF TRANSFUSION REACTIONS

- **Stop the transfusion immediately.**
- Contact the blood bank immediately to initiate double-checking of paperwork.
- Draw a CBC, direct antiglobulin test, LDH, haptoglobin, indirect bilirubin, free hemoglobin, PT/PTT, UA, and urine hemoglobin.
- Repeat type and screen and draw a blood culture. Send all untransfused blood back to the blood bank with attached tubing.

TRANSFUSION PRODUCTS

Table 9.30 lists common types of transfusion products and their applications.

PLATELET TRANSFUSION THRESHOLD

The criteria for determining the platelet transfusion threshold are controversial but are as follows:

- A bleeding patient with a platelet count < 50,000.
- CNS bleeding with a platelet count < 100,000.
- Major surgery with a platelet count < 50,000.
- Asymptomatic with a platelet count < 10,000.

TABLE 9.30. Types of Transfusion Products

Product	Distinguishing Features	Use
Whole blood	Contains RBC and plasma.	Massive blood loss, as from trauma. Graft-versus-host disease.
Packed RBCs	Each unit of packed RBCs raises hemoglobin 1 g/dL.	Most patients who require RBC transfusion.
Washed RBCs	RBCs with plasma removed.	Prior allergic reactions, as seen in **IgA deficiency.**
Irradiated RBCs	Irradiation.	**Allogeneic stem cell transplant to prevent graft-versus-host disease.**
Leukocyte-depleted (leukoreduced) RBCs	Deplete donor leukocytes with WBC filter; costly.	Patients awaiting transplant; CMV-seronegative patients to prevent CMV transmission; patients with a prior transfusion reaction.
Random donor platelets	Pooled platelets from six donors. Each "six pack" should raise platelet count by 30,000–50,000/µL.	Most patients who need platelet transfusion.
Single-donor platelets	Platelets are extracted from a single donor by apheresis. Each unit should bump platelets by 30,000–50,000/µL.	Patients who are alloimmunized.
FFP	All clotting factors, but high fluid volume.	To correct coagulopathy of liver disease or excess warfarin.
Cryoprecipitate	Factor VIII, fibrinogen, and vWF.	**Use in DIC if fibrinogen is < 100 mg/dL.** Associated with a **high risk of transmitting infection** because it is not heat inactivated.

TABLE 9.31.   Malignant vs. Reactive Adenopathy

	FAVORS MALIGNANT	FAVORS REACTIVE
Patient characteristics	Smoker; older age.	Age < 40.
Size	Larger.	Lesions < 1 cm are almost always benign.
Consistency	Hard, matted, nontender, fixed.	Rubbery, mobile, tender.
Location	Supraclavicular (Virchow's node); periumbilical (Sister Mary Joseph's nodule).	Inguinal nodes up to 2 cm are normal.

KEY FACT

A firm, nontender left supraclavicular lymph node is Virchow's node and is a clue to GI or intrathoracic malignancy.

KEY FACT

Common causes of generalized lymphadenopathy include lymphoma, HIV, EBV, mycobacterial infection, SLE, and drug reactions (eg, phenytoin).

KEY FACT

In a patient with cirrhosis and new blistering skin lesions over sun-exposed hands and over the face, consider porphyria cutanea tarda.

Miscellaneous Hematology

LYMPHADENOPATHY

The 1° goal is to distinguish **malignant** from **reactive** adenopathy (see Table 9.31).

PORPHYRIAS

A variety of disorders that have in common genetic **defects in heme synthesis.** Two types may present in adults: acute intermittent porphyria and porphyria cutanea tarda.

Acute Intermittent Porphyria

- Caused by a defect in **porphobilinogen deaminase. Autosomal dominant;** most common in women in their 20s.
- Sx/Exam: Look for attacks of **abdominal pain, psychosis, and possibly SIADH,** triggered by menses, alcohol, caffeine, or meds (barbiturates, phenytoin, sulfonamides, estrogens).
- Dx: Look for excess **aminolevulinic acid or porphobilinogen in the urine.**
- Tx: **Avoid triggers;** use carbohydrates or IV heme to abort attacks.

VITAMIN DEFICIENCIES

Table 9.32 outlines common vitamin deficiencies and their associated disorders.

TABLE 9.32. **Common Vitamin Deficiencies**

Vitamin	Deficiency	Clinical Symptoms
A (retinol)		Night blindness, conjunctival xerosis, Bitot's spots (white spots on conjunctiva), keratomalacia.
B₁ (thiamine)	Dry beriberi, wet beriberi	Peripheral neuropathy, Wernicke-Korsakoff syndrome, high-output CHF, vascular leak.
B₂ (riboflavin)		Cheilosis, angular stomatitis, glossitis, weakness, corneal vascularization, anemia.
Niacin	Pellagra	**D**ermatitis, **D**iarrhea, **D**ementia (then **D**eath)—the **3 (or 4) D's.**
B₆ (pyridoxine)		Peripheral neuropathy, seizures, anemia (may be precipitated by INH).
C (ascorbic acid)	Scurvy	Perifollicular hemorrhage, petechiae, bleeding gums, hemarthrosis, poor wound healing.
D		Osteomalacia in adults; rickets in children.
E (α-tocopherol)		Areflexia, ophthalmoplegia, ↓ proprioception.

NOTES

CHAPTER 10

Hospital Medicine

Miten Vasa, MD

Ellis A. Johnson, MD, MPH

Robert L. Trowbridge, MD

Venous Thromboembolic Disease

A 30-year-old woman develops a lower extremity DVT one month following a cesarean section. She has had no previous venous thromboembolic events. She returns to the clinic after six months of anticoagulation with warfarin. Should warfarin be continued?

No. The patient had her first thrombotic event with transient risk factors (post-partum, following surgery). Therefore, it is appropriate to discontinue anticoagulation therapy after 3–6 months at a therapeutic INR.

KEY FACT

Almost all PE patients have dyspnea, pleurisy, or tachypnea, and the absence of all three argues against the diagnosis.

KEY FACT

In a patient with a PE, syncope is an ominous symptom, as it may represent a hemodynamically massive PE with impending cardiogenic shock.

KEY FACT

The results of the D-dimer, V/Q scan, and CT scan must be interpreted in conjunction with the pretest clinical probability.

PULMONARY EMBOLISM (PE)

The mortality rate for untreated venous thromboembolic disease exceeds 15%. Risk factors include **prior thromboembolic disease, malignancy, recent surgery, immobility, inherited thrombophilia, certain medications** (eg, OCPs, HRT), **tobacco use,** stroke, and **obesity.**

SYMPTOMS/EXAM

- There are no specific signs or symptoms for PE.
- **Dyspnea and pleurisy** are each seen in > 50% of cases.
- Less common are hemoptysis, fever, and cough.
- **Tachypnea, rales, tachycardia,** and a **loud P2** may be seen.

DIAGNOSIS

- **Clinical gestalt** is a powerful predictor of the likelihood of PE (see Table 10.1).
- The **modified Wells criteria** (see Table 10.2) more precisely refine the clinical gestalt:
  - **Wells score ≤ 4:** PE is unlikely. A low Wells score and a normal D-dimer rule out PE.
  - **Wells score > 4:** Further testing for PE is indicated.
- D-dimer:
  - Most useful for excluding PE in low-risk patients (ie, those with a modified Wells score ≤ 4) when levels are low or normal. The negative predictive value is high in these patients.
  - **The specificity of an elevated D-dimer is poor** (∼ 50%), as there are many reasons D-dimers may be elevated, particularly in older, hospitalized patients.

TABLE 10.1. Accuracy of Clinical Gestalt in Determining the Likelihood of PE[a]

CLINICAL LIKELIHOOD	ACTUAL INCIDENCE
Low (< 20%)	9%
Moderate (20–80%)	30%
High (> 80%)	68%

[a] According to the Prospective Investigation of Pulmonary Embolism Diagnosis (PIOPED) study.

TABLE 10.2.   Modified Wells Criteria for Pulmonary Embolism[a]

Clinical Findings That Increase Risk	Points
Clinical symptoms of DVT (leg swelling, pain with palpation)	3.0
Other diagnosis less likely than PE	3.0
Heart rate > 100	1.5
Immobilization (≥ 3 days) or surgery in the previous four weeks	1.5
Previous DVT/PE	1.5
Hemoptysis	1.0
Malignancy	1.0

[a]Scores > 4: PE is likely; scores ≤ 4: PE is unlikely.

- **Troponin:** May be elevated.
- **ABGs:** Respiratory alkalosis with an ↑ alveolar-arterial oxygen gradient is classically seen, although ABGs may be normal.
- **ECG:**
  - Nonspecific anterior T-wave inversions and sinus tachycardia are the most common ECG findings.
  - Evidence of new right heart strain—eg, a new RBBB, right axis deviation, and the combination of an S wave in lead I and a Q wave with an inverted T wave in lead III (**S1Q3T3**)—is less common but more suggestive of PE.

KEY FACT

Three clinical findings more specific for a massive PE are an ↑ P2, an S3 gallop, and cyanosis.

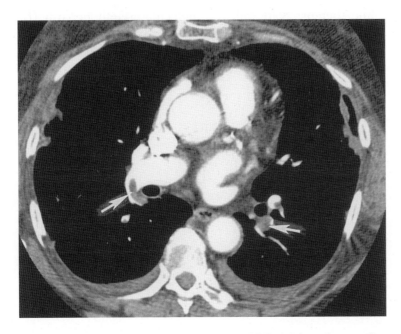

FIGURE 10.1.   CT angiogram demonstrating bilateral filling defects due to pulmonary emboli (arrows). (Reproduced with permission from Chen MY et al. *Basic Radiology.* New York: McGraw-Hill, 2004, Fig. 4-56C.)

TABLE 10.3.   **Pros and Cons of Diagnostic Tests in Pulmonary Embolism**

MODALITY	PROS	CONS	COMMENTS
V/Q scan	Noninvasive; results are well characterized.	Often not available after normal business hours; frequently nondiagnostic.	Performs best when baseline CXR is normal.
CT angiography	Specific; may reveal alternative diagnosis; better availability than V/Q in most hospitals.	Risk of contrast dye nephropathy; uncertain sensitivity, especially for smaller thrombi.	Sensitivity is < 90%; a ⊖ CT angiogram does not rule out PE.
Pulmonary angiography	The gold standard.	Most invasive; requires local expertise.	Perform only if other tests fail to establish the diagnosis.

KEY FACT

A V/Q result of "high probability for PE" is virtually diagnostic of PE when clinical suspicion is high. Similarly, "normal" or "low-probability" V/Q scans rule out PE when clinical suspicion is low. "Intermediate-probability" V/Q scans can never rule in or rule out PE.

KEY FACT

A D-dimer test is more useful in **ruling out** PE when normal; an elevated D-dimer is not specific for PE.

- **CXR:** Often shows nonspecific pleural effusion or atelectasis. Two rare findings suggest PE:
    - **Hampton's hump:** A pleural-based density representing pulmonary infarction.
    - **Westermark's sign:** Radiolucency distal to a pulmonary embolus due to oligemia.
- **Lower extremity venous Doppler ultrasound:** A thrombus is present in approximately 30% of PE cases.
- **CT angiogram:** See Figure 10.1 and Table 10.3.
- **Ventilation-perfusion (V/Q) scanning:** See Figure 10.2 and Tables 10.3 and 10.4.
- **Pulmonary angiogram:** See Table 10.3.

TREATMENT

- **First-line therapy:** Start with **low-molecular-weight heparin (LMWH)** (eg, enoxaparin 1 mg/kg SQ q 12 h) in stable patients. *or 1.5 mg/kg q24°*
- **Second-line therapy:** Give **IV unfractionated heparin,** adjusted to maintain therapeutic anti-Xa or PTT.

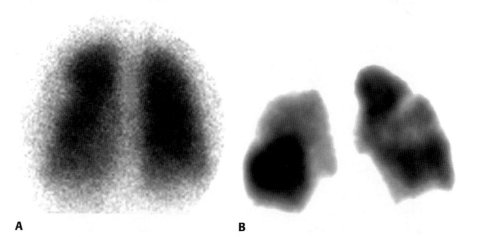

A   B

FIGURE 10.2.   **Lung scan for a 63-year-old woman who presented with idiopathic pulmonary embolism.** The lung scan showed normal ventilation (**A**) and multiple segmental perfusion defects (**B**), indicating a V/Q mismatch and a high probability of pulmonary embolism. (Reproduced with permission from Crawford MH. *Current Diagnosis & Treatment: Cardiology,* 3rd ed. New York: McGraw-Hill, 2009, Fig. 26-4.)

TABLE 10.4. **Probability of PE Based on V/Q Results and Clinical Probability**

V/Q Scan Result	High Clinical Probability	Intermediate Clinical Probability	Low Clinical Probability
High	95[a]	86	56
Intermediate	66	28	15
Low	40	15	4
Normal perfusion	0	6	2

[a]That is, 95% of patients with a high-probability V/Q scan and a high clinical probability were found to have a PE on angiography.

- Once the patient is adequately anticoagulated with heparin, **warfarin** should be started. Dual therapy should overlap for 4–5 days.
- The **duration of therapy** is somewhat controversial but should consist of at least 3–6 months of warfarin therapy with a goal INR of 2–3 for an initial provoked (reversible) episode.
  - Longer therapy is reserved for patients with idiopathic events or with risk factors for thrombophilia; recurrent events require lifelong anticoagulation.
  - For a full discussion of anticoagulants, refer to the Hematology chapter.
- Other treatment options are as follows:
  - **Factor Xa inhibitors** (eg, fondaparinux): Alternatives to LMWH in most clinical settings.
  - **Direct thrombin inhibitors:** Most commonly used in patients with heparin-induced thrombocytopenia, in whom standard heparin and LMWH are contraindicated. _ex argatroban_
  - **IVC filters:** Reserved for patients with contraindications to anticoagulation (see Table 10.5) and for those with recurrent events despite adequate anticoagulation. IVC filters ↓ the risk of PE in the short term (up to two weeks) but are associated with an ↑ incidence of recurrent lower extremity DVTs at two years.
  - **Thrombolysis** is controversial but is supported in the setting of massive PE (ie, for those with refractory hypotension due to PE).
  - **Surgical or catheter thrombectomy:** Last-ditch options for patients with hemodynamic compromise who fail or are not candidates for thrombolysis.

KEY FACT

LMWH and fondaparinux are superior to warfarin for the treatment of PE in patients with active cancer, but they are contraindicated in CKD.

KEY FACT

The two main indications for IVC filters in patients with PE are failed anticoagulation or a contraindication to anticoagulation.

TABLE 10.5. **Contraindications to Anticoagulation**

Absolute	Relative
Hemorrhagic stroke	Recent internal bleeding (within six months)
Active internal bleeding	Prior hemorrhagic stroke
Suspected aortic dissection	Thrombocytopenia
	CNS mass lesion (especially renal cell carcinoma and melanoma)

DEEP VENOUS THROMBOSIS (DVT)

Risk factors for DVT are the same as those for PE.

SYMPTOMS/EXAM

- **Pain, swelling,** or **erythema** of the affected extremity is most common.
- A **palpable cord** and low-grade **fever** are less commonly seen.
- Most thrombi occur in the **lower extremities,** although upper extremity thrombosis is increasing in frequency coincident with the use of long-term central venous catheters.
- Rarely, **phlegmasia cerulea dolens** (complete venous obstruction resulting in a painful, swollen, and bluish extremity) may be seen.

DIAGNOSIS

- **Compression/duplex ultrasonography:** Most common, and has a sensitivity and specificity of > 95%. Slightly less effective for thrombosis in the calf veins or above the inguinal ligament or for recent clots; consider repeat testing in 3–5 days if results are ⊖ but there is high clinical suspicion.
- **D-dimer:** As with PE, D-dimer is useful only when clinical suspicion is low, in which case a ⊖ D-dimer can rule out DVT or PE.

TREATMENT

Treatment is as outlined above for PE, with the following additional notes:

- **Outpatient therapy** should be an option only for patients who meet the following criteria:
  - Clinical stability with normal vital signs.
  - A low risk of bleeding.
  - Normal or near-normal renal function.
  - Adequate outpatient follow-up to ensure compliance and to monitor for complications.
- **Thrombolytic therapy** may result in fewer long-term complications (postphlebitic syndrome) at the expense of an ↑ risk of bleeding. Consider in patients (especially younger patients) with massive DVT, including phlegmasia cerulea dolens. IV therapy is equivalent to catheter-directed therapy.

PREVENTION

- Hospitalized medical and surgical patients are at risk for venous thromboembolic disease. Prophylaxis should thus be considered in all hospitalized patients.
- Although many regimens are effective, appropriate medications and doses vary according to the specific clinical scenario (see also Table 10.6):
  - **SQ "minidose" heparin:** Usually 5000 U SQ BID-TID.
  - **SQ LMWH or thrombin inhibitors:** Given at lower doses than those used for full anticoagulation—eg, enoxaparin 40 mg SQ daily; dalteparin 5000 U SQ daily; fondaparinux 2.5 mg SQ daily.
- **Elastic stockings** (thromboembolic disease stockings, or TEDS) and **sequential compression devices (SCDs)** may be used.
- Prophylaxis can be stopped in high-risk orthopedic patients who are discharged on anticoagulation once they are able to fully bear weight and ambulate (approximately 2–3 weeks postoperatively).

KEY FACT

Average-risk surgical patients (those without additional major risk factors) and medical inpatients should receive DVT prophylaxis with unfractionated heparin, LMWH (eg, enoxaparin, dalteparin), or fondaparinux. Use nonpharmacologic therapy (eg, TEDS, SCDs) if anticoagulation is contraindicated.

KEY FACT

Orthopedic patients or surgery patients with other major risk factors for DVT should be treated with LMWH or fondaparinux (or SCDs if anticoagulants are contraindicated).

TABLE 10.6. Selected Methods for the Prevention of Venous Thromboembolism

Risk Group	Recommendations for Prophylaxis
General surgery[a]	
Low risk	Early ambulation.
Moderate risk	Elastic stockings (ES), low-dose unfractionated heparin (LDUH),[c] LMWH, or intermittent pneumatic compression (IPC) + early ambulation if possible.
High risk	LMWH or fondaparinux is first line, in combination with IPC or ES. Second-line agents are warfarin or adjusted-dose IV unfractionated heparin + IPC or ES.
Orthopedic surgery	
Elective total hip or knee replacement surgery or hip fracture surgery	LMWH or fondaparinux is first line, in combination with IPC or ES. Second-line agents are warfarin or adjusted-dose IV unfractionated heparin + IPC or ES.
Neurosurgery	
Intracranial neurosurgery	LMWH or LDUH + IPC or ES.
Acute spinal cord injury	Same as above.
Trauma patients with an identifiable risk factor for thromboembolism	LMWH; IPC or ES if there is a contraindication to LMWH. Consider duplex ultrasound screening in very high risk patients. IVC filter insertion is appropriate if proximal DVT has been identified and anticoagulation is contraindicated.
Medical patients	
Most medical patients with expected length of stay > 3 days[b]	SQ LDUH, LMWH, or fondaparinux. Nonpharmacologic therapy with ES or IPC if anticoagulation is contraindicated.

[a]**Low risk:** Minor procedures, age < 40, and no clinical risk factors. **Moderate risk:** Minor procedures with additional thrombosis risk factors; age 40–60 and no other clinical risk factors; major operations with age < 40 and no additional clinical risk factors. **High risk:** Major operation; age > 40 or with additional risk factors.

[b]Especially patients with cancer, CHF, or severe pulmonary disease.

[c]LDUH 5000 U SQ q 8–12 h starting 1–2 hours before surgery.

(Adapted with permission from Tierney LM et al. *Current Medical Diagnosis & Treatment,* 44th ed. New York: McGraw-Hill, 2005: 283.)

Acute Pain Management

A 70-year-old man with metastatic lung cancer is hospitalized for severe pain of the hip and chest wall from bony metastases. The pain is not controlled with ibuprofen, acetaminophen, or oxycodone-acetaminophen, but it is adequately controlled with a continuous morphine sulfate infusion at a rate of 1 mg/hr, with breakthrough doses of IV morphine sulfate at a rate of 2 mg/hr. What would be an appropriate home regimen for this patient?

Controlled-released oral morphine sulfate (72 mg divided up 2–3 times daily) with immediate-release oral morphine sulfate (5–10 mg/hr) as needed. Dosages are based on equianalgesic conversion of IV to oral requirements—ie, morphine 10 mg IV = morphine 30 mg PO. When converting to a different opiate, however, you should factor in the incomplete cross-tolerance effect and consider decreasing the new opiate dose by 33–50% to start.

TABLE 10.7. **Opioid Loading Doses and Dosing Equivalency**

MEDICATION	COMMON TRADE NAMES	TYPICAL STARTING PARENTERAL DOSE (mg)	EQUIVALENT PO DOSE (mg)
Fentanyl	–	0.1	–
Hydromorphone	Dilaudid	1.5	7.5
Hydrocodone	Lortab, Vicodin	–	20
Oxycodone	Percocet, Percodan	–	20
Methadone	–	–	20
Morphine	Many	10	30
Meperidine	Demerol	75–100	–
Codeine	Many	–	200

KEY FACT

The lack of an adequate loading dose may result in frustrating efforts to "catch up" with the pain.

KEY FACT

IV-equivalent doses can be remembered as differing by roughly a factor of 10 (ie, fentanyl is 10 times as strong as hydromorphone, which is 10 times as strong as morphine, which is 10 times as strong as meperidine).

Several basic principles guide the management of acute pain in the hospitalized patient:

- The patient's description of symptoms is the most reliable indicator of pain.
    - **Mild to moderate pain:** Try nonopioid treatments first.
    - **Severe pain:** First select an **appropriate parenteral loading dose** with repeat doses every 10–15 minutes until pain relief has been achieved (see Table 10.7). Patients with active pain should not be treated with PRN medications alone.
- **Adjunctive measures** should be considered in all patients. The use of **nonsteroidal agents** in conjunction with opioids may be especially effective for postoperative pain. TCAs and gabapentin may also be effective for neuropathic pain.

Delirium

An 80-year-old woman with mild dementia, CAD, hypertension, hyperlipidemia, and type 2 DM undergoes an evaluation following surgical repair of a left hip fracture. Preoperatively she was on metoprolol, lisinopril, HCTZ, ASA, simvastatin, glipizide, and lorazepam as needed for sleep. On postoperative day 2, she is confused, agitated, and unable to focus attention on conversation or follow commands, and she is rambling incoherently. She is afebrile, and her vital signs and physical exam are unremarkable. What are the next steps in evaluating this patient's postoperative delirium?

Obtain an ECG, a CXR, and a metabolic panel, and review medications that can cause delirium as well as potential causes of postoperative delirium. After this initial evaluation, haloperidol or another antipsychotic can be considered for sedation. Behavioral and environmental interventions are also indicated, but restraints should be avoided. Empiric antibiotics, brain imaging, or LP can be pursued if indicated.

Occurs in up to 30% of hospitalized elderly patients. Patients often have multiple risk factors, including the following:

- **Underlying medical conditions:** Infection, fever, depression, dementia, substance abuse, pain, metabolic derangement.
- **Multiple medications:** Opioids, anticholinergics, benzodiazepines.
- **Other:** Advanced age, male gender, alterations in the sleep-wake cycle.

SYMPTOMS/EXAM

- Characterized by an **alteration in consciousness and cognition with rapid onset over hours to days.**
- **Symptoms wax and wane.**
- **Cognitive dysfunction:** Patients may be easily distracted and paranoid.

DIAGNOSIS

- Conduct a detailed physical exam, a review of the medication list, and appropriate lab studies (eg, electrolytes, serum calcium, TSH, UA, and CXR in the setting of new pulmonary findings).
- **CT of the head** is rarely useful, but consider in patients who are anticoagulated or have a history of trauma.
- **LP** should be performed only in the rare patient in whom there is clinical suspicion for meningitis.

TREATMENT/PREVENTION

- **Behavioral and environmental interventions** (eg, a quiet, supportive environment with orientation cues, nutrition, adequate sleep, hydration, regular mobility, and hearing aids/eyeglasses) can prevent up to one-third of delirium cases.
- **Pharmacologic treatment:**
  - When given in low doses, **haloperidol** can be effective as a second-line therapy.
  - Second-generation antipsychotic agents (**risperidone, olanzapine, quetiapine**) may be associated with ↑ mortality and should be prescribed with caution.

GI Prophylaxis in the Hospitalized Patient

Coagulopathy and **respiratory failure necessitating mechanical ventilation for at least 48 hours** are the most powerful risk factors for stress-related hemorrhage. Indications for prophylaxis are as follows (see also Table 10.8):

- **Coagulopathy: Platelet count < 50,000; INR > 1.5.**
- **Respiratory failure necessitating mechanical ventilation for at least 48 hours.**
- A history of ulceration or bleeding in the past year.
- Two or more of the following: sepsis, an ICU stay of > 1 week, glucocorticoid therapy, or an occult GI bleed for > 6 days.

KEY FACT

Although "hyperactive" delirium is more common, be aware of "hypoactive" delirium in the elderly.

KEY FACT

Potential causes of postoperative delirium include hyponatremia, severe hyperglycemia, severe anemia, hypoxemia, infection, unstable coronary syndrome, pneumonia, and CNS-altering medications (eg, opioids, benzodiazepines, anticholinergics).

KEY FACT

Avoidance of unnecessary medications and medical devices is key to preventing and treating delirium.

KEY FACT

Mechanical ventilation for > 48 hours and coagulopathy are the two most important risk factors for stress ulcer formation.

TABLE 10.8. Prophylaxis for GI Bleeding

TREATMENT	PROS	CONS
Sucralfate	Effective; reduces bleeding by 50%.	Interferes with the absorption of multiple medications; requires frequent dosing. Must be administered PO or through a feeding tube.
H$_2$ receptor blockers	As effective as sucralfate and easier to use; can be given IV or PO.	May be associated with an ↑ risk of nosocomial pneumonia.
PPIs	Likely as effective and easy to use as H$_2$ blockers.	Not as well studied for this purpose as the others; may ↑ the risk of nosocomial pneumonia and *C difficile* infection.
Enteral feeding	May ↓ bleeding risk.	Not as well studied for this purpose.

Perioperative Management

PREOPERATIVE CARDIAC EVALUATION

A 72-year-old woman with a history significant for type 2 DM (for which she takes insulin), pulmonary vascular disease, and previous CABG surgery is evaluated one week before elective infrainguinal peripheral vascular surgery for claudication. Her creatinine level is normal, and her urine shows no microalbuminuria. Which medication would ↓ her in-hospital perioperative cardiovascular risk and 30-day mortality rate?

This patient has two cardiac risks: CAD and DM requiring insulin. Thus, she would benefit from a perioperative β-blocker such as atenolol, which would ideally be started a week before surgery.

KEY FACT

Exercise treadmill testing, dipyridamole-thallium scintigraphy, and dobutamine stress echocardiography, when normal, predict a low risk of perioperative cardiac complications.

Cardiac disease is a frequent cause of perioperative morbidity and mortality, with 50,000 patients developing perioperative MIs each year. **Preoperative cardiac risk assessment** is therefore mandatory in all patients undergoing noncardiac surgery.

■ Risk assessment can be accomplished through use of a validated **risk prediction score** (see Table 10.9).

TABLE 10.9. Revised (Simplified) Cardiac Risk Index

RISK FACTOR	INTERPRETATION
Add one point for each risk factor: ■ Higher-risk surgery (thoracic, abdominal, or major vascular operation above the inguinal ligament) ■ Ischemic heart disease ■ CHF ■ Diabetes requiring insulin ■ Cerebrovascular disease (a history of stroke or TIA) ■ Renal insufficiency (Cr > 2)	The risk of major complications is 0.4%, 0.9%, 7%, and 11% for 0, 1, 2, and 3 or more points, respectively.

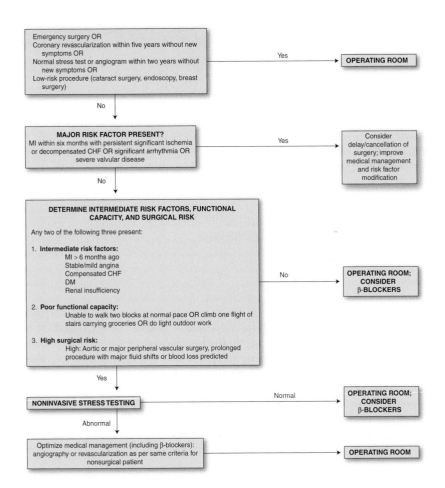

FIGURE 10.3.   Algorithm for further cardiac evaluation and intervention.

- Assessment of cardiac risk involves evaluation of three elements: **patient-specific variables, exercise capacity, and surgery-specific risk** (see Figure 10.3).
- The role of ischemia evaluation prior to noncardiac surgery is evolving. A recent study of patients undergoing vascular surgery at ↑ risk for perioperative cardiac events did just as well with a strategy of optimal medical management without further testing (ie, β-blockers) as they did with a strategy involving noninvasive testing.
- Patients considered for noninvasive ischemia testing independent of the planned noncardiac surgery should generally undergo such testing only if the test result might lead to coronary revascularization.
- In patients with known CAD who cannot exercise but have a high risk of cardiac complications by clinical assessment, dobutamine stress echocardiography is the preferred test.
- **Perioperative β-blockade:**
  - β-blockers may ↓ the risk of MI in patients undergoing major noncardiac surgery who are at ↑ risk (ie, those with a Revised Cardiac Risk Index ≥ 2; see Table 10.9) but may ↑ mortality (by increasing the risk of stroke, hypotension, and bradycardia) if such patients are not titrated appropriately to heart rate and BP.
  - Patients with no risk factors are at low risk, and β-blockers may have limited benefit or may be harmful.
  - When a β-blocker is given, β$_1$-cardioselective agents (eg, metoprolol or atenolol) should be used.

KEY FACT

"Prophylactic" CABG or angioplasty/stenting should not be done preoperatively unless it is likely to ↑ long-term survival.

KEY FACT

To recall the Revised Cardiac Risk Index, remember high-risk surgery, DM on insulin, and the "4 C's": **C**AD, **C**HF, **C**VA, and **C**KD.

KEY FACT

Patients considered for noninvasive ischemia testing should generally undergo such testing only if the test result might lead to coronary revascularization—ie, if they have new symptoms or worsening of symptoms suggestive of active CAD.

PREOPERATIVE PULMONARY EVALUATION

The major risk factors for perioperative pulmonary complications are as follows:

- **Surgical factors:** Surgery near the diaphragm (chest or abdominal surgery), head and neck surgery, prolonged surgery, and use of general anesthesia (vs. spinal/epidural).
- **Patient factors:**
    - Patients classified as American Society of Anesthesiologists (ASA) class ≥ 2.
    - Those with chronic lung disease, an abnormal chest exam or radiograph, a history of a prior stroke, or functional dependence.
    - Those who have smoked within the prior year or have had > 2 drinks of alcohol per day in the last two weeks.
    - Chronic steroid use.

PREVENTION

Preventive measures are as follows:

- **Smoking cessation:** Can significantly ↓ the risk of complications if completed at least two months preoperatively.
- **Incentive spirometry, including deep breathing exercises:** May ↓ the risk of complications; should be taught to the patient preoperatively.
- **Selective NG decompression:** Effective in preventing postoperative pulmonary complications after abdominal surgery in patients with nausea, vomiting, or abdominal distention.
- **Optimization of chronic lung disease.**

TABLE 10.10. Pre- and Postoperative Management of Chronic Disorders

CONDITION	POTENTIAL COMPLICATIONS	PREOPERATIVE MANAGEMENT	POSTOPERATIVE MANAGEMENT
DM, on insulin as outpatient	Hypo- and hyperglycemia, DKA, infection.	Give 50% of usual long-acting insulin on the morning of surgery with a glucose drip (the exception being glargine, which should be given at the usual dose the evening before surgery).	Strongly consider insulin drip titrating to normoglycemia; otherwise restart long-acting insulin with supplemental short-acting insulin (rapid titration of long-acting insulin).
DM, not on insulin	Hypo- and hyperglycemia; nonketotic hyperosmolar state; lactic acidosis (from metformin).	Omit oral hypoglycemic and metformin the day before surgery.	Consider insulin drip; use regularly scheduled short-acting insulin if needed and restart oral agent once able.
Chronic steroid use (especially greater than the equivalent of 20 mg prednisone × 3 weeks)	Adrenal crisis (rare).	Continue the usual dose.	Can usually give chronic dose; consider "stress-dose" steroids for longer/major surgeries (hydrocortisone 100 mg q 8 h × 2–3 days).
Liver disease	Mortality, hemorrhage, infection.	Optimize treatment of underlying complications; high morbidity and mortality for Child-Pugh Class C patients.	Optimize treatment of underlying complications.

- **Pulmonary function testing:** Not routinely useful in guiding treatment, but can yield an indication of the severity of underlying disease, and may help evaluate unexplained pulmonary symptoms.
- **ABG analysis** is not routinely necessary.
- **Antibiotics** should not be given routinely.

PERIOPERATIVE MANAGEMENT OF CHRONIC MEDICAL CONDITIONS

Table 10.10 lists guidelines for the perioperative management of chronic conditions.

Nutrition in the Hospitalized Patient

A 40-year-old alcoholic man is admitted to the hospital for pancreatitis. According to his friends, he had been drinking liquor all day for several weeks and eating only salty foods. During his hospitalization, he develops sepsis from a pancreatic abscess and requires drainage, vasopressor support, and mechanical ventilation. The patient is then started on total parenteral nutrition (TPN), 2000 calories daily in 2 L. For what condition is the patient at high risk after TPN is started?

Refeeding syndrome with high-carbohydrate loads in severely malnourished patients results in a dramatic ↑ in insulin levels, causing glucose, potassium, phosphate, and magnesium to shift into cells. The severe hypophosphatemia that results can lead to CHF, respiratory failure, rhabdomyolysis, cell dysfunction, seizures, and coma. Thus, phosphate levels should be closely monitored in severely malnourished patients. These patients need aggressive electrolyte supplementation.

> **KEY FACT**
>
> Poor perioperative glycemic control is associated with a higher incidence of infection as well as with delayed wound healing.

Nutritional options for hospitalized patients are summarized in Table 10.11.

TABLE 10.11.   **Indications for Enteral Feeding, TPN, and PPN**

	INDICATIONS	PROS	CONS
Enteral feeding	Nutritional needs cannot be met through oral feeding and supplements.	Less invasive; lower incidence of infectious complications. Preserved mucosal immunity and bowel integrity. More rapid transition to regular oral feeding.	Requires a functional GI tract; necessitates tube placement. Associated with an ↑ incidence of aspiration, although the risk may be lower with jejunal than with gastric tubes.
TPN	Long-term need (> 1–2 weeks) for supplemental or replacement nutrition; inability to use the GI tract.	Long-term therapy is possible.	The need for maintenance of central venous access can lead to catheter-related complications (2–3%). Catheter-related thromboses; metabolic complications (see Table 10.12).
PPN	Short-term need (< 1–2 weeks) for supplemental or replacement nutrition; inability to use the GI tract.	Does not require central venous access.	Effective only as a short-term option (1–2 weeks). Large-volume infusion.

TABLE 10.12.   **Metabolic Complications of TPN**

COMPLICATION	TREATMENT
Abnormal LFTs	↓ carbohydrate load; reconfigure the balance between fats, carbohydrates, and amino acids.
Acalculous cholecystitis (4% with long-term TPN)	Surgery.
Elevated BUN	Assess volume status; if adequate, ↓ the infusion rate and/or amino acid load.
Hyperglycemia	Frequent glucose checks; addition of insulin to TPN.
Micronutrient deficiencies (zinc, selenium, vitamin B_{12}, copper)	Regular supplementation.
Refeeding syndrome (hypophosphatemia, hypokalemia, hypomagnesemia)	Consider decreasing the infusion rate; electrolyte supplementation.

> **KEY FACT**
>
> Agents **not** bound by activated charcoal include lithium, ethanol/methanol/ethylene glycol, hydrocarbons, and heavy metals such as iron.

> **KEY FACT**
>
> The combination of an **elevated** anion gap and an **elevated** osmolar gap suggests the ingestion of ethanol, methanol, or ethylene glycol. The combination of a **normal** anion gap and an **elevated** osmolar gap suggests the ingestion of isopropyl alcohol.

> **KEY FACT**
>
> Liver enzymes and INR may be normal when a patient presents within 12 hours of a potentially lethal acetaminophen ingestion. Maintain a low threshold to initiate treatment with *N*-acetylcysteine.

Overdose/Toxic Ingestion

A 70-year-old suicidal man with a history of alcoholism is brought to the ICU following the ingestion of an unknown quantity of unspecified OTC pills. He is unresponsive and intubated; has diffuse crackles on lung exam; and is tachypneic, tachycardic, and febrile. Labs are as follows: Na 147 mEq/L, Cl 108 mEq/L, HCO_3 14 mEq/L, BUN 29 mg/dL, Cr 1.5 mg/dL, glucose 65 mg/dL, and serum osmolarity 319 mOsm/L. What substance is this patient most likely to have ingested, and how should his overdose be treated?

Salicylate overdose, which presents with altered mental status, hyperthermia, respiratory alkalosis, anion-gap metabolic acidosis, intravascular volume depletion, hypoglycemia, and noncardiogenic pulmonary edema. Treat with activated charcoal and gastric lavage; IV sodium bicarbonate infusion to alkalinize the urine in order to enhance salicylate excretion; and, because this is a severe toxicity (severely altered mental status), hemodialysis.

General guidelines for overdose and toxic ingestion are as follows (see also Tables 10.13 and 10.14):

- **Supportive care,** including volume/electrolyte repletion, is the mainstay of treatment.
- **Airway protection,** including endotracheal intubation if necessary.
- Screen all patients for **coingestions** for which there is a specific antidote or treatment (eg, acetaminophen, ASA).

TABLE 10.13. Comparison of Methods for Removing Toxins

Method	Pros	Cons
Activated charcoal with cathartics ("gut dialysis")	Binds most medications; safe.	Not effective for lithium, iron, alcohols, or hydrocarbons; must be given immediately. Contraindications include altered mental status, nausea, and bowel obstruction.
Gastric lavage	Can remove undigested pill fragments.	↑ risk of aspiration. Intubate prior to lavage if mental status is impaired. Useful only within the first 1–4 hours after ingestion.
Emetics (eg, ipecac)	Useful only when implemented < 1 hour after ingestion (if at all).	↑ risk of aspiration. **Avoid in most adults.**
Urine alkalinization to a pH > 7 with IV sodium bicarbonate	↑ the excretion of **ASA, TCAs, and phenobarbital.**	Ineffective for all other ingestions.
Hemodialysis	Effectively clears salicylates, digoxin, and toxins that are not bound by charcoal (lithium, methanol, ethylene glycol, isopropyl alcohol).	Invasive; not effective for removing benzodiazepines, opiates, or TCAs.
Charcoal hemoperfusion	Highly effective for digoxin, theophylline, and salicylates.	Invasive.

TABLE 10.14. Characteristics and Treatment of Common Ingestions

Substance	Manifestations	Lab Tests	Treatment	Comments
Acetaminophen	Initially presents with nausea and vomiting. An asymptomatic interval is followed by recurrent nausea, abdominal pain, and jaundice. Stages are as follows: ■ **Stage I (< 24 hours):** Nausea, malaise, lethargy, diaphoresis. ■ **Stage II (24–72 hours):** ↑ AST and ALT; ↓ stage I symptoms. ■ **Stage III (> 72 hours):** Altered mental status, bleeding, renal failure; LFTs peak. ■ **Stage IV:** Recovery stage possible.	Elevated acetaminophen level as a function of time of ingestion; > 150 µg/dL at four hours indicates the need for treatment. LFTs begin to rise within 12 hours, peaking at 4–6 days. AST and ALT may be markedly elevated (> 10,000 IU). PT is most indicative of prognosis (a PT < 90 predicts an 80% survival rate). Renal failure is seen in up to 50% of cases with hepatic failure.	Treat with **activated charcoal** if the patient presents within four hours of ingestion, if the level at that time is > 250 µg/mL, or if delayed absorption is suspected. Treatment-based nomogram. **N-acetylcysteine** (140-mg/kg load followed by 70 mg/kg q 4 h × 17 doses). Also available IV. **Immediate transfer to a liver transplant center** for progressive coagulopathy, acidosis, or liver failure.	N-acetylcysteine is most effective within 10 hours but may be effective significantly later. Chronic alcoholics are at risk for hepatotoxicity at lower doses of acetaminophen.

(continues)

TABLE 10.14.   Characteristics and Treatment of Common Ingestions *(continued)*

SUBSTANCE	MANIFESTATIONS	LAB TESTS	TREATMENT	COMMENTS
Aspirin	Nausea and vomiting; tinnitus; GI bleeding and volume depletion; mental status changes. Noncardiogenic pulmonary edema. Hyperthermia.	**Anion-gap metabolic acidosis with concomitant respiratory alkalosis. Elevated PT.** Elevated serum salicylate. Hepatotoxicity, hypoglycemia.	Activated charcoal and gastric lavage. **Sodium bicarbonate** to alkalinize serum and urine to promote renal elimination. **Hemodialysis** in the setting of severe acidosis, altered mental status, or levels > 80–100 mg/dL.	The threshold for hemodialysis should be lowered to 60 mg/dL for chronic ingestion.
Digoxin	GI symptoms, visual disturbance, confusion, bradycardia. Prolonged PR segment and "scooping" ST segment along with arrhythmias.	Hyperkalemia (potassium level correlates with the degree of acute toxicity). Hypokalemia may be seen in chronic toxicity. Digoxin levels.	Atropine for bradycardia. Activated charcoal is effective if given within 6–8 hours of ingestion. Digoxin-specific Fab fragments for K > 5 mEq/dL, hemodynamic instability, life-threatening arrhythmias, severe bradycardia, or a digoxin level of > 10 ng/mL.	Verapamil, diltiazem, erythromycin, and tetracycline can ↑ digoxin levels.
Cyanide	Almond odor breath, headache, tachycardia, tachypnea, pulmonary edema. Cherry-red cyanosis is a late finding. Can progress to seizures, renal failure, hepatic necrosis, hypotension, coma, and arrhythmias.	Bright red venous blood. Cyanide levels. Severe metabolic acidosis with an elevated anion gap and lactate level. ↓ arterial-venous oxygen gradient.	Resuscitate, ABCs, decontaminate, activated charcoal. Three steps: (1) amyl nitrate inhalation; (2) 3% sodium nitrite IV; (3) sodium thiosulfate IV.	The first two steps create methemoglobinemia to displace cyanide from hemoglobin so that the third step can inactivate cyanide.
Organophosphate	↑ salivation, miosis, nausea, vomiting, diarrhea, abdominal cramps, chest tightness, weakness.		Decontaminate; give atropine PRN for moderate to severe symptoms; 2-protopam (2-PAM) IV.	
Lithium	Altered mental status progressing to encephalopathy or coma. Tremor, seizures, hyperreflexia, clonus, parkinsonism. Vomiting and diarrhea.	Elevated serum lithium level. Toxicity may occur at low levels with chronic administration.	Volume repletion; consider alkalinization of urine. Dialysis for a lithium level of > 4 mEq/L (> 2.5 mEq/L if the patient is significantly symptomatic) or in the setting of concomitant renal failure.	Levels may "rebound" after dialysis and require repeat dialysis. Not bound by activated charcoal.

TABLE 10.14. **Characteristics and Treatment of Common Ingestions** *(continued)*

Substance	Manifestations	Lab Tests	Treatment	Comments
SSRIs	Somnolence, agitation; nausea, vomiting, tachycardia.	None.	Supportive care.	Rarely fatal. There is an ↑ risk of serotonin syndrome with mixed ingestions.
TCAs	**"Mad as a hatter, red as a beet, dry as a bone, blind as a bat, hot as a hare"**—ie, altered mental status; flushed, dry mouth; dilated pupils.	Widened QRS (> 0.12). Tachycardia. Prolonged PR and QT intervals. Pronounced R wave in aVR (> 3 mm). AV block and ventricular dysrhythmias.	Activated charcoal; consider gastric lavage (because anticholinergic effects may delay gastric emptying, consider up to 12 hours following ingestion). **IV sodium bicarbonate** boluses may ameliorate cardiotoxicity. Lidocaine but not procainamide for ventricular dysrhythmia; norepinephrine or epinephrine (not dopamine) for hypotension.	Maintain a low threshold for admission (especially for patients with anticholinergic symptoms and signs). Pronounced R waves in aVR may be most predictive of cardiac complications.
Methanol	Altered mental status, seizures, nausea, vomiting, visual disturbances, blindness.	Anion-gap metabolic acidosis. Elevated osmolar gap ($osm_{measured}$ $- osm_{calculated}$). Elevated serum methanol level.	If the patient presents within 1–2 hours of ingestion, use gastric lavage. Charcoal is ineffective. **Mild cases:** Sodium bicarbonate and IV **fomepizole.** **Severe cases: Immediate hemodialysis** (ie, with a level of > 50 mg/dL or an osmolar gap > 10; with severe acidosis; or with mental status changes/seizures).	Mortality is > 80% with seizures or coma. The lethal dose is 75–100 mL.
Ethylene glycol	Same as methanol. Oxalate crystals in the urine (see Figure 10.5). Fluorescence of urine with Wood's lamp. Acute renal failure.	Anion-gap metabolic acidosis. Elevated osmolar gap ($osm_{measured}$ $- osm_{calculated}$). Elevated serum ethylene glycol.	Treatment is the same as that for methanol, except hemodialysis is appropriate for ethylene glycol levels > 20 mg/dL.	The lethal dose is 100 mL.

(continues)

TABLE 10.14.   **Characteristics and Treatment of Common Ingestions** *(continued)*

SUBSTANCE	MANIFESTATIONS	LAB TESTS	TREATMENT	COMMENTS
Isopropyl alcohol (eg, rubbing alcohol)	Altered mental status progressing to coma; ataxia; hypotension 2° to myocardial depression.	Elevated osmolar gap ($osm_{measured}$ − $osm_{calculated}$). Lack of metabolic acidosis. Ketonuria.	If the patient presents within 1–2 hours of ingestion, treat with gastric lavage. **Hemodialysis** for coma or for a plasma isopropanol level > 400 mg/dL; also consider for hypotension as well as with concomitant hepatic or renal dysfunction.	The lethal dose is 150 mL.
Carbon monoxide	Headache, altered mental status, seizures, coma. Also nausea and abdominal pain. Poisoning can cause long-term CNS impairment, cognitive deficiencies, and personality/ movement disorders.	**Elevated carboxy-hemoglobin saturation** on ABG (values may normally be up to 15% in smokers). Toxicity is seen when level is > 15–30%. Pulse oximetry and Po_2 may be normal.	**High-flow O_2 via an endotracheal tube** for severe cases. Hyperbaric oxygen if immediately available for severe poisoning (persistent neurologic deficits, syncope, seizures, or coma) as well as for pregnant patients (controversial).	Cherry-red lips are infrequently seen. Po_2 and pulse oximetry may be falsely reassuring.

Acute Complications of Substance Abuse

A 22-year-old male college student is brought to the ER from a party and is found to be febrile, hypertensive, tachycardic, and combative. While in the ER, he has a witnessed generalized tonic-clonic seizure that lasts approximately three minutes. His pupils are dilated. What is the diagnosis, and how should he be treated?

Cocaine intoxication (sympathomimetic syndrome). The patient's hypertension, tachycardia, fever, agitation, and seizure should all respond to benzodiazepines.

KEY FACT

Overdoses of anticholinergics and stimulants cause dilated pupils, tachycardia, hypertension, agitation, and fever. To differentiate the two, look for warm, dry skin due to anticholinergics vs. clammy skin from stimulants.

Table 10.15 delineates guidelines for treating acute complications associated with the ingestion of controlled substances.

TABLE 10.15.   Manifestations and Treatment of Acute Complications of Substance Abuse

Substance	Manifestations	Lab Tests	Treatment	Comments
Gamma-hydroxybutyrate (GHB)	Somnolence and respiratory depression; bradycardia; muscle twitching and seizures.	None.	Consider activated charcoal if ingestion was very recent. Supportive care.	Most patients spontaneously recover within six hours.
Opioids	Somnolence followed by respiratory depression and coma. Constricted pupils, hypotension, bradycardia, apnea, hypothermia. Pulmonary edema and aspiration are possible. Meperidine and tramadol may cause seizures.	⊕ urine toxicology screen (except methadone and tramadol).	Supportive care. Naloxone 0.4–1.0 mg PRN (the effect of naloxone lasts only two hours, and repeated doses may be necessary).	Fentanyl may require very high doses of naloxone. Patients should be observed for at least 24 hours (or longer for methadone coingestion). Screen for coingestion (many opioids, such as Tylox and Percocet, are compounded with acetaminophen).
Cocaine	Agitation, palpitations, chest pain. Tachycardia, hypertension. Myocardial ischemia/infarction. Stroke.	Toxicology screen. Always obtain an ECG to assess for ischemic changes.	Benzodiazepines.	Avoid β-blockers with myocardial ischemia. If a β-blocker is used for hypertension, a vasodilating agent should be added.
Amphetamines (including MDMA)	Agitation, tachycardia, hypertension, hyperthermia, seizures, rhabdomyolysis.	Elevated CK with rhabdomyolysis. Hyponatremia may accompany MDMA ingestion.	Benzodiazepines. Specific treatment of complications (cooling and neuromuscular paralysis for hyperthermia; hydration and alkalinization for rhabdomyolysis).	Avoid β-blockade.
Ethanol	Disinhibition, agitation, slurred speech. Somnolence progressing to stupor with respiratory depression and coma.	Elevated blood alcohol level.	Supportive care. Attention to nutritional deficiencies in chronic alcoholics. Screen for coingestions.	
PCP (phencyclidine)	Agitation, psychosis, and nystagmus that may be in any direction (including rotatory).	May not be detected by a standard urine toxicology screen; request specific test.	Supportive care.	Patients on PCP are prone to sudden violent outbursts.

Withdrawal Syndromes

ETHANOL WITHDRAWAL

The mortality rate from ethanol withdrawal is approximately 5% and results primarily from the hemodynamic instability seen in delirium tremens (DTs).

SYMPTOMS/EXAM

- Symptoms of tremulousness and anxiety usually begin 2–3 days after the last drink. Withdrawal seizures almost always occur within 36 hours of stopping drinking.
- DTs usually occur several days after the last drink and include **hypertension, tachycardia, agitation, and hyperthermia.**
- Some patients experience **alcoholic hallucinosis**—auditory or tactile hallucinations that occur with an otherwise clear sensorium.

TREATMENT

- **Benzodiazepines** (eg, lorazepam or diazepam) are the cornerstone of treatment for withdrawal symptoms as well as for withdrawal seizures.
    - **Symptom-triggered schedules:** Administer benzodiazepines as directed by the Clinical Institute Withdrawal Assessment for Alcohol Scale (CIWA) score. May result in the use of lower doses of medications than other schedules, but requires frequent reassessment.
    - **Fixed schedules:** Provide regular benzodiazepines regardless of symptoms. May result in oversedation.
- **β-blockers, clonidine, and carbamazepine:** May be useful adjuncts, but their use should not supplant the role of benzodiazepines.
- All patients should receive **thiamine** supplementation.

KEY FACT

In the treatment of alcohol withdrawal, β-blockers may mask the signs of withdrawal and do not prevent seizures or DTs, so use them only with concomitant benzodiazepines.

KEY FACT

Symptom-triggered protocols to treat alcohol withdrawal (eg, the CIWA protocol) have been well studied and result in lower doses of benzodiazepines used, but they require frequent reassessment.

Hypertensive Urgency and Emergency

A 68-year-old man with a history of hypertension, hyperlipidemia, peripheral vascular disease, and CAD with a stent placed one year ago presents to the ER six hours after sudden onset of headache, nausea, vomiting, and chest pain radiating to his back. He is on metoprolol, atorvastatin, and ASA, and he had a normal stress test two months ago. His BP is 220/120 mm Hg in both arms; other vital signs are normal, and he is diaphoretic. He has an S4 gallop and crackles at both bases. His ECG shows LVH with a strain pattern and ST depressions in the lateral leads. What is the diagnosis, and what are the drugs of choice for treatment?

Dissecting aortic aneurysm. The goal is to ↓ BP to prevent end-organ damage, but not to the degree that it might cause cerebral, cardiac, and renal ischemia due to autoregulation. IV labetalol followed by sodium nitroprusside are the drugs of choice.

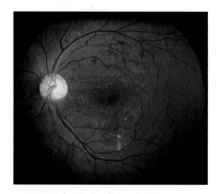

FIGURE 10.4. Flame hemorrhages of hypertensive retinopathy. The left eye of this African American patient with poorly controlled hypertension has a darkly pigmented choroid, a normal variant that darkens the entire photograph. There are multiple flame hemorrhages within the plane of the nerve fiber layer as well as several "cotton wool" spots (nerve fiber layer infarctions). (Reproduced with permission from LeBlond RF et al. *DeGowin's Diagnostic Examination,* 9th ed. New York: McGraw-Hill, 2009, Plate 23.)

Hypertensive **emergency** occurs when an elevated BP leads to **active end-organ damage** that is likely to result in death or serious morbidity in the absence of immediate treatment. Hypertensive **urgency** occurs with severe hypertension (> 220/120) **without end-organ complications.**

SYMPTOMS/EXAM

- Systolic BP is usually > 220 mm Hg; diastolic BP is usually > 120 mm Hg. The BP level tolerated may depend on the chronic baseline BP.
- **Funduscopic exam** may reveal papilledema and flame hemorrhages (see Figure 10.4).
- **Hypertensive encephalopathy** is marked by nausea/vomiting, headache, confusion, lethargy, and/or irritability.
- Focal neurologic deficits suggest **intracranial hemorrhage.**
- Severe chest pain radiating to the back and differential pulses in the upper extremities may occur with **aortic dissection.**
- **Ischemic chest pain** may be present as an individual process or as a complication of dissection.
- **Heart failure** features.

DIFFERENTIAL

Poorly controlled essential hypertension is most common, but consider other 2° causes (see Table 10.16).

KEY FACT

Hypertensive emergencies may occur at BPs that are not considered "critically" high.

KEY FACT

Poorly controlled essential hypertension is by far the most common cause of hypertensive urgency/emergency.

TABLE 10.16. Secondary Etiologies of Hypertension

CONDITION	KEY FEATURES IN ADDITION TO HYPERTENSION	DIAGNOSIS	TREATMENT
Rebound hypertension after antihypertensive meds are stopped	History of chronic therapy with oral clonidine or β-blockers.	Based on the history.	Restart chronic medications.
Cocaine or methamphetamine use	Agitation, tachycardia, dilated pupils.	Urine toxicology screen.	**Benzodiazepines.** **Avoid β-blockers** (cause unopposed alpha effects and may worsen symptoms).
Pheochromocytoma	Palpitations, headache, weight loss.	24-hour urine metanephrines and catecholamines or plasma free metanephrines.	Volume replacement; then **phenoxybenzamine first.** Add β-blockers later to prevent unopposed alpha effects when β-blockers are given alone.
Hyperthyroidism	Tachycardia, weight loss, tremors.	↓ TSH.	See the Endocrinology chapter.
Hypercortisolism	Weight gain, abdominal striae, buffalo hump, moon facies.	1-mg dexamethasone suppression test or 24-hour urine cortisol.	Based on the cause of excess cortisol; see the Endocrinology chapter.
Hyperaldosteronism (eg, Conn's syndrome)	Low potassium.	For 1° hyperaldosteronism (Conn's), plasma aldosterone to plasma renin ratio > 25.	Based on the cause of excess aldosterone; see the Endocrinology chapter.
Scleroderma renal crisis	Taut skin, CREST features.	Clinical, based on features of scleroderma. ANA and anti-SCL-70 antibodies are typically present.	**ACEIs.**

TABLE 10.17. **Medications for Hypertensive Emergency**

MEDICATION	PROS	CONS
Nitroprusside	Highly effective; easily titrated; predictable BP response. Short acting.	May cause nausea and vomiting. Thiocyanate toxicity is possible, especially in patients with renal or hepatic insufficiency.
Fenoldopam	Useful in renal failure; predictable BP response.	May cause nausea, headache, and reflex tachycardia. ↑ intraocular pressure (avoid with glaucoma).
Labetalol	Excellent for hyperadrenergic states.	May precipitate bronchospasm and heart block.
Enalapril	Easily transitioned to oral therapy.	Response may be extreme in high renin states. Use with care in renal insufficiency. Can cause hyperkalemia.
Nicardipine	Potent antihypertensive.	Avoid with dissection and myocardial ischemia.
Hydralazine	Useful in pregnancy.	May cause reflex tachycardia. Avoid with dissection and myocardial ischemia.

KEY FACT

In a young patient with refractory or severe hypertension, palpitations, and headache, consider pheochromocytoma and order 24-hour urine metanephrines and catecholamines or plasma free metanephrines.

KEY FACT

Mean arterial pressure should be lowered by no more than 20–25% within the first hour. BP should subsequently be lowered to a level of approximately 160/100 mm Hg over the ensuing 4–6 hours.

KEY FACT

Rapid-acting oral or sublingual nifedipine should be avoided, as it may lower BP too drastically and precipitate stroke.

DIAGNOSIS

Evaluate further if symptoms suggest a complication or an unusual etiology (see Table 10.17):

- **CT of the head** in patients with mental status changes or focal neurologic deficits to exclude intracranial hemorrhage.
- **MRI** in hypertensive encephalopathy may demonstrate **posterior reversible leukoencephalopathy syndrome (PRES),** white matter edema in the parietal and occipital areas (see Figure 10.5).
- **Emergent transesophageal echocardiography or thoracic CT** in suspected aortic dissection.
- **Electrocardiography** in patients with suspected myocardial ischemia.

TREATMENT

- **Pharmacologic** treatment is dictated by the specific end-organ complications (see Table 10.18).
- **Hypertensive emergency: BP should be lowered within one hour,** and parenteral agents are almost always necessary.
  - **The immediate goal is not normotension,** as a dramatic reduction in BP can overwhelm the cerebral autoregulatory mechanism, causing ischemic stroke.
  - A ↓ in mean arterial pressure up to 20–25% or a ↓ in diastolic BP to < 120 mm Hg over the first several hours is an accepted guideline.
- **Hypertensive urgency: Oral medications are most useful,** and BP may be controlled at a more leisurely rate. Outpatient treatment is appropriate in most instances. **Captopril** and **clonidine** are particularly effective.

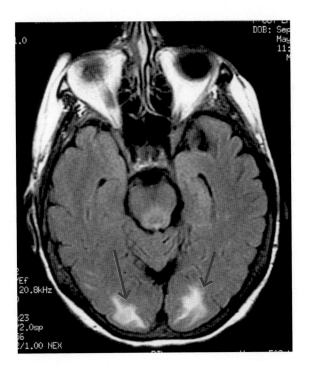

FIGURE 10.5. **Posterior reversible leukoencephalopathy.** Transaxial MR image from FLAIR sequence shows signal hyperintensity in the subcortical white matter of both occipital lobes (arrows). (Reproduced with permission from Ropper AH, Samuels MA. *Adams & Victor's Principles of Neurology,* 9th ed. New York: McGraw-Hill, 2009, Fig. 43-1.)

TABLE 10.18.   **Medications for Specific Complications of Hypertensive Emergency**

INDICATION	DRUGS OF CHOICE	CONTRAINDICATED
Aortic dissection	Nitroprusside and labetalol	Nicardipine, hydralazine
Pulmonary edema	Nitroprusside, nitroglycerin	
Myocardial ischemia/ infarction	Nitroglycerin, labetalol	Nicardipine, hydralazine
Hypertensive encephalopathy	Labetalol, nicardipine	Nitroprusside
Eclampsia	Labetalol, hydralazine	Enalapril
Acute renal failure	Fenoldopam, labetalol	
Scleroderma hypertensive crisis	ACEIs	

Syncope

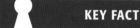 A 75-year-old man with a history of CAD, DM, hypertension, and hyper-lipidemia experienced a one-minute episode of syncope while getting out of his car. He noticed diaphoresis and palpitations before the episode but states that he was not incontinent. He has not started any new medications in the past few months and is not taking a diuretic. His exam is normal, and his ECG shows an old bifascicular block. An exercise stress test, an echocardiogram, and 24-hour Holter monitoring are all normal. What is the next step in the evaluation of his syncope?

A continuous loop recorder. Long-term (≥ 30-day) event monitoring is warranted if the suspicion of an arrhythmia is still high after inpatient telemetry and outpatient Holter monitoring are found to be normal. With CAD and a bifascicular block, arrhythmia should be strongly suspected. The one-year cardiac mortality and sudden death rates are higher in cardiac than in noncardiac or idiopathic syncope.

Defined as a transient loss of consciousness and postural tone; accounts for 3% of all ER visits and up to 6% of all hospital admissions. The frequency of common etiologies of syncope are as follows (see also Table 10.19):

- **Cardiac:** 18%.
- **Neurologic:** 10%.
- **Vasovagal:** 24%.
- **Orthostatic:** 8%.
- **Medications:** 3%.
- **Unknown:** 37%.

SYMPTOMS/EXAM

- The history and physical exam establish a diagnosis in almost 50% of patients with syncope. However, specific findings are dependent on the underlying etiology, and knowledge of the differential diagnosis is critical (see Table 10.19).
- Situational syncope includes syncope associated with vagal stimulation—eg, straining, micturition, defecation, cough, and occasionally swallowing (cold liquids).

DIAGNOSIS

Other than a history and physical, additional testing should be individualized. Consider additional testing in those with risk factors for an adverse outcome (eg, patients > 45 years of age, those with a history of CHF or a ventricular arrhythmia, and those with an abnormal ECG).

- **Orthostatic vital signs:** When moving the patient from a supine to an upright position results in a ↓ in systolic BP of ≥ 20 mm Hg, an ↑ of ≥ 20 beats in HR, or the reproduction of symptoms, consider orthostatic hypotension.
- **ECG:** Look for evidence of ischemia, arrhythmia, new bundle branch block, or a prolonged QT interval.
- **Echocardiogram:** Look for structural heart disease. Consider in patients with a history of heart disease, those with an abnormality on physical exam or ECG, or elderly patients.

TABLE 10.19.   Differential Diagnosis of Syncope

MECHANISM	SUGGESTIVE FEATURES
Orthostatic hypotension	A history of presyncope upon standing; advanced age; a drop in BP (systolic BP by $\geq$ 20 mm Hg or diastolic BP by $\geq$ 10 mm Hg) upon standing.
Medication related	Diuretics, antihypertensives, polypharmacy.
Autonomic insufficiency	Features of parkinsonism plus autonomic dysfunction suggest multiple-system atrophy.
Neurally mediated (**vasovagal**, vasomotor, neurocardiogenic, situational)	Preceded by nausea, flushing, diaphoresis, and tachycardia. Autonomic symptoms often persist upon awakening. Occurrence during emotional stress or pain or in specific situations (eg, while coughing, micturating, or defecating).
Carotid sinus hypersensitivity	A specific type of neurally mediated syncope seen in older patients, classically provoked by neck stretching (eg, to loosen a tight collar, while shaving, from a tumor or dissection, or while looking over the shoulder when driving a car in reverse).
Cardiac arrhythmia (tachyarrhythmia, bradyarrhythmia)	No premonitory symptoms or residual symptoms upon awakening; history of cardiovascular disease.
Valvular heart disease (aortic stenosis, pulmonic stenosis)	Characteristic murmur on exam.
Myocardial ischemia/infarction	Associated chest pain.
Hypertrophic obstructive cardiomyopathy	Characteristic systolic murmur that decreases with squatting and increases with Valsalva.
Aortic dissection	Chest pain radiating to the back; differential pulses in upper extremities.
PE	Pleurisy; dyspnea; history of venous thromboembolism.
Atrial myxoma	Tumor plop on auscultation.
Migraine	Subsequent headache.
Vertebrobasilar insufficiency (VBI)	Tinnitus, dysarthria, diplopia; focal neurologic findings. It is highly unusual to have VBI as a cause of syncope in the absence of other brainstem findings.
Seizures	Postictal state, incontinence, slow recovery (> 5 minutes), prodromal aura.
Psychiatric	Signs and symptoms of psychiatric disease. Diagnosis of exclusion.

- **Holter monitoring:** Use when the patient has symptoms that suggest arrhythmia (eg, a cluster of spells, sudden loss of consciousness, palpitations, use of medications associated with arrhythmia, known heart disease, an abnormal ECG). **Loop recorders and event monitors** ↑ the yield.
- **Tilt-table testing:** Use in patients with normal hearts and relatively infrequent syncope, nondiagnostic Holter monitoring, or symptoms that suggest vasovagal spells (eg, warmth, nausea) but lack an obvious precipitating event.

KEY FACT

Testing for neurologic disease with CT and MRI is very low yield in syncope in the absence of specific neurologic signs and symptoms.

- **Carotid sinus massage with cardiac monitoring:** Should be completed in older patients with no readily identifiable cause of syncope or in those with symptoms suggestive of carotid sinus hypersensitivity. A **three-second pause is diagnostic** and may indicate the need for pacemaker insertion.
- **CT and MRI** of the head are rarely indicated unless there was concomitant head trauma. **EEG** is useful only when seizures are suspected.

TREATMENT

- Treatment is directed at the underlying condition.
- **Guidelines for hospital admission** are as follows:
  - **Definite admission:** Evidence of acute coronary syndrome, stroke, or arrhythmia; a history of CAD, heart failure, or ventricular arrhythmia; evidence of heart failure or valvular disease.
  - **Possible admission:** Patients > 70 years of age; those with exertional or frequent syncope, orthostasis, or injury due to a syncopal episode.

KEY FACT

In a patient with syncope, the first priority is to search for a cardiac cause, as patients with cardiogenic syncope are at ↑ risk for sudden death.

Community-Acquired Pneumonia (CAP)

A 65-year-old nonsmoking man with a chronic productive cough and a history of severe pneumonia 20 years ago presents with a cough, fever, and yellow-green sputum production. He reports that he usually requires antibiotics once or twice yearly, when his sputum production ↑ or gets darker and his cough becomes worse than his baseline. On exam, he is found to be febrile with coarse breath sounds at the right lung base, and a CXR shows a patchy right lower lobe infiltrate where four years ago there were nonspecific ↑ markings on CXR. The patient also has leukocytosis and bandemia. What organism should be covered in the selection of an empiric regimen for this patient?

Pseudomonas aeruginosa is more likely in patients with bronchiectasis (chronic productive cough after a severe pneumonia; chronic CXR changes), especially in those who have received multiple antibiotic regimens.

The sixth leading cause of death in the United States.

SYMPTOMS/EXAM

- Fever, dyspnea, and cough productive of purulent sputum are most commonly seen.
- **Pleuritic chest pain** and **chills/rigors** are also possible.
- Patients who are immunocompromised, reside in an institution, have recently been hospitalized, or are at risk for aspiration should be considered separately (see the section on health care–associated pneumonia).

DIAGNOSIS

- **CXR:** Shows an infiltrate, but radiographic findings cannot predict the microbiologic cause (see Figure 10.6). False-⊖ results have been reported in patients who are dehydrated on admission.
- **Sputum Gram stain and culture:** Although only marginally predictive of microbiology, these are recommended for inpatients and can be considered in outpatients as well. **Accurate only if there are < 10 epithelial cells per low-power field.**

KEY FACT

Certain historical features may suggest a specific microbiologic etiology for community-acquired pneumonia, but none is adequately specific to establish a diagnosis.

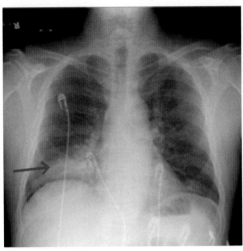
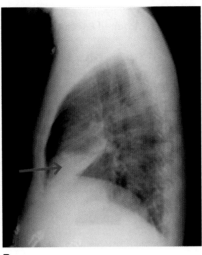

A   **B**

FIGURE 10.6. **Community-acquired pneumonia.** Frontal (**A**) and lateral (**B**) radiographs show airspace consolidation in the right middle lobe (red arrows) in a patient with community-acquired pneumonia. (Reproduced, with permission, from USMLERx.com.)

- **Blood cultures:** Provide reliable data and may allow for the tailoring of antimicrobial therapy. ⊕ in approximately 10% of cases.
- **Other:** Tests for specific etiologies (see Table 10.20), including serologies for Q fever and psittacosis, culture and urine antigen testing for *Legionella*

TABLE 10.20. **Causative Organisms and Historical Features of Community-Acquired Pneumonia**

ORGANISM	CAUSE (%)	SUGGESTIVE HISTORICAL FEATURES
Streptococcus pneumoniae	20–60	Acute onset; often follows a URI; underlying COPD. Drug resistance is more likely in patients > 65 years of age; in those who have had β-lactam therapy in the last three months; and in the setting of EtOH abuse, immunosuppression, multiple comorbidities, and/or exposure to a sick child in day care.
Haemophilus influenzae	3–10	Often follows a URI; COPD.
S aureus	3–5	May follow influenza infection; cavitary disease.
Legionella spp.	2–8	Associated with exposure to humidifiers, hot tubs, or air-conditioning cooling towers. Pleuritic chest pain and pleural effusion are common; diarrhea, hyponatremia.
Klebsiella, other gram-⊝ rods	3–10	Associated with ethanol abuse, DM, residence in a nursing home, recent antibiotic use, and multiple comorbidities.
Mycoplasma pneumoniae	1–6	Commonly affects young adults in summer and fall; associated rash and bullous myringitis. CXR appears worse than symptoms suggest.
Chlamydia pneumoniae	4–10	Commonly affects young adults; pneumonia often occurs 2–3 weeks after a prolonged sore throat (biphasic pattern).
Q fever (*Coxiella burnetii*)	Rare	Exposure to livestock (cattle, goats, sheep); elevated LFTs.
Chlamydia psittaci	Rare	Exposure to birds, including parrots, pigeons, and chickens; headache; temperature-pulse dissociation.

TABLE 10.21. Pneumonia Severity Index (PORT) Score for Risk Class Assignment of Community-Acquired Pneumonia

PATIENT CHARACTERISTIC	POINTS ASSIGNED
Demographic factor	
Men	Age
Women	Age − 10
Nursing home resident	+10
Coexisting illnesses	
Neoplastic disease	+30
Liver disease	+20
CHF	+10
Cerebrovascular disease	+10
Renal disease	+10
Physical exam findings	
Altered mental status	+20
RR ≥ 30/min	+20
Systolic BP < 90 mm Hg	+20
Temperature < 35°C or > 40°C	+15
Pulse ≥ 125/min	+10
Laboratory/x-ray findings	
Arterial pH < 7.35	+30
BUN > 30 mg/dL	+20
Sodium < 130 mmol/L	+20
Glucose ≥ 250 mg/dL	+10
Hematocrit < 30%	+10
Pao_2 < 60 mm Hg	+10
Pleural effusion	+10
Risk group (number of points)	Mortality rate
I (points not calculated)[a]	0–0.4%
II (≤ 70)	0.4–0.7%
III (71–90)	0–2.8%
IV (91–130)	8.2–9.3%
V (> 130)	27.0–31.1%

[a]Patients < 50 years of age without active neoplastic disease, liver disease, CHF, cerebrovascular disease, or renal disease, and who have normal or only mildly deranged vital signs and normal mental status, are placed into risk group I.

(Adapted with permission from Stone CK, Humphries RL. *Current Diagnosis & Treatment: Emergency Medicine,* 6th ed. New York: McGraw-Hill, 2008, Table 40-9.)

and pneumococcus, and IgM titers for *Mycoplasma*, should be obtained only when there is high clinical suspicion or severe CAP.

TREATMENT

■ **Outpatient therapy:** Appropriate in many patients. The **Pneumonia Severity Index** (see Table 10.21), devised by the Pneumonia Patient Out-

TABLE 10.22. **Criteria for Discharge in Community-Acquired Pneumonia**

CRITERION	COMPONENTS
Clinical stability	▪ Improvement in cough/dyspnea. ▪ O$_2$ saturation > 90%. ▪ Temperature < 37.8°C. ▪ Resolution of tachycardia. ▪ Resolution of tachypnea. ▪ Resolution of hypotension.
No evidence of complicated infection	For example, no extrapulmonary or pleural involvement.
Ability to tolerate oral medications	

comes Research Team (**PORT**), can help guide decisions regarding the need for hospitalization.

- Patients categorized as Class I, II, or III (≤ 90 points on the PORT scale) are at sufficiently low risk for death that they can be considered for outpatient treatment or for an abbreviated course of inpatient care.
- Class IV and V patients should be hospitalized.
- **Antibiotic treatment:** Largely empirical, covering typical and atypical agents. Appropriate choices include the following:
    - Extended-spectrum fluoroquinolones (eg, moxifloxacin, levofloxacin).
    - A third-generation cephalosporin plus a macrolide.
    - A β-lactam/β-lactamase inhibitor combination plus a macrolide.
    - In **severe CAP requiring treatment in the ICU,** consider "double coverage" for *Pseudomonas* (ie, two antibiotics with antipseudomonal activity).
    - **Prompt initiation of antimicrobial therapy** (within eight hours of presentation) has a significant beneficial effect on mortality.
- **Early conversion from parenteral to oral therapy** should be considered in patients with decreasing leukocytosis, improvement in cough/dyspnea, and no fever for at least eight hours. This can usually be done within three days of starting treatment.
- Patients may be **discharged** without delay at the time of conversion to oral therapy as long as they meet discharge criteria (see Table 10.22).
- **Duration of treatment** varies from one to two weeks.
- **Repeat CXR** is not indicated during hospitalization except when complications (eg, pleural effusion) are suspected. A follow-up film to ensure clearing and to assess for underlying processes in 4–6 weeks is appropriate, especially in smokers and older patients.
- **Pneumococcal vaccine:** All patients with CAP should receive this prior to discharge unless already vaccinated.

KEY FACT

Age is often the largest contributor to the Pneumonia Severity Index score. Anyone who is > 70 years of age with abnormal vital signs or labs should probably be treated in the hospital.

KEY FACT

There is no benefit to observing patients in the hospital after conversion to oral therapy once they have met the criteria for clinical stability.

Health Care–Associated Pneumonia (HCAP)

Defined as pneumonia that developed in a nonhospitalized patient who:

- Was hospitalized in an acute care facility for > 48 hours within three months of developing the pneumonia.
- Resides in a long-term care facility **and**

- Received IV antibiotics, chemotherapy, or wound care within one month prior to the pneumonia **or**
- Attended a hospital or a hemodialysis clinic within the past month.

DIAGNOSIS/TREATMENT

- It is important to differentiate HCAP from CAP because their etiologies, treatment, and prognoses differ.
- Organisms to consider include enteric gram-$\ominus$ organisms (particularly in the elderly), *S pneumoniae*, *S aureus* (including MRSA), and *H influenzae*.
- Empiric treatment for HCAP involves deciding if the patient is at risk for infection from a multidrug-resistant (MDR) organism. **Risk factors for MDR infections** are as follows:
  - Receipt of antibiotics within the preceding 90 days.
  - Current hospitalization of ≥ 5 days' duration.
  - A high frequency of antibiotic resistance in the community or in the specific hospital unit.
  - Immunosuppressive disease and/or therapy.
- **Empiric regimen for HCAP without concern for resistant organisms:** Choose one of the following: ceftriaxone, ampicillin-sulbactam, piperacillin-tazobactam, a respiratory fluoroquinolone, or ertapenem.
- **Empiric three-drug regimen for HCAP with concern for resistant organisms:** Includes an antipseudomonal (cephalosporin, a carbapenem, piperacillin-tazobactam, aztreonam) + another antipseudomonal (a fluoroquinolone or aminoglycoside) + MRSA coverage (vancomycin, linezolid) in the setting of high local incidence or risk factors for MRSA.

Environmental (Accidental) Hypothermia

Risk factors for environmental hypothermia include **advanced age, trauma, alcohol or drug use, cognitive impairment,** and **psychiatric disease. Cold water exposure is common.**

SYMPTOMS/EXAM

Symptoms based on severity are as follows:

- **Mild hypothermia:** Temperatures 32–35°C (82–90°F). **Tachycardia, tachypnea, and shivering** are seen.
- **Moderate and severe hypothermia:** Temperatures < 28–32°C (< 82°F). Lethargy, irritability, and confusion are common. **Loss of shivering, bradycardia, hypotension, respiratory depression,** and **coma** may develop. Look for Osborn waves (see Figure 10.7).

DIFFERENTIAL

Environmental (accidental) exposure, occult sepsis, myxedema, adrenal insufficiency, hypopituitarism, DKA, hepatic failure.

DIAGNOSIS

- **Laboratory abnormalities** include metabolic acidosis, hypo- and hyperglycemia, DIC, hyperkalemia, and hyperamylasemia.
- ECG may show **Osborn or J waves** (notching of the terminal aspect of the QRS complex, best seen in lead V_4), **slow atrial fibrillation, and prolonged cardiac intervals** (see Figure 10.7).

KEY FACT

Residence in a cold climate is not mandatory for hypothermia to develop.

KEY FACT

Temperatures < 32°C (< 82°F) or Osborn waves on ECG imply moderate or severe hypothermia. Shivering stops, and bradycardia and respiratory depression occur.

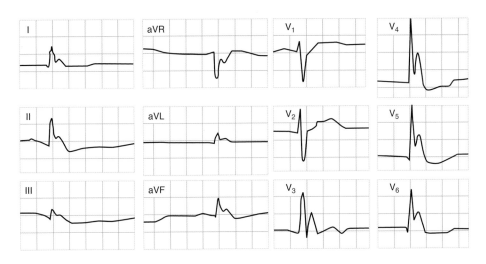

FIGURE 10.7.   Osborn wave in hypothermia.

TREATMENT

Limit movement and manipulation of the patient; unnecessary stimulation (eg, central lines, NG tubes, pacemakers) can result in ventricular dysrhythmias. The treatment of accidental hypothermia is summarized in Table 10.23.

TABLE 10.23.   Rewarming Techniques in Accidental Hypothermia

METHOD	DESCRIPTION	INDICATIONS	COMMENTS
Passive external rewarming	Removal of wet clothes; coverage with blankets.	Mild hypothermia.	Limited efficacy.
Active external rewarming	Warmed blankets (including hot air blankets over the torso only); warmed baths.	Mild hypothermia.	Rewarming the extremities can cause **paradoxical lowering of core temperature** because of the return of chilled blood from the extremities.
Active internal or core rewarming[a]	Warmed IV fluids; warmed humidified air.	Moderate and severe hypothermia.	Widely available; limited efficacy.
	Extracorporeal blood rewarming via cardiopulmonary, arteriovenous, or venovenous bypass.	Moderate and severe hypothermia; cardiac arrest.	The most effective technique, but invasive. Also requires the application of specialized knowledge and equipment.
	Peritoneal/pleural lavage with warmed fluids.	Moderate and severe hypothermia.	Useful when extracorporeal techniques are not available.

[a]The decision to proceed with invasive active internal rewarming is individualized to the patient and dependent on both temperature and clinical manifestations. Noninvasive measures may suffice for most patients with moderate hypothermia.

Acute Exacerbations of Asthma

Intercurrent infection, especially viral, is the most common cause. Bacterial infections, environmental exposure to smoke or allergens, GERD, medical noncompliance, and use of certain medications (NSAIDs, β-blockers) are also potential factors.

Symptoms/Exam

- Presents with **dyspnea, wheezing, coughing,** and **chest tightness.**
- Fever and purulent sputum usually represent a complicating process such as pneumonia.
- Indicators of a severe asthma exacerbation include the following (each presents individually in < 50% of cases):
    - Absence of wheezing with poor air movement
    - Tachypnea (> 30 breaths/min)
    - Tachycardia (> 130 bpm)
    - Pulsus paradoxus (> 15 mm Hg)
    - Accessory respiratory muscle use
    - Altered mental status

Diagnosis

- **Peak expiratory flow rate (PEF):** Most predictive of the severity of the exacerbation; should guide therapy as well as all decisions regarding disposition.
- **ABG analysis:** Reserved for those with a severe ↓ in PEF or suspected hypoventilation; usually shows a ↓ P_{CO_2} unless the patient is developing ventilatory failure.
- **CXR:** Usually normal; necessary only when a 2° process is suspected.

Treatment

Treatment should proceed as outlined below (see also Table 10.24):

- **Systemic corticosteroids:** The mainstay of treatment; ↓ the need for hospitalization and the subsequent relapse rate when begun immediately. Oral and IV preparations are equally effective.
- **Inhaled corticosteroids (ICS):** Currently the mainstay for chronic maintenance therapy, although some advocate it to treat acute exacerbations. Higher doses have been implicated in increasing pulmonary infections as well as oral thrush and dysphonia. However, ICS have little if any effect on the pituitary-adrenal axis and are much less likely than oral steroids to contribute to cataracts, glaucoma, fractures, and easy bruising.

TABLE 10.24. **Treatment of Acute Asthma Exacerbations**

All Patients	Selected Patients	Not Useful or Harmful
Oral or IV corticosteroids	Antibiotics	Theophylline
Inhaled bronchodilators	O_2	Injected bronchodilators
	Mechanical ventilation	Chest physiotherapy
	? Noninvasive mechanical ventilation	Mucolytic agents
		Magnesium

- **Inhaled bronchodilator therapy:**
  - **Combination therapy** (β_2-agonists and ipratropium bromide): Should be given to all patients with moderate to severe exacerbations.
  - **Drug delivery:** Equivalent to handheld metered-dose inhalers (MDIs) and nebulizer therapy, although the latter may be more effective in patients who have difficulty using inhalers or are in respiratory distress.
- **Methylxanthines:** No longer recommended, as they add no benefit to the above therapy.
- **Antibiotics:** Generally **unnecessary**; reserve for patients with evidence of an underlying bacterial infection. If administering antibiotics, consider a macrolide, as *M pneumoniae* and *C pneumoniae* are identified in roughly 5% of asthma exacerbations.
- **O$_2$ therapy:** Should be provided to keep O$_2$ saturations above 90%.
- **Noninvasive ventilation or endotracheal intubation and mechanical ventilation:** Reserve for patients who do not respond to the above therapies and continue to experience severe airflow obstruction. Indications for mechanical ventilation include the following:
  - Persistent hypercapnia
  - Altered mental status
  - Progressive and persistent acidemia (pH < 7.30)
  - Respiratory fatigue
- The efficacy of **noninvasive mechanical ventilation** is not well established.

COMPLICATIONS

Risk factors for death in asthma exacerbations are as follows:

- Previous severe exacerbations/ICU admissions/intubation.
- More than two hospitalizations or three ER visits in the past year.
- Use of corticosteroids or > 2 canisters of β_2-agonist MDIs per month.
- Difficulty in perceiving the presence or severity of airflow obstruction.
- Low socioeconomic status.
- Illicit drug use.
- Serious comorbidities.

NOTES

CHAPTER 11

Infectious Diseases

Anuj Gaggar, MD, PhD
José M. Eguía, MD, MPH

Infectious Disease Clinical Syndromes

MENINGITIS

A 34-year-old homeless man presents with confusion and is found on MRI to have enhancement of his basal cisterns. An LP shows ↑ protein, a lymphocytic predominance, and low glucose. How should this patient be treated while cultures are pending?

Treatment should consist of rifampin, INH, pyrazinamide, and ethambutol +/– steroids. Basilar meningitis is commonly seen with TB or fungal meningitis. A lymphocytic-predominant CSF in the setting of TB risk factors makes TB meningitis the most likely diagnosis. Given its high morbidity, TB meningitis should be treated empirically before a definitive diagnosis is made.

May be acute or chronic. Etiologies are as follows:

- **Acute meningitis: Acute neutrophilic meningitis** is caused by bacteria (see Table 11.1).
- **Chronic meningitis:**
  - Characterized by symptoms lasting from weeks to months with persistent CSF pleocytosis (usually lymphocytic).
  - Etiologic agents include TB (40%), atypical mycobacteria, *Cryptococcus* (7%), *Coccidioides, Histoplasma, Blastomyces,* 2° syphilis, Lyme disease, and Whipple's disease. The etiology is frequently unknown (34%). Noninfectious causes include CNS or metastatic neoplasms

TABLE 11.1. Initial Antimicrobial Therapy for Purulent Meningitis of Unknown Cause

Age Group	Common Microorganisms	Empiric Antibiotics—First Choice[a,b]	Severe Penicillin Allergy
Adults 18–50 years of age	*Streptococcus pneumoniae, Neisseria meningitidis.*	Ceftriaxone/cefotaxime +/– vancomycin.	Chloramphenicol + vancomycin.
Adults > 50 years of age	*S pneumoniae, Listeria monocytogenes,* gram-⊖ bacilli.	Ceftriaxone/cefotaxime + ampicillin +/– vancomycin.	Chloramphenicol (*N meningitidis*) + TMP-SMX (*Listeria*) + vancomycin.
Impaired cellular immunity (or alcohol abuse)	*S pneumoniae, L monocytogenes,* gram-⊖ bacilli (*Pseudomonas*).	Ceftazidime + ampicillin +/– vancomycin.	TMP-SMX + vancomycin.
Post-neurosurgery or post–head trauma	*S pneumoniae, S aureus,* gram-⊖ bacilli (including *Pseudomonas*).	Ceftazidime + vancomycin (for possible MRSA).	Aztreonam or ciprofloxacin + vancomycin.

[a]Steroids (dexamethasone 10 mg q 6 h × 2–4 days) may be added for patients who present with acute community-acquired meningitis that is likely to have been caused by *S pneumoniae.*

[b]Doses for meningitis are higher than those for other indications: ceftriaxone 2 g IV q 12 h, cefotaxime 2 g IV q 4 h, vancomycin 1 g IV q 8 h, ampicillin 2 g IV q 4 h, or ceftazidime 2 g IV q 8 h.

(Adapted with permission from Tierney LM et al. *Current Medical Diagnosis & Treatment,* 44th ed. New York: McGraw-Hill, 2005: 1251.)

(8%), leukemia, lymphoma, vasculitis, sarcoid, and subarachnoid or subdural bleeds.
- **Chronic neutrophilic meningitis:** May be caused by *Nocardia*, *Actinomyces*, *Aspergillus*, *Candida*, SLE, or CMV in advanced AIDS.
- **Chronic eosinophilic meningitis:** Associated with *Coccidioides*, parasites, lymphoma, and chemical agents.
- **Chronic meningitis and cranial nerve palsies:** Caused by Lyme disease, syphilis, sarcoid (CN VII—Bell's palsy), and TB (CN VI—lateral rectus palsy).
- **Aseptic meningitis:**
  - Usually viral with a benign course. Treat with nonspecific supportive care.
  - Associated with enteroviruses and arboviruses in the late summer and early fall and with mumps in the spring.
  - Also associated with HSV-2 (if recurrent, known as Mollaret's meningitis) as well as with HIV (often acute). Unlike HSV-1 encephalitis, HSV-2 meningitis has a benign course, but treatment and/or suppression can be considered.
  - Less common but treatable causes include 2° syphilis (penicillin), Lyme disease (ceftriaxone), and leptospirosis (doxycycline).

KEY FACT

Common medications that can cause aseptic meningitis include TMP-SMX, IVIG, NSAIDs, and carbamazepine.

SYMPTOMS/EXAM

- Presents with **fever,** headache, neck stiffness, altered mental status (ranging from mild lethargy to confusion, stupor, and coma), and alterations in speech and behavior.
- Atypical presentations are more likely in neonates, young children, and the elderly.

DIAGNOSIS/TREATMENT

- **Fulminant presentation (< 24 hours) or ill-appearing patients:** Give antibiotics **within 30 minutes;** give dexamethasone along with or prior to antibiotics. Then perform a history and physical and obtain a CT/MRI (if indicated) and an LP.
- Obtain a head CT/MRI before LP if a mass lesion is suspected (eg, in the setting of papilledema, coma, seizures, focal neurologic findings, or immune compromise).
- CSF Gram stain sensitivity is 75% (60–90%); CSF culture sensitivity is 75% (70–85%) for bacterial meningitis (see Table 11.2). Sensitivity is unchanged if antibiotics are administered < 4 hours before culture.

KEY FACT

A low glucose concentration in the CSF is commonly seen in bacterial and TB etiologies of meningitis. A high protein may not be helpful diagnostically.

PREVENTION

- **N *meningitidis* chemoprophylaxis:**
  - Give to household contacts, roommates, or cellmates; those with direct contact with the patient's oral secretions (kissing, sharing utensils, endotracheal intubation, suctioning, day care contacts if < 7 days); and special cases (immunocompromised patients, outbreaks).
  - Also indicated for index patients who are not treated with a cephalosporin (penicillins and chloramphenicol do not reliably penetrate the nasal mucosa). Possible regimens include rifampin 600 mg PO BID × 4 doses, ciprofloxacin 500 mg PO × 1 dose, or ceftriaxone 250 mg IM × 1 dose.
- **N *meningitidis* vaccine (serotypes A, C, Y, and W-135, not B):** Appropriate for epidemics as well as for military recruits, pilgrims to Mecca, and travelers to the African Sahel (meningitis belt), Nepal, and northern India. May also be given to college freshmen living in dormitories, asplenic pa-

TABLE 11.2. CSF Profiles in Various CNS Diseases

DIAGNOSIS	RBCs (PER μL)	WBCs (PER μL)	GLUCOSE (mg/dL)	PROTEIN (mg/dL)	OPENING PRESSURE (cm H$_2$O)	APPEARANCE
Normal[a]	< 10	< 5	~ 2/3 of serum	15–45	10–20	Clear
Bacterial meningitis	Normal	↑ (PMNs)	↓	↑	↑	Cloudy
Aseptic/viral meningitis, encephalitis	Normal	↑ (lymphs)[b]	Normal	Normal or ↑	Normal or ↑	Usually clear
Chronic meningitis (TB, fungal)	Normal	↑ (lymphs)[b]	↓	↑	↑	Clear or cloudy
Spirochetal meningitis (syphilis, Lyme disease)	Normal	↑ (lymphs)[b]	Normal	↑	Normal or ↑	Clear or cloudy
Neighborhood reaction[c]	Normal	Variable	Normal	Normal or ↑	Normal or ↑	Usually clear
SAH, cerebral contusion	↑↑	↑	Normal	↑↑	Normal or ↑	Yellow or red

[a]Traumatic tap usually yields 1 WBC/800 RBCs and 1 mg protein/1000 RBCs.

[b]May have PMN predominance in early stages.

[c]May be seen with brain abscess, epidural abscess, vertebral osteomyelitis, sinusitis/mastoiditis, septic thrombus, and brain tumor.

tients, and those with terminal complement (C5–C9) and properdin deficiencies.

- ■ *H influenzae* **type b chemoprophylaxis:** Give rifampin to household contacts of unvaccinated children < 4 years of age; also consider for day care contacts.
- ■ *H influenzae* **type b vaccine:** Routine childhood immunization; consider in adult patients with asplenia.

ENCEPHALITIS

A 45-year-old man undergoing chemotherapy presents with confusion of five days' duration. His vital signs and basic labs are unremarkable except for a low-grade fever, and on exam he is noted to be agitated and acting inappropriately. His MRI shows enhancement around his temporal lobes. What is the next best test to diagnose this patient's condition?

CSF HSV PCR. This patient presents with symptoms of encephalitis and has temporal lobe involvement, which is classically seen in HSV. The next step would be to perform an LP, which may show a high RBC count from brain necrosis; an HSV PCR from the CSF can then be conducted to make the diagnosis. Note that the PCR may be ⊖ early in disease and may turn ⊕ on subsequent LPs.

HSV and arboviruses (eg, **West Nile virus,** eastern and western equine virus, St. Louis virus) are the most common causes of encephalitis in the United States. Patients may report travel (Japanese B virus), a tick bite (Rocky Mountain spotted fever, Lyme disease, ehrlichiosis), or an animal bite (rabies). Postinfectious cases are seen 1–3 weeks after URI, measles infection, or smallpox vaccination.

SYMPTOMS

Presentation is similar to that of meningitis (see above).

EXAM

- Exam reveals focal neurologic signs, including motor weakness, accentuated DTRs, hemiparesis, cranial nerve palsies (especially CN III and CN VI), and seizures.
- A rash may be seen with Lyme disease, Rocky Mountain spotted fever, and VZV; weakness and flaccid paralysis may be seen with West Nile virus.

DIFFERENTIAL

Brain abscess, 1° or 2° brain tumor, subdural hematoma, SLE, drugs/toxic encephalopathy.

DIAGNOSIS

The 1° goal is to **distinguish HSV from other causes.**

- CSF findings are usually abnormal but nonspecific. **RBCs** may be seen in HSV encephalitis.
- EEG shows diffuse slowing of brain waves. **HSV encephalitis may localize to the temporal lobes** with highly characteristic slow-wave (2- to 3-Hz) complexes.
- MRI with gadolinium shows multifocal lesions (white matter demyelination may be seen in postinfectious cases). Temporal lobe involvement is seen with HSV.
- Acute and convalescent serologies depending on the suspected etiology (eg, **fourfold** rise in serum antibodies against St. Louis virus).
- Special CSF testing for specific arboviral IgM antibodies. **PCR for HSV is sensitive and specific in most studies.**

TREATMENT

- Supportive care (antipyretics, antiseizure medications, lowering of ICP, mechanical ventilation); IV acyclovir for HSV and VZV.
- The effect of steroids or IVIG on postinfectious encephalitis is unclear.

COMPLICATIONS

Patients with HSV encephalitis have high mortality (70%) and serious sequelae, especially if treatment is delayed. Arboviral infections are largely subclinical except for eastern equine virus, which has > 50% mortality in infants and older adults but is the least common.

KEY FACT

Encephalitis that develops in the summer or fall is often due to arboviruses. In late spring or early summer, think of tick-borne infections. In the winter or spring, think of measles, mumps, and HSV.

KEY FACT

Encephalitis preceded by flaccid paralysis is a clue to West Nile virus, which affects anterior horn cells.

ENDOCARDITIS

> A 65-year-old man with a congenital bicuspid aortic valve presents with fever and is found to have *S aureus* bacteremia with an aortic valve vegetation. He is hemodynamically stable and placed on the appropriate antibiotics. On hospital day 5, he develops weakness, and an ECG reveals AV dissociation. What is the next best step in this patient's management?
> Surgical valve repair. This patient has developed third-degree heart block, which can be a complication of aortic valve endocarditis with perivalvular extension. It is an indication for surgical management of the infected valve.

Infection of the heart valves. Classified as **native valve endocarditis (NVE)** or **prosthetic valve endocarditis (PVE)**. IV drug users are a special population at risk, particularly for tricuspid valve endocarditis (see Table 11.3).

Symptoms

- **Acute bacterial endocarditis:** High fever (80%), chills, and embolic phenomena; often there is no murmur.
- **Subacute endocarditis:** Has an **indolent course;** presents with **nonspecific symptoms** such as low-grade fever, chills, night sweats, malaise, weight loss, anorexia, and more immunologic manifestations.

Exam

- Presents with fever, a regurgitant heart murmur, **Osler's nodes** ("**OUCH**ler's" nodes—painful nodules on the finger and toe pads), **splinter hemorrhages** (reddish-brown streaks in the proximal nail beds), **petechiae** (especially conjunctival and mucosal), **Janeway lesions** (nontender hemorrhagic macules on the palms and soles), and **Roth's spots** (see the Dermatology chapter for images).
- Patients with right-sided disease may develop right-sided heart failure or pulmonary findings, including pleuritic chest pain, cough, and radiographic abnormalities (multiple septic pulmonary emboli and pleural effusions).

Differential

Atrial myxoma, marantic endocarditis (nonbacterial thrombotic endocarditis, seen in cancer and chronic wasting diseases), Libman-Sacks Endocarditis

TABLE 11.3. Etiologies of Endocarditis

Type	Etiology
NVE	Viridans streptococci, other streptococci, *S aureus,* enterococci.
PVE	*Staphylococcus epidermidis, S aureus.*
IV drug use	*S aureus.*
"Culture-⊖" endocarditis	Recent antibiotic use. **HACEK organisms: H**aemophilus, **A**ctinobacillus, **C**ardiobacterium, **E**ikenella, **K**ingella. ***Candida*** and ***Aspergillus:*** IV drug users, long-term indwelling catheters, immunosuppressed. **Rare causes:** *Chlamydia psittaci,* the "ellas" (*Bartonella, Legionella, Brucella, Coxiella*), Whipple's disease.

(seen in **SLE**; involves autoantibodies to heart valve), acute rheumatic fever, suppurative thrombophlebitis, catheter-related sepsis, renal cell carcinoma, carcinoid syndrome.

DIAGNOSIS

- **Labs:** Leukocytosis with left shift, mild anemia, ↑ ESR. UA may show proteinuria, **microscopic hematuria,** and RBC casts.
- **Blood cultures** are critical in establishing a diagnosis and are ⊕ in 85–95% of cases. It is recommended that **three sets** of blood cultures be taken at least **one hour apart** (before antibiotics).
- **Echocardiography:** Transthoracic echocardiography (TTE) has 60–75% sensitivity; transesophageal echocardiography (TEE) has 95% sensitivity. Both are 95% specific.
- **Duke criteria:** A **definitive diagnosis** can be made with the following:
  - **Pathologic criteria:** A ⊕ valve culture or histology.
  - **Clinical criteria:** Two major, one major plus three minor, or five minor criteria.
    - **Major criteria:** ⊕ blood cultures (two or more sets drawn at separate sites and times) and either a **new regurgitant murmur** or an **oscillating vegetation on echocardiogram.**
    - **Minor criteria: Predisposing conditions (valvular heart disease or IV drug use), fever, embolic disease** (pulmonary or intracranial infarcts, mycotic aneurysm, conjunctival hemorrhages, Janeway lesions), **immunologic phenomena** (glomerulonephritis, Osler's nodes, Roth's spots, RF), and a ⊕ **blood culture** not meeting the major criteria.
- According to the Duke criteria, a diagnosis of endocarditis is **possible** with **one major plus one minor or three minor clinical criteria.**

TREATMENT

- **NVE (empiric):** Typically started with vancomycin plus gentamicin. Adjust antibiotics on the basis of culture results and treat for 4–6 weeks.
- **PVE (empiric):** Vancomycin plus rifampin plus gentamicin. Adjust antibiotics on the basis of culture results and treat for six weeks.
- **Persistent fever after one week of appropriate antibiotic therapy** raises concern for a perivalvular or myocardial abscess or a septic embolic focus.
- **The reappearance of fever** after initial defervescence suggests septic emboli, drug fever, interstitial nephritis, or, less commonly, the emergence of resistant organisms.

PREVENTION

- **Antibiotic prophylaxis** is recommended for prosthetic heart valves, patients with a history of infective endocarditis, those with cyanotic heart disease (unrepaired or within six months after repair), or heart transplant recipients with valvulopathy.
- **Procedures for which prophylaxis is recommended** include dental extractions and periodontal procedures; incision or biopsy of respiratory mucosa (eg, tonsillectomy, transbronchial biopsy); and procedures on infected skin or musculoskeletal structures (eg, abscess drainage). Prophylaxis may also be reasonable for patients with enterococcal UTIs who will have invasive urinary procedures.
  - **Dental procedures:** PO amoxicillin, IV ampicillin, or IV/PO clindamycin 30–60 minutes before the procedure.
  - **Procedures on infected skin or musculoskeletal structures:** PO cephalexin or IV nafcillin or cefazolin 30–60 minutes before the procedure. For severe penicillin allergy or suspected MRSA, use clindamycin or vancomycin.

KEY FACT

Streptococcus bovis and *Clostridium septicum* endocarditis/bacteremia are seen in patients with bowel pathology and should prompt upper and lower GI endoscopies.

KEY FACT

PR prolongation in a patient with endocarditis may suggest conduction abnormalities due to an aortic valve ring abscess.

KEY FACT

Indications for surgery during active infection include refractory CHF (has 50% mortality if surgery is delayed), valvular obstruction, myocardial abscess, perivalvular extension (new conduction abnormalities), persistent bacteremia, fungal endocarditis, and most cases of PVE.

COMPLICATIONS

- **CHF:** Caused by valvular destruction or myocarditis. **The most common cause of death due to endocarditis.**
- **Embolic phenomena:** Mycotic aneurysms, infarcts, or abscesses in the CNS, kidney, coronary arteries, or spleen. Right-sided disease usually causes pulmonary emboli but may also cause systemic emboli with a **patent foramen ovale** (as indicated by a ⊕ bubble study on echocardiogram).
- Arrhythmias and heart block.
- Myocardial or perivalvular abscess (especially with *S aureus*); may extend to cause pericarditis and tamponade.

FEVER OF UNKNOWN ORIGIN (FUO)

A **temperature of > 38.3°C** (100.9°F) that lasts at least **three weeks** and remains undiagnosed despite evaluation for **more than two outpatient visits** or **three hospital days**. Etiologies vary depending on the patient's age, immune status, and geographic location. In the United States, infection (33%), cancer (25%), and, to a lesser extent, autoimmune diseases (13%) are responsible for most identified cases. Infection is likely if the patient is older or from a developing country, as well as in the setting of nosocomial, neutropenic, or HIV-associated FUO. Etiologies can be broadly categorized as follows:

- **Infectious: TB, endocarditis,** and **occult abscesses** are the most common infectious causes of FUO in immunocompetent patients. Consider 1° HIV infection or opportunistic infections due to unrecognized HIV.
- **Neoplastic: Lymphoma** and **leukemia** are the most common cancers causing FUO. Other causes include hepatoma, renal cell carcinoma, and atrial myxoma.
- **Autoimmune:** Adult Still's disease, SLE, cryoglobulinemia, polyarteritis nodosa, giant cell (temporal) arteritis/polymyalgia rheumatica (more common in the elderly).
- **Miscellaneous:** Other causes of FUO include drug fever, hyperthyroidism or thyroiditis, Crohn's disease, Whipple's disease, familial Mediterranean fever, recurrent pulmonary embolism, retroperitoneal hematoma, and factitious fever.
- In roughly 10–15% of cases, the cause is not diagnosed. **Most of these cases resolve spontaneously.**

KEY FACT

FUO is most commonly due to unusual presentations of common diseases rather than to rare diseases.

EXAM

Repeated physical exams may yield subtle findings in the fundi, conjunctivae, sinuses, temporal arteries, and lymph nodes. Heart murmurs, splenomegaly, and perirectal or prostatic fluctuance/tenderness should be assessed.

DIAGNOSIS

- **History:** Ask about immune status, cardiac valve disorders, drug use, travel, TB exposure history, exposure to animals and insects, occupational history, all medications (prescription, OTC, and herbals), sick contacts, and a family history of fever.
- **Labs/imaging:**
    - Obtain routine labs, blood cultures (with the patient off antibiotics; hold culture bottles for two weeks), CXR, and PPD. If indicated, obtain cultures of other body fluids (sputum, urine, stool, CSF) as well as a blood smear (eg, for malaria, babesiosis) and an HIV test.
    - Echocardiography for vegetations; CT/MRI (eg, of abdomen or pelvis) if neoplasms or abscesses are suspected.

- Use more specific tests selectively (ANA, RF, viral cultures, antibody/antigen tests for viral and fungal infections).
- Invasive procedures are generally low yield except for temporal artery biopsy in the elderly, liver biopsy in patients with LFT abnormalities, and bone marrow biopsy for HIV.

TREATMENT

- If there are no other symptoms, treatment may be deferred until a definitive diagnosis is made.
- Broad-spectrum antibiotics if the patient is severely ill or neutropenic.

INFECTIOUS MONONUCLEOSIS

Caused by the Epstein-Barr virus (EBV). Commonly seen in late adolescence and early adulthood, particularly in college or military populations. The clinical course is generally benign, with patients recovering in 2–3 weeks.

SYMPTOMS

- Presents with the triad of **fever, sore throat** (may be severe), and **generalized lymphadenopathy,** often with an abrupt onset.
- Patients may have a viral-like prodrome as well as retro-orbital headache or abdominal fullness (from hepatosplenomegaly).

EXAM

- Exam reveals lymphadenopathy (especially of the posterior cervical nodes), pharyngitis, and splenomegaly.
- A maculopapular rash occurs in 10% of patients (especially in those given ampicillin), and palatal petechiae may be seen. RUQ tenderness is more common than hepatomegaly.

DIFFERENTIAL

- **CMV:** Consider if there was a recent blood transfusion. Symptoms are usually systemic; sore throat and lymphadenopathy are uncommon. Diagnose with a ⊕ CMV IgM.
- **Acute toxoplasmosis:** Presents with nontender head and neck lymphadenopathy and mild lymphocytosis. Diagnose with *Toxoplasma* IgM and IgG seroconversion.
- **1° HIV infection:** Fever, lymphadenopathy, pharyngitis, maculopapular rash, and, less commonly, aseptic meningitis.
- **HAV or HBV:** Characterized by markedly ↑ AST and ALT.
- **Syphilis.**
- **Rubella:** A prominent rash begins on the face and progresses to the trunk and extremities. Has a shorter course (only several days).
- **Streptococcal pharyngitis:** Presents with fever, tender submandibular or anterior cervical lymphadenopathy, and pharyngotonsillar exudates with no cough. Splenomegaly is not seen. Diagnose with a rapid streptococcal test and throat culture if the antigen test is ⊖.

DIAGNOSIS

- Labs reveal neutropenia (mild left shift); **atypical lymphocytes** (see Figure 11.1) in 70% of cases (WBC count 12,000–18,000 and occasionally 30,000–50,000/μL); thrombocytopenia; and mildly ↑ LFTs.
- **Heterophile antibodies** (Monospot test) are found in 90% of cases (may initially be ⊖ and then turn ⊕ in 2–3 weeks). Other EBV serologies are rarely needed.

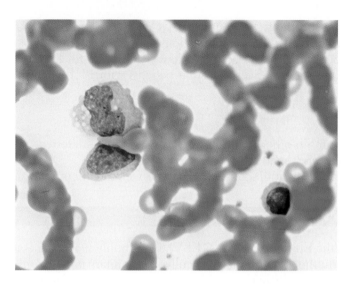

FIGURE 11.1. **Atypical lymphocytosis in a patient with infectious mononucleosis.** These reactive T lymphocytes are large with eccentric nuclei and bluish-staining RNA in the cytoplasm. (Reproduced with permission from Fauci AS et al. *Harrison's Principles of Internal Medicine,* 17th ed. New York: McGraw-Hill, 2008, Fig. 174-2.)

- Anti-VCA IgM is ⊕ at presentation; anti-EBNA and anti-S antibodies are ⊕ in 3–4 weeks. Anti-VCA IgG antibodies are ⊕ if patients were previously exposed. Cold agglutinins are found in 80% of cases after 2–3 weeks.

TREATMENT

No treatment is necessary in the majority of cases. Steroids are used on rare occasions for tonsillar obstruction, severe thrombocytopenia, autoimmune hemolytic anemia, and CNS complications.

COMPLICATIONS

Autoimmune hemolytic anemia (< 3%). Splenic rupture is rare but may occur in weeks 2–3 (patients should avoid contact sports and heavy lifting). Meningoencephalitis is rare, and patients usually recover completely.

OSTEOMYELITIS

A 47-year-old Asian man presents with lower back pain. Plain films show possible loss of vertebral height in the thoracic spine, and an MRI reveals enhancement of adjacent vertebral bodies with sparing of the intervening disk space. What is the most likely diagnosis?

Tuberculous osteomyelitis (Pott's disease). Pyogenic osteomyelitis usually has involvement of the disk space between adjacent vertebral bodies; the finding of disk sparing is more classic for spinal TB. A biopsy may be useful in showing granulomas or may grow AFB. Adjunctive testing with PPD and CXR may also be used to make the diagnosis. RIPE therapy (rifampin, INH, pyrazinamide, and ethambutol) is the treatment of choice.

Spread may be contiguous (80%) or hematogenous (20%). **Local spread** occurs in diabetics and in patients with vascular insufficiency, prosthetic joints, decubitus ulcers, trauma, and recent neurosurgery. **Hematogenous spread** affects IV drug users, those with sickle cell disease, and the elderly. Categorized as follows:

- **Etiologic agents:**
    - Common agents include *S aureus* and, to a lesser extent, coagulase-⊖ staphylococci (prosthetic joints or postoperative infections), streptococci, anaerobes (bites, diabetic foot infections, decubitus ulcers), *Pasteurella* (animal bites), *Eikenella* (human bites), and *Pseudomonas* (nail punctures through sneakers).
    - Other causes include *Salmonella* (sickle cell disease), *Mycobacterium tuberculosis* (foreign immigrants, HIV), *Bartonella* (HIV), and *Brucella* (unpasteurized dairy products).
- **Location:** *Pseudomonas* affects the sternoclavicular joint and symphysis pubis (in IV drug users); *Brucella* affects the sacroiliac joint, knee, and hip. TB affects the lower thoracic vertebrae (Pott's disease).

SYMPTOMS/EXAM

- **Contiguous spread:** Local redness, warmth, and tenderness; patients are afebrile and are not systemically ill.
- **Hematogenous spread:** Sudden fever; pain and tenderness over the affected bone. May present only with pain (but no fever).
- **Vertebral osteomyelitis with epidural abscess:** Spinal pain followed by radicular pain and weakness.
- **Prosthetic hip and knee infections:** May present only as pain on weight bearing.

DIAGNOSIS

- **Probing to bone (diabetic patients):** Approximately 66% sensitive and 85% specific (PPV 89%).
- **Plain radiographs:** May initially look normal and then reveal bony erosions or periosteal elevation ≥ 2 weeks after infection (see Figure 11.2).

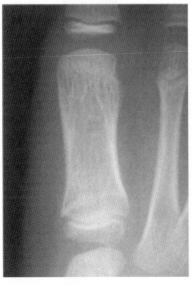
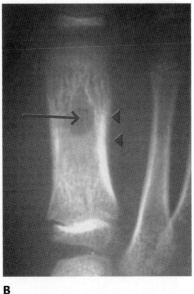
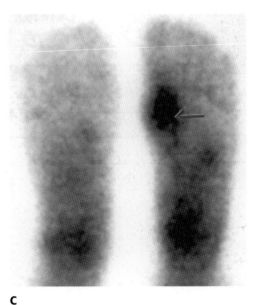

A   **B**   **C**

FIGURE 11.2.   Acute osteomyelitis. (A) Radiograph of the right foot first metatarsal following puncture injury, with no foreign body and no evidence of osteomyelitis. **(B)** Follow-up radiograph reveals interval development of focal lucency (red arrow) and periosteal reaction (red arrowheads) consistent with acute osteomyelitis. **(C)** Planar image from a bone scan obtained at the same time as Image B shows increased radiotracer uptake in the region of the first metatarsal of the right foot (red arrow), confirming osteomyelitis. (Reproduced with permission from Skinner HB. *Current Diagnosis & Treatment in Orthopedics,* 4th ed. New York: McGraw-Hill, 2006, Fig. 8-8A, C, and D.)

Less helpful in trauma or diabetic/vascular patients with neuropathy (frequent stress fractures).

- **CT scans.**
- **MRI:** Approximately 90% sensitive and specific (can show abnormal marrow edema and enhancement and surrounding soft tissue infection). Especially useful for diagnosing vertebral osteomyelitis (see Figure 11.3).
- **Nuclear scans:** Three- or four-phase studies with technetium-99 are preferred. Most useful for distinguishing bone from soft tissue inflammation when the diagnosis is ambiguous.
- **Microbiology:** Obtain bone culture at debridement or by needle aspiration; sinus tract cultures are not reliable. With hematogenous osteomyelitis, blood cultures may obviate the need for bone biopsy.

TREATMENT

- After debridement of necrotic bone (with cultures taken), empiric antibiotics should be chosen to cover the likely pathogens (see above).
- IV antibiotics should be given for 4–6 weeks, although oral quinolones may be equally effective in some circumstances.
- The choice of agent should be guided by microbiology. In patients who are not candidates for definitive therapy, long-term suppressive antibiotics may be used.
- Surgery is indicated for spinal cord decompression, bony stabilization, removal of necrotic bone in chronic osteomyelitis, and reestablishment of vascular supply.

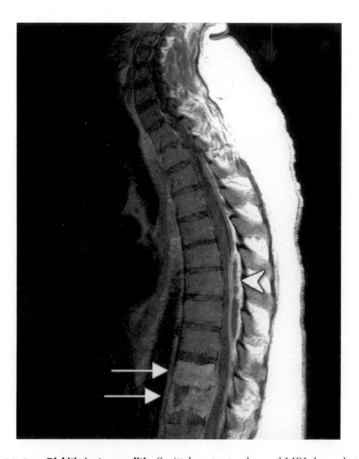

FIGURE 11.3. Diskitis/osteomyelitis. Sagittal contrast-enhanced MRI shows destruction of a lower thoracic intervertebral disk with abnormal enhancement throughout the adjacent vertebral bodies (arrows) and a posterior rim-enhancing epidural abscess (arrowhead) in the spinal canal. (Reproduced with permission from Tintinalli JE et al. *Tintinalli's Emergency Medicine: A Comprehensive Study Guide,* 6th ed. New York: McGraw-Hill, 2004, Fig. 305-5.)

PREVENTION

Diabetics with neuropathy (detected by the 10-g monofilament test) should be taught to examine their feet on a daily basis and should be examined by a clinician at least once every three months.

COMPLICATIONS

Vertebral osteomyelitis with epidural abscess; chronic osteomyelitis.

PYELONEPHRITIS

Caused by the same bacteria as those responsible for uncomplicated UTI (eg, *E coli*). With the exception of *S aureus*, most cases are caused by organisms ascending from the lower urinary tract; *S aureus* is most frequently hematogenous and produces intrarenal or perinephric abscesses. Renal struvite stones (staghorn calculi) are frequently associated with recurrent UTI due to urease-producing bacteria (*Proteus*, *Pseudomonas*, and enterococci).

SYMPTOMS

Presents with flank pain and fever. Patients often have lower urinary tract symptoms (dysuria, urgency, and frequency) that sometimes occur 1–2 days before the upper tract symptoms. They may also have nausea, vomiting, or diarrhea.

EXAM

Exam reveals fever, CVA tenderness, and mild abdominal tenderness.

DIFFERENTIAL

Renal stones, renal infarcts, cholecystitis, appendicitis, diverticulitis, acute prostatitis/epididymitis.

DIAGNOSIS

UA shows pyuria and bacteriuria and may also exhibit hematuria or WBC casts. CBC reveals leukocytosis with left shift. Urine culture is usually ⊕, and blood culture may be ⊕ as well. Imaging is not required to make a diagnosis of pyelonephritis.

 KEY FACT

Fever and WBC casts on UA are seen in pyelonephritis but not in cystitis.

TREATMENT

- Fluoroquinolone × 7 days or ampicillin plus gentamicin or ceftriaxone × 14 days.
- Radiologic evaluation for complications may be useful in patients who are severely ill or immunocompromised; those who are not responding to treatment; or those in whom complications are likely (eg, pregnant patients, diabetics, and those with nephrolithiasis, reflux, transplant surgery, or other GU surgery).
- Radiographs can detect stones, calcification, masses, and abnormal gas collections, or they may look normal.
- Ultrasound is rapid and safe.
- Contrast-enhanced CT is most sensitive (see Figure 11.4) but may affect renal function.

COMPLICATIONS

- Perinephric abscess should be considered in patients who remain febrile 2–3 days after appropriate antibiotics; UA may be normal and cultures ⊖. Patients are treated by percutaneous or surgical drainage plus antibiotics.
- Intrarenal abscesses (eg, infection of a renal cyst) < 5 cm in size usually respond to antibiotics alone.

 KEY FACT

Patients with diabetes may develop emphysematous pyelonephritis, which usually requires nephrectomy and is associated with a high mortality rate.

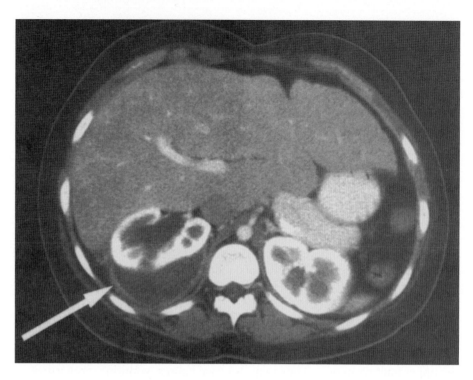

FIGURE 11.4. **Perinephric abscess.** Acute right pyelonephritis complicated by a right perinephric abscess (arrow). (Reproduced with permission from Tanagho EA, McAninch JW. *Smith's General Urology,* 17th ed. New York: McGraw-Hill, 2008, Fig. 13-4.)

Sexually Transmitted Diseases (STDs)

GENERAL CHARACTERISTICS

Table 11.4 outlines STDs that result in genital ulcers as well as urethral or cervical discharge. Refer to the Women's Health chapter for further discussion of STDs, cervical cancer screening, and chlamydia screening.

SYPHILIS

 A 33-year-old HIV-⊕ man presents with new visual complaints. He is referred to an ophthalmologist, who notes bilateral chorioretinitis. The patient has a ⊖ PPD, a CD4 count of 430 cells/mm³, and an RPR of 1:64. His only previous RPR was taken 18 months ago and was nonreactive. How should this patient be treated?

He should be treated with a 14-day course of IV penicillin for neurosyphilis. Having a ⊕ RPR with the most recent ⊖ RPR taken > 1 year ago would place this patient in the category of late latent syphilis, but the finding of ocular involvement qualifies this as neurosyphilis. As such, the patient should be treated with a full 14-day course of IV penicillin.

Caused by the spirochete *Treponema pallidum.*

TABLE 11.4.   Diagnosis and Treatment of Selected STDs

DISEASE	PATHOGEN	CLINICAL PRESENTATION	DIAGNOSIS	TREATMENT OPTIONS
CAUSES OF GENITAL ULCERS				
Chancroid	*Haemophilus ducreyi*	A **painful** erythematous papule evolving into a pustule that erodes into an **ulcer with purulence.** Also presents with **marked lymphadenitis (buboes).**	Gram stain shows small gram-⊖ rods in parallel alignment ("school of fish"); culture, PCR.	**Drain buboes.** **Azithromycin 1 g PO × 1** or ceftriaxone IM, ciprofloxacin, or erythromycin.
HSV	Human herpes simplex virus 1 or 2	**Painful** multiple vesicular or ulcerative lesions. Reactive lymphadenopathy is common.	Tzanck smear shows multinucleated giant cells (50% sensitivity); culture, DFA, PCR, IgG ELISA.	**Acyclovir 400 mg PO TID or 200 mg PO 5ID × 7–10 days,** or famciclovir or valacyclovir. Consider suppressive or episodic treatment for recurrent infection.
Granuloma inguinale	*Klebsiella granulomatis* (formerly known as *Calymmato- bacterium granulomatis*)	**Painless, progressive ulcerative lesions without regional lymphadenopathy. Beefy-red ulcers** bleed on contact. Rare in the United States; endemic in tropical regions.	Culture is low yield. Biopsy shows dark-staining Donovan bodies. PCR is available.	**Doxycycline 100 mg PO BID × ≥ 3 weeks until all lesions have completely healed.** Alternative regimens include azithromycin, ciprofloxacin, erythromycin, or TMP-SMX × ≥ 3 weeks until all lesions have completely healed.
Lymphogranuloma venereum	*Chlamydia trachomatis* (serovar L1, L2, or L3)	A **painless,** small ulcer at the site of inoculation. Also presents with **large, tender, fluctuant inguinal lymphadenopathy (buboes).** Rectal disease may result in hemorrhagic proctocolitis. Strictures and fistulae may form.	Culture is low yield; serology is most commonly used. PCR is available.	**Drain buboes.** **Doxycycline 100 mg PO BID** or erythromycin × 21 days.
Syphilis	*Treponema pallidum*	A **painless** solitary ulcer (rarely multiple). May have painless, rubbery lymphadenopathy.	Darkfield microscopy; DFA of tissue. RPR/VDRL confirmed by FTA-ABS (RPR/VDRL may take 12 weeks to turn ⊕).	**For 1° syphilis:** **Benzathine penicillin G 2.4 million U IM × 1.** For penicillin-allergic patients, give doxycycline 100 mg PO BID × 14 days or tetracycline 500 mg PO QID × 14 days.

(continues)

TABLE 11.4. **Diagnosis and Treatment of Selected STDs** *(continued)*

DISEASE	PATHOGEN	CLINICAL PRESENTATION	DIAGNOSIS	TREATMENT OPTIONS
		CAUSES OF URETHRITIS AND CERVICITIS		
Gonococcal (GC)	*Neisseria gonorrhoeae*	Purulent discharge. May have **pharyngitis, proctitis, and PID.** Disseminated GC infection is associated with two syndromes: (1) fever, tenosynovitis, and painful vesiculopustular skin lesions or (2) purulent arthritis without skin lesions.	Gram stain of urethral or cervical swab shows intracellular gram-⊖ diplococci (see Figure 11.5). Culture on Thayer-Martin media, nucleic acid amplification test (NAAT), DNA probe.	Ceftriaxone 125 mg IM × 1 or cefixime PO × 1 **plus treatment for chlamydia if chlamydial infection is not ruled out.**[a]
Nongonococcal (NG)	***C trachomatis*** (less common pathogens include *Mycoplasma genitalium,* HSV, *Trichomonas vaginalis,* and *Ureaplasma urealyticum*)	**Mucoid or watery discharge; dysuria.** Other syndromes include proctitis, epididymitis, and PID. Has a known association with postinfectious reactive arthritis.	**Urethritis:** Mucopurulent or purulent discharge; Gram stain of urethral secretions shows > 5 WBCs/hpf plus leukocyte esterase on first-void urine. ***C trachomatis:*** NAAT on the urethra, vagina, or urine; culture.	Azithromycin 1 g PO × 1 or doxycycline 100 mg PO BID × 7 days.

[a] Quinolones are no longer recommended by the CDC for treatment of GC infections in the United States owing to high rates of resistance.

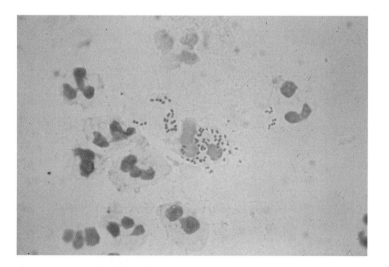

FIGURE 11.5. **Gonococcal urethritis: Gram stain of *Neisseria gonorrhoeae.*** Multiple gram-⊖ diplococci are seen within PMNs as well as in the extracellular areas of a smear from a urethral discharge. (Reproduced with permission from Wolff K et al. *Fitzpatrick's Color Atlas & Synopsis of Clinical Dermatology,* 5th ed. New York: McGraw-Hill, 2005: 906.)

SYMPTOMS/EXAM

- 1° syphilis:
    - Usually presents with a chancre (see Figure 11.6), a single painless papule that erodes to form a clean-based ulcer with raised/indurated edges (may be multiple or atypical for HIV-⊕ patients or minimal for those with previous syphilis).
    - Also presents with **regional nontender lymphadenopathy.** The incubation period is three weeks (ranging from three days to three months). The chancre resolves in 3–6 weeks, but lymphadenopathy persists.
- 2° syphilis:
    - Presents with a **maculopapular rash** that may include the palms and soles; **condylomata lata** in intertriginous areas (painless, broad, grayish-white to erythematous plaques that are highly infectious); **alopecia** (see Figure 11.7); or a **mucous patch** (condylomata lata on the mucosa).
    - **Systemic symptoms** include low-grade fever, malaise, pharyngitis, laryngitis, lymphadenopathy (especially epitrochlear), anorexia, weight loss, arthralgias, headache, and meningismus (aseptic meningitis).
    - Occurs 2–8 weeks after the 1° chancre, but may overlap.

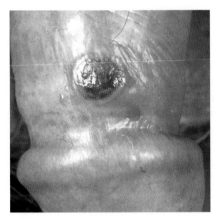

A

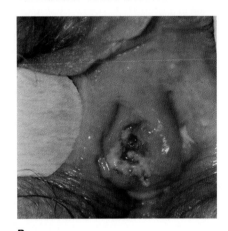

B

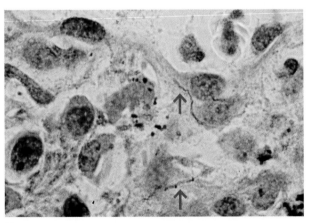

C

FIGURE 11.6.   **Syphilis.** (A) Male and (B) female genital chancres, respectively, in primary syphilis infection. (C) Silver stain of sample from a chancre showing spiral-shaped spirochetes (arrows). (Reproduced with permission from Wolff K et al. *Fitzpatrick's Dermatology in General Medicine,* 7th ed. New York: McGraw-Hill, 2008, Figs. 200-2, 200-5, and 200-1.)

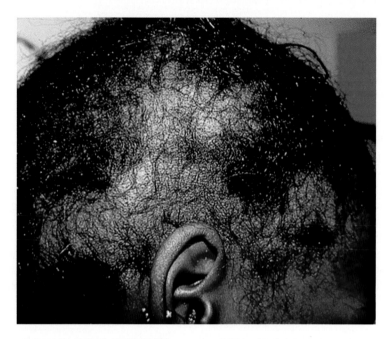

FIGURE 11.7. Alopecia of 2° syphilis. Hair loss may be one of the only cutaneous manifestations of 2° syphilis that may present either as patchy, "moth-eaten" alopecia or as generalized thinning. (Reproduced with permission from Wolff K et al. *Fitzpatrick's Dermatology in General Medicine*, 7th ed. New York: McGraw-Hill, 2008, Fig. 200-19.)

- **Latent syphilis:** ⊕ serology but no current symptoms.
    - **Early latent** (< 1 year): Characterized by a fourfold ↑ in antibody titer; associated with a known history of 1° or 2° syphilis and an infected partner.
    - **Late latent** (> 1 year or unknown duration): One-third of patients progress to 3° syphilis.
- **3° syphilis:**
    - May include **aortitis** (aneurysm rupture is the leading cause of death from syphilis) or destructive **gummas** (bone, skin, mucocutaneous areas).
    - **Neurosyphilis** is usually asymptomatic (CSF findings include a WBC count of > 5, ↑ protein, low glucose, and a ⊕ CSF-VDRL). CNS symptoms include **tabes dorsalis** (demyelination of the posterior columns leading to a wide-based gait and foot slap), **Argyll Robertson pupil** (an irregular, small pupil that accommodates but does not respond to light), and meningovascular syphilis (subacute encephalopathy with multifocal ischemic infarcts).
    - Occurs 1–20 years after initial infection.

DIFFERENTIAL

Table 11.5 outlines the differential diagnosis of lesions on the palms and soles. The differential of genital ulcer disease is as follows:

- 1° syphilis.
- HSV.
- Chancroid (*H ducreyi*).
- **Lymphogranuloma venereum** (*C trachomatis* serovars L1–L3).

TABLE 11.5. **Differential Diagnosis of Lesions on the Palms and Soles**

Disease	Cause	Lesion Features	Distribution
Rocky Mountain spotted fever	*Rickettsia rickettsii*	Macules, then petechiae (see Figure 11.8).	Begins on the wrists and ankles; then spreads centrally; then affects the palms and soles late in the disease course.
2° syphilis	*T pallidum*	Reddish-brown, copper-colored papules; never vesicular (see Figure 11.9).	Condylomata lata or mucous patches on mucosa.
Erythema multiforme	Drug reaction, HSV, or *Mycoplasma* infection	Target lesions (see Figure 11.10).	Symmetric over the elbows, knees, palms, and soles. May become diffuse and involve the mucosa.
Acute meningococcemia	*N meningitidis*	Blanching macules; then gun-metal-gray petechiae and purpura (see Figure 11.11).	Begins on the distal extremities; then spreads to the trunk and "pressure spots" over hours.
Smallpox	Orthopoxvirus	Deep, round, tense vesicles and pustules.	Starts on the face and extremities; then moves to the trunk (centrifugal).
Endocarditis	*Staphylococcus, Streptococcus,* others	Janeway lesions are painless, hemorrhagic macules (see Figure 11.12). Osler's nodes are subcutaneous, tender, pink or purplish nodules.	Janeway lesions appear on the palms and soles. Osler's nodes are found on the pads of digits.
Hand-foot-and-mouth disease	Coxsackie A16 virus	Tender vesicles.	Peripheral and in the mouth. Outbreaks occur within families.
Rat-bite fever	*Streptobacillus moniliformis*	Maculopapules or purpura.	May be more severe at the joints of the arms and legs.
Atypical measles	Paramyxovirus (in patients who received killed virus vaccine from 1963 to 1967)	Maculopapules; may be hemorrhagic.	Most marked on the extremities. Typical measles has a central distribution (face/chest).

- Granuloma inguinale, donovanosis (*K granulomatis*).
- Trauma, excoriation (eg, zippers, scabies).
- **Other:** Psoriasis, Behçet's disease, Reiter's syndrome, lichen planus.

DIAGNOSIS

- Direct visualization of motile spirochetes by darkfield microscopy from condylomata lata or mucous patches.
- **VDRL and RPR:** Nontreponemal, nonspecific antibody tests are useful for screening (detect antibodies that cross-react with beef cardiolipin). The **prozone effect** may be seen in 2° syphilis or pregnancy (high antibody titers produce ⊖ tests that become ⊕ as the sample is diluted). The sensitivity of VDRL/RPR is 70% in 1° syphilis and 99% in 2° syphilis. False ⊕s have a titer of ≤ 1:8.

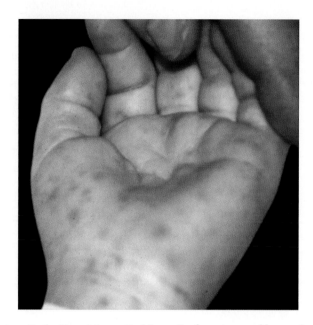

FIGURE 11.8. **Rocky Mountain spotted fever.** Erythematous and hemorrhagic macules and papules are seen on the wrists of a young child. (Reproduced with permission from Wolff K, Johnson RA. *Fitzpatrick's Color Atlas & Synopsis of Clinical Dermatology,* 6th ed. New York: McGraw-Hill, 2009, Fig. 26-1.)

- **FTA-ABS and MHA-TP:** Specific treponemal antibody tests that are used to confirm VDRL and RPR. Antibodies remain ⊕ for life (patients are "serofast").
- Patients at high risk of developing neurosyphilis should undergo LP and have a **CSF-VDRL** test. CSF-VDRL is specific but not sensitive for neurosyphilis (sensitivity 30–70%).
- **LP:** Indicated for patients with neurologic symptoms, a serum RPR ≥ 1:32, current aortitis or gummas, and previous treatment failure. LP for all HIV-⊕ patients has been recommended by some but is controversial.

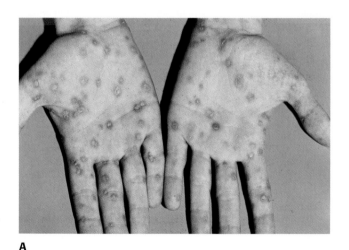

A

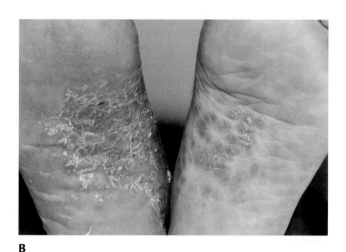

B

FIGURE 11.9. **2° syphilis.** Characteristic lesions can be seen on the palms (**A**) and soles (**B**). (Reproduced with permission from Wolff K et al. *Fitzpatrick's Dermatology in General Medicine,* 7th ed. New York: McGraw-Hill, 2008, Fig. 200-12.)

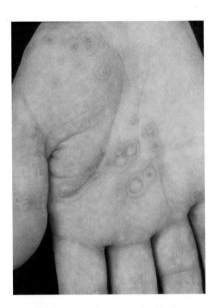

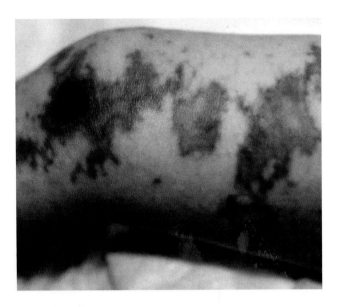

FIGURE 11.10. **Erythema multi-forme.** Typical target lesions are seen on the palm. (Reproduced with permission from Wolff K et al. *Fitzpatrick's Dermatology in General Medicine,* 7th ed. New York: McGraw-Hill, 2008, Fig. 38-2.)

FIGURE 11.11. **Acute meningococcemia.** (Reproduced with permission from Wolff K et al. *Fitzpatrick's Color Atlas & Synopsis of Clinical Dermatology,* 6th ed. New York: McGraw-Hill, 2009, Fig. 24-51.)

TREATMENT

- Think of syphilis as **early** (1°, 2°, early latent), **late** (late latent or 3°), or **neurosyphilis.**
  - Patients with **early syphilis** should receive benzathine penicillin G 2.4 MU IM × 1 or doxycycline or ceftriaxone. Failures occur with azithromycin (especially if the patient is infected with HIV).
  - Those with **late syphilis** should receive benzathine penicillin G 2.4 MU IM q week × 3 or doxycycline.
  - Patients with **neurosyphilis** require penicillin G 3 MU IV q 4 h × 10–14 days.

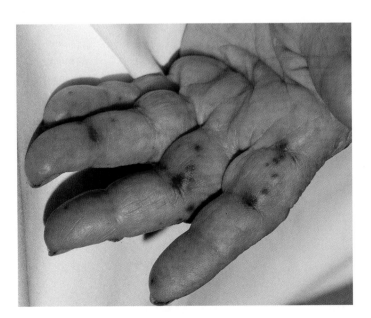

FIGURE 11.12. **Janeway lesions in endocarditis.** (Reproduced with permission from Wolff K et al. *Fitzpatrick's Color Atlas & Synopsis of Clinical Dermatology,* 6th ed. New York: McGraw-Hill, 2009, Fig. 24-46.)

- Pregnant women who are allergic to penicillin should be desensitized and treated with penicillin to prevent congenital syphilis.
- Repeat RPR or VDRL at 3, 6, 12, and 24 months; titer should ↓ **at least fourfold** 6–9 months after the treatment of 1° or 2° syphilis. If the test remains ⊕ after that time period, it suggests treatment failure, reinfection, or HIV.
- Treat again if clinical signs persist or recur or if the VDRL/RPR titer does not ↓ **fourfold.**
- **Jarisch-Herxheimer reactions** are commonly seen in the first 24 hours of treatment and are characterized by low-grade fever, headache, myalgias, malaise, and new skin lesions. They are thought to be due to cytokine release and may be seen following the treatment of other spirochetal illnesses (eg, Lyme disease, relapsing fever). Treat with antipyretics.

Skin and Soft Tissue Infections

SOFT TISSUE INFECTIONS

Table 11.6 outlines the etiology, clinical presentation, and treatment of common soft tissue infections.

TABLE 11.6. Common Soft Tissue Infections

ORGANISM	PATIENT CHARACTERISTICS	SOURCE OF ORGANISM	CLINICAL FEATURES	TREATMENT (EXAMPLES)
Group A streptococcus and occasionally groups B, C, and G	Normal.	Skin flora.	Cellulitis, erysipelas.	Dicloxacillin, cephalexin, clindamycin (penicillin if documented strep only).
S aureus	Same as above.	Same as above.	Furunculosis, abscess, cellulitis.	Same as above.
Vibrio vulnificus, other *Vibrio* spp.	Cirrhosis.	Shellfish or seawater exposure.	Hemorrhagic bullae, septic shock.	Ceftazidime, doxycycline.
Mycobacterium marinum	Normal.	Fish tanks.	Nonhealing ulcer, nodular lymphangitis.	Rifampin plus ethambutol, TMP-SMX.
Mycobacterium fortuitum	Normal.	Nail salon foot baths.	Furuncles.	Excision.
Pseudomonas, Aeromonas	Normal.	Hot tubs, freshwater exposure.	***Pseudomonas:*** Folliculitis. ***Aeromonas:*** Spreading cellulitis.	Quinolones.
Pseudomonas	Neutropenia.	—	Ecthyma gangrenosum (hemorrhagic bullae that ulcerate; see Figure 11.13).	Quinolones.

TABLE 11.6. **Common Soft Tissue Infections** *(continued)*

Organism	Patient Characteristics	Source of Organism	Clinical Features	Treatment (Examples)
Noninfectious agents	IBD, RA.	–	Pyoderma gangrenosum (a pustule/nodule that ulcerates).	Steroids.
Erysipelothrix	Fishermen, crab handlers.	–	Hands, fingers.	Penicillin, ampicillin, quinolone.
Bacillus anthracis	Hide tanners and wool workers (postal workers).	Soil (bioterrorism agent).	Nonpainful ulcer/eschar, extensive edema.	Doxycycline, quinolones.
Francisella tularensis (tularemia)	Trappers and skinners of wild rodents.	Ticks, rabbits.	Regional lymphadenopathy, pneumonia.	Doxycycline, streptomycin.
Pasteurella, Capnocytophaga	Normal.	Animal bites or scratches.	**Pasteurella:** Rapidly progressing cellulitis. **Capnocytophaga:** DIC, sepsis in asplenic and cirrhotic patients.	Amoxicillin/clavulanate.
Sporothrix schenckii	Gardeners, rose handlers.	Thorned plants.	Nodular lymphangitis.	Itraconazole.
Pityriasis rosea	After a viral URI, patients develop a "herald patch" followed by a generalized eruption.	–	Round, pink scaling patches; "Christmas tree" distribution on the back.	UV light; topical steroids and antihistamines for itching.

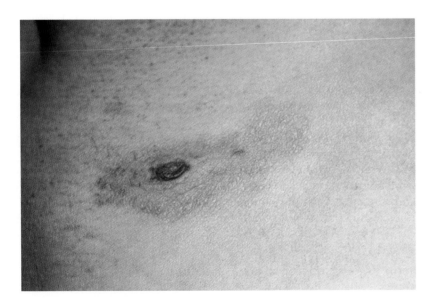

FIGURE 11.13. **Ecthyma gangrenosum.** Hemorrhagic bullae evolve from erythematous plaques, both of which are shown here. (Reproduced with permission from Lichtman MA et al. *Williams Hematology,* 8th ed. New York: McGraw-Hill, 2010, Fig. 123-13.)

TOXIC SHOCK SYNDROME (TSS)

Usually affects healthy individuals; associated with **exotoxins** released by certain strains of *S aureus* or group A streptococci (rarely groups B, C, or G). May cause a concurrent infection (osteomyelitis, occult abscesses, erysipelas, necrotizing fasciitis or myositis) or simply colonize a mucosal, postoperative, or burn-wound surface.

- **Streptococcal TSS:** Commonly associated with invasive infections.
- **Staphylococcal TSS:** Associated with menses and with the use of hyperabsorbable tampons that have now been withdrawn from the market ("menstrual TSS"). Most cases are now nonmenstrual TSS due to vaginal or surgical wound colonization.

SYMPTOMS/EXAM

- Staphylococcal or streptococcal isolation, evidence of end-organ damage (renal insufficiency, coagulopathy, abnormal LFTs), rash, ARDS, generalized edema or effusions, soft tissue necrosis.
- Staphylococcal TSS also requires fever and a diffuse macular rash that may subsequently desquamate (especially on the palms and soles). Other features include vomiting, diarrhea, severe myalgias, and confusion.
- Streptococcal TSS may be preceded by an influenza-like prodrome or by increasing pain at a deep site of infection.
- TSS is rarely preceded by streptococcal pharyngitis.

DIFFERENTIAL

Gram-⊖ septic shock, Rocky Mountain spotted fever, leptospirosis, measles, DVT.

DIAGNOSIS

- Routine labs, including CK.
- Vaginal examination.
- Cultures of blood, wounds, and vaginal mucosa.
- Evaluate for invasive streptococcal infection or occult staphylococcal infection.

TREATMENT

- Aggressive hydration and surgical debridement of deep-seated streptococcal infection and necrotic tissue are critical. Administer empiric broad-spectrum antibiotics.
- If the appropriate organism is isolated, narrow therapy to penicillin plus clindamycin (for streptococci) or nafcillin/oxacillin (vancomycin for MRSA) and perhaps clindamycin (for staphylococci).
- Clindamycin is added because it may ↓ toxin production and is active against organisms in the stationary phase; the cell wall–acting penicillins are most effective against rapidly growing bacteria. Consider adding IVIG.

COMPLICATIONS

Death (in 30% of streptococcal or 3% of staphylococcal TSS), gangrene of the extremities, ARDS, CKD.

Bioterrorism Agents

Table 11.7 outlines infectious agents that could potentially be used in acts of bioterrorism.

TABLE 11.7. Potential Bioterrorism Agents

Agent/Disease	Clinical Findings	Syndrome	Differential	Initial Diagnostic Testing	Immediate Infection Control	Treatment
Inhalational anthrax	Nonspecific flulike illness followed by abrupt onset of fever, chest pain, and dyspnea without CXR findings of pneumonia; progression to shock and death in 24–36 hours.	Acute respiratory distress with fever.	Pulmonary embolism, dissecting aortic aneurysm.	CXR with widened mediastinum; gram-⊕ rods in blood.	Standard precautions.	Ciprofloxacin, doxycycline, penicillin.
Pneumonic plague	Apparent severe community-acquired pneumonia, but with hemoptysis, cyanosis, GI symptoms, and progression to shock and death in 2–4 days.	Acute respiratory distress with fever.	Community-acquired pneumonia, hantavirus pulmonary syndrome, meningo-coccemia, rickettsial disease.	Gram-⊖ rods or coccobacilli with a "safety pin" appearance in sputum, blood, or lymph nodes.	Standard and droplet precautions.	Ciprofloxacin, doxycycline, gentamicin, streptomycin.
Smallpox	Severe flulike prodrome followed by a generalized papular rash that begins on the face and extremities and uniformly progresses to vesicles and pustules, headache, vomiting, back pain, and delirium.	Acute rash with fever.	Varicella (chickenpox), disseminated herpes zoster, monkeypox.	Clinical diagnosis.	Standard, droplet, airborne, and contact precautions.	Supportive care.
Viral hemorrhagic fever (eg, Ebola)	Fever with mucosal bleeding, petechiae, thrombocytopenia, and hypotension.	Acute rash with fever.	Meningo-coccemia, malaria, typhus, leptospirosis, TTP, HUS.	Clinical diagnosis.	Standard and contact precautions.	Supportive care.

(continues)

TABLE 11.7. Potential Bioterrorism Agents *(continued)*

Agent/Disease	Clinical Findings	Syndrome	Differential	Initial Diagnostic Testing	Immediate Infection Control	Treatment
Tularemia	Fever, rigors, headache, myalgia, coryza, and sore throat followed by substernal discomfort, dry cough, pleuritis, or pneumonitis.	Influenza-like illness.	Influenza, atypical pneumonia, SARS, anthrax, smallpox, plague, Q fever.	CXR with infiltrate, hilar adenopathy, or effusion; small gram-⊖ coccobacilli in sputum or blood.	Standard precautions.	Ciprofloxacin, doxycycline, gentamicin, streptomycin.
Cutaneous anthrax	A pruritic maculopapule that ulcerates by day 2, progressing to vesicles and a painless black eschar with extensive nonpitting edema.	Localized ulcer and extensive edema.	Staphylococcal lymphadenitis, ecthyma gangrenosum.	Gram-⊕ rods in vesicle fluid.	Standard precautions.	Ciprofloxacin, doxycycline, penicillin.

(Adapted from the California State Department of Health, Sacramento, CA, and the Centers for Disease Control and Prevention, Atlanta, GA.)

KEY FACT

Patients are usually afebrile in toxin-mediated food-borne illness.

Food-Borne Illnesses

Table 11.8 outlines the causes and treatment of food-borne illness, grouped according to incubation period.

TABLE 11.8. Causes of Food-Borne Illness

Disease/Associations	Agent	Symptoms	Treatment
INCUBATION PERIOD < 2 HOURS: LIKELY TOXIN OR CHEMICAL AGENT			
Ciguatera (grouper, snapper)	Neurotoxin from algae that grow in tropical reefs.	Perioral paresthesias and shooting pains in the legs; bradycardia/hypotension if severe.	Emetics/lavage; IV fluids.
Scombroid (tuna, mahi-mahi, mackerel)	Histamine-like substance in spoiled fish.	Burning mouth/metallic taste; flushing, dizziness, headache, GI symptoms; urticaria/bronchospasm if severe.	Antihistamines.
MSG poisoning ("Chinese restaurant syndrome")	Acetylcholine.	Burning sensation in the neck/chest/abdomen/extremities; sweating, bronchospasm, tachycardia.	No treatment.

TABLE 11.8. **Causes of Food-Borne Illness** *(continued)*

Disease/Associations	Agent	Symptoms	Treatment
Incubation Period 2–14 Hours: Likely Toxin			
S aureus (dairy, eggs, mayonnaise, meat products)	Preformed heat-stable enterotoxin.	Vomiting, epigastric pain.	No treatment.
Bacillus cereus	Preformed toxin (like *S aureus*) or sporulation and toxin production in vivo (like *C perfringens*).	Vomiting, epigastric pain, diarrhea.	No treatment.
Clostridium perfringens (frequently from reheated meats, stews, gravies)	Toxin is released after heat-resistant clostridial spores germinate in the intestines.	Lower GI symptoms.	No treatment.
Incubation Period > 14 Hours: Bacteria, Viruses			
Campylobacter (most common)		Fever, diarrhea.	Ciprofloxacin or azithromycin.
Salmonella		Same as above.	Same as above.
Shigella	Shiga toxin.	Same as above.	Same as above.
Enteroinvasive *E coli*		Same as above.	Same as above.
Yersinia		Same as above.	TMP-SMX or ciprofloxacin.
Vibrio parahaemolyticus (undercooked seafood)		Same as above.	No treatment.
Enterohemorrhagic *E coli* O157:H7 (undercooked ground beef, contaminated produce)	Shiga toxin.	Usually afebrile; bloody diarrhea; HUS in 5% of cases.	No antibiotics (may ↑ risk of HUS).
Enterotoxigenic *E coli* ("traveler's diarrhea")	Enterotoxins.	Usually afebrile; diarrhea.	Ciprofloxacin.
Norovirus (cruise ship and nursing home outbreaks)		Usually afebrile; vomiting, headaches, diarrhea.	No treatment.

Tick-Borne Illnesses

GENERAL CHARACTERISTICS

Table 11.9 outlines the predominant tick-borne diseases in the United States.

TABLE 11.9. Clinical Presentation and Treatment of Tick-Borne Diseases

DISEASE AND ORGANISM	TICK	LOCATION	CLINICAL FEATURES	TREATMENT	COMMENTS
Babesiosis (*Babesia microti*)	*Ixodes*	Coastal New England and Long Island (overlaps with Lyme disease and human granulocytic anaplasmosis). Less common: Upper Midwest and West Coast.	Asymptomatic to fever, hepatosplenomegaly, and jaundice. **Less common:** Petechiae or ecchymoses. **Hemolytic anemia** and **thrombocytopenia**. ***Babesia* parasites look like *Plasmodium falciparum*** signet-ring ('headphone") forms. Less common: Intracellular forms may look like classic **"Maltese cross"** tetrads (see Figure 11.14).	Most cases are self-limited, so no treatment is needed. If treatment is warranted, give clindamycin + quinine or atovaquone + azithromycin; exchange transfusion in the setting of profound hemolysis or parasitemia.	Suspect coinfection with ***Borrelia burgdorferi* (Lyme disease)** and/ or ***Anaplasma phagocytophilum* (human granulocytotropic anaplasmosis)** given similar geographical exposure.
Lyme disease (*Borrelia burgdorferi*)	*Ixodes scapularis* or, less commonly, *Ixodes pacificus*	Coastal New England, Long Island, mid-Atlantic, upper Midwest (overlaps with babesiosis and human granulocytic anaplasmosis) Less common: West Coast.	**Erythema migrans** is seen in early disease. If left untreated, facial nerve palsy and AV block may be seen. Arthritis and chronic neurologic symptoms are seen in late disease.	**Early disease:** Doxycycline or amoxicillin × 14–21 days. **Late disease:** Doxycycline, amoxicillin, or ceftriaxone for up to 28 days.	Coinfection/ alternative diagnosis with **babesiosis** possible.

TABLE 11.9. **Clinical Presentation and Treatment of Tick-Borne Diseases** *(continued)*

DISEASE AND ORGANISM	TICK	LOCATION	CLINICAL FEATURES	TREATMENT	COMMENTS
Human granulocytic anaplasmosis (HGA) (*Anaplasma phagocytophilum*)	*I scapularis*	Northeast and upper Midwest (overlaps with Lyme disease and babesiosis).	Flulike symptoms in the spring and summer, including fever. Labs show **leukopenia, thrombo-cytopenia**, and ↑ **LFTs**. **Morulae** (Latin for mulberries), a cluster of organisms in WBCs, are seen on a peripheral blood **buffy-coat smear.**	Doxycycline.	A high fever (uncommon in Lyme) together with **leukopenia, thrombocytopenia**, and ↑ **LFTs** may suggest coinfection with HGA in patients with Lyme disease.
Human monocytic ehrlichiosis (HME) (*Ehrlichia chaffeensis*)	Lone Star tick	Southern states such as Arkansas and Missouri (overlaps with Rocky Mountain spotted fever).	Flulike symptoms in the spring and summer, including fever. Labs reveal **leukopenia, thrombo-cytopenia**, and ↑ **LFTs**. Less commonly seen are **morulae** in peripheral blood **buffy-coat smear.**	Doxycycline.	Called "spotless" Rocky Mountain spotted fever because of epidemiologic and clinical overlap.
Rocky Mountain spotted fever (*Rickettsia rickettsii*)	Mainly *Dermacentor* spp. (dog ticks)	Mid-Atlantic and South Central states (overlaps with HME).	Flulike symptoms, including fever. A centripetal rash follows (first affects wrists and ankles; then spreads centrally).	Doxycycline.	**Not** commonly found in the Rocky Mountain states.

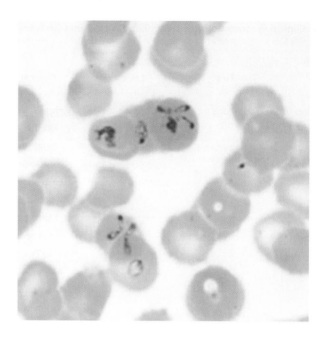

FIGURE 11.14. Babesiosis on a blood smear. Note the "Maltese cross" tetrads, which are pathognomonic for *Babesia*. (Courtesy of the Centers for Disease Control and Prevention, Atlanta, GA.)

LYME DISEASE

 An 18-year-old man returned from a one-day hike in Missouri and discovered an 8-mm tick on his leg, which he removed. One day later, he developed an erythematous rash around the tick bite and presented to his primary care physician for evaluation. What is the proper course of action?

None. Several features of this exposure make this rash unlikely to be Lyme disease. The tick described is large and is thus more likely to be a Lone Star tick than an *Ixodes* tick (which is small). In addition, the tick was attached for < 24 hours, making transmission of *Borrelia* less probable. Also, the rash is presenting one day later, a finding that is unusual for a typical erythema chronicum migrans rash, which takes 3–7 days to appear. Finally, the Midwest is not a typical endemic area of Lyme disease. This is likely another tick-borne rash and will not require treatment or prophylaxis.

> **KEY FACT**
>
> The rash of early Lyme disease, erythema migrans, is often missed and resolves in 3–4 weeks without treatment.

A tick-borne illness caused by *Borrelia burgdorferi* (found in the Northeast, mid-Atlantic, and upper Midwest more than the West). Prevalence is based on the distributions of the tick vectors *Ixodes scapularis* (found in the Northeast and upper Midwest) and *Ixodes pacificus* (found in the West). Transmitted primarily by nymphal stages that are active in late spring and summer. Requires tick attachment for > 24 hours.

SYMPTOMS/EXAM

- **Early localized infection:** Occurs one week (3–30 days) after the tick bite. Presents with **erythema migrans** (60–80%), which appears as an expanding red lesion with "bull's eye" central clearing on the thigh, groin, or axilla (see Figure 11.15). Often accompanied by fever, myalgias, and lymphadenopathy.

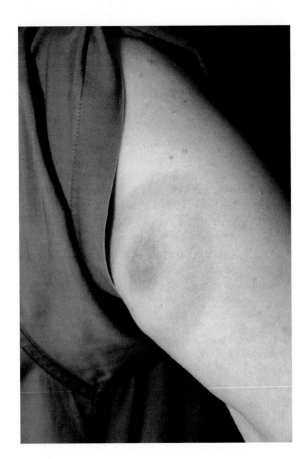

FIGURE 11.15.   Erythema chronicum migrans seen in Lyme disease. Note the classic "bull's eye" lesion, which consists of an outer ring where the spirochetes are found, an inner ring of clearing, and central erythema due to an allergic response at the site of the tick bite. (Courtesy of James Gathany, Public Health Image Library, Centers for Disease Control and Prevention, Atlanta, GA, as published in McPhee SJ et al. *Current Medical Diagnosis & Treatment 2010.* New York: McGraw-Hill, 2010, Plate 32.)

- **Early disseminated infection:**
  - Occurs days to weeks after onset of the initial erythema migrans lesion. Skin lesions are like erythema migrans but are smaller and often multiple.
  - Neurologic involvement may include cranial neuritis (CN VII palsy is most common and may be bilateral), peripheral neuropathy, and/ or aseptic meningitis. Cardiac abnormalities include AV block (rarely requiring a permanent pacemaker), myopericarditis, and mild left ventricular dysfunction.
  - Migratory **myalgias, arthralgias, fatigue,** and malaise are common during this phase.
- **Late Lyme disease:**
  - Occurs months to years later in untreated patients. Arthritis may develop in large joints (commonly the knee; shows PMN predominance) or small joints. Attacks last weeks to months **with complete remission between recurrences** and become less frequent over time.
  - Chronic neurologic findings include subacute encephalopathy (memory, sleep, or mood disturbances) and peripheral sensory polyneuropathy (pain or paresthesias; abnormal EMG).
- **Congenital Lyme disease:** Cases of congenital transmission resulting in fetal death have been reported.

KEY FACT

Lyme disease may present as asymmetric oligoarticular arthritis, frequently of the knee or other large joints.

DIAGNOSIS

The testing strategy depends on the pretest probability of disease (per the American College of Physicians 1997 guidelines):

- **High likelihood (> 80%, eg, erythema migrans in an endemic area):** Clinical diagnosis is sufficient. Serology is often ⊖ in early disease and is not needed to confirm the diagnosis.
- **Low likelihood (< 20%, eg, nonspecific complaints with no objective findings):** Serologic testing is not indicated, and patients should not be treated (⊕ results will likely be false ⊕s).
- **Intermediate likelihood (20–80%, eg, some typical findings and residence in an endemic area):** Combine ELISA with a confirmatory Western blot (as with HIV). In the first month of symptoms, test IgM and IgG antibodies in acute and convalescent sera; later, test only IgG antibodies.
- Patients with neuroborreliosis usually have a ⊕ serum serology. CSF antibody testing is not necessary.
- PCR of plasma and tissue (but not CSF) is sensitive, but no guidelines exist.

TREATMENT

- **Early Lyme disease:** Doxycycline or amoxicillin × 14–21 days. In the presence of meningitis, radiculopathy, or third-degree AV block, treat with ceftriaxone × 14–28 days (or, alternatively, doxycycline). Treatment response for early Lyme disease is excellent.
- **Late Lyme disease:** Treat arthritis with doxycycline or amoxicillin × 28 days. Treat late neurologic disease with ceftriaxone × 14–28 days; response may be slow and incomplete.

PREVENTION

Patients in endemic areas with a tick that is partially engorged or attached for > **24 hours** may benefit from doxycycline PO × 1 dose. Testing of ticks for infectious organisms is not recommended. Lyme disease vaccine is no longer available.

COMPLICATIONS

- Some patients may have treatment-resistant (autoimmune) arthritis for months to years despite appropriate antibiotics. *B burgdorferi* DNA is not found in the joint, and patients do not respond to antibiotics.
- Following appropriately treated Lyme disease, some patients may develop poorly defined, subjective complaints (myalgias, arthralgias, fatigue, memory impairment). **These patients do not benefit from repeated or prolonged antibiotic treatment.** The most common reason for apparent antibiotic failure in Lyme disease is misdiagnosis.

ROCKY MOUNTAIN SPOTTED FEVER

A tick-borne illness caused by *Rickettsia rickettsii*. The vector is the *Dermacentor* tick, which needs to feed for only 6–10 hours before injecting the organism (a much shorter attachment time than for Lyme disease). Most commonly found in the mid-Atlantic and South Central states (**not** the Rocky Mountain states). The highest rates are seen in late spring and summer and in children and men with occupational tick exposures.

KEY FACT

Ixodes scapularis bites can lead to coinfection with Lyme disease, human granulocytic anaplasmosis, and/or babesiosis.

KEY FACT

Patients with a tick attached for < 24 hours do not need treatment for Lyme disease.

SYMPTOMS/EXAM

- **Initial symptoms (seven days after a tick bite)** are fever, myalgias, and headaches.
- A maculopapular rash (found in 90% of cases) starts four days later and progresses to petechiae or purpura. The rash first appears on the wrists and ankles and then spreads centrally and to the palms and soles.
- Patients may develop severe headache, irritability, and even delirium or coma.

DIFFERENTIAL

Meningococcemia, measles, typhoid fever, ehrlichiosis (HME or HGA), viral hemorrhagic fevers (eg, dengue), leptospirosis, vasculitis.

DIAGNOSIS

- Diagnosis is made clinically (symptoms and signs plus recent tick bite); treatment should be started as soon as Rocky Mountain spotted fever is suspected.
- Diagnosis can be made by biopsy of early skin lesions or confirmed retrospectively by serologic testing.
- Labs may show thrombocytopenia, ↑ LFTs, and hyponatremia. The Weil-Felix test (for antibodies cross-reacting to *Proteus*) is no longer considered reliable.

TREATMENT

Doxycycline, chloramphenicol (for pregnant or doxycycline-allergic patients).

COMPLICATIONS

Pneumonitis, pulmonary edema, renal failure, and death after 8–15 days.

Travel Medicine

GENERAL GUIDELINES

Most cases of fever in returned travelers are due to common illnesses such as influenza, viral URI, pneumonia, and UTI. Life-threatening infections that are treatable if diagnosed early include falciparum malaria, typhoid fever, and meningococcemia (consider these in all returned travelers with fever).

SYMPTOMS/EXAM

- **Careful travel history:** Determine the countries visited, urban vs. rural locales, accommodation type, immunizations, chemoprophylaxis, and sexual history.
- **Specific exposures:** Determine if there was freshwater contact (leptospirosis, schistosomiasis) or exposure to unpasteurized dairy (brucellosis), mosquitoes (malaria, dengue), ticks (rickettsial diseases, tularemia), or sick contacts (meningococcus, TB, viral hemorrhagic fevers).
- Examine for lymphadenopathy, maculopapular rash (dengue, leptospirosis, acute HIV, acute HBV), eschars at the site of a tick bite (rickettsial disease), and splenomegaly (malaria, typhoid, brucellosis).

KEY FACT

Think of Rocky Mountain spotted fever and start treatment early in patients with a recent tick bite (especially in the mid-Atlantic or South Central states) along with fever, headache, and myalgias followed by a rash that starts on the wrists/ankles and spreads centrally.

KEY FACT

The most common travel-related infections are malaria, typhoid fever, hepatitis, dengue, and amebic liver abscess.

> **KEY FACT**

Dengue fever ("break-bone fever") is a cause of a fever in a returning traveler with fevers for 5–7 days, headache, myalgias, and arthralgias, followed by fatigue for up to several weeks.

> **KEY FACT**

For fever after recent travel (< 21 days), consider malaria, typhoid fever, dengue, leptospirosis, rickettsial illnesses, and meningococcemia. For longer incubation periods (> 21 days), consider non-falciparum malaria, TB, hepatitis, amebic liver abscess, acute HIV, and brucellosis.

> **KEY FACT**

Treat traveler's diarrhea with hydration, antimotility agents (avoid in dysenteric cases), and antibiotics to shorten disease duration (ciprofloxacin × 1–3 days; azithromycin).

DIFFERENTIAL

- **Malaria** (see below).
- **Typhoid fever:** Presents with fever, malaise, and abdominal discomfort, often without GI symptoms. Exam reveals splenomegaly, pulse-temperature dissociation, and evanescent rose spots. Diagnose by blood cultures growing *Salmonella*; treat with ciprofloxacin or levofloxacin. Vaccine is 70% effective.
- **Hepatitis:** HAV and HEV are transmitted by the fecal-oral route and may have nonspecific prodromes. HBV and HCV are transmitted by sexual contact, shared needles, or blood transfusions.
- **Dengue:** Endemic in equatorial and subtropical areas. Patients have abrupt onset of fever, retro-orbital headache, and myalgias. Exam shows a blanching rash. Treatment is supportive.
- **Leptospirosis:** Recent outbreaks have affected eco-travelers in Hawaii and Indonesia. May be biphasic, with fever, chills, and headache that resolve but are followed 1–3 days later by conjunctivitis, a maculopapular rash, hepatosplenomegaly, and aseptic meningitis. Severe cases (Weil's syndrome) have jaundice, renal failure, pulmonary hemorrhage, and hypotension. Treat with penicillin or doxycycline (patients may get **Jarisch-Herxheimer reactions**).
- **Rickettsial illnesses:** Include Mediterranean spotted fever and African tick typhus. Fever, headaches, myalgias, eschars, and maculopapular rashes spread from the trunk outward to the palms and soles (unlike rashes in Rocky Mountain spotted fever, which spread inward). Treat with doxycycline.
- **Amebiasis (*Entamoeba histolytica*):** May cause bloody dysentery or liver abscesses. Diagnose by stool microscopy showing cysts or trophozoites with ingested RBCs. Colonoscopy shows typical flask-shaped ulcers. Serologic tests are 95% sensitive for diagnosing liver abscess. Treat with metronidazole followed by paromomycin to eradicate stool cysts. **Amebic liver abscesses do not require drainage.**
- **Acute schistosomiasis: Swimmer's itch** refers to multiple pruritic, papular lesions at the entry site of a fluke that often appear 24–48 hours following exposure. It may result from infection with human or nonhuman species. **Katayama fever** is an immunologic reaction to the organism that may occur 4–8 weeks following infection, resulting in acute onset of fever, myalgias, arthralgias, dry cough, and diarrhea with associated diffuse lymphadenopathy and hepatosplenomegaly.
- **Acute HIV and other STDs.**
- **Traveler's diarrhea:** Caused by enterotoxigenic *E coli* (> 50%), *Campylobacter*, and, to a lesser extent, *Shigella*, *Salmonella* (< 15% each), and parasites (*Giardia*, *Entamoeba*, *Cryptosporidium*). Onset is usually within one week of arrival, with watery diarrhea lasting 2–4 days; patients are **usually afebrile.** Dysentery with bloody diarrhea and fever may be seen with *Shigella* or *Entamoeba*.

DIAGNOSIS

- Routine tests include CBC, liver and renal chemistries, UA, and CXR.
- Evaluate the differential for eosinophilia; obtain thick and thin blood smears for malaria (may need to repeat every 8–12 hours for two days). Blood cultures for typhoid fever and meningococcus; stool for culture and ova/parasites.

PREVENTION

- Avoid untreated water, ice cubes, undercooked foods ("boil it, cook it, peel it, or forget it"), stray or wild animals, swimming in freshwater, and insect bites (use insect repellents containing 30–35% DEET or permethrin to coat mosquito netting or clothes).
- Malaria prophylaxis (see below).
- **Safe-sex counseling.**
- **Regular adult immunizations:** Tetanus, diphtheria, measles/mumps/rubella (MMR), and polio vaccinations should be up to date. Influenza and pneumococcal vaccine is appropriate for some adults; hepatitis B vaccine should be given to sexually active adults and health care workers.
- **Vaccines for most travelers to developing countries:** Hepatitis A and typhoid (for rural areas). Consider immune globulin (for hepatitis A in travelers leaving < 2–3 weeks after vaccination), meningococcus (for Nepal, sub-Saharan Africa, and pilgrims to Mecca), Japanese encephalitis (for rural China and southern Asia), yellow fever (required by certain countries), and rabies.
  - **Live attenuated vaccines (avoid during pregnancy or if immunosuppressed):** MMR, **oral** polio, **oral** typhoid, yellow fever, and oral cholera (not recommended for use).
  - **Egg-based vaccines:** Influenza, yellow fever.

MALARIA

> A 24-year-old woman develops a high fever with night sweats four days after returning from a two-week vacation to Thailand. She does not have diarrhea, nausea, chest pain, or shortness of breath and complains only of fatigue and chills. Her exam is notable for a temperature of 40°C (104°F), and her labs show a hematocrit of 28%. She had no freshwater exposure in Thailand but did have several mosquito bites and did not take any prophylaxis while there. What is the most likely diagnosis, and what test could confirm this?
>
> *Plasmodium falciparum* malaria, which can be confirmed with a thick and thin smear. Epidemiologic data show that most travelers who develop a fever within < 1 week of their return usually have falciparum malaria or dengue fever, both of which can be found in Asia. In this patient, however, the lack of malaria prophylaxis, the low hematocrit (from lysis of RBCs), and the absence of the prominent myalgias/arthralgias seen in dengue make malaria the most likely etiology.

A common cause of fever in the tropics and in returned travelers or immigrants. *Plasmodium falciparum* is the most dangerous species and has a high prevalence in sub-Saharan Africa. Other species include *Plasmodium vivax, malariae,* and *ovale.* Malaria is transmitted by *Anopheles* mosquitoes or is acquired congenitally, through blood transfusions, or from stowaway mosquitoes ("airport malaria"). Nonimmune individuals (eg, young children, visitors, migrants returning to the tropics after living in nonendemic areas) and pregnant women are at risk for severe disease.

SYMPTOMS/EXAM

- Fever, chills, malaise, headache, myalgias, and GI symptoms occur primarily when parasitized RBCs burst open, eventually leading to cyclic symptoms every 48 or 72 hours.

- Signs include hemolytic anemia, splenomegaly, hypoglycemia, thrombocytopenia, transaminitis, indirect hyperbilirubinemia, and hemoglobinuria ("blackwater fever").
- Illness usually occurs 1–2 weeks after infection with *P falciparum*, but incubation may be longer for other species.
- Nephrotic syndrome due to immune complexes is most common with *P malariae*. Relapsing illness may be seen after months or years with *P vivax* and *P ovale* because these have dormant liver stages or hypnozoites.
- Mature *P falciparum* parasites (schizonts) bind to vascular endothelium, leading to capillary obstruction and ischemia. If left untreated, this can lead to hypoglycemia, cerebral malaria (seizures, coma), nephritis, renal failure, and pulmonary edema. Falciparum malaria also leads to high rates of parasitized RBCs, causing severe anemia.

DIAGNOSIS

- **Order blood smears in all febrile travelers or returned immigrants from endemic areas.** Giemsa- or Wright-stained **thick and thin smears** are the best diagnostic tests.
- ***P falciparum* must be distinguished from other species** (see Figure 11.16) because it requires hospital admission and is the only species with significant drug resistance. *P falciparum* is usually characterized by > 1% parasitized RBCs, > 1 parasite/RBC, banana-shaped gametocytes, and a lack of mature schizonts. It is also associated with travel to Africa, severe disease, and symptoms that occur within two months of travel.
- ***P vivax* is as widespread as but generally less virulent than *P falciparum*** (see Figure 11.17). ***P malariae*** and ***P ovale*** are much less common causes of malaria.

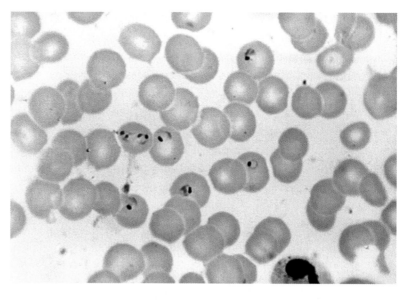

FIGURE 11.16. **Falciparum malaria on a thin blood smear.** Young signet-ring-shaped parasites are seen for all species of *Plasmodium*, but only *P falciparum* shows multiple parasites within a single RBC. (Courtesy of Steven Glenn, Public Health Image Library, Centers for Disease Control and Prevention, Atlanta, GA, as published in McPhee SJ et al. *Current Medical Diagnosis & Treatment 2010.* New York: McGraw-Hill, 2010, Plate 112.)

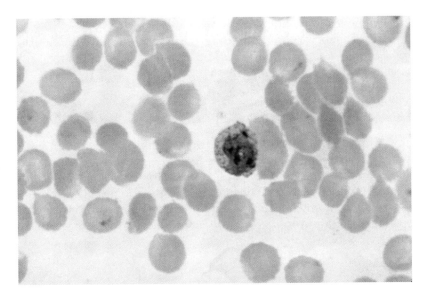

FIGURE 11.17.   **Vivax malaria on a thin blood smear.** Blood smear showing *Plasmodium vivax* schizonts. (Courtesy of Steven Glenn, Public Health Image Library, Centers for Disease Control and Prevention, Atlanta, GA, as published in McPhee SJ et al. *Current Medical Diagnosis & Treatment 2010.* New York: McGraw-Hill, 2010, Plate 114.)

TREATMENT

- **P vivax, P ovale, and P malariae:** Treat with chloroquine. *P vivax* and *P ovale* should also be treated with primaquine to eradicate chronic liver stages (if patients have normal G6PD levels).
- **P falciparum:**
  - **Assume chloroquine resistance** (unless acquired in Central America, Haiti, or the Middle East) and treat with quinine plus doxycycline, quinine plus sulfadoxine/pyrimethamine (Fansidar), Fansidar alone, mefloquine, or atovaquone/proguanil (Malarone). Artesunate and artemisinin compounds are the fastest-acting malaricidal agents but are unavailable in the United States.
  - **Repeat blood smears at 48 hours** to document a > 75% ↓ in parasitized RBCs. Exchange transfusion may be used for severe malaria or in the presence of > 15% parasitemia.

PREVENTION

- Avoid mosquito bites (use bed netting, window screens, insecticides, and insect repellents with 30–35% DEET).
- **Chloroquine is effective in Central America, Haiti, and parts of the Middle East.** For most other areas, the CDC recommends mefloquine or atovaquone/proguanil. For Southeast Asia (the Thai-Burmese and Thai-Cambodian border areas), use doxycycline or atovaquone/proguanil, as resistance to all other antimalarials is common.

COMPLICATIONS

- In the United States, IV quinidine is often used because IV quinine may be unavailable.
- Primaquine may lead to severe hemolytic anemia, so screen for G6PD deficiency before using it.
- Adverse effects of mefloquine include irritability, bad dreams, GI upset, and, to a lesser extent, seizures and psychosis.

KEY FACT

P **V**ivax and P **O**vale may lead to **V**ery **O**ld infections, presenting months or years after individuals leave an endemic area. Be sure to include primaquine at the end of treatment regimens to eradicate the chronic liver stages.

- Doxycycline leads to photosensitivity and GI upset.
- During pregnancy, chloroquine is safe, and quinine, sulfadoxine/pyrimethamine, and doxycycline may be used despite potential fetal risks because morbidity and mortality are so high.

STRONGYLOIDES

KEY FACT

Consider hyperinfection with *S stercoralis* in patients with vague abdominal complaints or fleeting pulmonary infiltrates plus eosinophilia, or in immunosuppressed patients who develop systemic gram-⊖ or enterococcal infection.

Infection with the helminth *Strongyloides stercoralis* is endemic in warm climates such as the southeastern United States, Appalachia, Africa, Asia, the Caribbean, and Central America. Unlike most other parasitic worms, *Strongyloides* can reproduce in the small intestine, leading to a high worm burden. Hyperinfection (autoinfection) and dissemination are seen in hosts with deficient cell-mediated immunity (eg, AIDS, chronic steroids, organ transplants, leukemia, lymphoma).

SYMPTOMS/EXAM

- **Normal hosts:**
  - May be asymptomatic or present with vague epigastric pain, nausea, bloating, diarrhea, or weight loss due to malabsorption.
  - Serpiginous papules or urticaria ("larva currens") may be seen around the buttocks, thighs, and lower abdomen as larvae migrate from the rectum and externally autoinfect the host.
- **Immunocompromised hosts:**
  - Hyperinfection or disseminated strongyloidiasis can develop. Worms leave the GI tract and travel to the lungs and elsewhere.
  - Patients present with fever, severe abdominal pain, dyspnea, productive cough, hemoptysis, and local symptoms (eg, CNS, pancreas, eyes).

DIFFERENTIAL

Local enteric disease mimics PUD, sprue, or ulcerative colitis. Hyperinfection resembles overwhelming bacterial or fungal sepsis.

DIAGNOSIS

- Stool or duodenal aspirates can be tested for ova and parasites. In hyperinfection, larvae may be seen in sputum, bronchoalveolar lavage (BAL), CSF, and urine. Paradoxically, **eosinophilia is prominent in normal hosts with disease but is uncommon in patients with hyperinfection. Serology is available.**
- CXR shows transient (normal host) or diffuse, persistent pulmonary infiltrates (hyperinfection).

TREATMENT

Thiabendazole, albendazole, or ivermectin. Discontinue steroids and other immunosuppressive agents.

COMPLICATIONS

Ileus or small bowel obstruction can result from enteric worms. Hyperinfection and tracking of enteric bacteria (gram-⊖ rods, enterococci) can lead to bacteremia, meningitis, UTI, or pneumonia.

Immunocompromised Hosts

A 42-year-old woman who underwent a lung transplant one year ago is being evaluated for a new lung nodule. A CT-guided lung biopsy grows weakly acid-fast bacteria in a branching-rod pattern. What is the treatment of choice for this patient?

TMP-SMX. This immunocompromised patient has a nodule that is growing *Nocardia*, a gram-⊕ branching bacterium that is weakly acid fast. The treatment of choice for this is TMP-SMX.

ASPLENIA-RELATED INFECTIONS

Postsplenectomy sepsis has a short viral-like prodrome followed by abrupt deterioration and shock. Encapsulated organisms involved include *S pneumoniae* (> 50%), *N meningitidis*, and *H influenzae*. Other organisms include *Capnocytophaga* (dog or cat contact), *Salmonella* (sickle cell anemia), *Babesia*, and malaria (more fulminant).

PREVENTION

- **Vaccinate** against *S pneumoniae*, *H influenzae* type b (unvaccinated older individuals), and *N meningitidis*. Vaccinate ≥ 2 weeks before elective splenectomy or > 2 weeks after surgery.
- Give a supply of antibiotics to be taken as **self-administered therapy** for fever (eg, amoxicillin to be taken at the onset of fever, followed by immediate evaluation in urgent care). **Daily prophylaxis** for a defined period (eg, penicillin for 3–5 years following splenectomy) is recommended for children but not adults.

FEBRILE NEUTROPENIA

See the Oncology chapter.

HUMAN IMMUNODEFICIENCY VIRUS (HIV)

A 23-year-old man presents to his primary care physician with fever, pharyngitis, and adenopathy. On history, he reports an unprotected sexual encounter that occurred two weeks ago. If this is 1° HIV, what testing should be done?

HIV viral load or p24 antigen. The combination of fever, pharyngitis, and adenopathy is a common presentation, but among the possible diagnoses, 1° HIV should not be excluded. Inasmuch as an antibody response would take at least 1–3 months to develop, a viral load would constitute the best test with which to diagnose acute HIV so soon after an exposure.

Risk factors include unprotected sexual intercourse, IV drug use, maternal infection, needlesticks, and mucosal exposure to body fluids; also at risk are patients who received blood products before 1985. Prognostic factors are CD4 count and HIV RNA viral load. CD4 count measures the degree of immune compromise and predicts the risk of opportunistic infections; viral load measures HIV replication rate, gauges the efficacy of antiretrovirals, and predicts CD4 count decline.

SYMPTOMS/EXAM

- **1° HIV infection:** May be asymptomatic. Acute retroviral syndrome presents 2–6 weeks after initial infection with fever, sore throat, lymphadenopathy, and a truncal maculopapular rash or mucocutaneous ulcerations. Other signs and symptoms include myalgias, arthralgias, diarrhea, headache, nausea, vomiting, weight loss, aseptic meningitis, and thrush.
- **Chronic HIV infection:** Fatigue, fevers, night sweats, diarrhea, persistent lymphadenopathy, and weight loss. Suspect in patients with thrush, oral hairy leukoplakia, herpes zoster, seborrheic dermatitis, oral aphthous ulcers, or recurrent vaginal candidiasis.

DIFFERENTIAL

Acute retroviral syndrome resembles infectious mononucleosis, acute CMV infection, aseptic meningitis, and syphilis.

DIAGNOSIS

- **ELISA/enzyme immunoassay (EIA) and rapid HIV antibody tests:** Detect antiviral antibodies; used to diagnose HIV. Usually ⊕ by **three months** after initial infection. Because false-⊕ results may occur (especially in low-risk populations being screened), confirm by **Western blot.**
- **HIV RNA viral load:** Not approved by the FDA for **diagnosing** HIV. Has high sensitivity even in patients who have not yet developed antibodies. False-⊕ results may occur, usually in the form of a low copy number (eg, < 10,000 copies/mL); true-⊕ results in antibody-⊖ patients with acute infection are usually > 100,000 copies/mL.
- **p24 core antigen:** Highly specific but less sensitive (85–90%) and less readily available than HIV viral load. Approved by the FDA for diagnosing acute HIV.

TREATMENT

- Current recommendations are to **start HIV treatment in all patients who are symptomatic. Treatment of asymptomatic patients should be started when the CD4 count is < 500 cells/mm³;** treatment is also recommended at all CD4 counts during **pregnancy** as well as for **HIV-associated nephropathy** and **hepatitis B coinfection.**
- Consider initiating antiretrovirals in patients with acute retroviral syndrome.
- Use three drugs—usually two nucleoside analogs (AZT, 3TC, d4T, ddI, abacavir, tenofovir, emtricitabine) plus (1) a non-nucleoside analog (nevirapine or efavirenz), (2) a protease inhibitor that may be ritonavir "boosted" (fosamprenavir, indinavir, nelfinavir, saquinavir, atazanavir, or lopinavir/ritonavir), or (3) an integrase inhibitor (raltegravir). Protease inhibitors can have significant drug interactions.
- **During pregnancy, women should be offered standard therapy** in the form of two nucleoside reverse transcriptase inhibitors (including AZT) plus nevirapine or a protease inhibitor. Consider starting after 10–14 weeks of gestation to minimize the risk of teratogenicity. **Efavirenz is contraindicated during pregnancy.**

KEY FACT

Do not use HIV viral load as a factor in deciding when to initiate antiretroviral therapy.

COMPLICATIONS

Progressive immunosuppression from HIV leads to opportunistic infections and malignancies. Prophylactic measures against some of these conditions are outlined in Table 11.10.

TABLE 11.10.   Prophylaxis Against AIDS-Related Opportunistic Infections

PATHOGEN	INDICATIONS FOR PROPHYLAXIS	MEDICATION	COMMENTS
Pneumocystis jiroveci pneumonia (PCP)	CD4 count < 200 or a history of oral thrush. Prophylaxis may be stopped if CD4 count is > 200 for ≥ 3 months on highly active antiretroviral therapy (HAART).	TMP-SMX, dapsone, pentamidine nebulizers, or atovaquone.	Single-strength tablets of TMP-SMX are effective and may be less toxic than double-strength tablets.
Mycobacterium avium complex (MAC)	CD4 count < 50. Prophylaxis may be stopped if CD4 count is > 100 for ≥ 3 months on HAART.	Azithromycin, clarithromycin, rifabutin.	Azithromycin can be given once weekly. Rifabutin can ↑ hepatic metabolism of other drugs.
Toxoplasma	CD4 count < 100 and *Toxoplasma* IgG ⊕. Prophylaxis may be stopped if CD4 count is > 200 for ≥ 3 months on HAART.	TMP-SMX or dapsone + pyrimethamine or atovaquone.	Covered by all PCP regimens except pentamidine and dapsone monotherapy.
Mycobacterium tuberculosis	PPD > 5 mm; history of a ⊕ PPD that was inadequately treated; close contact with a person with active TB.	INH sensitive: INH × 9 months (include pyridoxine).	For INH-resistant strains, use rifampin or rifabutin +/− pyrazinamide.
Candida	Frequent or severe recurrences.	Fluconazole or itraconazole.	
HSV	Frequent or severe recurrences.	Acyclovir, famciclovir, valacyclovir.	
Pneumococcus	All patients.	Pneumococcal vaccine.	Some disease may be prevented with TMP-SMX, clarithromycin, and azithromycin. Repeat when CD4 count is > 200.
Influenza	All patients.	Influenza vaccine.	
HBV	All susceptible patients (ie, hepatitis B core antibody ⊖).	Hepatitis B vaccine (three doses).	
HAV	All susceptible patients at ↑ risk for HAV infection or with chronic liver disease (eg, chronic HBV or HCV).	Hepatitis A vaccine (two doses).	IV drug users, men who have sex with men, and hemophiliacs are at ↑ risk.

HIV-RELATED OPPORTUNISTIC INFECTIONS

Table 11.11 outlines common HIV-related opportunistic infections with treatment guidelines.

TABLE 11.11. **Diagnosis and Treatment of Opportunistic Infections in HIV/AIDS**

Disease	Clinical Presentation	Diagnosis	1° Therapy	Alternative Therapy	Other
Pneumocystis jiroveci pneumonia (PCP)	Nonproductive cough, fever, and dyspnea. Symptoms often progress over weeks. CD4 count is often < 200.	CXR frequently shows bilateral interstitial infiltrates but may be normal. Hypoxia with ambulation; ↑ LDH. Confirm with organism seen on silver-stained sputum sample or bronchoscopy.	TMP-SMX. If P_{O_2} is < 70 mm Hg at room air, add prednisone.	Pentamidine or dapsone + TMP or primaquine + clindamycin or atovaquone.	Maintenance therapy should be continued following initial therapy.
Mycobacterium avium complex (MAC)	Fever, night sweats, weight loss, fatigue, diarrhea, abdominal pain. Diffuse lymphadenopathy and hepatosplenomegaly may be seen. CD4 count is often < 50.	Pancytopenia, ↑ alkaline phosphatase, low albumin. CT of the abdomen may reveal diffuse lymphadenopathy and hepatosplenomegaly. Diagnosed by culture of the organism from a sterile site (blood or lymph node).	Clarithromycin + ethambutol +/− rifabutin.	Azithromycin + ethambutol +/− rifabutin.	Maintenance therapy should be continued following initial therapy.
Toxoplasma gondii encephalitis	Fever, headache, altered mental status, seizure, and/or focal neurologic changes. Presentation may be very subtle. CD4 count is often < 100.	Head CT with contrast or MRI with ring-enhancing lesions (often multiple). *Toxoplasma* IgG is ⊕ in 95% of patients. LP may be normal or may show ↑ protein and mononuclear pleocytosis.	Pyrimethamine + sulfadiazine.	Pyrimethamine + clindamycin or TMP-SMX or pyrimethamine + atovaquone.	Leucovorin should be given with pyrimethamine. Steroids should be given only if there is mass effect from intracranial lesions.

TABLE 11.11. **Diagnosis and Treatment of Opportunistic Infections in HIV/AIDS** *(continued)*

Disease	Clinical Presentation	Diagnosis	1° Therapy	Alternative Therapy	Other
Cryptococcus neoformans	**Meningitis:** Headache, malaise, nausea, fever, visual changes, cranial nerve deficits, meningismus. Often subacute. **Pneumonia:** May be asymptomatic or present with pulmonary symptoms. CD4 count is often < 100.	**CSF:** High opening pressure, elevated protein, low glucose, and lymphocytosis. Twenty-five percent of patients may have normal studies. ⊕ CrAg; CSF culture ⊕. **Blood:** ⊕ CrAg; blood cultures ⊕.	**Induction:** Amphotericin B plus flucytosine × 14 days. **Consolidation:** Fluconazole 400 mg QD × 10 weeks. **Maintenance:** Fluconazole 200 mg QD indefinitely.	Liposomal amphotericin B plus flucytosine or fluconazole plus flucytosine.	May require multiple LPs to relieve high ICP. Chronic maintenance therapy may be discontinued after the completion of treatment with a CD4 count of > 100 for six months on HAART.
CMV	**Retinitis:** Painless loss of vision, floaters. **Esophagitis:** Odynophagia. **Colitis:** Diarrhea (watery or bloody), abdominal pain. CD4 count is often < 50.	**Ophthalmologic exam:** Large plaques with perivascular exudates and hemorrhages. **Endoscopy:** Hemorrhages, ulcerations; 10% are normal. Confirm with biopsy.	Ganciclovir.	Valganciclovir, foscarnet, or cidofovir. Consider intraocular ganciclovir implants for severe retinitis.	Ganciclovir may cause bone marrow suppression. CMV may also cause pneumonitis, myelitis, or encephalitis.
Crypto-sporidiosis	Persistent watery diarrhea; occasional nausea, vomiting, and/or fever. Can cause HIV cholangiopathy. CD4 count is < 100.	Must request stool exam for cryptosporidia (modified AFB, trichrome, or DFA); not seen on standard O&P exam.	Initiation of HAART is the only treatment shown to have benefit.	Possible benefit from nitazoxanide.	Symptomatic relief with antimotility agents and electrolyte repletion. Cholangiopathy requires ERCP and HAART.

Hospital Infections

CATHETER-RELATED INFECTIONS

Include catheter-related bloodstream infections (CRBSIs) as well as exit-site, tunnel, and pocket infections. The most commonly isolated etiologic agents are coagulase-⊖ staphylococci, *S aureus*, enterococci, and *Candida albicans*.

SYMPTOMS/EXAM

- **Clinical findings are unreliable.** Fever and chills are sensitive but not specific findings. Inflammation and purulence around the catheter and bloodstream infection are specific but not sensitive.

- Risk factors for complicated *S aureus* bacteremia (eg, endocarditis, osteomyelitis, or septic thrombophlebitis) include community acquisition, skin findings suggesting acute systemic infection, persistent fever at 72 hours, and ⊕ follow-up blood culture results at 48–96 hours.
- **Blood cultures:** Obtain two sets of cultures, at least one of which is drawn percutaneously. Compare **time to positivity;** if the blood culture drawn through a catheter becomes ⊕ > 2 hours before the peripheral blood culture, CRBSI is suggested.
- **Catheter cultures:** Should be performed only if CRBSI is suspected. The **semiquantitative (roll plate) method,** in which the catheter tip is rolled across an agar plate, is most commonly used. A **colony count of > 15** following overnight incubation suggests catheter-related infection.

TREATMENT

- **Catheter removal** is indicated in most cases of **nontunneled** CRBSI. For **tunneled catheters and implantable devices,** consider removal in the setting of severe illness or documented infection (**especially S aureus, gram-⊖ rods, or Candida**) or if complications occur.
- **Initial antibiotic therapy:** Treatment is usually **empiric** with vancomycin (to cover MRSA).
- **Duration of treatment:** Patients with **uncomplicated bacteremia** should be treated for **10–14 days;** those with **complicated infections** (eg, persistently ⊕ blood cultures after catheter removal, endocarditis, septic thrombophlebitis, osteomyelitis) should be treated for **4–6 weeks.**

COMPLICATIONS

Septic thrombophlebitis, infective endocarditis, septic pulmonary emboli, osteomyelitis, or other complications due to septic emboli.

CLOSTRIDIUM DIFFICILE COLITIS

Risk factors for *C difficile* colitis include antibiotic use (particularly clindamycin, cephalosporins, and ampicillin), cancer chemotherapy, bowel surgery, and multiple-organ failure. Diarrhea usually occurs after **one week** of antibiotic therapy but may arise up to **ten weeks** later.

SYMPTOMS/EXAM

Presents with diarrhea (**watery** much more often than **bloody**), abdominal pain and distention, fever, and **leukocytosis.**

DIFFERENTIAL

Antibiotic side effects without *C difficile*, neutropenic enterocolitis/**typhlitis,** IBD, ischemic bowel, laxatives/stool softeners.

DIAGNOSIS

- **Fecal WBCs and stool cultures are not useful.**
- **Detection of C difficile toxins:** Toxin assays are **necessary** because 5% of healthy patients and 25% of hospitalized patients have *C difficile* in their stools, but only one-third have toxin-mediated disease.
- **Cytotoxin assay:** Stool supernatant is directly applied to cell culture. Cell lysis suggests the presence of toxin.
- **EIA for C difficile toxin:** The most frequently used test. Has lower sensitivity than cytotoxin assay, but sensitivity ↑ with repeat testing.
- **Radiographs are often normal** but may show colonic distention and thickening ("thumbprinting" may be seen on plain abdominal films). CT scans

often show marked colonic wall thickening and pericolonic inflammatory changes.

- **Endoscopy** shows friable, edematous colonic mucosa with raised yellow plaques (pseudomembranes); specific but not sensitive.

TREATMENT

- **Stop antibiotics** if possible.
- Avoid antidiarrheal agents and opiates.
- Contact isolation.
- Hand hygiene using **soap and water** (alcohol-based products do not kill spores).
- For **mild** disease, give **PO** or IV **metronidazole** (PO is preferred). For **severe** disease (eg, pseudomembranes seen on endoscopy, treatment in the ICU, age > 60 years, fever, albumin level < 2.5 mg/dL or WBC >15,000 cells/mm³), give PO vancomycin (**IV vancomycin is not effective**).
- The **relapse** rate is 15%, with relapses usually occurring **within two weeks** of treatment cessation.
- For first-time recurrences, treat again with the same regimen.
- For refractory cases, consider tapering or pulse-dosing PO vancomycin treatment, rifaximin, cholestyramine (binds toxin), IVIG, or fecal transplants (instillation of normal feces in the patient's colon to repopulate with normal flora).
- For severe cases, surgical colectomy is sometimes necessary

COMPLICATIONS

Ileus, toxic megacolon, perforation (all may be accompanied by a ↓ in diarrhea); hemorrhage, sepsis.

INFECTION CONTROL PRECAUTIONS

Isolation and barriers are used to prevent the transmission of microorganisms from patients to other patients, visitors, or health care workers (see Table 11.12).

KEY FACT

Diarrhea that arises during antibiotic treatment may also be caused by adverse drug effects (amoxicillin, amoxicillin/clavulanic acid, erythromycin).

KEY FACT

For mild *C difficile* colitis, give PO or IV metronidazole (PO is preferred). For severe disease, give PO vancomycin.

TABLE 11.12. Infection Control Measures

PRECAUTION	PREVENTS TRANSMISSION OF	BARRIERS TO BE USED	SHOULD BE USED FOR (EXAMPLES)
Standard	Transient flora from patients or surfaces.	Hand washing; gloves for contact with all body fluids and mucosa. Face shields and gowns if splashes of body fluids are possible.	Everybody!
Airborne	Droplet nuclei (≤ 5 μm) or dust particles that remain suspended for long distances.	Negative-pressure rooms and use of surgical masks when transporting patients. Health care workers should use fitted N-95 masks. Consider face shields.	TB, measles, SARS, vesicular rashes (chickenpox, zoster, smallpox).
Droplet	Large droplets that travel < 3 feet and are generated by coughing, sneezing, talking, suctioning, or bronchoscopy.	Private rooms and use of surgical masks when patients are transported. Health care workers should use surgical masks.	Meningococcal or *H influenzae* meningitis, influenza, pertussis.
Contact	Direct and indirect contact.	Private rooms (patients may be grouped together); limit patient transport. Dedicated equipment (eg, stethoscopes). Health care workers should use gowns and gloves for all patients.	Some fecally transmitted infections (HAV, *C difficile*), vesicular rashes (chickenpox, zoster, smallpox), SARS.

MNEMONIC

To remember gram-⊕ cocci–

The Grapes of Staph (like The Grapes of Wrath):

Staphylococci are frequently seen in grapelike clusters.

Strep = strip:

Streptococci are often seen in long strips or chains.

MNEMONIC

To remember gram-⊕ rods–

Bad ChORal ACTs Need CLOSe and PROPer LISTening

Bacillus
CORynebacterium
ACTinomyces
Nocardia
CLOStridium
PROPionibacterium
LISTeria

MNEMONIC

To remember lactose-fermenting gram-⊖ rods–

SEEK Carbs

Serratia
E coli
Enterobacter
Klebsiella
Citrobacter

Specific Microbes

MICROBIOLOGY PRINCIPLES

Gram-⊕ Cocci

- In clusters (sometimes chains or pairs): *Staphylococcus*.
- Coagulase ⊕: *S aureus*.
- Coagulase ⊖: Examples include *S epidermidis* and *S saprophyticus*.
- In chains or pairs: *Streptococcus*.
- Lancet-shaped pairs: *S pneumoniae* (see Figure 11.18).
- In pairs: *Enterococcus*.

Gram-⊕ Rods

- Large with spores: *Bacillus, Clostridium*.
- Small, pleomorphic (diphtheroids): *Corynebacterium, Propionibacterium*.
- Filamentous, branching, beaded:
  - Aerobic: *Nocardia*.
  - Anaerobic: *Actinomyces*.
  - Other: *Listeria, Lactobacillus, Erysipelothrix*.

Gram-⊖ Cocci

- In pairs (diplococci): *N gonorrhoeae, N meningitidis, Moraxella (Branhamella) catarrhalis*.
- Other: *Acinetobacter*.

Gram-⊖ Rods

- Enterobacteriaceae (lactose fermenters): *E coli, Serratia, Klebsiella, Enterobacter, Citrobacter*.
- Nonfermenters: *Proteus, Serratia, Edwardsiella, Salmonella, Shigella, Morganella, Yersinia, Acinetobacter, Stenotrophomonas, Pseudomonas*.
- Anaerobes: *Bacteroides, Fusobacterium*.
- Fusiform (long, pointed): *Fusobacterium, Capnocytophaga*.
- Other: *Haemophilus*.

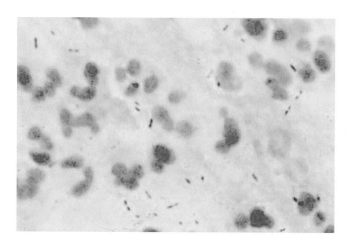

FIGURE 11.18.   Pneumococcal pneumonia. This Gram-stained sputum sample shows many neutrophils and lancet-shaped gram-⊕ cocci in pairs and chains, indicating infection with *S pneumoniae*. (Reproduced with permission from Fauci AS et al. *Harrison's Principles of Internal Medicine,* 17th ed. New York: McGraw-Hill, 2008, Fig. 128-2.)

Acid-Fast Bacteria

- Mycobacteria, including TB and leprosy.
- *Nocardia* (weakly or partially acid-fast).

ACTINOMYCES VS. NOCARDIA

Table 11.13 contrasts the clinical presentation, diagnosis, and treatment of *Actinomyces* infections with that of *Nocardia* infections.

BARTONELLA

A gram-⊖ rod. *Bartonella henselae* is transmitted by kittens or feral cats, *Bartonella quintana* by body lice. Clinical manifestations vary depending on (1) the transmitted species and (2) the immune status of the host. *B henselae* can cause **cat-scratch disease**, bacillary angiomatosis, and peliosis hepatis (multiple blood-filled cysts within the liver). *B quintana* infection may result in **trench fever, bacteremia, endocarditis,** bacillary angiomatosis, and peliosis hepatis.

SYMPTOMS/EXAM

- **Cat-scratch disease (*B henselae*; immunocompetent patients):** Presents with fever, malaise, a papule or pustule at the site of the cat scratch or bite, and regional adenopathy (usually in the head, neck, or axillae).
- **Bacillary angiomatosis and peliosis hepatis (*B henselae* and *B quintana*; AIDS patients):** The skin nodules of bacillary angiomatosis are friable, red-to-purplish lesions that may ulcerate. Peliosis hepatis produces fever, weight loss, abdominal pain, and hepatosplenomegaly; imaging shows hypodense, cystic, blood-filled structures in the liver, spleen, or lymph nodes. May be a cause of fever of unknown origin (FUO) in AIDS patients.
- **Trench fever (*B quintana*; immunocompetent patients):** Relapsing febrile paroxysms last up to five days each and are sometimes accompanied by headache, myalgias, hepatosplenomegaly, and leukocytosis. Seen in the homeless and in those from war-torn regions.

KEY FACT

Actinomycosis can spread without regard to tissue planes. It commonly presents with a "lumpy jaw" or draining fistula and is diagnosed by sulfur granules in a pathology specimen.

TABLE 11.13.   Diagnosis and Treatment of *Actinomyces* and *Nocardia* Infections

	ACTINOMYCES	**NOCARDIA**
Gram stain	Gram-⊕, branching rod.	Gram-⊕, branching rod.
Acid-fast stain	⊖.	Weakly AFB ⊕.
Pathology	Sulfur granules and draining sinuses.	Abscess.
Infected host	Immunocompetent; poor dentition or IUD user.	Immunocompromised.
Sites of infection	Mandible, lung, abdomen/pelvis.	Lung, CNS, skin.
Treatment	Penicillin × 6–12 months.	TMP-SMX × 3–6 months.

KEY FACT

In a patient with AIDS who has FUO, purple skin lesions that resemble Kaposi's sarcoma, and cystic lesions in the liver and spleen, suspect bacillary angiomatosis. Treat with macrolides.

DIFFERENTIAL

- **Cat-scratch disease:** TB, atypical mycobacterial infection, toxoplasmosis, brucellosis, sporotrichosis, tularemia, plague, leishmaniasis, histoplasmosis, infectious mononucleosis.
- **Bacillary angiomatosis:** Kaposi's sarcoma, pyogenic granuloma.
- **Trench fever:** Endocarditis, TB, typhoid fever.

DIAGNOSIS

- Blood cultures (not sensitive), serologic tests.
- Lymph node aspirate in cat-scratch disease may show sterile pus.
- Lymph node biopsy shows granulomas that may coalesce to form stellate necrosis. Warthin-Starry silver stain demonstrates bacilli.

TREATMENT

- Erythromycin, azithromycin, doxycycline.
- Cat-scratch disease usually resolves in several months and may not require treatment other than needle aspiration for symptom relief.

FUNGAL INFECTIONS

See Figure 11.19 for typical forms of fungi that might be seen in tissues examined by histopathology. Common fungal infections are discussed below.

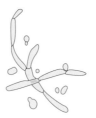

Candida albicans

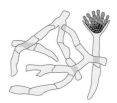

Aspergillus fumigatus

Endemic mycoses:

Cryptococcus neoformans

Blastomyces dermatitidis

Paracoccidioides brasiliensis

Histoplasma capsulatum

Coccidioides immitis

FIGURE 11.19. Characteristic forms of fungi in human tissue (37°C). (Reproduced with permission from Bhushan V, Le T. *First Aid for the USMLE Step 1: 2005.* New York: McGraw-Hill, 2005: 191.)

Candidiasis

> A 37-year-old man is admitted to the hospital for progressive chest pain and odynophagia. His exam is notable for some oral plaques and wasting. A rapid HIV test returns ⊕, and a CD4 count is 130 cells/mm³. What is the most appropriate therapy for this patient?
>
> Fluconazole. This patient with advanced HIV likely has esophageal candidiasis, most likely caused by *C albicans*. His CD4 count is too high to be associated with CMV disease, and the presence of oral lesions consistent with *Candida* makes this diagnosis most likely. It should be noted that most patients with candidal esophagitis do not have oral lesions.

The opportunistic yeast *Candida* is a commensal found on the skin, GI tract, and female genital tract. **Superficial infection** is especially common among diabetics. Risk factors for **deep or disseminated infection** include **immune compromise** (HIV, malignancy, neutropenia, or steroids), multiple or prolonged **antibiotic** treatment, and **invasive procedures**. *C albicans* is the most common cause.

SYMPTOMS/EXAM/DIAGNOSIS

- **Candiduria:** Yeast in urine **usually represents colonization** and not infection. Seen in patients with Foley catheters or antibiotic use. Diagnose infection by detecting pyuria or yeast in urine casts; treat if the patient is symptomatic or neutropenic, has undergone renal transplantation, or is awaiting urinary tract procedures.
- **Intertrigo ("diaper rash"):** Pruritic vesiculopustules rupture to form macerated or fissured beefy-red areas at skin folds. Satellite lesions may be present. Seen in both immunocompetent and immunosuppressed patients.
- **Oral thrush:** Presents with burning sensations of the tongue or mucosa with white, **curdlike patches that can be scraped away to reveal a raw surface.** Seen in patients with AIDS or malignancy or in those who use inhaled steroids for asthma. Diagnosis can be confirmed with a KOH prep or Gram stain.
- **Candidal esophagitis:** Presents with dysphagia, odynophagia, and substernal chest pain. Seen in patients with AIDS, leukemia, and lymphoma. Diagnosed by the endoscopic appearance of white patches or from biopsy showing mucosal invasion. May occur concurrently with HSV or CMV esophagitis.
- **Candidemia and disseminated candidiasis:** Diagnosed through cultures of blood, body fluids, or aspirates. Mortality is 40%. Candidemia may lead to endophthalmitis (eye pain, blurred vision), osteomyelitis, arthritis, or endocarditis.
- **Hepatosplenic candidiasis:** Presents with fever and abdominal pain that emerge as neutropenia resolves following bone marrow transplantation. Associated with a high mortality rate. Diagnosed by ultrasound or CT imaging showing abscesses. Blood cultures are frequently ⊖.

> **KEY FACT**
>
> All patients with candidemia should have an ophthalmologic exam to rule out candidal endophthalmitis.

TREATMENT

- **Candiduria:** Most cases do not need treatment.
- **Intertrigo and oral thrush:** May be treated with **topical antifungals** (nystatin, clotrimazole, or miconazole creams, or nystatin suspension swish and swallow).

- **Esophagitis and other deep or disseminated infections:** Systemic therapy with fluconazole, amphotericin, voriconazole, or caspofungin.
- Replace vascular catheters at a new site (do not exchange over a wire!).
- *C albicans* is usually susceptible to fluconazole. Patients who have been on fluconazole prophylaxis may have resistant *C albicans* or non-albicans species (eg, *Candida glabrata*, *Candida krusei*) and should initially be treated with an echinocandin (eg, caspofungin) until guided by susceptibility testing.

COMPLICATIONS

Patients with persistent candidemia after catheter removal may have peripheral septic thrombophlebitis or septic thrombosis of the central veins.

Aspergillosis

Aspergillus fumigatus and other species are widespread in soil, water, compost, potted plants, ventilation ducts, and marijuana.

SYMPTOMS/EXAM

- **Allergic bronchopulmonary aspergillosis (ABPA):** Presents with episodic bronchospasm, fever, and brown-flecked sputum. Seen in patients with underlying asthma or CF. CXR shows patchy, fleeting infiltrates and lobar consolidation or atelectasis. Central bronchiectasis may be a late finding. Labs show eosinophilia, ↑ serum IgE, and ⊕ serum IgG precipitins.
- **Aspergilloma of the lungs or sinus:** May be asymptomatic or present with hemoptysis, chronic cough, weight loss, and fatigue. Seen in patients with previous TB, sarcoidosis, emphysema, or PCP. CXR and CT may show a rim of air around a fungus ball in a preexisting pulmonary cavity. Labs show ⊕ serum IgG precipitins.
- **Invasive aspergillosis:**
  - Presents with dry cough, pleuritic chest pain, and persistent fever with a new infiltrate or nodule despite broad-spectrum antibiotics. Seen in patients with prolonged neutropenia, advanced AIDS, diabetes, and chronic granulomatous disease as well as in those on high-dose steroids or immunosuppressants.
  - **Imaging:** CXR and CT may show wedge-shaped lesions from tissue infarction, an **air-crescent sign** from cavitation of a necrotic nodule, or a **halo sign** of a necrotic nodule with surrounding hemorrhage.
  - **Labs:** The *Aspergillus* galactomannan assay is approved for diagnosis in patients with hematologic malignancies and following bone marrow transplantation. IgG precipitins and blood cultures are rarely ⊕. In high-risk patients, ⊕ sputum or bronchial washing cultures are strongly suggestive, but definitive diagnosis requires a biopsy demonstrating tissue invasion.
  - **Patients are often severely ill, and empiric antifungal therapy may be reasonable in high-risk patients.**

DIFFERENTIAL

- **ABPA:** TB, CF, lung cancer, eosinophilic pneumonia, bronchiectasis.
- **Aspergilloma:** Invasive aspergillosis.
- **Invasive aspergillosis:** Aspergilloma, cavitating lung tumor, nosocomial *Legionella* infection.

TREATMENT

- **ABPA:** Systemic corticosteroids plus itraconazole × 8 months improves lung function and ↓ steroid requirements.

- **Aspergilloma:** Surgical excision for massive hemoptysis. Antifungals play a limited role.
- **Invasive aspergillosis:** Voriconazole, amphotericin, or caspofungin.

COMPLICATIONS

- **ABPA:** Bronchiectasis, pulmonary fibrosis.
- **Aspergilloma:** Massive hemoptysis; contiguous spread to the pleura or vertebrae.
- **Invasive aspergillosis:** High mortality, especially in bone marrow and liver transplant patients.

Cryptococcosis

A 23-year-old man with untreated HIV and a CD4 count of 55 cells/mm³ presents with headache and malaise. His head CT is normal, and an LP reveals an opening pressure of 25 mm Hg, a WBC count of 8 (30% PMNs), a glucose level of 55 mg/dL, and a protein level of 79 mg/dL. What test is likely to make the diagnosis?

CSF cryptococcal antigen (CrAg). The presence of headache and an ↑ CSF opening pressure in a patient with advanced HIV should be diagnosed as cryptococcal meningitis until proven otherwise. The CSF can often appear relatively normal, but a high suspicion for cryptococcal meningitis should remain.

Cryptococcus neoformans is an encapsulated budding yeast found worldwide in soil, bird (pigeon) droppings, and eucalyptus trees. Risk factors for the disease are HIV-related immunosuppression, Hodgkin's disease, leukemia, and steroid use. *C neoformans* is the most common fungal infection in AIDS patients (usually associated with a CD4 count of < 100 cells/mm³) and is the most common cause of fungal meningitis in all patients. *Cryptococcus gattii* has emerged in the Pacific Northwest and British Columbia as a cause of cryptococcal infections, especially in patients who are immunocompetent.

SYMPTOMS/EXAM

- **Meningitis:** Mental status changes, headache, nausea, cranial nerve palsies. **HIV patients usually lack obvious meningeal signs.**
- May also cause atypical pneumonia (pulmonary infection is usually asymptomatic) or skin lesions (umbilicated papules resembling molluscum contagiosum), or may involve the bone, eye, or GU tract.
- *C gattii* is more likely than *C neoformans* to present as a cryptococcoma (nodule) in the lung, brain or muscle.

DIFFERENTIAL

Meningitis due to TB, neurosyphilis, toxoplasmosis, coccidioidomycosis, histoplasmosis, HSV encephalitis, meningeal metastases.

DIAGNOSIS

- **LP:** Patients often have high opening pressure, low glucose, high protein, and lymphocytic pleocytosis. **Patients with more advanced immunosuppression may have a bland CSF profile even with meningitis.** India ink or Gram stain of CSF (see Figure 11.20) may show budding yeast with a thick capsule (both are < 50% sensitive).

> **KEY FACT**
>
> Cryptococcemia (a ⊕ serum CrAg or blood culture) indicates disseminated disease even with a normal LP.

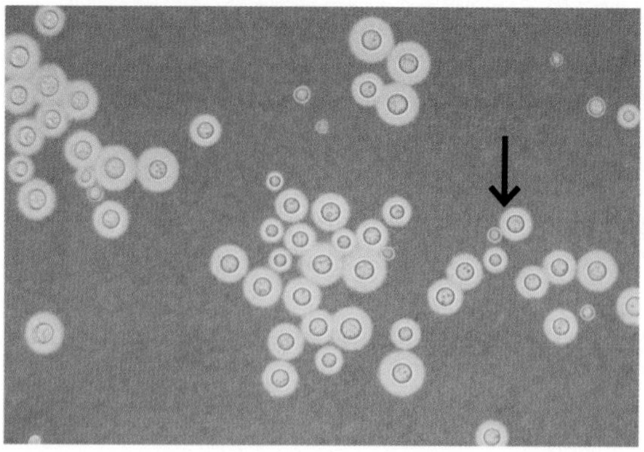

FIGURE 11.20. ***Cryptococcus neoformans.*** India ink preparation demonstrating budding yeast (arrow) and thick, translucent polysaccharide capsules outlined by the dark India ink particles. (Courtesy of Dr. L. Haley, Public Health Image Library, Centers for Disease Control and Prevention, Atlanta, GA, as published in Levinson W. *Review of Medical Microbiology and Immunology,* 10th ed. New York: McGraw-Hill, 2008, Color Plate 38.)

KEY FACT

Unlike what is typically seen in bacterial meningitis, HIV patients with cryptococcal meningitis often have minimal symptoms and a bland CSF.

- **Polysaccharide CrAg in serum or CSF:** Serum CrAg is > 99% sensitive in AIDS patients with meningitis but is less sensitive in non-AIDS patients. CSF CrAg is only 90% sensitive. A serum CrAg titer of > 1:8 indicates active disease.
- **Fungal culture** of blood, CSF, urine, sputum, or BAL.
- **Imaging:** CT or MRI may show hydrocephalus or may occasionally reveal nodules (cryptococcomas).

Treatment

- **HIV-⊖ patients:** For mild to moderate lung disease, treat with oral fluconazole × 6–12 months. For meningitis, cryptococcemia, or severe lung disease, treat with amphotericin plus 5-flucytosine × 2 weeks followed by oral fluconazole for at least 10 weeks.
- **HIV-⊕ patients:**
  - For mild to moderate lung disease, treat with fluconazole daily.
  - For severe lung disease, treat with amphotericin until symptoms are controlled and then with fluconazole.
  - For meningitis, give **induction/consolidation therapy** with amphotericin plus 5-flucytosine × 2 weeks followed by oral fluconazole daily × 10 weeks.
  - Patients with HIV need **long-term maintenance therapy** with oral fluconazole. It may be reasonable to stop prophylaxis if the CD4 count ↑ to > 200 for > 6 months in response to antiretrovirals.
  - **Repeat LP** until symptoms resolve in patients with coma or other signs of ↑ ICP.

KEY FACT

Serum CrAg titers are not useful for monitoring response to treatment for meningitis in immunosuppressed patients. CSF CrAg titers should ↓ during successful treatment.

Complications

A poorer prognosis for meningitis is seen in patients with abnormal mental status, those > 60 years of age, and those with evidence of high organism load or lack of immune response (as indicated by cryptococcemia, a high initial CrAg titer in CSF or serum, high CSF opening pressure, < 20 WBCs in CSF, low glucose, and a ⊕ India ink stain).

Coccidioidomycosis

A 47-year-old African American construction worker in central California presents with recent development of widespread cutaneous nodules. Exam reveals many raised, slightly painful nodules throughout the upper and lower extremities, and a biopsy shows spherules on pathology. What is the likely diagnosis?

This patient has disseminated coccidioidomycosis and should be treated with systemic antifungals such as fluconazole. Risk factors for dissemination include non-Caucasian ethnicity, particularly African American or Filipino ethnicity. Skin biopsy may show spherules, and this patient's outdoor exposure in central California makes coccidioidomycosis more likely.

Coccidioides immitis is found in the arid **southwestern United States,** central California, northern Mexico, and Central and South America. It is found in soil, and outbreaks occur after earthquakes or dust storms. Risk factors include exposure to soil and the outdoors (construction workers, archaeologists, farmers).

SYMPTOMS/EXAM

- 1° infection ("valley fever," "desert rheumatism"):
    - Usually presents with self-limited flulike symptoms, fever, dry cough, pleuritic chest pain, and headache, often accompanied by **arthralgias, erythema nodosum, or erythema multiforme.** CXR may be normal or may show unilateral infiltrates, nodules, or thin-walled cavities.
    - Some patients (5%) may develop chronic pneumonia, ARDS, or persistent lung nodules.
- **Disseminated disease (1%):** Chronic meningitis, skin lesions (papules, pustules, warty plaques), osteomyelitis, or arthritis.

DIFFERENTIAL

Atypical pneumonia, TB, sarcoidosis, histoplasmosis, blastomycosis.

DIAGNOSIS

- **Serologic tests** (complement fixation assays); titers ≥ 1:32 indicate more severe disease and a higher risk of dissemination.
- **Histology** may show giant **spherules** in infected tissues.
- **Cultures** of respiratory secretions or aspirates of bone and skin lesions may grow the organism (alert the laboratory if the diagnosis is suspected; *Coccidioides* is highly infectious to lab workers).

TREATMENT

- Treatment may not be necessary for acute disease but may be reasonable in patients at risk for dissemination.
- Fluconazole, itraconazole, or amphotericin should be given for disseminated disease.

COMPLICATIONS

Disseminated disease is more common in nonwhites, pregnant women, and patients with HIV, diabetes, or immunosuppression.

Histoplasmosis

Histoplasma capsulatum is found in the **Mississippi** and **Ohio River valleys.** The organism is found in moist soil and in bat and bird droppings. Risk factors include exploring caves and cleaning chicken coops or attics.

SYMPTOMS/EXAM

- **1° infection: Most patients are asymptomatic.** However, patients may present with fever, dry cough, and substernal chest discomfort. CXR may show patchy infiltrates that become nodular or exhibit multiple small nodules and hilar or mediastinal adenopathy. Some patients may develop chronic upper lobe cavitary pneumonia or mediastinal fibrosis (dysphagia, SVC syndrome, or airway obstruction).
- **Disseminated disease:** Presents with **hepatosplenomegaly,** adenopathy, **painless palatal ulcers,** meningitis, and pancytopenia from bone marrow infiltration. Patients with HIV may develop colonic disease (diarrhea, perforation or obstruction from mass lesions).

DIFFERENTIAL

Atypical pneumonia, influenza, coccidioidomycosis, blastomycosis, TB, sarcoidosis, lymphoma.

DIAGNOSIS

- **Urinary antigen test** is most useful in HIV/AIDS patents with disseminated disease.
- **Histology with silver stain** of bone marrow, lymph node, or liver.
- Cultures of blood or bone marrow are ⊕ in immunosuppressed patients with disseminated disease.
- Serologic tests (complement fixation and immunodiffusion assays) are often ⊕ in immunocompetent patients.

TREATMENT

- Treatment is not needed for acute pulmonary disease.
- Itraconazole or amphotericin for chronic cavitary pneumonia, mediastinal fibrosis, or disseminated histoplasmosis.

COMPLICATIONS

Severe or disseminated disease is more common in patients infected with a large inoculum and in elderly, immunosuppressed, and HIV patients.

Blastomycosis

Blastomyces dermatitidis is found in the **central United States** (as is *Histoplasma*) as well as in the upper Midwest and Great Lakes regions. Risk factors include exposure to woods and streams.

SYMPTOMS/EXAM

Acute pneumonia. May lead to warty, crusted, or ulcerated **skin lesions** or to osteomyelitis, epididymitis, or prostatitis.

DIAGNOSIS

Microscopy and culture of respiratory secretions; biopsy or aspirate material shows large yeast with **broad-based budding.**

TREATMENT

Itraconazole or amphotericin for all infected patients.

HANTAVIRUS

- First identified in the southwestern United States. Infection follows inhalation of **aerosols of dried rodent urine, saliva, or feces.**
- **Sx/Exam:** The disease begins as a nonspecific **febrile syndrome** (sudden fever, myalgias) with **rapid progression** to respiratory failure/ARDS and shock. Patients have leukocytosis, hemoconcentration, and thrombocytopenia.
- **Dx:** Diagnose by serology or by immunohistochemical staining of sputum or lung tissue.
- **Tx: Ribavirin** has been used experimentally, but mortality remains 50%.

NONTUBERCULOUS (ATYPICAL) MYCOBACTERIA

Nontuberculous (atypical) mycobacteria are natural inhabitants of water and soil. They can cause clinical disease in both immunocompetent and immunocompromised patients and are often difficult to diagnose and treat.

SYMPTOMS/EXAM

- *Mycobacterium avium:* Most frequently presents as **cavitary upper lobe lesions** (as with *M tuberculosis*) in patients with underlying pulmonary disease (COPD). However, otherwise normal hosts can develop **midlung nodular bronchiectasis** ("Lady Windermere syndrome"). In HIV/AIDS patients, a systemic disease with fever, abdominal pain, lymphadenopathy, and hepatosplenomegaly is most frequently seen.
- *Mycobacterium kansasii:* Primarily a pulmonary pathogen presenting in a manner **similar to *M tuberculosis*.** Patients may or may not be immunocompromised and often have underlying lung disease.
- *Mycobacterium marinum:* The 1° presentation consists of **skin ulcers** and **nodular lymphangitis** in patients with exposure to freshwater and saltwater, including marine organisms, swimming pools, and fish tanks.
- **Rapidly growing mycobacteria (*Mycobacterium abscessus, fortuitum,* and *chelonae*):** *M abscessus* is the most virulent of these pathogens, causing **nodular or cavitary pulmonary disease** and often causing **skin or soft tissue infections.** Disseminated or localized skin and soft tissue infections are the most common clinical manifestation of *M fortuitum* (associated with nail salons) and *M chelonae.*

DIFFERENTIAL

- **Cavitary or nodular lung disease:** *M tuberculosis,* endemic mycoses (coccidioidomycosis, histoplasmosis, blastomycosis, paracoccidioidomycosis), *Nocardia,* aspergillosis, neoplasms.
- **Skin ulcers or nodular lymphangitis:** *Sporothrix schenckii, Nocardia brasiliensis, M marinum, Leishmania braziliensis, Francisella tularensis.*

DIAGNOSIS

- **Pulmonary disease: All three of the following criteria** must be satisfied:
  - **Clinical criteria:** Compatible signs and symptoms (cough, fatigue, fever, weight loss) with reasonable exclusion of other diseases.
  - **Radiographic criteria:** CXR with persistent or progressive infiltrates with cavitation and/or nodules or CT with multiple small nodules or multifocal bronchiectasis.
  - **Bacteriologic criteria:** Three ⊕ cultures with ⊖ AFB smears **or** two ⊕ cultures with one ⊕ AFB smear **or** a single bronchoscopy or tissue biopsy with growth from a sterile site.
- **Nodular lymphangitis:** A ⊕ culture from biopsy.

KEY FACT

Think of pulmonary *Mycobacterium avium–intracellulare* in an elderly, nonsmoking woman with cough, malaise, and midlung nodular bronchiectasis on CXR.

TREATMENT

Treatment requires multiple drug regimens for prolonged courses of therapy. Many of these organisms (particularly the rapidly growing mycobacteria) are resistant to multiple antimicrobial agents. Consultation with a specialist is recommended.

COMPLICATIONS

Pulmonary disease can result in progressive lung cavitation and destruction with dissemination. Skin and soft tissue disease can be locally destructive or lead to disseminated infection.

TUBERCULOSIS (TB)

> A 35-year-old woman who emigrated from India 10 years ago has a PPD as part of her routine physical and is found to have 20 mm of induration. She feels well and has no fever, cough, or weight loss but notes that she received the BCG vaccine as a child. What are the next appropriate steps for this employee?
>
> Rule out active disease (eg, with a CXR) and then treat for latent tuberculosis infection (LTBI) or active disease if this is noted on CXR. Her BCG status does not affect the decision to treat, as it is not clear when the conversion occurred.

In the United States, *Mycobacterium tuberculosis* is most commonly found among the disadvantaged (homeless, malnourished, crowded living conditions) and in immigrants from developing countries.

SYMPTOMS/EXAM

- **1° TB:** Usually asymptomatic with no radiographic signs, but 5% of patients (usually infants, elderly, and the immunosuppressed) develop **progressive 1° infection.**
- **LTBI:** Patients are infected (and are usually skin test ⊕) but do not have symptoms of active disease. Bacilli are contained by granuloma-forming T cells and macrophages.
- **Active TB/reactivation disease:** Approximately 10% of LTBI patients develop active disease, **5% within the first two years of infection** and 5% over the rest of their lives. **Risk factors for reactivation** include recent infection (within two years), HIV, hematologic malignancy, immunosuppressive medications (eg, steroids, especially > 15 mg prednisone daily), diabetes, illicit drug use, silicosis, and gastrectomy.
- **Pulmonary TB:** Presents with subacute cough (initially dry and then productive, sometimes with blood-streaked sputum) as well as with malaise, fever, sweats, and weight loss. Exam is normal or reveals apical rales, rhonchi, or wheezing.
- **Extrapulmonary TB:** Lymphatic (painless cervical lymph node swelling) and pleural disease are most common. Other sites of infection may be seen, especially in patients with advanced HIV. Fever may be seen with more extensive disease.
- Figure 11.21 shows the evolution of pulmonary TB from initial infection to reactivation.

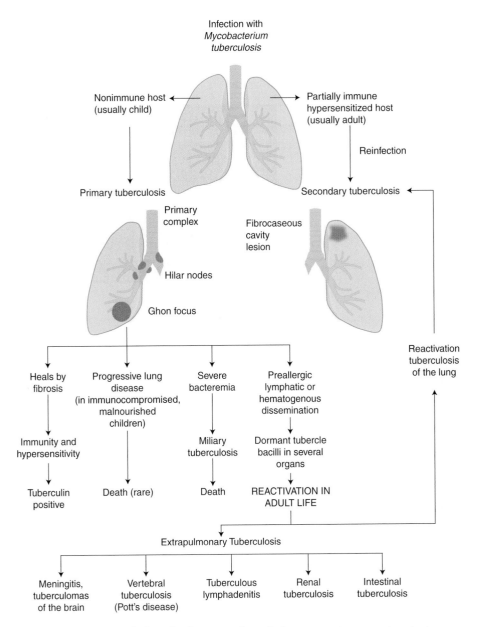

FIGURE 11.21. **Evolution of pulmonary tuberculosis.** (Modified with permission from Chandrasoma P, Taylor CR. *Concise Pathology*, 2nd ed. Originally published by Appleton & Lange. Copyright © 1995 by The McGraw-Hill Companies, Inc.)

DIFFERENTIAL

Pneumonia or lung abscess (bacterial, fungal, PCP), malignancy (of the lung or elsewhere), Crohn's disease (for GI TB), UTI (renal TB may yield a "sterile pyuria"), HIV infection, colonization by atypical mycobacteria (in patients with underlying emphysema or bronchiectasis).

DIAGNOSIS

- **Radiographic findings in active pulmonary TB** show infiltrates, nodules (including hilar), cavities (especially the apical or posterior segments of the upper lobes or the superior segments of the lower lobes), and calcifications (see Figure 11.22). **Advanced HIV patients and the elderly may have normal or atypical radiographs.**

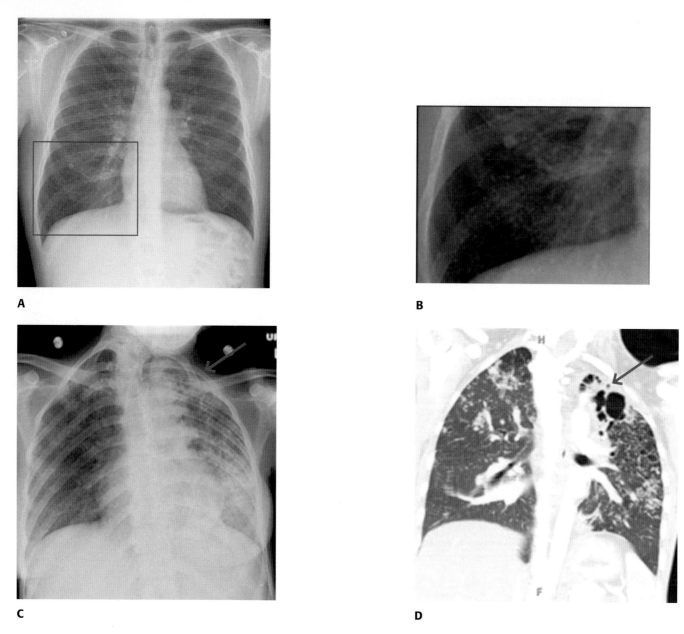

FIGURE 11.22. **Pulmonary tuberculosis.** (A) Frontal CXR demonstrating diffuse, 1- to 2-mm nodules due to miliary TB. (B) A zoomed-in view corresponding to the area delineated by the red box in Image A. (C) Frontal CXR demonstrating left apical cavitary consolidation (red arrow) and patchy infiltrates in the right and left lung in a patient with reactivation TB. (D) Coronal reformation from a noncontrast chest CT in the same patient as Image C, better demonstrating left apical cavitary consolidation (red arrow) and other areas of parenchymal abnormality corresponding to the endobronchial spread of TB. (Reproduced with permission from USMLERx.com.)

- **Sputum smears** are most sensitive in patients with cavitary disease (see Figure 11.23). Bacilli are visualized by acid-fast (Ziehl-Neelsen, Kinyoun) or fluorochrome (rhodamine-auramine) stain.
- **Cultures** of sputum, blood, or tissue are the **gold standard** but may take weeks to months to grow. Sensitivities help guide treatment.
- **Nucleic acid amplification and/or hybridization tests** are adjuncts to smear and culture that are approved by the FDA for rapid identification of TB in respiratory smears (not extrapulmonary sites). Not available in all laboratories.
- For extrapulmonary disease, **histopathology** shows granulomas with caseating necrosis; AFB stains may show bacilli. For pleural TB, biopsy of the pleura showing granulomas is more sensitive than pleural fluid culture.

- **Tuberculin skin testing** identifies patients with latent or active infection but is not 100% sensitive or specific; false ⊖s are seen in elderly, malnourished, and immunosuppressed patients as well as in those with overwhelming TB infection. A blood test that measures the release of α-interferon from lymphocytes in response to PPD is also available for the diagnosis of LTBI.
- The **Quantiferon-TB Gold assay** measures the release of γ-interferon in whole blood in response to stimulation by synthetic peptide mixtures simulating two proteins secreted by *M tuberculosis*. This test is approved for the diagnosis of LTBI and TB disease. It has a sensitivity similar to that of PPD but ↑ specificity, and it does not require a follow-up visit for reading (as is required by PPD skin testing).

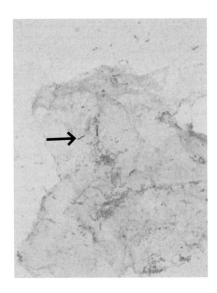

FIGURE 11.23. *Mycobacterium tuberculosis* **on AFB smear.** (Courtesy of the Centers for Disease Control and Prevention, Atlanta, GA, as published in Fauci AS et al. *Harrison's Principles of Internal Medicine,* 17th ed. New York: McGraw-Hill, 2008, Fig. 158-1.)

TREATMENT

- Hospitalized patients with suspected active TB should be placed in **respiratory isolation.** Cases should be reported to public health authorities.
- For most cases of TB, the CDC recommends starting **treatment with four drugs;** INH, rifampin, pyrazinamide, and ethambutol are most commonly used. Modify once susceptibility results are available. Ethambutol may be omitted if the transmitted organism is known to be fully susceptible.
- In patients on protease inhibitors, non-nucleoside reverse transcriptase inhibitors, itraconazole, methadone, or other medications metabolized by the liver, **rifabutin** may be used instead of rifampin because it is associated with less cytochrome P-450 induction.
- Steroids may be helpful for meningitis and pericarditis.
- **Strongly consider using directly observed therapy** to maximize compliance. Treat most adults for six months. Patients with HIV/AIDS or miliary/meningeal disease are sometimes treated longer.

PREVENTION

- **Screening and treatment of LTBI:** Patients who are at risk for reactivation disease should be screened regardless of age ("a decision to screen is a decision to treat"). The Mantoux tuberculin skin test measures **induration** (not erythema) transversely on the forearm 2–3 days after intradermal injection of tuberculin; a visible wheal must be seen at the time of injection. ⊕ skin tests should be followed by a CXR to rule out active pulmonary disease. Table 11.14 outlines CDC guidelines governing tuberculin skin test positivity.
- The CDC recommends treatment of LTBI (formerly called "prophylaxis") in HIV-⊖ persons with INH QD or BIW × 9 months or with rifampin QD × 4 months. The use of combination rifampin/pyrazinamide for two months has been associated with severe and fatal hepatitis and should be avoided.
- New health care workers and others who will be tested repeatedly should have **two-step testing,** with a repeat skin test after 1–3 weeks if they are initially ⊖ (≤ 10 mm). If the second test is ⊕, it is likely due to a boosting response, and the person is considered a "reactor" but not a "recent converter." A **skin-test conversion** indicating recent infection is defined as an ↑ of ≥ 10 mm of induration within a two-year period. **Anergy testing** is not recommended. **Previous BCG vaccination** should be disregarded, as persistent reactivity is unlikely after > 10 years.

COMPLICATIONS

- Treatment failure is usually due to medication nonadherence (> 95% of cases).
- While patients are on treatment, **monitor monthly for clinical symptoms.** Consider **monthly LFTs** for those with baseline liver disease. In the pres-

KEY FACT

You should not consider previous BCG vaccination status when interpreting a reactive PPD.

KEY FACT

Because of potential drug interactions, HIV patients on protease inhibitors should receive **rifabutin** instead of rifampin for the treatment of TB.

TABLE 11.14. CDC Guidelines for Tuberculin Skin Test Positivity

≥ 5 MM OF INDURATION (FOR PATIENTS AT HIGHEST RISK OF REACTIVATION)	≥ 10 MM OF INDURATION	≥ 15 MM OF INDURATION (FOR PATIENTS AT LOWEST RISK OF REACTIVATION)
HIV. Immunosuppression due to organ transplants or other medications (prednisone ≥ 15 mg/day for one month or more). Close contacts of TB cases. CXR with fibrotic changes consistent with prior TB.	Recent immigrants (≤ 5 years) from developing countries. Residents or established employees of jails, long-term care facilities, or homeless shelters. IV drug users. Patients with chronic illnesses such as silicosis, diabetes, CKD, leukemia, or lymphoma; head and neck or lung cancers; 10% weight loss; gastrectomy.	Patients with no risk factors for TB. New employees of high-risk institutions (at work entry).

ence of severe hepatitis (eg, AST and ALT five times greater than the upper limit of normal), discontinue all hepatotoxic drugs and reintroduce one at a time every 3–4 days while monitoring symptoms and LFTs.

- **Other baseline monitoring:** Visual acuity and color vision (patients on ethambutol), uric acid (pyrazinamide), and audiometry (streptomycin). Give **pyridoxine** (vitamin B_6) to HIV patients to ↓ the risk of INH-related peripheral neuritis.

VARICELLA-ZOSTER VIRUS (VZV)

1° infection causes chickenpox. Reactivation of latent infection leads to herpes zoster, or "shingles." Immunosuppressed patients can have more severe disease.

SYMPTOMS/EXAM

- **Chickenpox:** The incubation period is **10–20 days.** Presents with prominent fever, malaise, and a pruritic rash starting on the face, scalp, and trunk and spreading to the extremities. The rash is initially maculopapular and turns into vesicles ("dewdrops on a rose petal") and then into pustules that rupture, leading to crusts. **Multiple stages are present simultaneously.**
- **Herpes zoster:** Dermatomal tingling or pain followed by rash.

DIFFERENTIAL

- **Smallpox:** Lesions are deeper and painful; **all lesions occur at the same stage.**
- **Disseminated HSV:** Especially in the setting of a skin disorder; diagnose by culture.
- **Meningococcemia:** Petechiae, purpura, sepsis.

DIAGNOSIS

- Usually a clinical diagnosis.
- Confirm by scraping of lesions (culture or DFA staining for virus).
- Tzanck smear of vesicle base for multinucleate giant cells.
- PCR of CSF for CNS complications.

TREATMENT

- Acyclovir, valacyclovir, and **famciclovir** ↓ the duration and severity of disease and may prevent complications in adult chickenpox (if treated within **24 hours**) and shingles (if treated within **72 hours**).
- The addition of prednisone to acyclovir in immunocompetent patients with shingles may ↓ the risk of postherpetic neuralgia.
- Varicella-zoster immune globulin (**VariZIG**) may prevent complications in immunocompromised or pregnant patients.

PREVENTION

- **Chickenpox:** Vaccine can be given up to three days after exposure to patients with active lesions. **This live attenuated vaccine should not be given to immunosuppressed patients.**
- **Herpes zoster:** None. The effect of vaccine on risk of shingles is unknown.

COMPLICATIONS

- Chickenpox:
  - **Interstitial pneumonia** may occur, especially in pregnant women.
  - **Bacterial infections** (group A streptococcal infection).
  - **Encephalitis.**
  - **Transverse myelitis.**
  - Varicella may **disseminate** or be multidermatomal in immunosuppressed patients (HIV, steroids, malignancy).
  - **Reye's syndrome** (fatty liver, encephalopathy) may develop in children with chickenpox (or influenza) after taking **aspirin.**
- Herpes zoster:
  - **Postherpetic neuralgia** is most common in the elderly and may be prevented by starting antivirals **within 72 hours** of rash onset. The effect of steroids is less clear.
  - **Ophthalmic zoster** may lead to blindness; patients with lesions on the tip of the nose should have an ophthalmologic consult.
- **Ramsay Hunt syndrome:** Presents with vesicles on the ear, facial palsy, loss of taste on the anterior two-thirds of the tongue, and vertigo. Tinnitus/deafness may occur.

KEY FACT

The rash of smallpox starts on the face and extremities and moves to the trunk, where it is sparse. Generally, chickenpox rash also begins on the face and scalp and moves rapidly to the trunk, where it is denser, with relative sparing of the extremities.

NOTES

CHAPTER 12

Nephrology

Christina A. Lee, MD
Alan C. Pao, MD

Sodium Disorders

HYPONATREMIA

A 65-year-old healthy woman who is not on any medications presents with cough and dyspnea of five days' duration and is found to have right lower lobe pneumonia. Her exam is notable for a JVP of 8 cm, good skin turgor, moist mucous membranes, a normal cardiac exam, and crackles in the right lower lobe. Her labs are as follows: Na^+ 124 mEq/L, K^+ 4.1 mEq/L, Cl^- 85 mEq/L, HCO_3^- 29 mEq/L, BUN 13 mg/dL, and creatinine 1.1 mg/dL. Her serum osmolality is 260 mOsm/kg, urine Na 90 mEq/L, and urine osmolality 430 mOsm/kg H_2O. Her WBC count is 13.8 with PMN predominance. What is the most likely etiology of this patient's hyponatremia, and what would constitute first-line management?

Euvolemic hyponatremia due to SIADH. First, the patient has low serum osmolality (defined as < 280 mOsm/kg), confirming hypotonic hyponatremia. Second, she is euvolemic. Third, her urine osmolality is much greater than her serum osmolality, which suggests inappropriate ADH secretion, likely from her pneumonia. Treatment consists of free-water restriction; if the condition is refractory, consider demeclocycline or, alternatively, conivaptan, an AVP receptor antagonist.

KEY FACT

For the boards, you should be given the plasma osmolality, which should be the same as the calculated osmolality unless there is an osmolar gap due to alcohol ingestion.

KEY FACT

The vast majority of clinically significant hyponatremias will have a P_{osm} of < 280 mOsm/kg. The main reason to check plasma osmolality is to exclude pseudohyponatremia (severe hyperlipidemia, severe hyperproteinemia, hyperglycemia, or mannitol infusion).

KEY FACT

Psychogenic polydipsia and water intoxication are not associated with a normal P_{osm} (they have low P_{osm})!

SYMPTOMS/EXAM

- Symptoms are related to the rate and severity of the decline in Na^+.
- Can include nausea/vomiting, confusion, lethargy, seizures, and coma. May be asymptomatic.

DIFFERENTIAL

An algorithm for the evaluation and differential diagnosis of hyponatremia is given in Figure 12.1.

DIAGNOSIS

- **Step 1:** Determine plasma osmolality:

  Plasma osmolality $(P_{osm}) = (2 \times Na^+) + (BUN/2.8) + (glucose/18)$

- **Step 2:** For hypotonic hyponatremias, determine volume status:
  - On clinical exam, look for volume overload ($\uparrow$ JVP, S3 gallop, ascites, edema) or volume depletion (dry mucous membranes, flat JVP).
  - A **urine Na^+** (U_{Na+}) of < 10 mEq/L suggests hypovolemia.
  - A **fractional excretion of Na^+ (Fe_{Na+})** of < 1% is a more accurate predictor of low volume status than U_{Na+}:

  Fe_{Na+} = excreted Na^+/filtered Na^+ = $(U_{Na+} \times P_{Cr}) / (P_{Na+} \times U_{Cr})$

  where P_{Cr} = plasma creatinine, P_{Na+} = plasma sodium, and U_{Cr} = urine creatinine.
- **Step 3:** Measure urine osmolality. $U_{osm} > P_{osm}$ or $U_{osm} > 100$ **mOsm/kg** essentially rules out 1° polydipsia or a reset osmostat and reflects impaired renal water excretion.

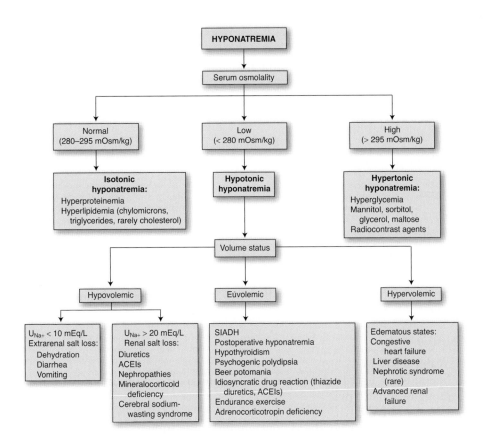

FIGURE 12.1. **Algorithm for the evaluation of hyponatremia.**

TREATMENT

- Fluid management depends on **volume status.**
    - **Hypervolemia:** Fluid restriction or diuretics.
    - **Euvolemia:** Fluid restriction.
    - **Hypovolemia:** Isotonic or hypertonic saline.
- The rate at which Na^+ should be corrected depends on how quickly it dropped and on the chronicity of the patient's symptoms.
    - **Acute symptomatic hyponatremia:** Na^+ should be ↑ until symptoms resolve (1–2 mEq/L/hr). If the patient has seizures, altered mental status, or other severe symptoms (eg, severe nausea, vomiting, headache), hypertonic (3%) saline is often required.
    - **Chronic symptomatic hyponatremia:** Na^+ should be ↑ more slowly (0.5–1.0 mEq/L/hr).
    - **Chronic asymptomatic hyponatremia:** No immediate correction is required; fluid management as outlined above often suffices.
- Treat the underlying cause.

 KEY FACT

To prevent central pontine myelinolysis, do not ↑ sodium more than 10–12 mEq/L over a 24-hour period.

SIADH

Remember the **"big three"** causes of SIADH: any CNS disorder, any pulmonary disorder, and medications (especially psychiatric medications such as chlorpropamide, TCAs, haloperidol, phenothiazine, and SSRIs).

 KEY FACT

The "big three" causes of SIADH: any CNS disorder, any pulmonary disorder, and medications (especially psych meds).

SYMPTOMS/EXAM

Presentation depends on the level of hyponatremia and the underlying cause of SIADH.

For euvolemic hyponatremias, urine osmolality can help distinguish SIADH (concentrated urine) from psychogenic polydipsia (dilute urine). SIADH has ↑ urine osmolality ($U_{osm} > 100$, $U_{Na} > 20$, or $U_{osm} > P_{osm}$), whereas psychogenic polydipsia has ↓ urine osmolality ($U_{osm} < 50$).

If SIADH is treated with normal saline, hyponatremia will worsen.

Conivaptan, an AVP receptor antagonist, is good for euvolemic hyponatremias. Vaptans may eventually replace demeclocycline in SIADH treatment.

DIFFERENTIAL

- CNS disorders:
  - **Head trauma:** SAH, subdural hematoma.
  - **Infection:** Meningitis, encephalitis, brain abscess.
  - **Other:** Tumors, CVA, MS.
- **Pulmonary disorders:** Small cell lung cancer, pneumonia, lung abscess, TB, pneumothorax.
- **Drugs:** Chlorpropamide, TCAs, haloperidol, phenothiazine, SSRIs.
- **Malignant neoplasia.**

DIAGNOSIS

- Diagnosis warrants a stepwise approach:
  - **Step 1:** Low P_{osm}.
  - **Step 2:** Euvolemia by physical exam.
  - $U_{osm} > P_{osm}$.
- **SIADH is a diagnosis of exclusion,** so other euvolemic causes of hyponatremia, including adrenal insufficiency (AI) and hypothyroidism, must be ruled out.

TREATMENT

- **Water restriction.**
- **Second-line agents:** Hypertonic saline and a loop diuretic for life-threatening hyponatremia.
- **Chronic SIADH:** Demeclocycline if fluid restriction is ineffective (impairs the kidney's ability to concentrate urine; induces nephrogenic DI). If demeclocycline does not work, consider conivaptan, an AVP receptor antagonist.

HYPERNATREMIA

 An 80-year-old bedridden woman with dementia presents with altered mental status of five days' duration. Exam reveals severely dry mucous membranes, lack of axillary sweat, and general confusion with an otherwise nonfocal neurologic exam. Her serum Na is 165 mEq/L, and her head CT is normal. What is the most likely etiology, and what would constitute first-line management?

The patient has a water deficit, as evidenced by hypernatremia. This is likely due to restricted access to water, which is common among bedridden elderly patients. First treat with normal saline to correct her hypovolemia, and then follow with hypotonic fluids (eg, ½ normal saline solution) to further correct her hypernatremia.

Hypernatremia is almost always due to free-water deficits (and only rarely to an ↑ in body sodium). Because hypernatremia leads to thirst, most patients who become hypernatremic have restricted access to water (eg, dementia patients who are bedridden).

SYMPTOMS/EXAM

- Usually occurs in the setting of ↓ access to water (eg, in dementia or in bedridden patients), as thirst protects against hypernatremia. Hyperosmolality results in cellular dehydration and **CNS symptoms** (lethargy, weakness, irritability, altered mentation, seizures, coma).
- **Volume depletion** presents as dry mucous membranes, hypotension, and low urinary output.

DIFFERENTIAL

Think of the differential in terms of volume status, as with the algorithm for hyponatremia:

- **Hypovolemic hypernatremia:** Renal losses (diuretics) vs. extrarenal losses (insensible losses from the skin, GI tract, or respiratory tract).
- **Euvolemic hypernatremia:** Central or nephrogenic DI. Suspect in a hypernatremic patient with copious dilute urine; see the Endocrine chapter for further details.
- **Hypervolemic hypernatremia (rare):** Mineralocorticoid excess (1° hyperaldosteronism) or hypertonic IV fluid administration.

DIAGNOSIS

- Based on clinical presentation.
- Measure U_{osm} (should be high in hypovolemia).
- **Water restriction test:** Urine remains inappropriately dilute in both central and nephrogenic DI.
- **DDAVP challenge test** (desmopressin, a type 2 vasopressin receptor agonist, is comparable to synthetic ADH): Urine becomes concentrated in central DI but not in nephrogenic DI.

TREATMENT

- Calculate free-water deficit:

$$\text{Deficit} = \text{normal body water} - \text{current body water} =$$
$$0.5 \times \text{body weight in kg} \left[(\text{plasma Na}^+ - 140) / 140 \right]$$

- Replace the calculated free-water deficit using hypotonic fluid so that the rate of correction does not exceed 0.5 mEq/L/hr (not to exceed 12 mEq/L in a 24-hour period).
- If the patient is hypotensive and volume depleted, isotonic saline should be used initially; hypotonic saline can be used once tissue perfusion is adequate.
- Check plasma sodium levels frequently to prevent overcorrection and cerebral edema.

Potassium Disorders

A 60-year-old woman with type 2 DM and hypertension has recurrent hyperkalemia (K$^+$ = 5.4–5.8 mEq/L). She is on lisinopril 10 mg and metformin 500 mg BID. She denies excess intake of high-potassium foods. Her urine potassium is 20 mEq/L, urine osmolality 570 mOsm/kg, serum osmolality 290 mOsm/kg, and serum potassium 6 mEq/L. What is the most likely cause of her hyperkalemia?

The transtubular K$^+$ gradient (TTKG) for this patient is 1.7. A TTKG value of < 5.0 reflects a defect in urinary K$^+$ excretion, which typically occurs with diseases associated with hypoaldosteronism. The most likely causes of hyperkalemia for this patient are the presence of DM (in the setting of type 4 RTA) and ACEI use, both of which can impair urinary K$^+$ excretion.

KEY FACT

Patients with DI have extremely dilute urine, with no change in urine output even if fluid intake is ↓. If U_{osm} is low in a hypernatremic patient, consider DI.

KEY FACT

Giving DDAVP to an individual with central DI should ↓ urine output and ↑ urine osmolality.

HYPERKALEMIA

SYMPTOMS/EXAM

May be asymptomatic or may present with symptoms ranging from muscle weakness to ventricular fibrillation (VF).

DIFFERENTIAL

- **High K⁺ dietary intake.**
- **Extracellular K⁺ shift:** Metabolic acidosis (often DKA), insulin deficiency, α-adrenergic blockade, rhabdomyolysis, tumor lysis syndrome, digitalis overdose, succinylcholine, periodic paralysis—hyperkalemic form.
- **Low urine K⁺ excretion:** Renal failure (common), ↓ effective circulating volume, hypoaldosteronism, K⁺-sparing diuretics. In HIV patients, consider high-dose TMP or pentamidine.
- **↓ renin-angiotensin system activity:** Hyporeninemic hypoaldosteronism, ACEIs, NSAIDs, cyclosporine, AI (commonly seen in HIV).

DIAGNOSIS

- Review the history, medications, and basic labs (chemistry panel with BUN, creatinine, and CK).
- Check an ECG as an indicator of severity.
    - **Mild:** Normal or peaked T waves.
    - **Moderate:** QRS prolongation or flattened P waves.
    - **Severe:** VF.
- Order additional labs if indicated:
    - **Tumor lysis syndrome:** High LDH, uric acid, and phosphorus; low calcium.
    - **Hypoaldosteronemic states:** Check **TTKG** (a value < 5 is suggestive of hypoaldosteronemic state):

$$TTKG = (U_{K+}/P_{K+}) / (U_{Osm}/P_{Osm})$$

where U_{K+} = urine potassium and P_{K+} = plasma potassium.

TREATMENT

- If ECG changes are present (life-threatening), first ↓ cardiac excitability. Give IV calcium gluconate and repeat every five minutes if ECG changes persist.
- **Shift K⁺ entry into cells:** Glucose and insulin, β₂-adrenergic agonists (eg, inhaled albuterol), NaHCO₃.
- **Remove excess K⁺:** Diuretics, cation exchange resin (Kayexalate), dialysis.

HYPOKALEMIA

SYMPTOMS/EXAM

- Symptoms usually occur when P_{K+} is < 2.5–3.0 mEq/L.
- Presents with muscle cramps, weakness, rhabdomyolysis, ileus, and arrhythmias.

DIFFERENTIAL

- **Low K⁺ dietary intake.**
- **Intracellular K⁺ shift:** Alkalemia, ↑ insulin availability, ↑ α-adrenergic activity, periodic paralysis (classically associated with thyrotoxicosis).
- **GI K⁺ loss:** Diarrhea.

KEY FACT

Suspect non-anion-gap metabolic acidosis (NAGMA) with ↓ serum HCO₃⁻ and ↑ Cl. A history of diarrhea points to GI bicarbonate loss; in the absence of diarrhea, consider RTA as the cause of NAGMA. The urine anion gap can confirm clinical suspicion.

KEY FACT

Distal (type 1) RTA presents with NAGMA, hypokalemia, **recurrent kidney stones** or hypercalciuria, and **alkaline urine pH** (urine pH is often > 6). Think Sjögren's syndrome and amphotericin. Treat with bicarbonate.

KEY FACT

In proximal (type 2) RTA (HCO₃⁻ wasting), urine is acidic when at a steady state but is initially alkaline (high). Think **multiple myeloma,** acetazolamide, and heavy metal poisoning. Treat associated diseases and institute Na⁺ restriction.

- **Renal K⁺ loss:** Diuretics, vomiting. Also consider mineralocorticoid excess (licorice ingestion, Cushing's disease) and Liddle's syndrome (consider in the setting of low K⁺, metabolic alkalosis, and hypertension).
- **Other:** Hypomagnesemia (always replete if present with low K⁺); Bartter's syndrome (acts like a loop diuretic; high urine Ca⁺), Gitelman's syndrome (acts like HCTZ; low urine Ca⁺).

DIAGNOSIS

- Review the history and medications.
- Check plasma renin and aldosterone levels if hyperaldosteronism is suspected.
- If the history includes hypokalemic periodic paralysis, check TSH.

TREATMENT

Replete KCl and magnesium.

Acid-Base Disorders

Figure 12.2 illustrates an overall approach toward the diagnosis and management of acid-base disorders.

METABOLIC ACIDOSIS

There are **two main categories** of metabolic acidosis: **anion gap and non–anion gap.** Refer to Figure 12.2 and the mnemonic **MUDPILES** for further details.

TREATMENT

See Table 12.1.

METABOLIC ALKALOSIS

Due to one of four main causes: volume depletion, chloride depletion, potassium depletion, or hyperaldosteronism. **Volume status and urine chloride** concentration (U_{Cl}) distinguishes these causes.

DIAGNOSIS/TREATMENT

- **If hypervolemic:** Points to 1° mineralocorticoid excess (1° **hyperaldosteronism** or hyperreninemia).
- **If euvolemic or hypovolemic:** Measure U_{Cl}.
  - U_{Cl} **is low** (< **10 mEq/L**): The kidney is trying to retain Na⁺ and Cl⁻, so urine Cl⁻ is low.
    - **GI loss:** Vomiting, NG suction, or chloride-losing diarrhea.
    - **Diuretics.**
    - **Gain of HCO₃⁻:** Intake of NaHCO₃ or antacids.
    - **Treatment:** NaCl infusion (thus also called "saline-responsive" alkalosis).
  - U_{Cl} **is high** (> **10 mEq/L**): Chloride-resistant metabolic alkalosis.
    - Active diuretic use.
    - Bartter's syndrome (like a loop diuretic).
    - Gitelman's syndrome (like HCTZ).
    - Magnesium deficiency.

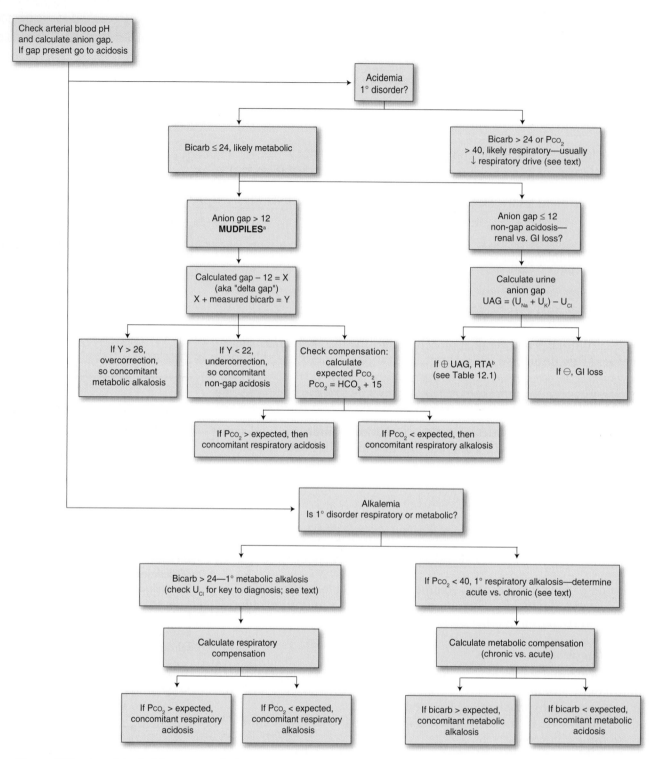

a. Measure BUN and creatinine, lactate, serum or urine ketones, and salicylate level.
   ■ Calculate the **osmolal gap** to rule out ingestion of an alcohol:
      Osm gap = measured osm − calculated osm
      Calculated osm = $(2 \times Na^+) + (BUN/2.8) + (glucose/18)$
   ■ **An osm gap > 20 indicates the ingestion of an alcohol:** Ethanol, methanol, ethylene glycol.

b. Diagnosis of specific RTA:
   ■ **If high serum K:** Type 4 RTA.
   ■ **If normal or low:** Look at the **urine pH.**
   ■ If > **5.5,** distal RTA.
   ■ If < **5.0,** proximal RTA (usually associated with glycosuria, low-grade proteinuria, or hypophosphatemia).

FIGURE 12.2. Approach to acid-base disorders.

TABLE 12.1. **Characteristics of Different Types of Renal Tubular Acidosis[a]**

	TYPE 1 (DISTAL)	TYPE 2 (PROXIMAL)	TYPE 4
Basic defect	↓ distal acidification.	↓ proximal HCO_3^- reabsorption.	Aldosterone deficiency or resistance.
Urine pH during acidemia	> 5.3.	Variable: Usually < 5.3, but can be high initially.	Usually < 5.3.
Plasma HCO_3^-, untreated	Very low (may be < 10 mEq/L).	Moderately low (14–20 mEq/L).	Usually > 15 mEq/L.
Plasma K^+	↓ or normal.	↓ or normal.	**High K^+.**
Nonelectrolytic complications	**Nephrocalcinosis and renal stones.**	Rickets or osteomalacia.	None.

[a] What had been called type 3 RTA is actually a variant of type 1 RTA.

(Adapted with permission from Rose BD, Post TW. *Clinical Physiology of Acid-Base and Electrolyte Disorders,* 5th ed. New York: McGraw-Hill, 2001: 613.)

RESPIRATORY ACIDOSIS

SYMPTOMS/EXAM

Presents with somnolence and altered mental status, depending on the severity of hypercapnia.

DIFFERENTIAL

- **Drugs:** Opiates, anesthetics, sedatives.
- **Other:**
    - Central sleep apnea; obstructed upper airway.
    - Impaired respiratory muscle or chest wall function.
    - Impaired alveolar gas exchange.

DIAGNOSIS

- An arterial pH of < 7.40 and an arterial P_{CO_2} of > 45 mm Hg suggest 1° respiratory acidosis.
- Calculate the alveolar-arterial oxygen gradient to distinguish intrinsic pulmonary from extrapulmonary disease (see the Pulmonary chapter for details).
- Compensation for acute vs. chronic respiratory acidosis:
    - **Acute:** For every 10-mm Hg ↑ in P_{CO_2}, plasma HCO_3^- ↑ 1 mEq/L.
    - **Chronic** (after 3–5 days): For every 10-mm Hg ↑ in P_{CO_2}, plasma HCO_3^- ↑ 3 mEq/L.

TREATMENT

- Correct the underlying disorder.
- Provide noninvasive ventilation (eg, BiPAP) or mechanical ventilation if necessary.

KEY FACT

Respiratory acidosis and respiratory alkalosis can **never** be present simultaneously; you can't hypoventilate and hyperventilate at the same time!

RESPIRATORY ALKALOSIS

SYMPTOMS/EXAM

- Presents with tachypnea, lightheadedness, and altered mental status.
- Can result in hypocalcemia, leading to paresthesias, circumoral numbness, and carpopedal spasms.

DIFFERENTIAL

- **CNS mediated:** Salicylate poisoning, pregnancy ($\uparrow$ progesterone), sepsis, neurologic disease.
- **Other:** Hypoxia, pulmonary disorders, mechanical overventilation.

DIAGNOSIS

- A pH of > 7.45 and a P_{CO_2} of < 35 constitute respiratory alkalosis.
- Compensation for acute vs. chronic respiratory alkalosis:
  - **Acute:** For every 10-mm Hg $\downarrow$ in P_{CO_2}, plasma HCO_3 $\downarrow$ 2 mEq/L.
  - **Chronic** (after 3–5 days): For every 10-mm Hg $\downarrow$ in P_{CO_2}, plasma HCO_3 $\downarrow$ 4 mEq/L.

TREATMENT

Correct the underlying disorder.

MIXED ACID-BASE DISORDERS

A 27-year-old woman with type 1 DM presents to the ER with intractable vomiting and abdominal pain. On exam, she is found to be tachypneic and hypovolemic. Her labs show the following levels: Na^+ 126 mEq/L, K^+ 5.2 mEq/L, Cl^- 75 mEq/L, HCO_3^- 15 mEq/L, BUN 65 mg/dL, creatinine 1.5 mg/dL, and glucose 567 mg/dL. Her ABGs reveal a pH of 7.52, a P_{CO_2} of 30 mm Hg, and a P_{O_2} of 260 mm Hg on room air. What is the patient's underlying acid-base disturbance?

A mixed acid-based disorder consisting of anion-gap metabolic acidosis (AGMA), metabolic alkalosis, and compensatory respiratory alkalosis. The AGMA is likely from DKA. Her HCO_3^- is much higher than expected for her degree of gap acidosis, indicating a concomitant metabolic alkalosis from severe vomiting. Finally, her low P_{CO_2} and tachypnea indicate respiratory alkalosis that is compensatory for DKA.

See Figure 12.2 for an algorithm of acid-base disorders.

TRIPLE ACID-BASE DISORDERS—THE "TRIPLE RIPPLE"

Defined as metabolic acidosis + metabolic alkalosis + respiratory acidosis or alkalosis. Classic causes are as follows:

- **Diabetic or alcoholic ketoacidosis:** Non-anion-gap and anion-gap metabolic acidosis (ketoacidosis), metabolic alkalosis (vomiting and hypovolemia), compensatory respiratory alkalosis.
- **Salicylate toxicity:** Anion-gap metabolic acidosis (from salicylic acid), metabolic alkalosis (vomiting), 1° respiratory alkalosis (salicylates directly stimulate the respiratory center).

NEPHROLITHIASIS

A 30-year-old man presents with sudden onset of colicky flank pain that radiates to the groin. He has no fever or peritoneal signs. His UA shows 0–2 WBCs/hpf, 10–30 RBCs/hpf, a urine specific gravity of 1.015, and ⊖ ketones. What is the likely diagnosis?

A kidney stone. Once the UA shows hematuria, the next step is to obtain a noncontrast CT to confirm the presence of a stone.

More common in men than in women. Eighty percent of stones are calcium oxalate.

Symptoms/Exam

- Presents with flank pain +/− radiation to the groin.
- Urinary frequency, urgency, and dysuria are also noted.
- Exam reveals microscopic or gross hematuria.

Diagnosis

- Collect and analyze the stone!
- Labs:
  - **UA:** To look for blood, assess urine pH, and rule out UTI.
  - **Plasma Ca⁺, phosphorus, uric acid, and electrolytes:** To assess renal function, acidosis, and hypokalemia.
  - **PTH level.**
- The gold standard is noncontrast spiral CT (see Figure 12.3). Plain x-rays capture calcium-containing stones but miss uric acid stones.

Treatment

- **Asymptomatic stones:** ↑ daily fluid intake.
- **Symptomatic stones:** Most will pass spontaneously with ↑ daily fluid intake. Consider calcium channel blockers and α-blockers to encourage passage.

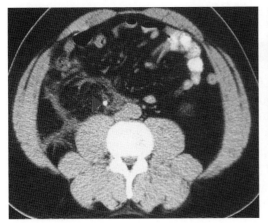
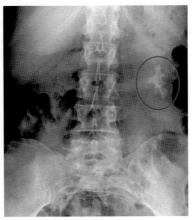

A **B**

FIGURE 12.3. Urinary calculi. (A) Transaxial image from a CT scan without IV contrast shows a right ureteral calculus (arrowhead) with surrounding inflammatory changes of the retroperitoneal fat. **(B)** Prone abdominal radiograph shows a right staghorn or struvite (Mg-NH₄-PO₄) stone filling the collecting system of the right kidney. (Image A reproduced with permission from Chen MY et al. *Basic Radiology*. New York: McGraw-Hill, 2004, Fig. 9-31. Image B reproduced with permission from USMLERx. com.)

TABLE 12.2. Types, Mechanisms, and Treatment of Kidney Stones

Type	Mechanisms and Disease Associations	Treatment[a]	Notes
Calcium oxalate	**Hypercalciuria:** Hyperparathyroidism, malignancy, granulomatous diseases. **Hyperoxaluria:** Short gut syndrome, IBD. **Hypocitraturia:** Metabolic acidosis from RTA, CKD, chronic diarrhea.	**Ca^{++} restriction is not helpful** (may lead to hyperoxaluria). Thiazides, potassium citrate.	Citrate is the 1° stone formation inhibitor.
Uric acid	**Acidic urine (pH < 5.5):** A diet high in animal protein. **Hyperuricosuria:** Gout, tumor lysis syndrome.	**Allopurinol, potassium citrate to alkaline urine.**	
Cystine	**Hypercystinuria:** Cystinuria.	Tiopronin (Thiola).	
Struvite (Mg-NH_4-PO_4)	**Alkaline urine (pH > 6.5):** UTI with urease-splitting organisms (eg, *Proteus mirabilis*).	Treat the underlying infection.	Recurrent UTIs may be due to a residual nidus of infection from the stone.
Medication related	Triamterene, acyclovir, indinavir.		

[a]In addition to large-volume water intake.

KEY FACT

Checking urine sodium or calculating Fe_{Na} is reliable only when the patient is oliguric and not taking diuretics.

KEY FACT

The differential diagnosis of ARF with a low Fe_{Na} (< 1%):
- Prerenal azotemia
- Glomerulonephritis
- Contrast nephropathy
- Rhabdomyolysis
- Early obstructive nephropathy

KEY FACT

NSAID-induced nephropathy may include the following:
- ARF from afferent arteriolar vasoconstriction in the setting of prerenal azotemia.
- AIN and minimal change disease.
- Analgesic nephropathy (papillary necrosis—chronic interstitial nephritis).

- Extracorporeal shock-wave lithotripsy or percutaneous nephrolithotomy is indicated for invasive stone removal. **A high volume of daily fluid intake and a metabolic workup are indicated for recurrent symptomatic stones.**
- Specific treatment guidelines are outlined in Table 12.2. Clues from the history are as follows:
  - **Recurrent UTIs:** Struvite stones.
  - **Prior malignancies:** Uric acid stones (tumor lysis).
  - **IBD:** Oxalate stones.

Acute Renal Failure (ARF)

APPROACH TO ARF

There is no consensus definition for ARF. Definitions may include a 25–50% ↑ in serum creatinine, a urine output < 0.5 mL/kg/hr for > 6–12 hours, and an ↑ in serum creatinine ≥ 0.3 mg/dL above baseline. Guidelines are as follows (see also Tables 12.3 and 12.4):

- Review the history of present illness. Look for a history that might indicate systemic infection (sepsis, ATN), recent aortic dissection or aortic repair (renal ischemia), or CT contrast administration (contrast nephropathy).
- Review medications for nephrotoxic drugs.
- Assess volume status.
- Obtain urine electrolytes to calculate Fe_{Na} (if oliguric).
- Examine urine sediment.
- Order a renal ultrasound to rule out obstruction and assess kidney size.

TABLE 12.3.   Etiologies of ARF

PRERENAL	INTRINSIC RENAL[a]	POSTRENAL
Volume depletion	**Tubular injury—acute tubular necrosis (ATN):**	Urinary tract obstruction
Circulatory shock	▪ Ischemia	
Severe CHF	▪ Contrast dye	
Severe cirrhosis (hepatorenal syndrome)	▪ Myeloma	
	▪ Heme pigment (rhabdomyolysis, hemolysis)	
	▪ Aminoglycosides	
	Interstitium—acute interstitial nephritis (AIN):	
	▪ **Allergic and drug reactions** (antibiotics, NSAIDs, COX-2 inhibitors)	
	▪ **Infections** (HIV, toxoplasmosis)	
	▪ **Autoimmune** (sarcoidosis, SLE)	
	Glomerular—glomerulonephritis (see separate section)	
	Cholesterol emboli syndrome	

[a]See the section on ARF for details on how to use urine sediment to guide the differential.

TABLE 12.4.   Differential Diagnosis of ARF

CAUSE OF ARF	SUGGESTIVE CLINICAL FEATURES	TYPICAL UA	CONFIRMATORY TESTS
PRERENAL			
	Evidence of true volume depletion or ↓ effective circulatory volume (eg, heart or liver failure); treatment with NSAIDs or ACEIs.	Hyaline casts; **Fe$_{Na}$ < 1%, U$_{Na}$ < 10 mmol/L;** high specific gravity.	Occasionally requires invasive hemodynamic monitoring. Rapid resolution of ARF occurs upon restoration of renal perfusion.
INTRINSIC RENAL—DISEASES INVOLVING LARGE RENAL VESSELS			
Renal artery thrombosis	Atrial fibrillation or recent MI; flank or abdominal pain.	Mild proteinuria; occasional red cells.	↑ LDH with normal transaminases; renal imaging. ultrasound, MRA, or CTA is usually done before renal angiogram.
Atheroembolism	Age > 50 years, **recent manipulation of the aorta,** retinal plaques, subcutaneous nodules, palpable purpura, **livedo reticularis, vasculopathy,** hypertension, anticoagulation.	Often normal; **eosinophiluria;** rarely, casts.	Eosinophilia, **hypocomplementemia,** skin biopsy, renal biopsy.
Renal vein thrombosis	Evidence of **nephrotic syndrome** (loss of anticoagulant proteins) or pulmonary embolism; flank pain.	Proteinuria, hematuria.	Renal ultrasound with Dopplers; renal venogram; CT scan.

(continues)

TABLE 12.4. **Differential Diagnosis of ARF** *(continued)*

CAUSE OF ARF	SUGGESTIVE CLINICAL FEATURES	TYPICAL UA	CONFIRMATORY TESTS
INTRINSIC RENAL—DISEASES OF SMALL VESSELS AND GLOMERULI			
Glomerulonephritis/ vasculitis	Variable; see "Glomerular diseases."	**Red cell or granular casts;** red cells, white cells, moderate proteinuria.	C3, C4, ANCA, anti-glomerular basement membrane (anti–GBM) antibody, ANA, ASO, anti-DNase, cryoglobulins, blood cultures, renal biopsy.
HUS/TTP	Compatible clinical history (eg, **recent GI infection,** cyclosporine, anovulants); fever, pallor, ecchymoses, neurologic abnormalities.	May be normal; red cells, mild proteinuria; rarely, red cell/ granular casts.	Anemia, thrombocytopenia, schistocytes on blood smear, ↑ LDH, renal biopsy.
Malignant hypertension	Severe hypertension with headache, CHF, retinopathy, neurologic dysfunction, papilledema.	Red cells, red cell casts, proteinuria.	LVH by echo/ECG; resolution of ARF with BP control.
INTRINSIC RENAL—ARF MEDIATED BY ISCHEMIA OR TOXINS (ATN)			
Ischemia	Recent sepsis, hemorrhage, hypotension (eg, cardiac arrest), surgery.	**Muddy brown granular or tubular epithelial cell casts;** $Fe_{Na} > 1\%$, $U_{Na} > 20$ mmol/L.	Clinical assessment and UA.
Exogenous toxins	**Recent IV contrast,** nephrotoxic antibiotics or anticancer agents; often coexists with volume depletion, sepsis, chronic renal insufficiency.	Same as above.	Same as above.
Endogenous toxins	Rhabdomyolysis. Massive hemolysis (blood transfusion). Tumor, myeloma, ethylene glycol ingestion.	Urine supernatant ⊕ for heme. Urine supernatant pink and ⊕ for heme. Urate crystals, dipstick-⊖ proteinuria, oxalate crystals, respectively.	Electrolyte derangements (hyperkalemia, hyperphosphatemia), ↑ circulating myoglobin, ↑ CK and uric acid. Electrolyte derangements, hyperuricemia, pink plasma ⊕ for hemoglobin. Labs consistent with tumor lysis; circulating or urinary monoclonal spike for myeloma; toxicology screen, acidosis, osmolal gap (for ethylene glycol).

TABLE 12.4. Differential Diagnosis of ARF *(continued)*

Cause of ARF	Suggestive Clinical Features	Typical UA	Confirmatory Tests
Intrinsic Renal— Acute Diseases of the Tubulointerstitium			
Acute interstitial nephritis (AIN)	Recent ingestion of drug and fever, rash, or arthralgias.	**White cell casts,** white cells (frequently **eosinophiluria**), red cells; rarely, red cell casts, proteinuria (occasionally nephrotic).	**Systemic eosinophilia,** skin biopsy of rash **(leukocytoclastic vasculitis),** renal biopsy. **Can lead to chronic interstitial nephritis.**
Acute bilateral pyelonephritis	Flank pain and tenderness, toxic, febrile.	Leukocytes, proteinuria, red cells, bacteria.	Urine and blood cultures.
Postrenal			
	Abdominal or flank pain; palpable bladder.	Frequently normal; hematuria if stones, hemorrhage, malignancy, or prostatic hypertrophy.	Renal ultrasound or CT scan.

(Adapted with permission from Fauci AS et al. *Harrison's Principles of Internal Medicine,* 17th ed. New York: McGraw-Hill, 2008, Table 273-2.)

TREATMENT

- Treat the underlying cause or remove the offending agent.
- Support renal function through dialysis if necessary (see the mnemonic AEIOU).
- There is **no role** for "renal-dose" dopamine.

SPECIFIC CAUSES OF ARF

A 70-year-old man with type 2 DM and dementia is admitted to the hospital after having been found unresponsive by his family. His vital signs in the ER were as follows: T 39.0°C (102°F), BP 70/40 mm Hg, HR 125 bpm, RR 24, and O_2 saturation 91% on room air. His physical exam revealed a tender abdomen, and a CT of the abdomen/pelvis with contrast showed ischemic bowel. The patient subsequently underwent a right-sided hemicolectomy with no complications. Two days postoperatively, his serum creatinine was noted to have risen from a baseline of 1.2 mg/dL to 2.7 mg/dL. Urine sediment showed muddy brown casts. What is the most likely etiology of his ARF?

ATN from a combination of sepsis/hypotension and contrast-induced nephropathy.

See Tables 12.5 and 12.6 and the sections that follow for details on the causes of ARF.

MNEMONIC

Indications for emergent dialysis—

AEIOU

Acidosis
Electrolytes—hyperkalemia
Ingestions—severe acidemia
Overload—pulmonary edema
Uremia

KEY FACT

Clues to UA:
- Muddy brown casts or renal tubular epithelial cells: ATN.
- Red cell casts or dysmorphic RBCs: Glomerulonephritis.
- WBC casts: AIN, pyelonephritis.
- Hyaline casts: Nonspecific.

TABLE 12.5. Prerenal Azotemia vs. ATN

	PRERENAL AZOTEMIA	ATN
Fe_{Na}	< 1%	> 1%
BUN/Cr	> 20:1	10–15:1
U_{osm}	High.	Similar to P_{osm}.
Urine sediment	Bland.	Muddy brown casts (see Figure 12.4).
Response to fluids	Rapidly improves.	Poor; may take 2–3 weeks for recovery, and up to several months. Often requires dialysis in the interim.

Urinary Tract Obstruction

Obstruction of > 2 weeks' duration is likely to cause permanent damage.

KEY FACT

Suspect contrast nephropathy in patients who have rising creatinine within 24–72 hours after contrast load. There is no specific treatment.

DIFFERENTIAL

- Neurogenic bladder.
- **Malignancies** (GU cancers, lymphoma, pelvic lymphadenopathy).
- Kidney stones, BPH.
- Retroperitoneal fibrosis (radiation, drugs such as bromocriptine, malignancies such as lymphomas and sarcomas, infections such as TB and histoplasmosis, surgery).

TABLE 12.6. Features of Contrast Dye Nephropathy and Rhabdomyolysis

	CONTRAST NEPHROPATHY	RHABDOMYOLYSIS
Risk factors	Underlying kidney disease. Diabetes. Concomitant use of ACEIs, ARBs, or NSAIDs. Volume depletion or sepsis.	Muscle trauma, ischemia, or inflammation. Toxins: Alcohol, cocaine, statins, reverse transcriptase inhibitors. Metabolic: Severe hypokalemia, hypophosphatemia. Genetic: McArdle's disease.
Other clinical features	Creatinine peaks 24–72 hours after dye load and then typically improves.	Serum CK > 5000 U/L. Urine dipstick is ⊕ for blood, but no RBCs are seen on microscopy. Other lab changes include hyperkalemia, hyperphosphatemia, hyperuricemia, and hypocalcemia.
Treatment	Isotonic crystalloid fluid 1.0–1.5 mL/kg/hr before and after contrast administration. The superiority of $NaHCO_3$ over NaCl is controversial. *N*-acetylcysteine. Dialysis is rarely needed.	Early, aggressive volume repletion. Urine alkalization with $NaHCO_3$ may help. Dialysis may be needed.
Notes	Unlike other ATNs, Fe_{Na+} is low (due to intrarenal vasoconstriction).	Urine dipstick is ⊕ for blood due to myoglobin pigments in urine.

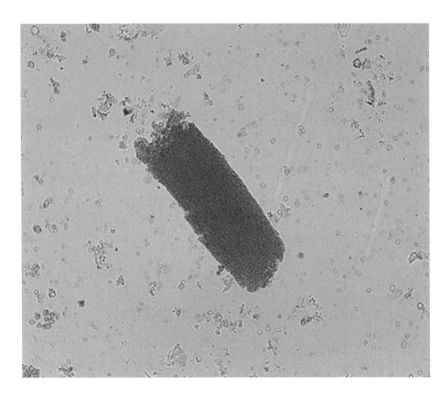

FIGURE 12.4. **Muddy brown cast.** (Courtesy of Rudy Rodriguez, MD.)

DIAGNOSIS

- Oliguria or anuria.
- Labs show moderately ↑ K^+, acidosis, and ↑ creatinine.
- Fe_{Na} is low (< 1%) early after obstruction and higher later in the course of disease.
- Foley catheter reveals a large postvoid residual.
- **Ultrasonography** reveals **hydronephrosis** (see Figure 12.5).

TREATMENT

- Relieve the obstruction.
- Volume repletion during postobstructive diuresis.

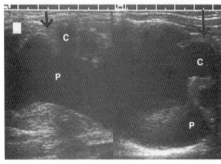

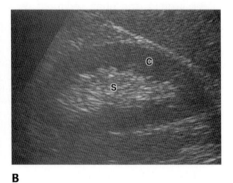

A   **B**

FIGURE 12.5. **Hydronephrosis.** (**A**) Ultrasound of a renal transplant shows severe hydronephrosis, with dilation of the renal pelvis (P) and the renal calyces (C). The overlying renal cortex is severely thinned (arrows). (**B**) Normal renal ultrasound for comparison. C = cortex; S = sinus fat. (Reproduced with permission from Tanagho EA, McAninch JW. *Smith's General Urology,* 17th ed. New York: McGraw-Hill, 2008, Fig. 6-22.)

Hepatorenal Syndrome (HRS)

Seen in severe liver disease with portal hypertension. Intense renal salt and water retention leads to oliguric or anuric renal failure.

DIAGNOSIS

- Look for advanced hepatic failure and portal hypertension.
- Serum creatinine >1.5 mg/dL, progressive over days to weeks.
- Additional features include the following:
    - No other obvious cause of renal failure; normal renal ultrasound; absence of hematuria (< 50 cells/hpf) and proteinuria (< 500 mg/24 hrs); no nephrotoxic drugs; no sepsis or signs of infection.
    - No improvement in renal function after volume expansion with **albumin** (1 g/kg) and diuretic withdrawal.
- A salt-avid state may be seen with very low urine sodium.

TREATMENT

- Albumin infusion.
- **Splanchnic vasoconstrictors:** Vasopressin analogs (terlipressin, ornipressin), midodrine, octreotide.
- Transjugular intrahepatic portosystemic shunt (TIPS).
- Renal replacement therapy as a bridge to liver transplantation. Liver transplantation is the treatment of choice.

Cholesterol Emboli Syndrome

See the Rheumatology chapter.

Glomerular Diseases

GLOMERULONEPHRITIS (NEPHRITIC)

> A 45-year-old woman with a history of diffuse joint pain is admitted to the hospital. She initially presented to the ER with severe peripheral edema and hypertension. Basic labs were notable for a BUN of 75 mg/dL, a creatinine of 3.7 mg/dL, an albumin level of 2.1 g/dL, and an ANA of 1:320. UA showed 3+ protein, and urine sediment revealed numerous dysmorphic RBCs. Serum complement levels were ↓. What is the most likely diagnosis?
> SLE with glomerulonephritis.

SYMPTOMS/EXAM

Presents with hypertension, edema, and oliguria +/– hematuria.

DIFFERENTIAL

See Figure 12.6 and Table 12.7.

DIAGNOSIS

- Urine microscopy shows **RBC casts** (see Figure 12.7).
- **Renal biopsy** is definitive.

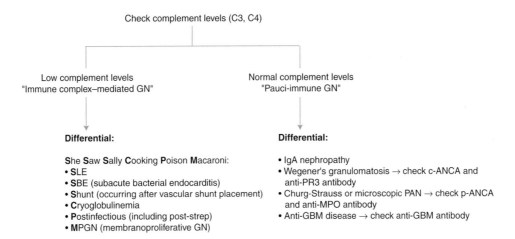

Check complement levels (C3, C4)

Low complement levels
"Immune complex–mediated GN"

Normal complement levels
"Pauci-immune GN"

Differential:

She Saw Sally Cooking Poison Macaroni:
- **S**LE
- **S**BE (subacute bacterial endocarditis)
- **S**hunt (occurring after vascular shunt placement)
- **C**ryoglobulinemia
- **P**ostinfectious (including post-strep)
- **M**PGN (membranoproliferative GN)

Differential:

- IgA nephropathy
- Wegener's granulomatosis → check c-ANCA and anti-PR3 antibody
- Churg-Strauss or microscopic PAN → check p-ANCA and anti-MPO antibody
- Anti-GBM disease → check anti-GBM antibody

FIGURE 12.6. **Differential diagnosis of glomerulonephritis.**

TABLE 12.7. **Subtypes of Glomerulonephritis**

SUBTYPE	RELEVANT SEROLOGIES	DISEASES
Immune complex	$\downarrow C_3, C_4$.	Membranoproliferative glomerulonephritis (MPGN), cryoglobulinemia. Postinfectious glomerulonephritis, SLE, subacute bacterial endocarditis. Shunt. IgA nephropathy, usually with normal C_3/C_4.
Pauci-immune	p-ANCA, c-ANCA. Normal complements.	Wegener's granulomatosis, Churg-Strauss syndrome, polyarteritis nodosa (PAN).
Anti-GBM	Anti-GBM antibodies. Normal complements.	Anti-GBM disease, Goodpasture's syndrome.

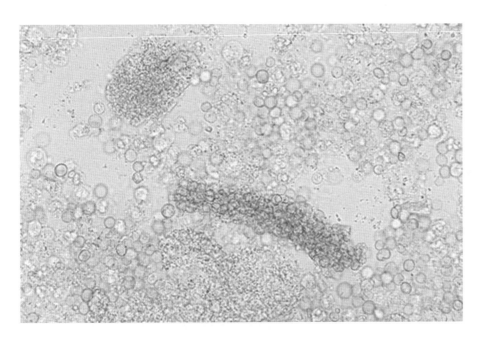

FIGURE 12.7. **Red blood cell cast.** (Courtesy of Rudy Rodriguez, MD.)

KEY FACT

Think of Wegener's glomerulonephritis when you see a patient with a history of sinusitis, pulmonary nodules, and dysmorphic RBCs or RBC casts with renal failure.

TREATMENT

See Tables 12.8 through 12.10.

NEPHROTIC SYNDROME

Can be 1° or 2° (due to a systemic cause). The most common 1° causes are **membranous nephropathy and focal segmental glomerulosclerosis.** The most common 2° cause is **DM.**

TABLE 12.8. **Immune Complex Glomerulonephritis**[a]

DISEASE	PRESENTATION	DIAGNOSIS	PATHOLOGY	TREATMENT
SLE	Any of the criteria for SLE (see Rheumatology chapter). Lupus nephritis can be the presenting feature.	Anti-dsDNA, anti-Sm antibodies ⊕.	Can be proliferative or membranous alone.	Steroids and cyclophosphamide depending on severity. End-stage renal disease (ESRD) occurs in 8–15% of cases.
Postinfectious	**Occurs 2–3 weeks after pharyngitis or skin infection.** Classically seen with streptococcal infection, but may be triggered by others.	↑ ASO and anti-DNase B antibodies ⊕.	Diffuse proliferative glomerulonephritis. EM reveals subepithelial "humps."	Renal failure typically resolves in six weeks. Only 5% of cases require dialysis acutely.
MPGN	**Cryoglobulin-related MPGN:** Arthralgias, palpable purpura, history of HCV infection. Microscopic hematuria with mild to heavy proteinuria. May be chronic or rapidly progressive.	⊕ cryoglobulins, RF. Check HBV, HCV, and HIV serologies. Check C3, C4.	Hypercellular glomerulus. EM shows subendothelial deposits.	Treat HCV-related disease and cryoglobulinemia with α-interferon alone or in combination with ribavirin (if kidney function is not severely impaired).
IgA nephropathy	More common in Asians and Hispanics. Episodic hematuria with or without proteinuria **(usually within 24 hours of URI).**	Renal biopsy. **Normal C3.**	IgA deposits in the mesangium and glomerular capillary wall.	**Mild disease:** ACEIs/ARBs. **Progressive disease:** Corticosteroids +/– alkylating agent. Ten to twenty percent of cases progress to ESRD. ↑ creatinine, proteinuria. Hypertension worsens the prognosis.
Endocarditis	Episodic hematuria with or without proteinuria (usually within 24 hours of URI).	Blood cultures, echocardiography. Check C3, C4.	May have renal impairment due to crescentic glomerulonephritis, cryoglobulinemia, ATN, or AIN.	Antibiotics. The general rule is that if endocarditis is cured, renal impairment will be cured.

[a]Most have ↓ C3 unless noted.

TABLE 12.9. **Pauci-immune/ANCA-Positive Glomerulonephritis**

DISEASE	PRESENTATION	DIAGNOSIS	PATHOLOGY	TREATMENT
Wegener's granulomatosis	Upper respiratory tract disease and nodular cutaneous lesions are common. Rapidly progressive glomerulo-nephritis (RPGN).	c-ANCA and anti–proteinase 3 (PR3) antibody ⊕. Renal biopsy.	Necrotizing small vessel vasculitis. Necrotizing crescentic glomerulonephritis.	Steroids with PO cyclophosphamide. Plasmapheresis.
Microscopic polyangiitis	Lower rate of upper respiratory tract than Wegener's. RPGN.	p-ANCA and anti-MPO antibody ⊕. Renal biopsy.	Same as above.	Steroids with PO cyclophosphamide.
Churg-Strauss syndrome	Asthma, allergic rhinitis, eosinophilia. Peripheral neuropathy (mononeuritis multiplex) common.	p-ANCA and anti-MPO antibody ⊕. Renal biopsy.	As above.	Steroids with PO cyclophosphamide.

SYMPTOMS/EXAM

Has the following clinical features:

- Anasarca/peripheral edema.
- Hypoalbuminemia (serum albumin < 3 g/dL).
- Hyperlipidemia.
- Proteinuria > 3.5 g/day.
- Hypercoagulability.

DIFFERENTIAL

- **Idiopathic or 1° nephrotic syndrome:** Has four subtypes (see also Table 12.11):
  - **Minimal change disease:** 2° causes include lymphoproliferative disease, drugs (particularly NSAIDs), and infection (syphilis, TB, HIV).
  - **Focal segmental glomerulosclerosis:** 2° causes include heroin, nephron loss (from hypertension, reflux nephropathy, or sickle cell disease), HIV (collapsing variant), obesity, and lymphomas.
  - **Membranous nephropathy:** 2° causes include gold, penicillamine, NSAIDs, HBV, HCV, captopril, and solid tumors (lung, kidney, breast, GI tract).

KEY FACT

Patients with nephrotic syndrome are hypercoagulable due to loss of anticoagulant proteins (eg, AT III, protein C, protein S) and thus have an ↑ incidence of venous and arterial thrombi.

KEY FACT

Minimal change disease can be caused by NSAIDs. Other inciting drugs are lithium, penicillamine, pamidronate, sulfasalazine, and γ-interferon.

TABLE 12.10. **Anti–Glomerular Basement Membrane Disease**

DISEASE	PRESENTATION	DIAGNOSIS	PATHOLOGY	TREATMENT
Goodpasture's syndrome	Pulmonary alveolar hemorrhage; dyspnea, cough. RPGN. May have ANCA-associated vasculitis.	Anti-GBM antibody ⊕. Renal biopsy.	Linear IgG deposition along GBM. Diffuse proliferative glomerulonephritis.	Corticosteroids + cyclophosphamide. Plasmapheresis.
Anti-GBM disease	RPGN alone.	Anti-GBM antibody ⊕. Renal biopsy.	Same; no pulmonary involvement.	Same.

TABLE 12.11.   1° Causes of Nephrotic Syndrome

Disease	Presentation	Pathology	Treatment	Clinical Course
Minimal change disease	Sudden onset with heavy proteinuria. More common in children.	Normal light microscopy. EM reveals epithelial foot process fusion.	Steroids.	Responds to steroids but often relapses. Renal failure is uncommon.
Focal segmental glomerulo-sclerosis	↑ in African Americans.	Focal segmental glomerulosclerosis.	Steroids, cyclosporine; cyclophosphamide.	Up to 50% develop ESRD within five years.
Membranous nephropathy	Can be 2° to HBV, HCV, syphilis; autoimmune (SLE); carcinomas. Predilection to clotting—renal vein thrombosis.	Thickened capillary loops with subepithelial "spikes." EM shows subepithelial deposits.	Observation with ACEIs/ ARBs if slow progression. Steroids; cyclosporine, tacrolimus, mycophenolate.	Twenty-five percent spontaneously remit. **"1/3 get better, 1/3 stay the same, 1/3 get worse."** Slow progression to renal failure.
MPGN	Can present with either nephritic or nephrotic features. Associated with HCV/ cryoglobulins, HBV, other infections, autoimmune (SLE).	Hypercellular glomerulus with lobular architecture. EM shows subendothelial deposits.	**Non-nephrotic:** Observe. **Nephrotic** or **worsening renal function:** Steroids.	Fifty percent die or progress to ESRD within five years of renal biopsy.

- **Membranoproliferative glomerulonephritis:** 2° causes include **HCV, SLE,** Sjögren's syndrome, and chronic infection (malaria, subacute bacterial endocarditis, chronic abscesses).
- **2° to systemic disease: DM nephropathy, amyloidosis,** multiple myeloma, HIV, HBV, drugs (especially NSAIDs) (see also Table 12.12).

DIAGNOSIS

- As above plus the following:
    - **UA:** In addition to proteinuria, oval fat bodies or **"Maltese crosses"** may be visualized under polarized light.
    - **24-hour urine protein:** The best way to quantify the extent of proteinuria. Calculate the spot urine protein-to-creatinine ratio (divide spot protein by creatinine to approximate 24-hour protein excretion in grams).
    - Renal biopsy is definitive.
- Additional labs to search for 2° causes include HbA_{1c}, SPEP/UPEP, and serologies for HBV, HCV, HIV, and syphilis.

TREATMENT

- **General measures:**
    - Control volume status and peripheral edema with loop diuretics.
    - Maintain good nutrition.
    - Give ACEIs to slow proteinuria.
    - Lipid lowering—generally target an LDL < 100 mg/dL.
- **Treat the underlying disease.**

TABLE 12.12. **2° Causes of Nephrotic Syndrome**

Disease	Presentation	Pathology	Treatment	Clinical Course	Notes
HIV-associated nephropathy	High viral load. Low CD4 count. **No peripheral edema.**	**Focal segmental glomerulo-sclerosis.** Large dilated tubular cysts.	Initiation of HAART. Steroids if there is evidence of interstitial nephritis.	If untreated, may progress to ESRD within a few months.	**Most common in African Americans and Hispanics.** Kidneys are large and echogenic on renal ultrasound.
Diabetic nephropathy	Onset 5–10 years after diagnosis in type 1 DM; more variable in type 2. **High prevalence of simultaneous DM retinopathy.**	Mesangial expansion. **Kimmelstiel-Wilson lesion (nodular glomerulo-sclerosis).** Tubulointerstitial fibrosis.	Glycemic control. Target LDL < 100 mg/dL. Target BP < 130/80 mm Hg.	Progresses from hyperfiltration to microalbuminuria to nephrotic to ESRD.	The leading cause of ESRD in the United States. **ACEIs/ARBs are first-line treatment.** BP control is very important in slowing GFR decline.
Multiple myeloma (light chain deposition disease)	**More severe renal failure with cast nephropathy.** May have tubular dysfunction, **Fanconi's syndrome** (glycosuria, aminoaciduria, phosphaturia, bicarbonaturia).	$\kappa > \lambda$ **light-chain involvement.** Glomerular or tubulointerstitial Congo-red stain (–) deposits.	See the Hematology chapter.	Higher creatinine is correlated with worse survival. Survival improves if stem cell transplantation is successful.	Monoclonal gammopathy on SPEP/UPEP. **Light chains will not be detected by urine dipstick for protein.**
Amyloidosis	May have heavy proteinuria of > 20 g/day. **AL (1°): Ig light chain deposition;** associated with multiple myeloma/ MGUS. **AA (2°):** Amyloid protein deposition; associated with **chronic inflammation and infection AF (familial):** Transthyretin mutation.	Amyloid fibril deposition. Glomerular or tubulointerstitial deposition. Congo-red stain (+) deposits.	**AL:** See Hematology chapter. **AA:** Control the underlying condition.	Mean survival in 1° amyloid is months.	

KEY FACT

In diabetes, ACEIs/ARBs can delay progression of proteinuria to overt nephropathy.

Essential Hypertension

See the Ambulatory Medicine chapter.

2° Hypertension

 A 24-year-old woman presents with persistent BPs in the 160s/80s since age 20. Her condition has been refractory to maximal doses of HCTZ, lisinopril, and metoprolol. She is not on OCPs or NSAIDs and denies the use of illicit drugs or alcohol. Her father had essential hypertension. Her exam reveals a normal BMI and cardiac exam and a continuous abdominal bruit. Her TSH, CBC, and creatinine are normal; K⁺ is 3.0 mEq/L. What is the most likely etiology of her refractory hypertension?

Renovascular hypertension from bilateral fibromuscular dysplasia, which can lead to 2° hyperaldosteronism, severe hypertension, and hypokalemia.

Comprises 5% of cases of hypertension.

SYMPTOMS/EXAM

Suspect a 2° cause of hypertension if:

- Age at onset is < 30 or > 50 years.
- Rapid onset of severe hypertension occurs in < 3–5 years.
- Hypertension is refractory to multiple medications.
- Spontaneous hypokalemia is seen.

DIFFERENTIAL

- **Renal:** Renovascular disease, renal parenchymal disease, polycystic kidney disease, Liddle's syndrome, syndrome of apparent mineralocorticoid excess, hypercalcemia.
- **Endocrine:** Hyper- or hypothyroidism, 1° hyperaldosteronism, Cushing's syndrome, pheochromocytoma, congenital adrenal hyperplasia (see also the Endocrinology chapter).
- **Drugs:**
    - **Prescription:** Estrogen, cyclosporine, steroids.
    - **OTC:** Pseudoephedrine, NSAIDs.
    - **Other:** Smoking, ethanol, cocaine.
- **Neurogenic:** ↑ ICP, spinal cord section.
- **Miscellaneous:** Aortic coarctation, obstructive sleep apnea, polycythemia vera.

DIAGNOSIS

- Diagnosed by the history, including medications and illicit substance use, and physical exam.
- See Table 12.13.

TABLE 12.13. **Tests for the Evaluation of 2° Hypertension**

Basic Tests	Special Screening Studies
TSH Hematocrit to screen for polycythemia vera Serum K⁺ ($\downarrow$ K⁺ suggests 1° aldosteronism) Serum creatinine and/or BUN for renal failure CXR to look for coarctation	**Renovascular disease:** ACEI radionuclide scan, renal duplex Doppler flow studies, or CT or MRI angiography. **Pheochromocytoma:** 24-hour urine assay for creatinine, metanephrines, and catecholamines, or plasma-free metanephrines and normetanephrines. **Cushing's syndrome:** Overnight dexamethasone suppression test or 24-hour urine cortisol and creatinine. **1° aldosteronism:** Plasma aldosterone-renin activity ratio.

TREATMENT

- Treat the underlying cause.
- See the Ambulatory Medicine chapter for a summary of antihypertensive medications.
- See the Hospital Medicine chapter for details on the treatment of hypertensive emergency.

RENOVASCULAR HYPERTENSION

$\downarrow$ renal blood flow causes $\uparrow$ renin and aldosterone levels, eventually resulting in hypertension (see Table 12.14). Fibromuscular dysplasia often occurs in younger patients, while atherosclerosis is the cause in older patients and in those with other atherosclerotic disease.

SYMPTOMS/EXAM

Clinical features include the following:

- Age at onset < 30 or > 50 years.
- Rapid onset in < 3–5 years.
- Severe hypertension despite an appropriate three-drug regimen, especially in patients with diffuse atherosclerotic disease.
- Flash pulmonary edema.
- Hypokalemia.
- Continuous abdominal bruit.
- $\uparrow$ in serum creatinine after initiation of ACEI treatment.

TABLE 12.14. **Causes of Renovascular Hypertension**

	Atherosclerosis (More Common)	Fibromuscular Dysplasia
Affected gender	Men and women	Women
Age	> 50	15–40
Total occlusion	Common	Rare
Ischemic atrophy	Common	Rare
Angioplasty	Less amenable	Highly amenable
Cure rate	Poor	Good

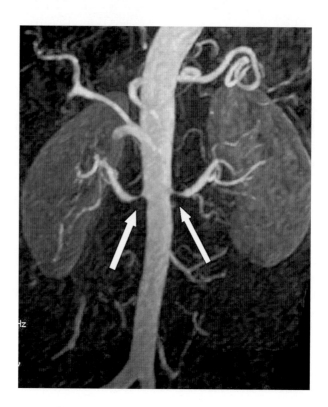

FIGURE 12.8. **Renal artery stenosis.** Coronal maximum-intensity projection (MIP) image from an MRA shows severe bilateral ostial narrowing of the renal arteries (arrows). (Reproduced with permission from Brunicardi FC et al. *Schwartz's Principles of Surgery,* 9th ed. New York: McGraw-Hill, 2010, Fig. 23-47.)

DIAGNOSIS

Imaging (duplex ultrasonography, MRA, CT angiography, angiography) reveals > 75% stenosis (see Figure 12.8). Sensitivity and specificity are operator dependent.

TREATMENT

- **Medical therapy:** Control cardiovascular risk factors; give antihypertensive medications. Revascularization is helpful only for hemodynamically significant stenosis.
- **Percutaneous transluminal angioplasty (PTA):** Effective for fibromuscular dysplasia.
- **PTA/stent:** May be effective for atherosclerotic patients.
- **Surgical intervention:** Benefit is unclear.

Chronic Kidney Disease (CKD)

Permanent loss of renal function or renal injury (albuminuria) of > 3 months' duration. **End-stage renal disease** is defined as permanent loss of renal function that requires renal replacement therapy; GFR is < 15 mL/min.

TREATMENT

- **Proteinuria** is the most important predictor of progression of renal disease.
- **ACEIs/ARBs are the drugs of choice.**

- **Hypertension:** Target BP < 130/80 mm Hg.
  - **First-line agents: ACEIs.**
  - **Second-line agents:** Diuretics (↑ Na⁺ retention in CKD patients).
- **Lipids:** Target LDL < 100 mg/dL.
- **Nutrition:** Protein restriction is controversial.

COMPLICATIONS

- **Anemia:**
  - Erythropoietin injections if hemoglobin is < 10 g/dL; a target hemoglobin of > 13 g/dL is associated with higher mortality.
  - Replete iron stores if ferritin is < 100 ng/mL or transferrin saturation (T_{sat}) is < 20% (IV iron can be used in hemodialysis patients).
- **Renal osteodystrophy** (see Figure 12.9): Phosphate control is typically initiated with a calcium-based phosphate binder ($CaCO_3$ or calcium acetate). 1,25-OH vitamin D (calcitriol) may be used to control PTH.
- **Hyperkalemia:** Dietary restriction, diuretics.
- **Acidosis:** $NaHCO_3$ supplementation to prevent ⊖ bone balance.
- **Pericarditis (can present as a rub, chest pain, or ECG abnormalities):** Initiate dialysis or ↑ dialysis dose.

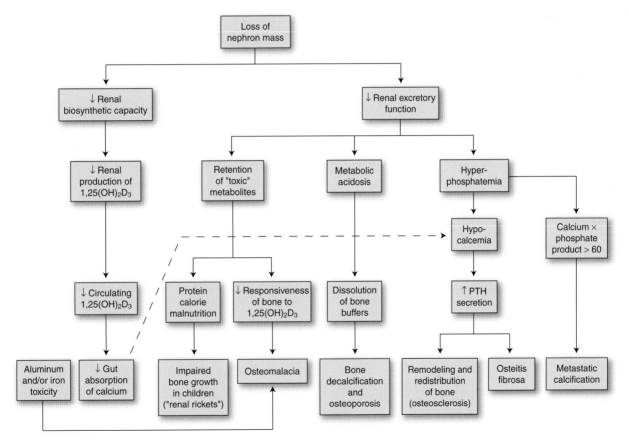

FIGURE 12.9. **Pathogenesis of bone disease in chronic kidney disease.** (Reproduced with permission from Wilson JD et al. *Harrison's Principles of Internal Medicine,* 12th ed. New York: McGraw-Hill, 1991.)

- **Dialysis-related problems:**
  - **Vascular catheter–related infections:**
    - *S aureus* is the most likely cause, followed by coagulase-$\ominus$ *Staphylococcus*.
    - Treat empirically with broad-spectrum antibiotics such as a third- or fourth-generation IV cephalosporin; add coverage for MRSA in the setting of high local prevalence.
    - Remove the catheter in the presence of a fungal infection, sepsis, endocarditis, or persistent bacteremia.
  - **Peritoneal catheter–associated peritonitis:**
    - *S aureus*, *S epidermidis*, and enteric gram-$\ominus$ rods are the dominant organisms.
    - Look for a cloudy appearance to peritoneal fluid, fever, or abdominal pain.
    - Diagnose with Gram stain (> 100 WBCs in peritoneal fluid) and culture of peritoneal fluid.
    - Treat with antibiotic infusion into the peritoneum. For severe cases, add IV antibiotics +/– catheter removal.
    - If culture grows fungus, anaerobes, or multiple organisms, suspect 2° peritonitis due to perforated abdominal viscus.

Genetic Disorders and Congenital Diseases of the Kidney

A 20-year-old man presents to an acute care clinic with severe arm and leg cramping of one week's duration. A review of systems reveals profound fatigue, chronic polyuria, and increasing nocturia. His BP is 105/65 mm Hg. He has tetany on exam, and his labs are notable for K^+ 2.9 mEq/L, Mg^{2+} 1.5 mg/dL, and metabolic alkalosis. His urine chloride concentration is normal. What is the most likely diagnosis?

Gitelman's syndrome.

Table 12.15 outlines genetic defects related to electrolyte balance. Table 12.16 presents the relationship of various genetic disorders to congenital diseases.

TABLE 12.15. Genetic Defects in Electrolyte Balance

SYNDROME	CLASSIC DEFECT	PRESENTATION
Bartter's syndrome	A defect in NaCl reabsorption in the thick ascending loop of Henle **(like furosemide).**	Renal salt wasting. Classically presents in childhood; a typical presentation would be a two-year-old child with persistently low potassium, an ↑ HCO_3^-, and normal serum magnesium without diuretic use. Normal/↓ BP.
Gitelman's syndrome	Defective Na^+/Cl^- cotransporter in the distal tubule **(like HCTZ).**	Renal salt wasting. A typical presentation would be an adult with persistently low potassium, an ↑ HCO_3^-, and ↓↓ magnesium who presents with cramps and tetany (from low potassium and magnesium). Normal/↓ BP.
Liddle's syndrome	↑ epithelial Na^+ channel activity in the collecting tubule.	**Renal salt retention.** Typified by an adult with persistently low potassium, an ↑ HCO_3^-, and **hypertension.** ↓ serum aldosterone levels.

TABLE 12.16. Genetic Disorders and Congenital Diseases of the Kidney

DISEASE	DEFECT	PRESENTATION	DIAGNOSIS	NOTES
Alport's syndrome	Type IV collagen of the GBM, cochlea, and lens.	**Hematuria,** nephritic-range proteinuria, progressive CKD. Sensorineural deafness, ocular defects.	Renal biopsy reveals a thickened GBM with splitting and splintering of the lamina densa.	Renal transplantation.
Autosomal dominant polycystic kidney disease (ADPKD)	PKD1 or PKD2 mutations.	Massive kidney enlargement due to multiple cyst formation; back/flank pain, kidney stones, hematuria. Hypertension; mitral valve prolapse; polycystic liver disease. Intracranial aneurysms (familial clustering).	Family history of ADPKD. The diagnosis depends on patient age, genotype, and the number of cysts on renal ultrasound.	ACEIs or ARBs for hypertension. Renal transplantation for ESRD.
Medullary sponge kidney	Collecting duct malformation leading to diffuse medullary cyst formation.	Asymptomatic or presents with hematuria, kidney stones, UTIs.	IVP. Retention of contrast media in the collecting ducts of the medulla, leading to a "bouquet of flowers" appearance. Ultrasound or CT may also be used (medullary nephro-calcinosis).	Benign clinical course.

NOTES

CHAPTER 13

Neurology

Miten Vasa, MD
Joey English, MD, PhD
S. Andrew Josephson, MD

Neurologic History and Exam

BASIC EXAM

The most important part of the workup of any neurologic disorder—and a critical element of any attempt to localize a lesion—is the history and physical exam. The history should focus on the following factors:

- Symptom onset:
  - **Acute onset (seconds to minutes):** Most likely caused by a **vascular event** (eg, stroke), a **seizure**, or a complicated **migraine.**
  - **Subacute onset (hours to days):** More likely caused by **infectious processes, inflammatory diseases,** or **autoimmune disorders** (eg, MS).
  - **Insidious onset (months to years):** More likely caused by slowly growing **structural lesions** (eg, tumors) or **neurodegenerative disorders.**
- **Age/gender:** In young patients, especially women, consider **autoimmune processes.** Neurodegenerative illnesses are more common in older patients.
- **Location of symptoms:** Classic symptoms of common neurologic disease processes by location are as follows:
  - **Myopathies (muscle): Symmetric proximal weakness** of all extremities.
  - **Neuromuscular junction: Fluctuating weakness** (eyes, proximal extremities) throughout the course of the day.
  - **Polyneuropathy: Symmetric distal sensory loss and weakness of all extremities,** often with ↓ or absent reflexes in affected areas.
  - **Myelopathy (spinal cord): Symmetric weakness of both legs (or both arms and both legs), sparing the face, along with bowel and bladder involvement.**
  - **Brainstem: Cranial nerve deficits, double vision, dysarthria, dysphagia, nystagmus.**
  - **Visual pathway:** Distinguishing **monocular from binocular defects** is key to localization between the cerebral hemisphere and eyes (see Figure 13.1).

COMA EXAM

The term *coma* refers to a condition in which patients are unresponsive, show no purposeful movement, and do not open their eyes to painful stimuli. It requires the impairment of either **both cerebral hemispheres** or the reticular activating system of the **brainstem.** It is generally caused by one of three processes:

- A **structural** problem affecting the **brainstem** (eg, mass effect with herniation, stroke).
- An **electrical** problem (ongoing seizure activity even if not clinically apparent—eg, nonconvulsive status epilepticus).
- A **metabolic** process (eg, anoxic brain injury, hepatic encephalopathy, severe electrolyte disturbances, infection).

SYMPTOMS/EXAM

- Evaluate brainstem function by checking cranial nerves (ie, pupillary response to light; extraocular movements of the eyes to either turning the head side to side ["doll's eyes"] or placing cold water in one ear) as well as corneal reflexes, gag reflex, cough reflex, and spontaneous respirations.

KEY FACT

In a comatose patient, the presence of "doll's eyes" or corneal reflexes means that brainstem function is still intact.

KEY FACT

Patients are comatose if they are "eyes closed and unresponsive."

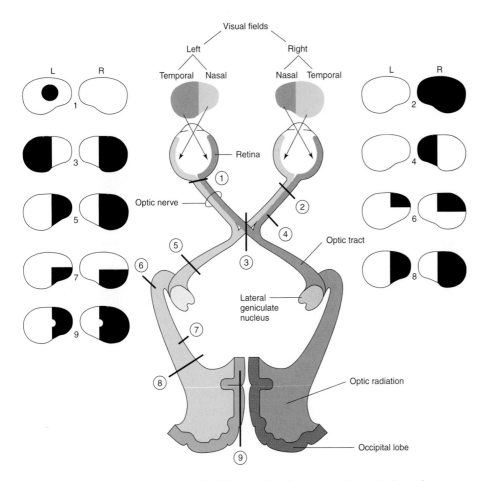

FIGURE 13.1.   Common visual field defects and their anatomic bases. 1. Central scotoma caused by inflammation of the optic disk (optic neuritis) or optic nerve (retrobulbar neuritis). 2. **Total blindness of the right eye** from a complete lesion of the right optic nerve. 3. **Bitemporal hemianopia** caused by pressure exerted on the optic chiasm by a pituitary tumor. 4. **Right nasal hemianopia** caused by a perichiasmal lesion (eg, calcified internal carotid artery). 5. **Right homonymous hemianopia** from a lesion of the left optic tract. 6. **Right homonymous superior quadrantanopia** caused by partial involvement of the optic radiation by a lesion in the left temporal lobe (Meyer's loop). 7. **Right homonymous inferior quadrantanopia** caused by partial involvement of the optic radiation by a lesion in the left parietal lobe. 8 and 9. **Right homonymous hemianopia** from a complete lesion of the left optic radiation with or without macular sparing resulting from a lesion such as a posterior cerebral artery occlusion.
(Reproduced with permission from Simon RP et al. *Clinical Neurology,* 7th ed. New York: McGraw-Hill, 2009, Fig. 4-7.)

- **Abnormal posturing** (see Figure 13.2) indicates large increases in ICP and/or impending herniation from severe brain injury, characterized by involuntary flexion or extension of the arms and legs.
- Motor response to central and peripheral pain is also critical, as asymmetric responses suggest a focal lesion.
- Patients with coma caused by a structural problem generally have **abnormal brainstem reflexes,** as their coma is caused by direct compression of the brainstem.
- Patients with metabolic or electrical coma typically have intact brainstem reflexes.

DIAGNOSIS/TREATMENT

- Focus on correctable problems, including easily detectable metabolic disorders (eg, hypoglycemia, drug overdose, electrolyte abnormalities, ure-

KEY FACT

Examination of brainstem reflexes differentiates the anatomic location of coma. If brainstem reflexes are abnormal, the lesion is in the brainstem.

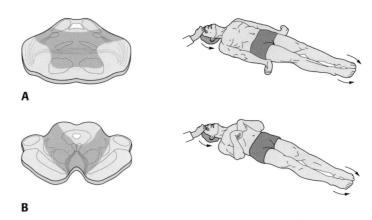

A

B

FIGURE 13.2. Decerebrate and decorticate postures. (A) Upper pontine damage. Damage to the lower midbrain and upper pons causes **decerebrate** posturing in which the lower extremities are extended with the toes pointed inward and the upper extremities are extended with the fingers flexed and the forearms pronated. The neck and head are extended. **(B) Upper midbrain damage.** Damage to the upper midbrain may cause **decorticate** posturing in which the upper limbs are flexed, the lower limbs are extended with the toes pointed slightly inward, and the head is extended. The prognosis is poor in both, although upper pontine damage carries a poorer prognosis than upper midbrain damage. (Reproduced with permission from Barrett KE et al. *Ganong's Review of Medical Physiology,* 23rd ed. New York: McGraw-Hill, 2010, Fig. 16-8.)

mia, liver failure) and structural problems (eg, subdural hematoma). Patients need urgent imaging of the brain as well as basic laboratory workup.
- Patients with unexplained coma should also have an EEG to rule out non-convulsive status epilepticus as well as CSF studies to rule out infectious causes of encephalopathy.

Neurodiagnostic Testing

LUMBAR PUNCTURE (LP)

- Patients with papilledema, focal neurologic signs, or immunosuppression should have imaging prior to LP to evaluate for mass effect and herniation risk. Imaging of the spine should precede LP in patients with spinal cord signs or symptoms.
- Coagulopathy is a contraindication to LP.

ELECTROENCEPHALOGRAPHY (EEG)

A tool for the investigation of seizure disorders, unexplained coma, metabolic encephalopathies, viral encephalitis, prion diseases, anoxic brain injury, and sleep disorders. Conditions with notable EEG findings include the following:

- **Metabolic encephalopathy:** Hepatic encephalopathy is the classic metabolic coma. The EEG typically shows generalized periodic triphasic waves.

- **HSV encephalitis:** The classic EEG finding consists of periodic lateralizing epileptiform discharges (PLEDs) originating over one or both temporal lobes.
- **Subacute sclerosing panencephalitis:** EEG typically shows a flat background punctuated by periodic generalized large-amplitude slow-wave discharges.
- **Prion disease:** EEGs in patients with Creutzfeldt-Jakob disease show periodic generalized sharp waves.

BRAIN IMAGING

- **Computed tomography (CT):** CT imaging of the brain is inferior to MRI for most studies but is the imaging study of choice for investigating acute hemorrhage (eg, SAH, epidural hematoma) and bone pathology (eg, skull or vertebral fractures).
- **Magnetic resonance imaging (MRI):** The best imaging modality for most diseases of the brain and spinal cord, including neoplastic, vascular, demyelinating, infectious, and structural diseases (eg, spondylosis of the spine).
- **Cerebral angiography:** The gold standard for investigating vascular abnormalities of the CNS, including stenosis, aneurysms, AVMs, and cerebral vasculitis. **Venography** is the gold standard for diagnosing venous sinus thrombosis.

ELECTROMYOGRAPHY/NERVE CONDUCTION STUDIES (EMG/NCS)

- **EMGs:** Examine spontaneous and voluntary muscle activity by using a needle electrode placed directly into the muscle. Useful for studying and differentiating radiculopathies (spinal root injuries), motor neuron disease, neuropathies, neuromuscular junction diseases, and myopathies.
- **NCS:** Obtained by stimulating peripheral nerves and recording either sensory or motor responses along the course of the nerve.

EVOKED POTENTIALS (EPs)

Obtained by measuring the time course of a specific CNS response to a given stimulus.

- **Visual EPs:** Generated by recording cortical response (using EEG electrodes) elicited by a visual stimulus. A delay in response suggests that the conduction velocity along the visual pathway is slow, often a sign of demyelination in the optic nerves (eg, in **MS**).
- **Brainstem and somatosensory EPs:** Useful for evaluating potential demyelinating lesions of the brainstem and dorsal columns of the spinal cord. Often used to obtain supportive evidence of CNS demyelination and can be helpful prognostically in hypoxic-ischemic encephalopathy.
- **Motor EPs:** Used for intraoperative monitoring during neurosurgical procedures involving the spinal cord or brainstem.

KEY FACT

The yield of electroencephalography in a patient with new-onset seizure is low, with only ~ 30% sensitivity. Sleep-deprived electroencephalography may have ↑ sensitivity but is seldom performed.

KEY FACT

Head CT detects ~ 95% of cases of acute intracranial hemorrhage (ICH) and is the imaging modality of choice to rapidly rule out intracranial bleed. For most other intracranial processes, MRI is superior to CT.

KEY FACT

Board exam questions may give you a clue to Guillain-Barré syndrome or chronic inflammatory demyelinating polyneuropathy by providing evidence of demyelination on nerve conduction studies.

KEY FACT

Evoked potentials are typically performed in patients being evaluated for demyelinating diseases such as MS or as a prognostic tool in the evaluation of a comatose patient.

Headache

Table 13.1 lists alarm symptoms in patients with headache, which should prompt further investigation (eg, imaging, basic labs, LP):

DIFFERENTIAL

See Table 13.1 and the entries below.

MIGRAINE HEADACHE

A 25-year-old woman presents with episodic left-sided headaches that have occurred a few times a month for the past year. The headaches usually resolve over 1–2 days and do not respond to decongestants, antihistamines, or acetaminophen, but they worsen with movement and improve when the patient rests in a quiet, dark room. Her mother has a history of similar headaches. Exam reveals facial tenderness on palpation. What is the most likely diagnosis?

Migraine without aura. Typical features include worsening of symptoms with movement, limitation of activities, photophobia, and phonophobia. Cluster headaches last < 2 hours and occur more often in men.

Roughly 10–20% of the U.S. population have experienced migraine headaches, with 80% of cases beginning before age 30. Most patients are **young women** (the female-to-male ratio is 3:1). **Ninety percent of patients have a strong family history.**

TABLE 13.1. Alarm Features in Patients with Headache

ALARM FEATURE	POTENTIAL URGENT DIAGNOSES
Abrupt-onset, severe headache	Intracranial bleed.
Visual complaints	Malignancy, infection, bleed, giant cell arteritis.
Fever	Meningitis, encephalitis, brain abscess.
Jaw claudication	Giant cell arteritis.
Worsening with Valsalva or cough	↑ ICP from malignancy or bleed.
Papilledema	↑ ICP from malignancy or bleed; pseudotumor cerebri.
History of malignancy	Brain metastasis.
Focal neurologic deficit or seizure	Bleed, malignancy, CNS infection.
Scalp tenderness	Zoster.
Onset of headache after age 40–50	Malignancy, CNS infection.

SYMPTOMS

- **Benign, recurrent headaches** that classically produce **unilateral pulsating pain** associated with symptoms such as **photophobia**, phonophobia, anorexia, **nausea**, and vomiting.
- Episodes typically last 4–72 hours, and patients often report improvement with resting in a **dark, quiet room.**
- Subtypes are as follows:
  - **Classic migraine (migraine with aura):** Occurs in 20% of patients. Neurologic symptoms occur before or during the headache. The most common auras are **visual**, including "fortification spectra" and scotomas (blind spots).
  - **Common migraine:** Most migraine patients do not have preceding auras.
  - **Migraine variants:** Named for associated focal neurologic deficits and/or vascular territories; include hemiplegic migraine, basilar migraine (involves brainstem symptoms such as ataxia, vertigo, and slurred speech), and ophthalmoplegic migraine (unilateral CN III palsy and pupillary abnormality).

EXAM

- Patients with classic and common migraines have **normal neurologic exams.**
- In patients with headache and focal neurologic deficits, a migraine variant remains a diagnosis of exclusion. These patients require workup for other causes of headache and focal deficits (eg, vascular events, infection, intracranial mass).

DIAGNOSIS

Based on the history, with a focus on the exact character of the headaches as well as the presence of a strong family history.

TREATMENT

- Management is divided into two categories: **abortive therapy** for the migraine itself (taken only at the time of the migraine) and **prophylactic therapy** for preventing future attacks (taken daily).
- **Prophylactic therapy** is given only to patients with frequent severe migraines (> 1 per week) and includes the following:
  - **Medications:** TCAs (eg, amitriptyline), β-blockers (eg, propranolol), calcium channel blockers (CCBs, eg, verapamil), and **antiseizure medications** (eg, valproic acid, topiramate).
  - **Behavioral measures:** Proper sleep hygiene and avoiding food triggers (eg, tyramine, nitrates, dairy products, xanthines).
  - **Menstrual migraine prophylaxis:** Low-dose estrogen therapy during menstruation, continuous estrogen therapy that is ↑ during menstruation, or oral magnesium.
- **Abortive therapy** includes the following:
  - **Triptans:** $5\text{-}HT_1$ serotonin receptor agonists (eg, sumatriptan, frovatriptan, eletriptan, naratriptan, almotriptan, rizatriptan, zolmitriptan) produce vasoconstriction. They **should not be used** in patients with vascular disease (eg, CAD, peripheral vascular disease) or in pregnant women.
  - **Ergotamines:** Also to be avoided in patients with vascular disease and in pregnant women.

MNEMONIC

Symptoms of migraines—

POUND

Pulsating
Oras (duration of 4–72 hours; *oras* in Spanish)
Unilateral
Nausea
Disabling

If four of five of the criteria are met, migraine is almost certainly the diagnosis.

KEY FACT

The typical migraine patient is a woman < 30 years of age with a unilateral headache associated with nausea or photophobia, a strong family history of migraines, a normal neurologic exam, and **no** preceding aura.

KEY FACT

Tension headache is usually a nonthrobbing, bilateral head pain that is generally not associated with nausea, vomiting, or prodromal visual disturbances.

■ **Other abortive agents:**

■ **Acetaminophen/butalbital/caffeine** (Fioricet): Butalbital is a barbiturate and has addictive properties.

■ **Isometheptene/dichloralphenazone/acetaminophen** (Midrin): Avoid in patients taking MAOIs.

■ **Antiemetics:** Prochlorperazine, promethazine.

CLUSTER HEADACHE

A 40-year-old man presents with a severe, throbbing left retro-orbital headache associated with left-sided rhinorrhea and ptosis. The headaches started three weeks ago and have occurred at 7 A.M. and 7 P.M. daily, lasting 30–60 minutes each. The patient had similar symptoms a year ago that lasted for six weeks. His vitals signs, funduscopic exam, and neurologic exam are normal. MRI of the brain and cervical spine are normal, as is his LP. What is the most likely diagnosis, and how should he be treated?

This patient has episodic cluster headache. Acute treatments to abort the attack include triptans, ergots, and high-flow O_2. Prednisone, anticonvulsants, or CCBs may also be indicated as prophylactic treatments for patients with frequent episodes.

Classically occurs in **young men** 20–40 years of age (the male-to-female ratio is 5:1). A family history of similar headaches is uncommon.

SYMPTOMS

■ The cardinal feature is **periodicity.** Headaches occur **many times daily** at **distinct times** over several weeks; onset with sleep is especially characteristic.

■ Immobility ↑ cluster headache pain (vs. migraines, in which symptoms are exacerbated by ↑ movement).

■ Clusters spontaneously remit for months to years before recurring, typically at the same time of year as previous attacks. **Alcohol** is a classic trigger.

■ Cluster headaches do not have auras. A typical attack is characterized by abrupt-onset, severe **unilateral periorbital pain** with associated **ipsilateral autonomic symptoms** (tearing of the eye and nares; rarely, Horner's). Headaches typically last 30–120 minutes.

EXAM

■ Patients are restless and agitated and often pace the room (vs. migraine patients).

■ Look for tearing, nasal discharge, and/or ptosis (eg, **Horner's**) ipsilateral to the location of eye pain.

DIFFERENTIAL

Clues to distinguish cluster headaches from migraines are shown in Table 13.2.

TABLE 13.2.   Cluster Headache vs. Migraine

	MIGRAINE	CLUSTER HEADACHE
Typical patient	Young woman	Young man
Triggered by alcohol	No	Yes
Periodicity	No	Yes
Aura	Yes (with classic form, ~ 20%)	No
Rhinorrhea, congestion	No	Yes
Response to O_2	No	Yes

TREATMENT

- As with migraines, treatment includes abortive and prophylactic therapies.
- **Prophylactic medications:**
  - Started once cluster headaches begin, but should not be used during remissions given that months to years may elapse between clusters.
  - Include **verapamil** (first-line prophylactic treatment for cluster headache), **prednisone** (a taper of oral steroids is often used at the beginning of a cluster), lithium, valproate, and methysergide.
- **Abortive therapy** includes the following:
  - O_2 **inhalation:** Give 5–10 L/min for 10–15 minutes.
  - **Intranasal lidocaine ointment:** Produces a block of the sphenopalatine ganglion and aborts the headache.
  - **Triptans:** Also useful for acute attacks.

TRIGEMINAL NEURALGIA (TIC DOULOUREUX)

A 70-year-old woman presents with a two-month history of severe, paroxysmal, stabbing right lower jaw pain that lasts for only a few seconds and is precipitated by eating, chewing, or brushing her teeth or even by a cold breeze. On exam, pain is elicited with light touch on the right lower gums, teeth, and jaw. Radiographs of the face and brain MRI are normal, as is a dentist's evaluation, and ESR is normal as well. What is the diagnosis and the most appropriate management course for this patient?

Trigeminal neuralgia; carbamazepine is the treatment of choice. Baclofen and other anticonvulsants can be useful as well.

A **unilateral** facial pain syndrome affecting middle-aged and elderly patients. Most commonly occurs in the sixth decade. Onset in young patients should raise suspicion for an underlying disorder (eg, MS, brainstem neoplasm).

KEY FACT

Suspect trigeminal neuralgia in a 50-year-old man with attacks of severe, unilateral electrical jaw pain triggered by light touch or shaving.

KEY FACT

In a patient with trigeminal neuralgia who is < 40 years of age or who has any neurologic deficits (including sensory deficits), brain imaging is warranted to exclude a mass lesion.

Symptoms

- Characterized by abrupt-onset, short-duration (seconds-long) episodes of severe, **unilateral, lancinating electrical pain,** typically **radiating along the jaw** in the distribution of the second and third divisions of CN V (the trigeminal nerve).
- Attacks are often **triggered by sensory stimuli** to the face (eg, touch, wind, shaving, chewing).

Exam

Neurologic exam is **normal.** Any abnormalities on exam, including sensory loss of the face in the distribution of the pain, suggests an alternative diagnosis (eg, mass lesions, infiltrative disease) and mandates further evaluation (eg, imaging, LP).

Treatment

Carbamazepine is first-line therapy. Alternatives include oxcarbazepine, valproate, phenytoin, baclofen, gabapentin, and benzodiazepines.

IDIOPATHIC INTRACRANIAL HYPERTENSION (PSEUDOTUMOR CEREBRI)

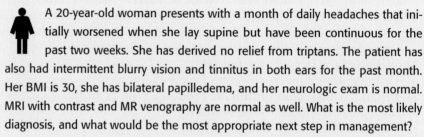

A 20-year-old woman presents with a month of daily headaches that initially worsened when she lay supine but have been continuous for the past two weeks. She has derived no relief from triptans. The patient has also had intermittent blurry vision and tinnitus in both ears for the past month. Her BMI is 30, she has bilateral papilledema, and her neurologic exam is normal. MRI with contrast and MR venography are normal as well. What is the most likely diagnosis, and what would be the most appropriate next step in management?

Pseudotumor cerebri, which typically affects obese young women, is the likely diagnosis. Several symptoms point to ↑ ICP, and normal imaging has excluded a mass lesion, hydrocephalus, or venous sinus thrombosis. An LP is needed to confirm ↑ CSF pressure, and an urgent ophthalmologic evaluation is needed, as is visual field monitoring. If the LP confirms the diagnosis, acetazolamide can be started to ↓ CSF production.

A headache syndrome related to chronically ↑ ICP. Classically seen in **young, obese women.** Associations have been noted with medications such as tetracycline derivatives, OCPs, steroids, and vitamin A as well as with disorders such as SLE, Behçet's syndrome, and uremia.

Symptoms

- Patients usually note a progressive **global headache** that intensifies when they lie flat, often worsening at night and **upon awakening.**
- Exacerbated by maneuvers that ↑ ICP (eg, Valsalva, cough, sneeze).
- ↑ ICP can produce **transient visual obscurations** (blurring or blackout of vision in either or both eyes for seconds), double vision from CN VI palsies, and/or progressive loss of peripheral vision. Total blindness can result.

Exam

Papilledema is the key finding (see Figure 13.3). Patients may also have ↓ visual acuity and/or **loss of peripheral vision.** Diplopia from CN VI palsies may result from ↑ ICP.

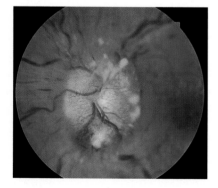

FIGURE 13.3. Papilledema. This obese young women with pseudotumor cerebri was misdiagnosed as a migraineur until funduscopy showed optic disk elevation, hemorrhages, and cotton-wool spots. (Reproduced with permission from Fauci AS et al. *Harrison's Principles of Internal Medicine,* 17th ed. New York: McGraw-Hill, 2008, Fig. 29-12.)

TABLE 13.3. Classic Case Presentations of Headache Syndromes

MIGRAINE	CLUSTER HEADACHE	TRIGEMINAL NEURALGIA	PSEUDOTUMOR CEREBRI
A 25-year-old woman resting uncomfortably in a dark, quiet room complains of unilateral head pain associated with nausea and photophobia. The headache was preceded by an aura of flashing colored lights.	A 32-year-old man pacing the ER has severe unilateral periorbital pain associated with tearing of the ipsilateral eye and nose. He has had three attacks per day over the past week, each occurring at the exact same time every day and lasting 20–40 minutes each. The headache began after the patient drank alcohol at a party.	A 58-year-old woman presents with attacks of brief, unilateral, severe electrical sensations radiating along the jaw.	A 22-year-old obese woman presents with a two-month history of progressive headaches. The headaches were initially associated with intermittent blurry vision but are now accompanied by a progressive ↓ in visual acuity.

DIFFERENTIAL

Table 13.3 outlines the presentation of various headache syndromes.

DIAGNOSIS

- Patients with headache and papilledema should first undergo **brain imaging,** preferably with MRI. In patients with pseudotumor, MRI is often normal.
- **MR venography** can exclude venous sinus thrombosis.
- **LP** should be performed with the patient in the lateral decubitus position, with pressure measured after the patient's legs are extended and relaxed. LP reveals an **opening pressure of > 200 mm H$_2$O,** normal protein and glucose, and no cells.

TREATMENT

- Based on lowering ICP. **Acetazolamide,** a carbonic anhydrase inhibitor that ↓ CSF production and ICP, is first-line therapy. Furosemide can also be used.
- Serial LPs, optic nerve fenestration, and permanent shunting of CSF are used for refractory cases.
- **Weight loss** is an important component of management in most patients.
- Serial **ophthalmologic evaluation** is mandatory for these patients, as visual loss can be severe and permanent.

MEDICATION REBOUND HEADACHE

- **Overuse of analgesic medications** (eg, acetaminophen, NSAIDs, butalbital/ASA/caffeine, isometheptene/dichloralphenazone, narcotics, triptans, ergotamines, barbiturates) for ≥ 2 days per week for headache syndromes can paradoxically produce refractory chronic daily headaches.
- **Tx:** Prophylactic medications are ineffective until patients have been weaned off the offending analgesic medications. Often requires a slow taper of the analgesic to prevent withdrawal symptoms.

KEY FACT

The term *papilledema* signifies optic disk edema resulting from ↑ ICP.

KEY FACT

An obese young woman with normal brain imaging who has global headaches that worsen with lying supine or with Valsalva most likely has idiopathic intracranial hypertension. Funduscopy that reveals papilledema and an LP with elevated opening pressure are additional clues.

The risk of a patient with a TIA developing a stroke within the next few days is estimated by the ABCD-2 score:

Age ≥ 60: 1 point.
Blood pressure ≥ 140/90 mm Hg at initial evaluation: 1 point.
Clinical features of TIA (unilateral weakness, 2 points; speech disturbance, 1 point).
Duration of symptoms (10–59 minutes, 1 point; ≥ 60 minutes, 2 points).
Diabetes mellitus: 1 point.

KEY FACT

TIA patients with an ABCD-2 score of 4–5 have a 4–6% risk of stroke, and those with a score of 6–7 have an 8–11% risk of stroke, at 2–7 days. Consideration should be given to hospitalization to help expedite the workup of these patients.

KEY FACT

Hypertension is the single most important risk factor for ischemic stroke.

Cerebrovascular Disease

Approximately 85% of strokes are ischemic (due to occlusion of arterial flow), with the remaining 15% caused by hemorrhage either in or around the brain (due to rupture of cerebral arteries or veins).

- A **stroke** is characterized by acute-onset focal neurologic deficits due to disruption of blood flow (by either occlusion or rupture) to a given area of the brain. By traditional definition, the neurologic deficits last > 24 hours. The residual deficit is related to underlying infarction of the brain.
- A **transient ischemic attack (TIA)** is fundamentally similar to stroke, but by traditional definition the deficits resolve within 24 hours. (In the overwhelming majority of TIAs, the deficits actually resolve in < 1 hour.) In TIAs, a region of the brain is briefly ischemic, but flow is restored before permanent infarction occurs.

ISCHEMIC STROKE

 A 70-year-old man with hypertension and hyperlipidemia was taken to the ER after he developed right upper extremity weakness and numbness. After going to bed at 10 P.M. the previous night, the patient awoke with these symptoms at 7 A.M. and arrived in the ER at 8 A.M. His BP is 170/89 mm Hg, and exam reveals left-sided neglect and a hemisensory deficit, a mild left central facial palsy, and left upper and lower extremity weakness. His CBC, coagulation studies, chemistry, and head CT are all normal. What is the most appropriate next step in this patient's management?

ASA therapy for acute ischemic stroke of the right MCA territory. With an unknown time of onset, this patient is not eligible for tPA, which is indicated only if therapy is started within four and one-half hours of symptom onset or when the patient was last known to be well. Early administration of ASA results in a modest ↓ in the risk of recurrent stroke in the short term and a slightly ↓ incidence of death and disability in the long term.

Caused by occlusion of arterial blood flow to the brain, which in turn is caused by either **extracranial embolism** of clot to the large intracranial vessels or **progressive thrombosis** of small intracranial arterioles. The nature of the focal neurologic deficits caused by strokes can first be divided into anterior or

TABLE 13.4. Strokes Affecting the Anterior Circulation

AFFECTED AREA	SIGNS/SYMPTOMS
Ophthalmic artery	Ipsilateral monocular vision loss (amaurosis fugax).
ACA	Contralateral leg weakness and sensory loss.
MCA	**Dominant hemisphere: Aphasia;** contralateral face/arm weakness and sensory loss; neglect; homonymous hemianopia. **Nondominant hemisphere:** Contralateral face/arm weakness and sensory loss; neglect; homonymous hemianopia.

posterior circulation symptoms (small vessel strokes are covered later in this section):

- **Anterior circulation** (see Table 13.4): Arise from the **internal carotid artery (ICA)** and include the **ophthalmic artery**, the **anterior cerebral artery (ACA)**, and the **middle cerebral artery (MCA)** (see Figure 13.4).
- **Posterior circulation** (see Table 13.5).

Embolic Stroke

A 20-year-old woman presents to the ER 10 hours after sudden onset of neck pain followed by vertigo, ataxia, slurred speech, and difficulty swallowing. Exam reveals right ptosis, anisocoria of the right pupil smaller than the left, nystagmus, right-sided dysmetria, and ↓ pain and temperature sensation on the right side of her face and the left side of her body. Her head CT is normal. What is the most likely diagnosis and the most appropriate next step in the evaluation of this patient?

Suspect spontaneous carotid or vertebral artery dissection as the etiology of stroke in a young patient with unexplained stroke and neck pain. This patient's symptoms point to vertebral artery dissection with localization to the right lateral medulla and right cerebellum. MRA is a sensitive diagnostic test for vertebral artery dissection as a cause of stroke. Initial treatment is often anticoagulation with heparin or LMWH.

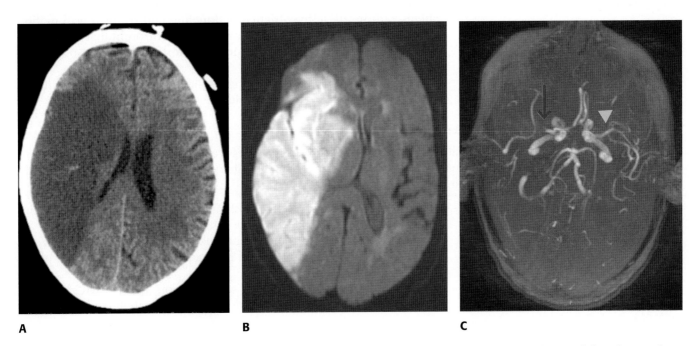

A   B   C

FIGURE 13.4.   Acute ischemic stroke. Acute left hemiparesis in a 62-year-old woman. **(A)** Noncontrast head CT with loss of gray and white matter differentiation and asymmetrically decreased size of the right lateral ventricle in a right MCA distribution (indicating mass effect). **(B)** Diffusion-weighted MRI with reduced diffusion in the same distribution, consistent with an acute infarct; **diffusion-weighted sequences are the most sensitive modality for diagnosing an acute ischemic infarct. (C)** MRA shows the cause: an abrupt occlusion of the proximal right MCA (arrow). Compare with the normal left MCA (arrowhead). (Reproduced with permission from USMLERx.com.)

TABLE 13.5.   Strokes Affecting the Posterior Circulation

AFFECTED AREA	SIGNS/SYMPTOMS
Posterior cerebral artery	Contralateral visual field deficits (homonymous hemianopia). Cortical blindness (Anton's syndrome) and paresthesias may also be seen.
Posterior inferior cerebellar artery (PICA)	Wallenberg's/lateral medullary syndrome[a]
Cerebellum	Vertigo, nystagmus, nausea, vomiting, ipsilateral incoordination.
Brainstem	**Basilar artery:** Oculomotor deficits and/or ataxia with "crossed" sensory/motor deficits of the face and body; stupor, coma. **Vertebral artery:** Lower cranial nerve deficits (dysphagia, dysarthria, tongue/palate deviation) and/or ataxia with crossed sensory deficits of the face and body, stupor, coma, and Wallenberg's syndrome.[a]

[a]Causes a constellation of vestibular symptoms (vertigo, diplopia, nystagmus, vomiting), ataxia, myoclonus, contralateral pain and temperature deficits from the body, ipsilateral pain and temperature deficits from the face, dysphagia, hoarseness, dysphonia, dysarthria, diminished gag reflex, and ipsilateral Horner's syndrome.

KEY FACT

Suspect cardiac emboli in a patient with ischemic strokes involving multiple vascular distributions.

KEY FACT

Think brainstem lesion if there are crossed symptoms such as a cranial nerve deficit with contralateral weakness or if vertigo, dysarthria, double vision, or ataxia is present.

Emboli most commonly arise from atherosclerotic plaques of the extracranial **ICA** or from the **heart**. Common sources include the following:

- **Atrial fibrillation (AF),** with clot arising in the left atrial appendage.
- **Valvular disease** (eg, endocarditis, prosthetic valves) is also associated with cardiogenic emboli.
- Patients with severe left ventricular dysfunction and regional wall motion abnormalities following MI can form **ventricular thrombi** that embolize.
- Severe atheromatous disease of the proximal **aortic arch** can also generate cerebrovascular emboli.
- **Paradoxical emboli** can arise from right-to-left shunting of venous thrombi and emboli across an atrial septal defect.

EXAM

Patients with embolic stroke need aggressive investigation of the potential embolic source to determine if specific intervention is warranted. Key points to direct workup are as follows:

- An embolic stroke involving the posterior circulation (cerebellum, brainstem, occipital lobes) is not caused by emboli from the carotid artery.
- **Amaurosis fugax** (acute transient monocular vision loss) is most commonly caused by cholesterol emboli from an atherosclerotic plaque of the **ipsilateral ICA** (see Figure 13.5).
- Embolic strokes involving the anterior circulation (ACA or MCA) can be 2° to either internal carotid emboli or cardiogenic emboli.

DIAGNOSIS/TREATMENT

See the discussion below.

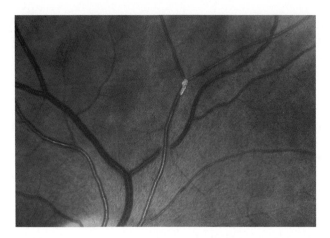

FIGURE 13.5. **Hollenhorst plaque lodged at the bifurcation of a retinal arteriole.** This finding proves that a patient is shedding emboli from the carotid artery, the great vessels, or the heart. (Reproduced with permission from Fauci AS et al. *Harrison's Principles of Internal Medicine,* 17th ed. New York: McGraw-Hill, 2008, Fig. 29-5.)

Thrombotic Stroke

A 60-year-old woman presents to the ER after awakening with vertigo, ataxia, and a headache. She has hypertension and stable angina and is on ASA, a statin, and metoprolol. On exam her BP is 168/90 mm Hg, and she has bidirectional nystagmus, gait ataxia, lethargy alternating with agitation, intractable hiccups, and dysmetria of the left upper and lower extremities. What is the most likely diagnosis?

Cerebellar infarction with classic symptoms of vertigo, ataxia, and headache along with developing signs of brainstem compression (intractable hiccups, altered mental status), indicating a need for more urgent intervention such as neurosurgical decompression.

Occurs when a small cerebral artery gradually occludes 2° to progressive local thrombosis. The classic vessels involved are the small penetrating terminal arterioles that supply the **brainstem** and the **deep structures of the cerebral hemispheres,** including the basal ganglia, thalami, and internal capsule. The internal capsule is of particular importance in that it contains the descending motor fibers. Occlusion of these small arterioles produces a discrete "**lacunar" infarct** of the small area of brain supplied by the terminal arteriole.

- **Lacunar infarcts:** Can have devastating effects despite their small size. The four classic "lacunar" strokes are as follows:
    - **Pure motor hemiparesis:** Presents with isolated weakness of the face, arm, and leg on one side of the body. Sensation is normal, and no "cortical signs" (eg, aphasia, visual field deficits) are present.
    - **Dysarthria–clumsy hand syndrome:** Essentially a variant of pure motor hemiparesis, with isolated slurred speech and unilateral hand weakness and incoordination.
    - **Ataxia hemiparesis:** Patients have mild weakness of the face, arm, and leg on one side associated with marked ataxia of the same side of the body.
    - **Pure sensory loss:** Patients have complete loss of sensation on one side of the body.

KEY FACT

Diffusion-weighted imaging (DWI) on MRI is the most sensitive modality for identifying acute ischemic strokes. Areas of restricted diffusion are bright on DWI sequences.

KEY FACT

The risk of brain herniation following an acute stroke is greatest in the first 24–72 hours, when cerebral edema peaks. In large MCA strokes, neurosurgical decompression may be indicated.

KEY FACT

In patients who survive the initial stroke, the leading causes of death are infection (UTI and aspiration pneumonia) and venous thromboembolism.

KEY FACT

In all patients with acute ischemic stroke, tPA should be considered if the stroke occurred within the past 3–4½ hours and there are no contraindications.

- **Other lacunar strokes:** The "named" brainstem strokes (eg, Wallenberg's; see Table 13.6) are typically caused by a small vessel lacunar stroke from thrombosis.

DIAGNOSIS

- **Imaging studies** are as follows:
  - **Brain:** A noncontrast head CT is the initial study of choice for acute stroke, primarily to evaluate for ICH. MRI is best for characterizing the location and size of ischemic strokes.
  - **Internal carotid:** Use Doppler ultrasound, CT angiography, or MRA of the extracranial carotid arteries to evaluate for significant (> 70%) ICA stenosis when an anterior circulation embolic stroke is suspected.
  - **Heart:** Transesophageal echocardiography (TEE) is superior to transthoracic echocardiography (TTE) for evaluating potential cardiac sources of emboli.
- **ECG:** The initial screening test for cardiac arrhythmias, especially AF or flutter.
- **Cardiac telemetry:** Monitoring patients on continuous cardiac telemetry for 24–48 hours can help detect paroxysmal AF.
- Patients < 50 years of age with unexplained embolic stroke should be evaluated for underlying hypercoagulable states (eg, antiphospholipid syndrome, antithrombin III, protein S and C deficiency, factor V Leiden mutation).

TREATMENT

- **Acute management of ischemic stroke** should include the following:
  - Serial neurologic exams to assess for deterioration and herniation.
  - Prevention of DVT/PE using prophylactic doses of LMWH.
  - Assessment of swallowing and measures to ↓ aspiration (eg, elevation of the head of bed; dietary modification to ↓ aspiration risk).
- Other medical therapy includes the following:
  - **tPA:** Only patients with acute ischemic stroke symptoms of < 3.0–4.5 hours' duration can receive IV thrombolysis with tPA. Other exclusions for tPA include coagulopathy (INR > 1.7), thrombocytopenia (platelets < 100,000), uncontrolled hypertension (systolic BP > 185 mm Hg), and prior ICH. The 1° risk of tPA treatment is ICH.
  - **Antiplatelet medications:** ASA is first line in the acute phase, but for 2° prevention, **clopidogrel and ASA/extended-release dipyridamole** are equally viable options.

TABLE 13.6. **Specific Brainstem Strokes**

NAME	LOCATION	SYMPTOMS
Wallenberg's syndrome	Lateral medulla	Ipsilateral loss of pain and temperature on the face. Contralateral loss of pain and temperature on the body. Ipsilateral Horner's, vertigo, slurred speech.
"Locked-in" syndrome	Pons	Intact mental status; quadriparesis; patients are able to do no more than move eyes up and blink.
Weber syndrome	Midbrain	Ipsilateral CN III palsy; contralateral hemiparesis.

- **Statins:** All ischemic stroke patients should receive a statin to ↓ stroke recurrence.
- **BP control:** In the first several days after an ischemic stroke, "**permissive hypertension**" should be allowed in order to maximize cerebral perfusion to the ischemic brain territory. Unless the patient is having ischemic chest pain or CHF, allow the BP to go as high as 220/110 mm Hg. After the first few days, if stroke symptoms are not progressing, initiate chronic antihypertensive therapy.
- **Anticoagulation with IV heparin or LMWH:** Generally to be avoided in acute ischemic stroke, although these agents may be given to patients with vertebral or carotid artery dissection.
- **Symptomatic internal carotid stenosis:** Patients with embolic stroke involving the anterior circulation who are found to have > 70% **stenosis** of the ipsilateral ICA benefit from **carotid endarterectomy.** It is most beneficial in the first few weeks after initial symptoms. **Carotid stenting** is another, less proven alternative.
- **Warfarin** therapy with a goal INR of 2–3 is the optimal treatment for patients with paroxysmal or chronic AF. In practice, specific identifiable cardiac sources of emboli (eg, left ventricular thrombus) are often treated with warfarin for 4–6 months.
- **Modification of 1° risk factors:** Long-term prevention of ischemic strokes rests primarily on aggressive control of hypertension, DM, and hyperlipidemia and on smoking cessation.

HEMORRHAGIC STROKE

A 40-year-old man is brought to the ER after his wife found him unresponsive when she returned home from work. He was behaving normally 10 hours ago, before she left for work. On exam, the patient is found to be in a deep coma and has normally reactive pupils. Head CT shows a small parenchymal hemorrhage in the right temporal lobe with extensive SAH but no significant brain edema. What is the most appropriate next step in determining the cause of the hemorrhage?

Conventional angiography, as the patient has an intracerebral (intraparenchymal) hemorrhage with an extensive subarachnoid (extraparenchymal) hemorrhage, which is the hallmark of a ruptured AVM but can occur with ruptured MCA aneurysms as well. Angiography not only establishes the diagnosis but helps plan treatment via endovascular coiling or the surgical clipping approach, ideally within 72 hours of symptoms.

As with ischemic stroke, focal symptoms in hemorrhagic stroke depend on the location of the hemorrhage. In contrast to ischemic stroke, intraparenchymal hemorrhages are usually associated with **headache** and rapid **deterioration in level of consciousness.**

- The leading cause of hemorrhagic strokes is **hypertension. Hypertensive hemorrhages classically occur in four subcortical structures: the basal ganglia, thalamus, cerebellum, and pons (part of the brainstem)** (see Figure 13.6).
- Intraparenchymal hemorrhages occurring within the cortex and underlying white matter (so-called **lobar hemorrhages**) can be caused by hypertension but raise suspicion for other etiologies, such as metastatic lesions, vascular abnormalities (eg, AVMs or aneurysms), hemorrhagic conversion

KEY FACT

The most common side effect of ASA/dipyridamole is headache, which usually resolves even if the patient continues the medication.

KEY FACT

The combination of clopidogrel and ASA/dipyridamole to treat stroke should be avoided because the risk of bleeding ↑ without a beneficial reduction in recurrent stroke.

KEY FACT

What diagnosis should you consider in an older patient who sustains a lobar hemorrhage and has no history of hypertension, and in whom brain imaging reveals no aneurysm or AVM? Cerebral amyloid angiopathy. Despite the name, these patients do **not** have systemic amyloidosis.

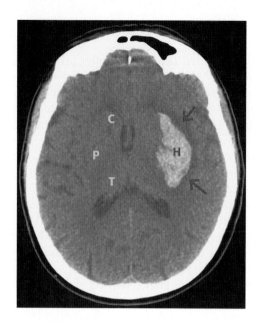

FIGURE 13.6. **Intracerebral hemorrhage.** Noncontrast head CT shows an intraparenchymal hemorrhage (H) and surrounding edema (arrows) centered in the left putamen, a common location for hypertensive hemorrhage. C, P, and T denote the normal contralateral caudate, putamen, and thalamus. (Reproduced with permission from Fauci AS et al. *Harrison's Principles of Internal Medicine,* 17th ed. New York: McGraw-Hill, 2008, Fig. 364-17.)

KEY FACT

Subarachnoid hemorrhages should raise suspicion for an underlying AVM or brain aneurysm.

KEY FACT

The risk of ICH ↑ with an INR of > 4.0 but may occur at a lower INR, especially in the elderly. The lack of a headache and a normal BP do not rule out hemorrhage. If CT shows an ICH, reversal of anticoagulation is indicated with fresh frozen plasma initially, followed by vitamin K.

of an ischemic stroke, infections (especially septic emboli), cocaine use, and cerebral amyloid angiopathy.

■ The American Heart Association does not recommend screening for aneurysms even among first-degree relatives of patients with SAH. Treatment of incidentally discovered unruptured aneurysms remains controversial.

TREATMENT

■ Largely supportive. **Cerebellar hemorrhages** should be considered a neurosurgical emergency, as swelling and herniation onto the brainstem can be lethal.

■ In the case of most other locations of ICH, evidence does not support urgent evacuation. A study of surgical evacuation vs. medical management for patients with ICH who appeared clinically stable up to 48 hours after onset showed no difference in mortality or functional outcomes.

COMPLICATIONS

Intraventricular hemorrhage is an ominous complication of ICH, and prompt ventricular drainage may ↓ ICP and improve outcome.

EXTRAPARENCHYMAL BLEEDS

The three types of extraparenchymal ICHs are **epidural, subdural,** and **subarachnoid.** The most common cause of all extraparenchymal ICHs is **head trauma.**

Epidural Hematomas

Typically caused by trauma to the side of the head, usually near the ear, resulting in injury to the **middle meningeal artery.** Such hematomas can expand rapidly, as they are produced by **arterial bleeding.**

SYMPTOMS

Although seen in < 25% of patients, the classic presentation is that of head trauma with brief (seconds to minutes) loss of consciousness followed by a **"lucid period"** in which mental status and level of alertness are normal for minutes to hours. This is then followed by a rapid decline in mental status.

DIAGNOSIS

Since the dura is tacked down to the skull at the suture lines, epidural bleeds will tamponade in a confined space and will not cross the sutures, leading to the characteristic **"lens-shaped"** hematoma on CT scan (see Figure 13.7A).

TREATMENT

Symptomatic epidural hematomas must be treated with urgent neurosurgical decompression.

Subdural Hematomas

Typically caused by head trauma that leads to a rapid deceleration of the skull (eg, MVAs) and subsequent shearing of the cerebral bridging veins as they travel through the subdural space into the draining venous sinuses. Most often seen in **elderly** who have **falls.** Spontaneous subdural hematomas may also occur, particularly in patients with underlying coagulopathy or thrombocytopenia.

SYMPTOMS

Can produce mass effect, which typically manifests as a progressive decline in mental status. May not have focal neurologic deficits.

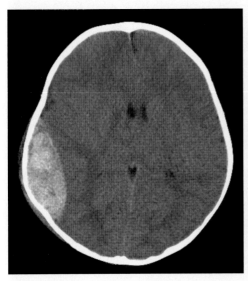
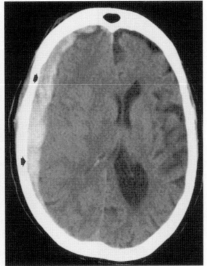

A   **B**

FIGURE 13.7.   **Acute epidural and acute subdural hematoma.** (**A**) Noncontrast CT showing a right temporal acute epidural hematoma. Note the characteristic **biconvex** shape. (**B**) Noncontrast CT demonstrating a right acute holohemispheric subdural hematoma. Note the characteristic **crescentic** shape. (Image A reproduced with permission from Doherty GM. *Current Diagnosis & Treatment: Surgery,* 13th ed. New York: McGraw-Hill, 2010, Fig. 36-8. Image B reproduced with permission from Chen MY et al. *Basic Radiology.* New York: McGraw-Hill, 2004, Fig. 12-32.)

DIAGNOSIS

Head CT reveals hematoma layering along the outer surface of the cerebral cortex (see Figure 13.7B). Must be in the differential of any elderly patient with dementia.

TREATMENT

As with epidural hematomas, symptomatic subdural hematomas require neurosurgical decompression.

Subarachnoid Hemorrhage (SAH)

The most common cause of nontraumatic SAH is a **ruptured intracranial aneurysm** (see Figure 13.8).

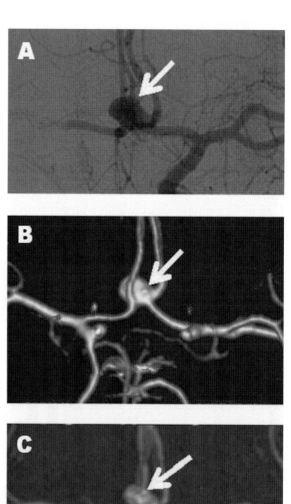

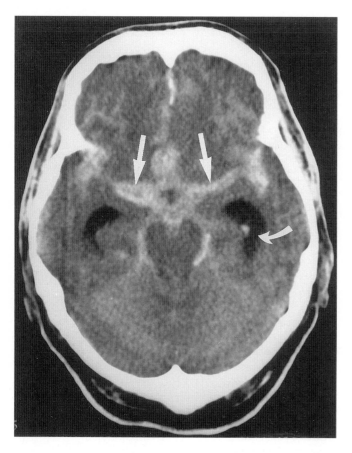

FIGURE 13.8. **Subarachnoid hemorrhage.** Noncontrast CT (left) showing SAH filling the basilar cisterns and sylvian fissures (straight arrows). The curved arrow shows the dilated temporal horns of the lateral ventricles/hydrocephalus. Coned-down images (right) from a catheter angiogram (**A**), a CT angiogram (**B**), and an MRA (**C**) show a saccular aneurysm arising from the anterior communicating artery (arrow). (Left image reproduced with permission from Tintinalli JE et al. *Tintinalli's Emergency Medicine: A Comprehensive Study Guide,* 6th ed. New York: McGraw-Hill, 2004, Fig. 237-4. Right image reproduced with permission from Doherty GM. *Current Diagnosis & Treatment: Surgery,* 13th ed. New York: McGraw-Hill, 2010, Fig. 36-6.)

Symptoms

Patients experience abrupt-onset severe headache ("**the worst headache of my life**," or "thunderclap" headache) that is often associated with nausea and vomiting. There may also be a ↓ level of consciousness and focal neurologic deficits.

Diagnosis

- Head CT is the initial imaging study of choice (see Figure 13.8). If CT is normal, perform an **LP** to look for **xanthochromia.**
- Patients with a confirmed SAH should then have conventional **cerebral angiography** to determine the presence, location, and anatomy of the aneurysm.

Treatment

The first priority is to secure the aneurysm as soon as possible, as the risk of rebleeding is significant in the first 48 hours. Currently, aneurysms are treated with either **endovascular coiling or neurosurgical clipping.**

Complications

- The major complications following SAH are related to **vasospasm** of the cerebral vessels. **Nimodipine,** which ↓ complications from vasospasm, is given to all patients with SAH and can be started on the first day and continued for three weeks. Vasospasm is also treated with "**triple-H therapy**" (Hypertension, Hypervolemia, and Hemodilution) with IV fluids and/or vasopressors in an effort to augment blood flow in areas of vasospasm.
- Transcranial Doppler is frequently used to identify subclinical vasospasm.
- Other complications include obstructive hydrocephalus and hyponatremia from **cerebral salt wasting.**

Seizures

A 20-year-old college student is brought to the ER from a party because he is febrile, hypertensive, tachycardic, and combative. He then has a generalized tonic-clonic seizure for about two minutes. His labs and head CT are normal. What is the most likely cause of his seizure, and what would be the most appropriate therapy?

Cocaine intoxication causing a sympathomimetic surge (tachycardia, hypertension, hyperthermia, mydriasis, agitation, and psychosis). The patient should receive sedation with lorazepam IV or IM to control agitation (↓ heart rate, BP, and temperature). Drug-induced seizures are usually self-limited and do not respond well to phenytoin, while haloperidol lowers the seizure threshold and should not be used for agitation in this patient.

A **seizure** is a paroxysmal neurologic event caused by abnormal, synchronous discharges from populations of cortical neurons. Symptoms can vary widely and can include overt convulsions, subtle alterations of consciousness (eg, staring spells), or simple sensations (eg, odd smells or sounds). **Epilepsy** is a condition in which patients have **unprovoked recurrent seizures.** The key step in diagnosis and treatment is to determine whether the initial seizure activity is **generalized** or **focal** in onset.

1° GENERALIZED SEIZURES

Originate with abrupt-onset, simultaneous, synchronized discharges of neurons throughout both cerebral hemispheres. Selected subtypes are as follows:

- **Tonic-clonic (grand mal):**
    - The most common generalized seizure type; typically seen in genetic epilepsy syndromes and in seizures arising from metabolic abnormalities (eg, hyponatremia, alcohol withdrawal, medications, CNS infections).
    - Begin with stiffening of the extremities (**tonic** phase), often associated with a guttural cry from contraction of the expiratory muscles, followed by rhythmic **clonic** jerking of the extremities.
    - Associated urinary incontinence, tongue biting, and postictal confusion are typically found.
- **Myoclonic:**
    - A **myoclonic jerk** is an abrupt, brief, single contraction of a muscle group that produces a quick contraction and movement. **Myoclonic seizures** are characterized by frequent but asynchronous, nonrhythmic, multifocal myoclonic jerks. Myoclonic jerks are most commonly seen with metabolic derangements (especially **uremia and after anoxia**) and **are usually not epileptic.**
    - **Atonic:** The epilepsy type that can most resemble syncope clinically. Characterized by the abrupt loss of all muscle tone associated with a brief loss of consciousness. Primarily seen with inherited forms of childhood epilepsy.

SYMPTOMS/EXAM

Although symptoms can vary, most generalized seizures are associated with a period of postictal confusion and lethargy generally lasting < 2–5 minutes.

DIAGNOSIS

- **Labs:** Routine evaluation of patients with new seizures includes metabolic labs, including electrolytes such as sodium and calcium, as well as screening for renal or liver dysfunction. LP should be considered when infection or inflammatory disease is a concern. Urine toxicology may detect unsuspected substance use (eg, cocaine, MDMA).
- **Imaging:** A brain MRI should be done to investigate for structural abnormalities, with particular attention paid to the temporal lobes.
- **EEG:** EEG obtained prior to and during a seizure may show symmetric and synchronous generalized epileptiform discharges at the onset.

TREATMENT

- "Broad-spectrum" anticonvulsants such as **valproic acid,** topiramate, and lamotrigine are considered first-line treatment for 1° generalized seizures.
- Two unique types of generalized epilepsy are **juvenile myoclonic epilepsy,** which is best treated with **valproic acid,** and **absence epilepsy,** which is classically treated with **ethosuximide.**

COMPLICATIONS

Table 13.7 outlines the side effects associated with common anticonvulsants used for seizure treatment. Other medication-related complications are as follows:

- **Anticonvulsants and OCPs:** Drugs that induce the liver cytochrome P-450 system (eg, phenytoin and carbamazepine) can lead to ↓ effective

KEY FACT

Pseudoseizures vary in presentation but can present with moaning, crying, and arrhythmic shaking of the body for > 10 minutes without loss of consciousness and with a normal EEG. Video or ambulatory EEG is the gold standard for diagnosis. Psychiatry should be consulted, as anxiety is often a major contributing factor. About 30% of patients have a history of epilepsy.

KEY FACT

Phenytoin and carbamazepine are **not** first-line agents for 1° generalized seizures and actually may exacerbate seizures in generalized epilepsy. Both also ↓ warfarin levels. These agents may be helpful when secondarily generalized tonic-clonic seizures are suspected (eg, from a mass lesion in the brain).

KEY FACT

Many anticonvulsants are associated with early osteoporosis, so early screening and prevention are key.

KEY FACT

Common acute toxicities of phenytoin include altered mental status and ataxia.

TABLE 13.7. **Classic Anticonvulsant Side Effects**

Drug	Side Effects
Phenytoin	Gum hyperplasia, ataxia, confusion, peripheral neuropathy, lymphoproliferative disorder, Stevens-Johnson syndrome (SJS), severe hypersensitivity syndrome.
Carbamazepine	Hyponatremia, lymphopenia, SJS, severe hypersensitivity syndrome. Induces its own metabolism; the initial dose can then become ineffective.
Valproate	Tremor, drowsiness, weight gain, hirsutism, thrombocytopenia, liver failure.

levels of other medications, including OCPs and warfarin. All female patients taking such anticonvulsants should be counseled to consider other means of birth control or use OCPs with high levels of estrogen.

- **Anticonvulsants and birth defects:** The use of anticonvulsants during pregnancy is associated with an ↑ risk of birth defects, particularly **neural tube defects.** All women of childbearing age who use anticonvulsants should be advised to take at least 4 mg/day of folate. Pregnant women with epilepsy should be treated with a single anticonvulsant at the lowest therapeutic dose; valproic acid is particularly teratogenic.

KEY FACT

If a patient taking phenytoin or carbamazepine develops transaminitis and rash (and possibly acute kidney failure and eosinophilia), suspect anticonvulsant hypersensitivity syndrome and stop the medication ASAP.

FOCAL (PARTIAL) SEIZURES

A 20-year-old woman with epilepsy asks if she can discontinue her carbamazepine. Her first generalized tonic-clonic seizure occurred at age 10 and was preceded by a complex focal seizure, with an EEG showing focal slowing in the right temporal lobe. The patient was treated with phenytoin but stopped after two months because she felt fatigued; she remained seizure free for a year until she had another generalized tonic-clonic seizure. Carbamazepine was then started, but she continued to have complex focal seizures until the dose was ↑. The patient has now been seizure free for one year. Her physical exam and brain MRI are normal. What is the most appropriate treatment option for this patient?

Continue carbamazepine at the current dose. Epileptic patients who are most likely to remain seizure free after medication withdrawal are those with no structural brain lesion, normal EEGs, a sustained seizure-free period (2–5 years), and no abnormalities on neurologic exam.

Much more common than 1° generalized seizures, focal seizures originate from a small, discrete focal lesion within the brain that gives rise to abnormal synchronized neuronal discharges. This activity may then spread to involve other areas of the brain. Subtypes are as follows:

- **Simple focal seizures:**
  - Focal seizures in which **no alteration of consciousness** is noted.
  - Initial symptoms depend on the location of the seizure focus and commonly include twitching/jerking of one side of the body (focal motor seizures) or sensations of strange smells or sounds.

KEY FACT

At least 30% of patients with epilepsy have depression, especially if seizures are uncontrolled, and depression is also a possible side effect of phenobarbital, phenytoin, valproate, levetiracetam, and topiramate. Suicide rates are also elevated, so TCAs should not be used for depression, as they lower seizure threshold. SSRIs and SNRIs are tolerated.

- **Complex focal seizures:**
  - Evolve from simple focal seizures as the initial focal seizure activity spreads to involve some but not all of both cerebral hemispheres. In fact, the **stereotypical warning or aura** that many patients report is simply the manifestation of the initial simple partial seizure.
  - As seizure activity spreads, patients develop an **impairment of consciousness** and **behavioral arrest,** during which they display stereotypical behaviors known as **automatisms** (eg, lip smacking, chewing, pulling at clothes).
  - In contrast to simple focal seizures, complex focal seizures are associated with postictal confusion and lethargy.
- **Complex focal seizures with 2° generalization:**
  - In many patients with prolonged complex focal seizures, seizure activity can ultimately spread to involve the entire cerebral cortex. The manifestation of the "2° generalization" of the initial focal seizure activity is usually generalized tonic-clonic activity.
  - Generalized seizures can thus be either **1°** (generalized seizure activity at onset) or **2°** (initial focal activity that spreads to involve the entire cortex).
- **Temporal lobe epilepsy:** The most common cause of simple and complex focal seizures is **temporal lobe pathology,** most commonly 2° to abnormalities of the **hippocampus.** Hippocampal sclerosis/calcification is seen on imaging. The classic auras of odd smells, sounds, or tastes are associated with temporal lobe epilepsy.

DIAGNOSIS

Given that focal seizures arise from focal lesions, brain imaging studies are typically abnormal; EEG often shows localized (ie, asymmetric) epileptiform activity. HSV encephalitis should be considered in patients with new-onset temporal lobe seizures.

TREATMENT

- **Medications:** Focal-onset seizures are best treated with anticonvulsants such as **phenytoin, carbamazepine,** phenobarbital, and valproic acid. Newer medications such as gabapentin, levetiracetam, lamotrigine, oxcarbazepine, and topiramate are also useful.
  - **Elderly patients** may be particularly sensitive to the cognitive, motor, and coordination side effects of phenytoin even if total levels are at therapeutic range.
  - **Gabapentin, lamotrigine,** and carbamazepine are equally effective at controlling partial-onset seizures in the elderly, but gabapentin and lamotrigine are better tolerated.
- **Vagal nerve stimulators:** Although their mechanism of action remains unclear, vagal nerve stimulators can ↓ the frequency of focal-onset seizures by 25% in patients with medically refractory seizures.
- **Surgery:** Patients with focal-onset seizures often have an identifiable brain lesion on imaging studies. This is particularly true of temporal lobe epilepsy 2° to hippocampal lesions. In patients with medically refractory seizures (ie, those with no response to three trials of medications), **surgical resection** of the causative lesion (eg, temporal lobectomy) can produce striking results, with up to 50–75% of patients becoming seizure free.

COMPLICATIONS

See Table 13.7 and the accompanying discussion.

KEY FACT

A patient with a generalized tonic-clonic seizure who is subsequently noted to have a postictal left hemiparesis—aka postictal **Todd's paralysis**—likely had a focal-onset seizure that began in the right hemisphere and secondarily generalized.

KEY FACT

In a patient who reports recurring odd smells, sounds, or tastes, suspect temporal lobe epilepsy and consider evaluating for HSV encephalitis.

STATUS EPILEPTICUS

Traditionally defined as (1) continuous seizure activity lasting > 30 minutes or (2) recurrent seizures without return of normal consciousness between seizures. Practically speaking, seizure activity lasting > 5 minutes is unlikely to remit spontaneously and carries the risk of permanent neuronal injury. Generally, ongoing or recurrent seizure activity lasting > 5 minutes is considered a medical emergency and is treated as status epilepticus.

TREATMENT

Treatment guidelines are as follows:

- ABCs.
- **Labs:** Draw a toxicology screen and labs for metabolic abnormalities (eg, glucose, sodium, calcium), but do not delay pharmacotherapy.
- **Pharmacologic:**
    - Administer thiamine and glucose.
    - Benzodiazepines are first-line anticonvulsants for status epilepticus. Give lorazepam 0.1 mg/kg IV at 1–2 mg/min.
    - Fosphenytoin IV loading dose (20 mg/kg) should then be started immediately even if seizures terminate with lorazepam.
    - If seizures persist, the next step is to give a second load of phenytoin or fosphenytoin using an additional 5- to 10-mg/kg IV load or move directly to the next step.
    - If seizures continue, the next step is to administer pentobarbital, midazolam, or propofol. Use of any of these medications typically requires continuous EEG recordings and mechanical ventilation.

> **KEY FACT**
>
> The treatment of choice for status epilepticus is IV lorazepam. For patients with prior status epilepticus, lorazepam administered by rectal gel may be helpful and can be administered by family members.

Movement Disorders

HYPOKINETIC DISORDERS

Parkinson's Disease

A 75-year-old woman presents with a left upper extremity tremor of two years' duration. She is left handed, and the tremor occurs both while she is walking and when she is at rest. She is now dropping things, and her handwriting has been affected. Over the past year she has also needed help with dressing. On exam, she has hypophonic speech, ↓ facial expression, slowness, rigidity, and ↓ arm swinging on the left side, but with normal balance. What is the most likely diagnosis and the most appropriate course of management?

Parkinson's disease with typical symptoms. Carbidopa/levodopa is first-line treatment in patients > 70 years of age with severe, limiting symptoms. COMT inhibitors and dopamine agonists (pramipexole or ropinirole) are second-line treatments in this age group.

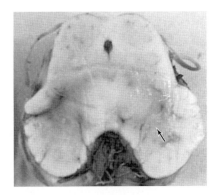

FIGURE 13.9.   Parkinson's disease. Midbrain of a 45-year-old woman with Parkinson's disease, showing depigmentation of the substantia nigra (arrow). (Reproduced with permission from Waxman S. *Clinical Neuroanatomy,* 26th ed. New York: McGraw-Hill, 2010, Fig. 13–9.)

An idiopathic progressive neurodegenerative disorder affecting the dopaminergic neurons of the substantia nigra (see Figure 13.9). Average age of onset is 60, and the male-to-female ratio is 1.5:1.

SYMPTOMS/EXAM

- The **cardinal features** are **resting tremor ("pill rolling"), bradykinesia, "cogwheel" rigidity,** and **postural instability.** Diagnosis requires the presence of at least two of these four symptoms.
- Symptoms typically begin **asymmetrically,** usually in one extremity. Gait and balance problems are typically not present early on. Cognition is preserved in idiopathic Parkinson's disease until late in the course. Thirty to forty percent of patients develop dementia.

DIFFERENTIAL

- Parkinson-plus syndromes present with parkinsonian features as well as with additional symptoms (see below).
- Other causes of parkinsonism include cerebrovascular disease; recurrent head trauma (eg, boxing), toxin exposure (including illicit drugs such as MPTP and heavy metals such as manganese), and antidopaminergic medications (eg, traditional antipsychotics, metoclopramide).

DIAGNOSIS

The diagnosis of idiopathic Parkinson's disease relies on the history and physical combined with response to levodopa. Young patients as well as those with atypical features should undergo further workup (eg, imaging studies, toxin screens).

TREATMENT

- **Medical:** Pharmacologic treatment includes the following:
  - **Levodopa/carbidopa:**
    - The gold standard for symptomatic treatment, and first-line treatment for patients > 70 years of age with new-onset Parkinson's disease and functional impairment.
    - A precursor of dopamine, levodopa is administered with carbidopa, a decarboxylase inhibitor that inhibits peripheral conversion of levodopa to dopamine.
    - Should be taken on an empty stomach to maximize absorption. Thirty percent of patients treated go on to develop psychosis and other psychiatric symptoms.
  - **Dopamine agonists:**
    - Direct agonists of D_2 dopamine receptors. Pramipexole or ropinirole can be used as initial monotherapy in patients < 70 years of age.
    - Slightly less effective than levodopa, but like COMT inhibitors, they are useful adjuncts for maintaining steady dopamine levels. Levodopa should be ↓ when the dosage reaches > 500 mg/day, if its effects are wearing off, or if dyskinesia appears. Can cause psychosis and impulse problems (eg, hypersexuality, gambling). Should be avoided in patients > 70 years of age or with dementia.
  - **COMT inhibitors:** Inhibition of this enzyme ↑ endogenous dopamine levels. Entacapone, tolcapone, and nitecapone are useful adjuncts as "levodopa extenders," decreasing the total dose of levodopa needed and providing more continuous dopamine receptor stimulation in late-stage disease if levodopa effects are wearing off. Can be hepatotoxic.
  - **MAO-B inhibitors:** Selegiline and rasagiline are examples, but they have a weak symptomatic effect and are generally added to levodopa to diminish motor fluctuations. Can cause sleep disturbance.

- **Anticholinergics:** Trihexyphenidyl and benztropine. Useful for tremor and rigidity in early stages or as an adjunct to levodopa in patients < 65 years of age (30% improvement is seen in 50% of patients). Can worsen psychosis.
- **Amantadine:** Not as potent as carbidopa/levodopa, and should not be used as first-line therapy in the elderly. As with anticholinergics, it improves tremor, bradykinesia, and rigidity but can worsen psychosis.
- **Atypical neuroleptic agents:**
  - **Clozapine:** Adjunctive therapy that suppresses the frequency of dyskinesia and can help with hallucinations.
  - **Quetiapine:** Can also help with psychosis, delusions, and paranoia.
  - These newer agents do not exacerbate parkinsonism (vs. neuroleptics such as haloperidol, which block D_2 dopamine receptors and are contraindicated).
  - **TCAs:** Can be used for nighttime sedation and associated depression.
- **Surgical:** Surgical treatment options primarily include deep brain stimulation of the globus pallidus interna nucleus or subthalamic nucleus of the basal ganglia.

Parkinson-Plus Syndromes

A 70-year-old man complains of lightheadedness, two episodes of fainting in the last year, imbalance, and frequent falls over the past two years. He also has urinary incontinence, constipation, and impotence. On exam, his BP is 120/80 mm Hg, and his pulse is 70/min while lying down and 85/55 mm Hg with no change in pulse while standing up. He has impaired gait, balance, and fine motor movements bilaterally along with mild rigidity. DTRs are brisk bilaterally, and extensor plantar response is present bilaterally. What is the most likely diagnosis?

Multiple-system atrophy (formerly known as Shy-Drager syndrome), which is characterized by orthostatic hypotension, neurogenic bladder, constipation, and impotence with gait-predominant parkinsonism and corticospinal tract signs. Progressive supranuclear palsy is also characterized by parkinsonism, but with vertical gaze palsy. These so-called Parkinson-plus syndromes respond poorly to levodopa.

A number of neurodegenerative diseases produce parkinsonian features along with a variety of other symptoms, including cognitive decline and cerebellar abnormalities (see Table 13.8). In general, Parkinson-plus syndromes respond poorly if at all to levodopa. A Parkinson-plus syndrome should thus be considered in **any patient who presents with parkinsonism associated with cerebellar or cognitive symptoms,** especially when the parkinsonian features do not respond to levodopa therapy.

KEY FACT

In a patient with features of Parkinson's who fails to improve with levodopa, suspect a Parkinson-plus syndrome.

KEY FACT

Combining selegiline with TCAs or SSRIs can potentially lead to serotonin syndrome.

KEY FACT

Think of progressive supranuclear palsy in a patient presenting with parkinsonian symptoms with dementia, deficits in vertical gaze (eg, inability to look down), and postural instability that is often unresponsive to levodopa.

KEY FACT

Treat Lewy body dementia with cholinergic medications (donepezil, galantamine, or rivastigmine) to alleviate the characteristic inattention, hallucinations, agitation, and fluctuating encephalopathy. Neuroleptics (eg, haloperidol and quetiapine) should be avoided, as they can cause severe parkinsonism and neuroleptic malignant syndrome in these patients.

TABLE 13.8. **Clinical Features of Parkinson-Plus Syndromes**

Syndrome	Key Features
Dementia with Lewy bodies	Cognitive decline; visual hallucinations; marked daily fluctuations in mental status due to cholinergic deficiency.
Progressive supranuclear palsy	Cognitive decline. Extraocular abnormalities, especially vertical gaze. Prominent rigidity of the entire body, leading to frequent falls.
Corticobasal degeneration	Cognitive decline; "alien limb" phenomenon; limb apraxia (inability to perform learned motor tasks such as brushing teeth or saluting).
Multiple-system atrophy	Encompasses a group of Parkinson-plus syndromes. Autonomic dysfunction, especially **orthostatic hypotension,** may occur early. Ataxia is common in the cerebellar form.

HYPERKINETIC DISORDERS

Huntington's Disease

A 30-year-old man presents with constant involuntary movements of his hands for the past year along with personality change of three years' duration. He has been forgetting things and making mistakes at work. He had an episode of depression in his 20s, and his father had a history of substance abuse, having left the family when the patient was a child. On exam, the patient is noted to have brief, brisk, irregular, and unpredictable involuntary movements fleeting from one body part to another. What is the most likely diagnosis? Huntington's disease with characteristic dancing-like chorea. The patient's age, chronicity, and associated cognitive and psychiatric changes suggest this diagnosis.

An **autosomal dominant** disorder characterized by progressive **chorea, dementia,** and **psychiatric** symptoms. Huntington's is a neurodegenerative disorder that particularly affects the caudate nucleus of the basal ganglia and is caused by a **polyglutamine (CAG) trinucleotide repeat expansion** in the Huntington gene on **chromosome 4.** This repeat can expand with successive generations, leading to the phenomenon of **anticipation**—earlier age of onset and more severe symptoms in successive generations.

DIAGNOSIS

- The clinical presentation combined with a strong family history suggests the disease.
- CT/MRI show marked **atrophy of the caudate nucleus** and exclude other structural abnormalities (see Figure 13.10).
- Genetic testing now provides definitive evidence of the trinucleotide (CAG) repeat expansion.

TREATMENT

- No treatment is currently available for the underlying disease process.
- Chorea can be treated symptomatically with neuroleptics (eg, haloperidol), dopamine-depleting agents (eg, reserpine, tetrabenazine), and GABAergic agents (eg, clonazepam).

KEY FACT

Huntington's disease may manifest earlier in successive generations within families—the so-called anticipation phenomenon—as a result of expansion of the trinucleotide CAG repeats.

KEY FACT

Genetic counseling is indicated for children of patients with Huntington's disease. For interested family members, testing for CAG repeats provides definitive evidence of Huntington's.

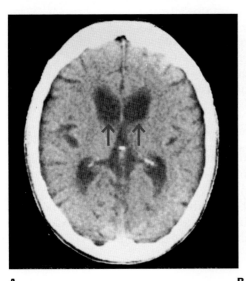 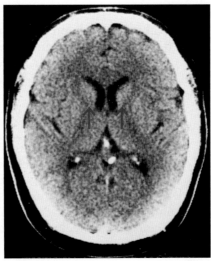

A **B**

FIGURE 13.10. **Cerebral and caudate nucleus atrophy in Huntington's disease.** (A) Non-contrast CT in a 54-year-old patient with Huntington's disease shows atrophy of the caudate nuclei (arrows) and diffuse cerebral atrophy with ex vacuo dilation of the lateral ventricles. (B) A normal 54-year-old subject (arrows on caudate nuclei). (Reproduced with permission from Ropper AH, Samuels MA. *Adams & Victor's Principles of Neurology,* 9th ed. New York: McGraw-Hill, 2009, Fig. 39-4.)

Wilson's Disease

An **autosomal recessive** disorder characterized by progressive neuropsychiatric symptoms and liver dysfunction. Copper deposition most prominently occurs in the liver and basal ganglia (specifically the lentiform nuclei) of the brain.

Symptoms/Exam

- Liver dysfunction is typically seen prior to neuropsychiatric illness (onset of liver disease occurs at 10–15 years of age); most patients present as adolescents and young adults.
- Patients have prominent extrapyramidal symptoms (tremor, dystonia, rigidity, bradykinesia) and cerebellar symptoms (ataxia, incoordination, slurred speech); common psychiatric symptoms include depression, psychosis, and personality changes.
- **Kayser-Fleischer rings,** greenish-brown rings along the limbus of the cornea from copper deposition, present in most patients with CNS symptoms; a **slit-lamp** evaluation is often necessary to detect them.

Diagnosis

- Diagnosis is supported by laboratory evidence of low serum copper and ceruloplasmin (a protein into which copper is normally incorporated in the hepatocyte) and high urinary copper.
- Liver biopsy reveals copper deposition.

Treatment

- **Penicillamine,** a copper-chelating agent, has classically been used to treat Wilson's disease, although side effects are common. In particular, a **myasthenia gravis syndrome** with titers of anti-ACh receptor antibodies can be induced by penicillamine therapy.
- Other treatment options include trientine and oral zinc.

KEY FACT

Consider Wilson's disease in young patients presenting with psychiatric disorders and liver abnormalities.

Essential Tremor

An idiopathic **postural and action tremor** that typically affects the **hands** and **head.** It is seen equally often in men and women, although hand tremor is most prominent in men and head tremor most prominent in women. Tremor onset may occur early between 35 and 45 years of age. Family history is often strongly $\oplus$.

SYMPTOMS

- In contrast to Parkinson's, essential tremor is not seen at rest but rather comes out with activity. The tremor is slightly faster than that of Parkinson's disease (8–10 Hz vs. 4–5 Hz).
- Most patients report a temporary but **striking improvement** in tremor with **alcohol** ingestion; conversely, physical and emotional stress exacerbates the tremor, as do medications such as caffeine and steroids.

EXAM

Postural tremor of the hands is tested by having patients maintain their arms fully extended from their bodies. In patients with essential tremor, strength is normal. In contrast to Parkinson's disease, no abnormalities in muscle tone are present.

DIAGNOSIS

Based on clinical features.

TREATMENT

The classic treatments are β-blockers (eg, **propranolol**) and **primidone.** Benzodiazepines and gabapentin have also been used when first-line treatments fail.

Tourette's Syndrome

A disorder characterized by **brief involuntary actions (motor and vocal tics)** and psychiatric disturbances. Onset typically occurs in adolescents < 18 years of age, with a **male-to-female ratio of 5:1.** Two-thirds of patients have some amelioration of symptoms in adulthood, but complete remission is rare.

SYMPTOMS/EXAM

- **Motor tics** can be simple (eg, eye twitching, blinking, shoulder shrugging) or complex (eg, mimicking another's actions, or **echopraxia**).
- **Vocal tics** can be simple sounds (eg, barking) or single words; classic vocal tics include **speaking obscenities (coprolalia)** and **mimicking another's speech (echolalia),** although neither is common. Tics are often exacerbated by physical or emotional stress.
- Associated neuropsychiatric disorders include **OCD and ADHD.**

DIFFERENTIAL

The differential for motor tics includes dystonia (see below) and ballismus.

TREATMENT

Neuroleptics (eg, haloperidol, risperidone), **clonidine,** and **benzodiazepines** (eg, clonazepam, diazepam) often help ↓ the frequency of tics.

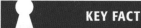
KEY FACT

In a patient with hand tremors that are most prominent when the arms are extended and improve with alcohol (and worsen with stress and caffeine), suspect essential tremor. The family history is usually $\oplus$, and head tremors may also occur. Treat with β-blockers first.

KEY FACT

There is an ↑ incidence of OCD and ADHD among patients with Tourette's.

Dystonia

- A syndrome characterized by repetitive, sustained contractions of agonist/antagonist muscles groups that typically produce painful **twisting/writhing movements** and/or **abnormal tonic postures** of the head or extremities.
- Can be focal or generalized. Focal dystonias most commonly include those that involve the musculature of the neck (**torticollis**), eyes (**blepharospasm**), and hands ("**writer's cramp**").
- Etiologies include inherited/genetic, neurodegenerative (eg, Huntington's, Wilson's, Parkinson's), rheumatologic (eg, SLE, antiphospholipid syndrome), metabolic (eg, thyroid disease), and toxin/medication related (eg, **neuroleptics**, OCPs).
- **Tx:** Treat **focal** dystonia with **selective injection of botulinum toxin** every 3–6 months for abnormal posture and associated pain. Other 1° treatments include trihexyphenidyl, clonazepam, or baclofen. For **generalized** dystonia, stop the offending medication and treat with **anticholinergics** such as benztropine or diphenhydramine acutely. Deep brain stimulation may be effective for refractory cases.

KEY FACT

Neuroleptics such as haloperidol can cause an acute dystonic reaction. Treat with anticholinergics.

Restless Leg Syndrome (RLS)

Uncomfortable paresthesias of the legs that are relieved by leg movement and worsen at night upon going to bed. Generally idiopathic, but also seen in patients with a wide variety of chronic illnesses (eg, Parkinson's, **anemia**, diabetes, COPD, thyroid disease, connective tissue diseases, neuropathies) and as a side effect of drugs (eg, caffeine, lithium, CCBs).

Symptoms/Exam

- Paresthesias are most severe when the legs are **at rest** (eg, while sitting or lying), especially at night as patients try to sleep. They are often described as "crawling" or "creeping" sensations and are **relieved by continued movement** of the legs.
- Patients may also have periodic limb movements of sleep (PLMS)—frequent stereotypical movements of the leg.
- Neurologic exam is normal unless RLS is related to an underlying neurologic disorder. NCS sometimes reveal a peripheral neuropathy.

Diagnosis/Treatment

- Before initiating treatment, it is essential to check serum iron studies. Oral iron therapy can alleviate symptoms and is recommended if serum ferritin levels are < 50 ng/mL.
- **Dopaminergic medications** administered before bedtime (eg, levodopa/carbidopa, pramipexole) are the **standard treatment** for RLS. Other useful agents include **benzodiazepines, narcotics,** and **gabapentin.**

KEY FACT

In patients with RLS, always check a serum ferritin level to assess for iron deficiency, a common reversible etiology.

Multiple Sclerosis (MS)

A 30-year-old woman comes to the clinic complaining of diplopia on lateral gaze in either direction that has worsened over the past week. Exam reveals paresis of the adducting eye with nystagmus of the abducting eye on horizontal gaze in either direction. MRI shows a hyperintense lesion on T2-weighted images within the pons as well as five hyperintense lesions in the cerebral white matter adjacent to the lateral ventricles. What is the diagnosis, and what long-term treatment should be considered?

The patient has bilateral internuclear ophthalmoplegia, which is a classic presentation for MS. Since there is no prior history of neurologic problems, this is a clinically isolated presentation of demyelination. MRI findings are typical. Treatment with interferon-β will ↓ the incidence of additional attacks in patients with monosymptomatic demyelination (including optic neuritis and myelopathy) who have multiple "silent" demyelinating lesions on brain MRI.

An autoimmune inflammatory disease affecting the myelin of the CNS. It is characterized by focal demyelinating plaques that occur at different times and locations within the CNS ("**separated in space and time**"). Typically affects the optic nerves, corpus callosum, periventricular white matter, brainstem, and spinal cord. Generally seen in **younger women**. Incidence ↑ with latitude of birth and is twice as high in patients of Northern European descent as in those of African descent.

SYMPTOMS

- In addition to focal abnormalities, patients often suffer from chronic **fatigue**.
- Symptoms are **exacerbated by heat and exercise** (the Uhthoff phenomenon); old deficits may also be worsened by underlying illness, especially infections such as UTIs or URIs.

EXAM

Classic lesions and exam findings include the following:

- **Optic neuritis:** Presents as unilateral subacute vision loss associated with pain with eye movement. Exam shows pallor of the optic nerve (may be normal in the acute setting), ↓ visual acuity, difficulty with color discrimination, and a **relative afferent pupillary defect** (also known as Marcus Gunn pupil; see Figure 13.11).
- **Internuclear ophthalmoplegia:** A demyelinating lesion of the medial longitudinal fasciculus in the brainstem. Patients complain of double vision when looking to one side; exam reveals inability to adduct the eye ipsilateral to the lesion during voluntary horizontal gaze. Adduction of the eye can be brought out by testing convergence, which remains normal.
- **Spinal cord:** Transverse myelitis symptoms (**paresthesias**, sensory level, bowel/bladder dysfunction, **UMN signs**) are common.
- **Lhermitte's sign** (electrical radiation down the spine elicited by neck flexion) is a classic finding and is likely related to dorsal column involvement.

KEY FACT

MS is a **clinical** diagnosis. The diagnosis is likely if patients report **two or more** clinically distinct episodes of typical neurologic symptoms.

KEY FACT

Internuclear ophthalmoplegia in a young woman is virtually diagnostic of MS.

KEY FACT

Consider MS in a young patient presenting with any of the following: subacute loss of vision; double vision when looking to one side; an electrical sensation running down the spine when the neck is flexed; subacute spinal cord symptoms (eg, paresthesias and bowel/ bladder dysfunction); and worsening of neurologic symptoms with heat or exercise.

Diffuse illumination

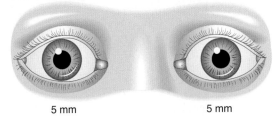

5 mm   5 mm

Light on normal eye

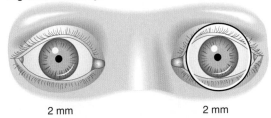

2 mm   2 mm

Normal reaction of both pupils

Light on eye with afferent defect

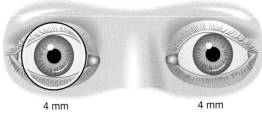

4 mm   4 mm

Decreased reaction of both pupils

FIGURE 13.11.   Afferent pupillary defect (Marcus Gunn pupil). (Reproduced with permission from Riordan-Eva P, Whitcher JP. *Vaughan & Asbury's General Ophthalmology,* 17th ed. New York: McGraw-Hill, 2008, Fig. 14-32.)

DIAGNOSIS

- **Clinical criteria:** No laboratory or imaging test is diagnostic for MS, and the diagnosis must therefore be based on clinical criteria. Definitive diagnosis requires evidence from the history and exam of at least two distinct attacks involving two separate CNS regions. Imaging and laboratory data support the diagnosis.
- **MRI:** MRI abnormalities are seen in > 90% of patients (see Figure 13.12). Most have multiple punctate/ovoid lesions involving the periventricular white matter ("Dawson's finger" lesions extending from the ventricles at right angles), **corpus callosum,** brainstem, and spinal cord. These are best seen on T2-weighted images. Acute "active" lesions enhance with gadolinium contrast.
- **CSF:** Typical findings include normal opening pressure, mild lymphocytic pleocytosis (5–40 WBCs/mm^3), normal glucose, and normal to mildly ↑ protein. Eighty percent of patients have > 2 **oligoclonal bands and an elevated CSF** IgG index, but neither is specific for MS.
- **EPs:** Occasionally used to obtain supportive evidence of demyelination if MRI and CSF results are inconclusive. For evaluation of MS, visual EPs are often used.

KEY FACT

MRI is the imaging modality of choice for MS but is used only to support the clinical diagnosis.

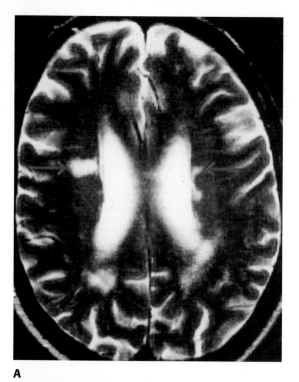

A

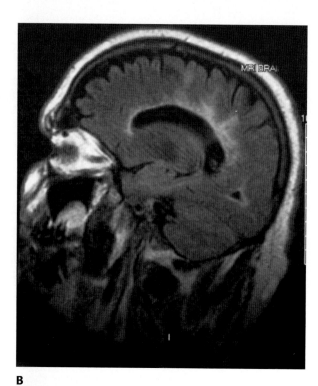

B

C

FIGURE 13.12.   Multiple sclerosis. T2-weighted MRI **(A)** and sagittal FLAIR image **(B)** show multiple MS plaques (arrows) in the periventricular matter oriented radially from the corpus callosum ("**Dawson's fingers**"). **(C)** Areas of demyelination of the white matter (arrows) in the frontal lobe of a 54-year-old man with multiple sclerosis. (Images A and B reproduced with permission from Ropper AH, Samuels MA. *Adams & Victor's Principles of Neurology,* 9th ed. New York: McGraw-Hill, 2009, Fig. 36-1. Image C reproduced with permission from Waxman SG. *Clinical Neuroanatomy,* 26th ed. New York: McGraw-Hill, 2010, Fig. 25-9.)

***T*REATMENT**

- **Disease-modifying therapies** include the following:
    - **β-interferon and glatiramer acetate—"ABC drugs"** (Avonex, Betaseron, Copaxone): These drugs have been shown to ↓ the frequency and severity of relapses in patients with relapsing-remitting MS. Table 13.9 outlines the administration of these drugs and delineates their potential side effects.

TABLE 13.9.   Administration and Side Effects of "ABC Drugs"

Drug	Administration	Side Effects
Interferon-β1a (Avonex)	Weekly IM	Flulike symptoms, depression.
Interferon-β1b (Betaseron)	QOD SQ	Flulike symptoms.
Glatiramer acetate (Copaxone)	Daily SQ	Flushing, chest tightness.

- **Glucocorticoids:** High-dose IV glucocorticoids (Solu-Medrol 1 g IV QD × 3–5 days), which are typically used to treat acute attacks and to address the presence of new enhancing lesions on MRI, appear to be superior to oral steroids (especially for treating optic neuritis), producing faster recovery. However, the administration of glucocorticoids has no effect on overall disease progression or long-term disability.
- **Mitoxantrone:** One of the few therapeutic options that slows progression of 2° progressive or severe relapsing-remitting MS. However, there is dose-related cardiotoxicity, and noninvasive cardiac imaging (echo or MUGA) is required before each dose.
- **Specific symptoms** are targeted with appropriate medications:
    - **Hyperreflexic bladder:** Oxybutynin.
    - **Fatigue:** Amantadine (first-line), modafinil.
    - **Paroxysmal symptoms** (eg, tonic spasms): Carbamazepine.
    - **Spasticity:** Baclofen, diazepam.

COMPLICATIONS

- Interferon-β is associated with an ↑ risk of spontaneous abortions and low birth weight. Women taking immunomodulatory treatment for MS should use effective contraception or, if they want to become pregnant, should stop therapy several months before attempting to conceive.
- During pregnancy, the frequency of MS relapses typically ↓ significantly in the third trimester, with a rebound ↑ in the first six months postpartum.
- First-degree relatives of a person with MS have a risk of disease 20–50 times greater than that of the general population.

> **KEY FACT**
>
> Corticosteroids help produce faster recovery in acute flares of MS but have no impact on overall disease progression or long-term disability. Most patients with optic neuritis have good recovery within six months with or without treatment. The decision to use corticosteroids depends on patient preference, the severity of the visual deficit, the health of the other eye, and vocational requirements.

> **KEY FACT**
>
> The only medications shown to ↓ the frequency and severity of relapses in patients with relapsing-remitting MS are β-interferon and glatiramer acetate.

Neuromuscular Junction Disorders

 A 60-year-old woman presents to the ER with a few weeks of intermittent ptosis of the left eye, diplopia, dysarthria, inability to swallow for the last two days, and shortness of breath. Her symptoms worsen with fatigue and improve with rest. Exam shows left ptosis, incomplete abduction of both eyes, weakness of the tongue and lower face, and weakness of the neck flexors, shoulder abductors, and hip flexors. Sensation and reflexes are normal. Her BMI is 22 and her FVC 1.6 L. What is the most likely diagnosis, and what is the appropriate treatment?

This patient is having a myasthenic crisis characterized by dysphagia that requires NG feeding and/or severe respiratory muscle weakness that necessitates ventilation. Plasmapheresis and IVIG are the treatments of choice.

MYASTHENIA GRAVIS (MG)

An **autoimmune** disorder that is usually caused by autoantibodies to the nicotinic ACh receptor (nAChR), resulting in impaired transmission at the neuromuscular junction. Occurs in **young women** (ages 20–30) and **older men** (ages 50–70). Associated with other autoimmune diseases, particularly **thyroid** disorders. May be precipitated by aminoglycosides, procainamide, β-blockers, stress, and infection.

SYMPTOMS

- The hallmark is **fluctuating, fatigable weakness** classically affecting the **eye muscles.**
- There are two forms:
  - **Ocular:** Isolated to the extraocular and eyelid muscles, yielding double vision and ptosis.
  - **Generalized:** Typically involves the ocular, facial, and proximal limb muscles, giving rise to ocular symptoms as well as to facial weakness, trouble swallowing and speaking, respiratory dysfunction, and limb weakness. Patients with ocular MG may progress to generalized MG.

EXAM

- **Ptosis,** often asymmetric, can be brought out by testing prolonged upgaze; an ice pack briefly placed on the eye will improve ptosis.
- **Extraocular muscle palsies** are typically seen on lateral gaze.
- **Easy fatigability** of proximal muscles with repeated strength testing.
- **Preserved DTRs** and sensation.

DIFFERENTIAL

- Lambert-Eaton myasthenic syndrome (see Table 13.10).
- **Drug-induced MG: Penicillamine** can cause a reversible antibody-⊕ MG syndrome.
- **Botulism:** Typically presents with cranial nerve palsies, including the extraocular muscles. Patients have CSF pleocytosis and often absent reflexes.

MNEMONIC

The 5 W's of myasthenia gravis:

Waxing and
Waning (fluctuating)
Weakness with
Work (fatigability), mostly in
Women

TABLE 13.10. Myasthenia Gravis vs. Lambert-Eaton Myasthenic Syndrome

CHARACTERISTIC	MYASTHENIA GRAVIS	LAMBERT-EATON MYASTHENIC SYNDROME
Antibody target channel	nAChR	Presynaptic voltage-gated calcium channel
Associated cancer	Thymoma	Small cell lung cancer
Eye muscle involvement	Yes	**No**
Autonomic symptoms	No	Yes
Reflexes	Normal	Hypoactive
Repetitive strength testing	Rapid fatigue	Initial improvement
Repetitive nerve stimulation	Decremental response	Initial enhancement

DIAGNOSIS

- **Anti-nAChR antibodies:** Present in > 80% of generalized MG and 50% of ocular MG cases.
- **Anti-MuSK antibodies:** Present in 20% of "seronegative" MG patients.
- **Tensilon test:** Tensilon (edrophonium), a short-acting AChE inhibitor, can give instantaneous improvement to an objectively weak muscle. Caution must be used, as it may precipitate cardiac arrhythmias. Falling out of favor as a diagnostic test.
- **EMG/NCS:** Direct testing of the muscle with EMG/NCS remains the **best test for MG.** Repetitive nerve stimulation reveals a **decremental** motor response, the correlate of clinical fatigability.

TREATMENT

- **Mild cases:** AChE inhibitors (eg, pyridostigmine) may be used but should be discontinued if the patient is on ventilator support, as the ↑ secretions ↑ the risk of aspiration.
- **Moderate to severe disease:** Treat with **immunomodulators** such as glucocorticoids, cytotoxic drugs (azathioprine), plasma exchange, and IVIG.
- **Thymectomy:** Patients require **chest imaging** to evaluate for thymic abnormalities, as 70% have hyperplasia and 10% have thymomas. Thymectomy is recommended for most patients < 60 years of age with generalized MG.

COMPLICATIONS

Myasthenic crisis:

- Presents with weakness with impending respiratory failure.
- It may be necessary to electively intubate the patient if **FVC** falls below 15 mL/kg.
- Plasmapheresis and IVIG both rapidly improve respiratory function and muscle strength, and either is the treatment of choice for myasthenic crisis.
- High-dose prednisone can transiently worsen symptoms in 30% of patients and may take several weeks before yielding clinical improvement, but it is safe if plasmapheresis is also being used for the initial treatment of crisis.

KEY FACT

The side effects of pyridostigmine include ↑ secretions and diarrhea; at high doses, weakness can occur that may mimic a myasthenic crisis.

KEY FACT

Myasthenia gravis is often associated with other autoimmune phenomena, such as thyroid disease, anemia from pure red cell aplasia, and thymomas.

Amyotrophic Lateral Sclerosis (ALS)

A 55-year-old woman presents with a six-month history of progressive left foot drop and slurred speech. On exam, she has weakness, fasciculations, and atrophy of the tongue, and her left foot is weak and atrophic with fasciculations. She has left ankle clonus and extensor plantar response with a normal sensory exam. What is the most likely diagnosis?

ALS is characterized by both upper motor neuron (UMN) signs (eg, hyperreflexia, spasticity, extensor plantar responses) and lower motor neuron (LMN) signs (eg, muscle atrophy, fasciculations, and weakness). Muscle weakness usually begins distally and asymmetrically in the upper or lower extremities or may be limited initially to the bulbar muscles, resulting in dysarthria and dysphagia.

KEY FACT

The hallmark of ALS is the combination of both upper and lower motor neuron signs and symptoms.

A progressive degenerative disease of the UMNs (arising in the motor cortex) and LMNs (arising in the brainstem and the anterior horn of the spinal cord). Affects males and females equally, with onset between 50 and 70 years of age. Life expectancy is 3–5 years, with death usually occurring 2° to aspiration pneumonia or respiratory failure. Five to ten percent of cases are familial. One genetic cause is autosomal dominant transmission of a mutation in the copper-zinc superoxide dismutase (SOD 1) gene on chromosome 21.

SYMPTOMS

- Presents with difficulty swallowing, nasal speech, "head drop" from weakness of the neck extensors, shortness of breath, "muscle twitches," muscle cramps, and progressive generalized weakness. Eye muscles are typically spared; bowel and bladder function is typically preserved.
- Frontotemporal dementia is common late in the disorder.

EXAM

- **UMN signs:** Spasticity (↑ muscle tone), hyperreflexia, ⊕ Babinski's sign.
- **LMN signs:** Atrophy (especially of the tongue and muscles of the hands); fasciculations (muscle twitches).

DIAGNOSIS

- **EMG/NCS** reveal evidence of widespread LMN injury (eg, fibrillations, **fasciculations**) and UMN injury that does not fall in a nerve root distribution. Sensory nerve studies are normal.
- **Spinal fluid** analysis is normal.
- **Cervical spine imaging** is normal.

TREATMENT

- **Riluzole,** a presumed glutamate antagonist, is the only FDA-approved medication for ALS. Improves survival by approximately six months.
- **Noninvasive positive-pressure ventilation** improves survival and should be considered if **FVC** falls to < 50% predicted.
- **Percutaneous gastrostomy tube placement** for patients with impaired swallowing and ↑ risk of aspiration.

Neuropathies

Table 13.11 reviews key features of common neuropathies.

POLYNEUROPATHIES

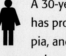

A 30-year-old man presents with numbness and tingling in both feet that has progressed over several days to gait instability, hand weakness, diplopia, and dyspnea. The symptoms started about a week after a viral illness. On exam, he cannot walk and is found to have proximal and distal weakness in the upper and lower extremities bilaterally, areflexia, and marked vibratory and position sense loss in the toes and fingers. What is the most likely diagnosis and the most appropriate treatment?

Guillain-Barré syndrome is characterized by proximal and distal weakness, distal sensory loss, autonomic symptoms, cranial nerve involvement, and respiratory failure in 25% of patients. Confirm with LP. Treatment is with IVIG or plasmapheresis.

TABLE 13.11. **Key Features of Common Neuropathies**

CLINICAL PRESENTATION	COMMON CAUSES	COMMENTS
Diabetic with sensory paresthesias in a "stocking glove" distribution	DM sensory polyneuropathy.	Often associated with retinopathy or nephropathy. Preventable with good glycemic control.
Wrist drop in an alcoholic who fell asleep while seated on a park bench	**Radial nerve mononeuropathy** from the arm hanging over the back of a bench (**"Saturday night palsy"**).	Usually improves with time and physical therapy.
Foot drop after prostatectomy or leg crossing	**Peroneal nerve mononeuropathy** from compression related to intraoperative positioning or leg positioning.	Same as above.
Weakness of right ankle dorsiflexion, then left hand extension, then other motor weakness	**Mononeuritis multiplex,** most commonly from **vasculitis** (eg, polyarteritis nodosa).	Biopsy of the affected nerve to confirm the diagnosis. Treat aggressively with anti-inflammatory or cytotoxic agents (eg, steroids, cyclophosphamide).
Impotence, orthostasis, dry mouth, and diarrhea	Autonomic neuropathy from diabetes, amyloid, porphyria, and many others.	When autonomic neuropathy is associated with parkinsonian features, think of multiple-system atrophy (does not respond as well to antiparkinsonian medications).
Bilateral lower extremity paresthesias with ascending weakness and areflexia	Demyelinating polyneuropathy: Guillain-Barré syndrome if acute; chronic inflammatory demyelinating polyneuropathy if chronic.	NCS show slowed conduction due to loss of myelin. Demyelination is often due to inflammation and is thus potentially reversible.
Paresthesias in a patient being treated for a ⊕ PPD; NCS show low amplitude	Axonal neuropathy from INH.	Treat with vitamin B_6 (pyridoxine).
Bilateral leg weakness, hyporeflexia, ↓ vibration sense, and macrocytosis	B_{12} deficiency.	Neurologic changes may not reverse with B_{12} treatment.
Fevers, altered mental status, and flaccid leg paralysis in late summer	West Nile virus, encephalomyelitis.	Flaccid weakness due to LMN injury from anterior horn cell injury.
A Brazilian man with areas of hypopigmented skin and loss of sensation over the distal extremity	Leprosy.	Eventually results in motor neuropathy (eg, claw hand or foot drop). Dapsone, in combination with other drugs, is the mainstay of treatment.

Guillain-Barré Syndrome (GBS)

A postinfectious autoimmune **acute demyelinating polyneuropathy.** Given the decline of polio, it is now the most common cause of acute flaccid paralysis. Look for prior GI illness caused by *Campylobacter jejuni,* as antibodies directed toward its bacterial lipopolysaccharide cross-react with peripheral nerve myelin.

KEY FACT

Miller-Fisher syndrome is a variant of GBS that produces ophthalmoplegia, ataxia, and areflexia of the upper extremities first. Anti-GQ1b antibodies support the diagnosis.

KEY FACT

Only 30% of patients with GBS report an antecedent illness.

KEY FACT

Critical illness polyneuropathy tends to occur in patients with multiorgan failure and sepsis and is characterized by generalized or distal flaccid paralysis, depressed or absent reflexes, ventilator dependence, distal sensory loss with sparing of cranial nerve function, and normal CSF studies.

SYMPTOMS

- Symptoms such as back pain or lower extremity paresthesias typically begin 1–2 weeks after the infection, followed by **symmetric weakness that begins in the feet** and gradually ascends over hours to days, in many cases leading to respiratory failure.
- Autonomic symptoms are prominent, and cardiac instability can be life-threatening.

EXAM

Cardinal features on exam are **areflexia** and **symmetric progressive weakness**.

DIAGNOSIS

- CSF shows "albuminocytologic dissociation"—**isolated elevated protein** with normal WBC counts.
- NCS reveal demyelinating changes (slow conduction velocities) of the proximal peripheral nerves.
- Serial PFTs with **maximum inspiratory force** and **FVC** are important for following diaphragmatic function, which often portends ventilatory failure.

TREATMENT

- Standard treatment is either **IVIG** or **plasmapheresis; steroids are not beneficial.** Mechanical ventilation should be considered when FVC falls to ≤ 15 mL/kg. Keep patients with autonomic symptoms on **cardiac telemetry.**
- Avoid IVIG in renal insufficiency, CHF, or IgA deficiency. Avoid plasmapheresis in those with labile BPs or infection.

Chronic Inflammatory Demyelinating Polyneuropathy (CIDP)

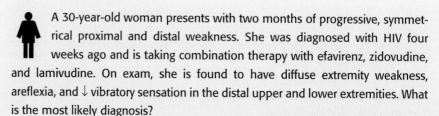

A 30-year-old woman presents with two months of progressive, symmetrical proximal and distal weakness. She was diagnosed with HIV four weeks ago and is taking combination therapy with efavirenz, zidovudine, and lamivudine. On exam, she is found to have diffuse extremity weakness, areflexia, and ↓ vibratory sensation in the distal upper and lower extremities. What is the most likely diagnosis?

CIDP is clinically similar to GBS initially except that symptoms progress for at least eight weeks. Like GBS, CIDP is characterized by proximal and distal weakness, areflexia, and distal sensory loss. In contrast, toxic neuropathies may also present acutely but are generally axonal and present with distal sensory loss and weakness with loss of the Achilles tendon reflexes only (rather than diffuse areflexia).

- A symmetric demyelinating disease of peripheral nerves that is characterized by proximal and distal weakness, areflexia, and distal sensory loss.
- **Sx/Exam:** Related to but distinct from **GBS**, as both share similar clinical and pathologic findings (including areflexia, weakness, ↑ CSF protein, and demyelination). CIDP, however, has **no associated antecedent illness** and evolves over **weeks to months**, often with a **relapsing and remitting** course.
- **Tx:** As for GBS, CIDP typically responds to IVIG or plasmapheresis.

Charcot-Marie-Tooth Disease (Hereditary Sensorimotor Neuropathy)

- Characterized by a strongly ⊕ family history; usually autosomal dominant. The most common inherited neurologic disorder. Life expectancy is normal despite morbidity from progressive weakness.
- **Sx/Exam:** Symptoms begin in the first and second decades, usually with distal weakness in the legs and clumsiness. Patients have **"inverted champagne bottle" legs;** high-arched feet (pes cavus) and hammer toes; progressive atrophy and weakness of the hands and feet; distal sensory loss; and ↓ or absent reflexes.
- **Tx:** No treatment is currently available.

Diabetic Neuropathy

- Diabetes is the most common cause of peripheral neuropathy in the United States. Ten percent of diabetics develop neuropathy, usually associated with retinopathy and nephropathy.
- **Sx/Exam:** Starts with paresthesias and pain in the feet and progresses to **stocking-glove distribution** of sensory and motor deficits. Can also affect autonomic nerves.
- **Tx:** Prevention depends on tight glycemic control. Neuropathic pain symptoms (burning, pain) can be treated with TCAs such as amitriptyline, SSRIs, or anticonvulsants such as gabapentin or carbamazepine.

Metabolic/Infectious Neuropathies

- Many insidious and chronic polyneuropathies are **metabolic** in nature, with common causes being nutritional deficiencies (eg, vitamin B_{12}), toxin exposure (eg, alcohol), and drug exposure (eg, vincristine, INH, dapsone).
- Many **infections** can also cause indolent polyneuropathies, including HIV and HSV; leprosy (Hansen's disease, caused by *Mycobacterium leprae*) remains one of the most common causes of polyneuropathy worldwide.

MONONEUROPATHIES

Carpal Tunnel Syndrome

- Caused by compression of the **median nerve** at the flexor retinaculum of the wrist. Risk factors include repetitive hand-finger activities such as typing.
- **Sx:** Classic symptoms include progressive wrist pain; awakening at night with hand numbness; and paresthesias and weakness of the thumb and index finger.
- **Exam:** Findings include the following:
    - **Atrophy of the thenar eminence** (the palmar muscle bulk at the base of the thumb), weakness of thumb opposition, and sensory abnormalities of the thumb and index finger.
    - **Phalen's sign:** Hyperflexion of the wrists leading to ↑ paresthesias.
    - **Tinel's sign:** Tapping over the median nerve at the level of the wrist eliciting electrical sensations along the thumb and index finger.
- **Dx:** NCS show median nerve abnormalities at the wrist.
- **Tx:** Options include immobilization with wrist splints, NSAIDs, local steroid injections, and surgical release at the wrist.

KEY FACT

Patients with carpal tunnel syndrome often have ↑ symptoms at night that are relieved by shaking or wringing of the hands.

Radial Nerve Palsy

- Typically results from acute injury to the nerve in the spiral groove of the humerus, most commonly by **fracture of the humerus** or direct compression of the nerve ("**Saturday night palsy**").
- **Sx/Exam:** The most prominent symptom is "**wrist drop**"; weakness of elbow extension (triceps) is also common.
- **Dx:** NCS help identify the exact location and extent of the injury.
- **Tx:** Treatment is mainly supportive. **Wrist splints** may temporarily restore function.

Ulnar Neuropathy

- An overuse injury commonly **caused by repetitive elbow flexion** leading to trauma or compression at the elbow, particularly near the medial epicondyle. Common among thin women.
- **Sx/Exam:** Paresthesias of the **fourth and fifth fingers** and weakness of the muscles that spread the fingers apart; in its most chronic form, resembles a "**claw hand**."
- **Tx: Splinting the elbow** at night is first-line treatment and is most helpful in conjunction with NSAIDs if there is pain. Surgical release or transposition of the nerve near the elbow is often tried but is not always beneficial.

Peroneal Nerve Compression

- **Sx/Exam:** Compression of the **peroneal nerve** near the fibular head produces a "**foot drop**" 2° to weakness of foot dorsiflexors, as well as paresthesias along the lateral aspect of the lower leg. Compression can be 2° to frequent leg crossing, trauma, or local masses (eg, cysts).
- **Tx:** Involves identifying the risk factors for compression, initiating physical therapy, and using an ankle-foot orthosis; surgery is occasionally needed when a local mass is identified as the etiology of compression.

Bell's Palsy

- An acute-onset, unilateral paralysis of CN VII (the **facial nerve**). Although a clear cause generally cannot be identified, HSV or its associated immune response is often implicated. Vesicles in the ear are a clue that VZV is the cause. Can also occur in Lyme disease and acute HIV.
- **Sx/Exam:**
  - **The upper and lower halves of one side of the face are affected**, resulting in inability to fully close the eye or move the mouth on that side (see Figure 13.13). By contrast, facial weakness from a central cause (eg, a stroke) typically spares the upper half of the face, producing unilateral lower facial weakness.
  - May also present with loss of taste, salivation, lacrimation, and hyperacusis.
  - **Ramsay Hunt syndrome** presents with unilateral facial paralysis associated with herpetic blisters in the external auditory canal.
- **Tx:**
  - Treatment of idiopathic Bell's palsy with **prednisone** shortens the course and improves function if started within seven days of onset of symptoms. Combined treatment with prednisone and acyclovir may enhance recovery (vs. treatment with prednisone alone), but recent studies have shown no clear benefit from the addition of antivirals; monotherapy with antivirals provides no benefit over placebo therapy.
  - Eye protection (artificial tears; use of an eye patch at night) is crucial for preventing corneal abrasions.

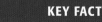

KEY FACT

If a patient presents with a facial droop, look for upper facial weakness. If the upper face is also weak, the lesion is peripheral (eg, Bell's palsy). If the upper face is normal, the lesion is central (eg, stroke).

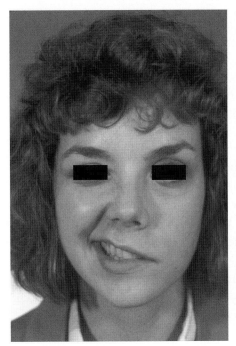 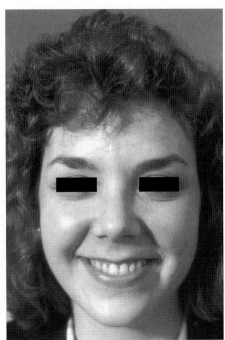

A   B

FIGURE 13.13. **Prototypic Bell's palsy.** (A) A 28-year-old female with acute-onset left facial paralysis involving the entire left face. She was treated with oral steroids. (B) The same patient following a full recovery two months after symptom onset. (Reproduced with permission from Lalwani AS. *Current Diagnosis & Treatment in Otolaryngology—Head & Neck Surgery,* 2nd ed. New York: McGraw-Hill, 2008, Fig. 68-1.)

TABLE 13.12. **Key Features of Neurologic Paraneoplastic Syndromes**

SYNDROME	KEY FEATURES	UNDERLYING CANCER	ASSOCIATED ANTIBODY
Lambert-Eaton myasthenic syndrome	Fluctuating muscle weakness that spares the eyes and improves on repetitive muscle testing. Autonomic symptoms are common, and reflexes are ↓.	Small cell lung cancer.	Anti-voltage-gated calcium channel.
Subacute cerebellar degeneration	Middle-aged women with subacute onset of slurred speech, ataxia, and limb incoordination.	Ovarian or breast cancer.	Anti-Yo (Purkinje cells).
Limbic encephalitis	Subacute behavioral problems, memory difficulties, and focal-onset seizures (see Figure 13.14). Resembles HSV encephalitis, but HSV is more acute in onset.	Small cell lung cancer.	Anti-Hu.
Sensory neuronopathy	Slowly progressive sensory loss that first affects the lower extremities. Exam shows areflexia and incoordination related to loss of proprioception.	Small cell lung cancer.	Anti-Hu.
Opsoclonus-myoclonus	**Opsoclonus:** Involuntary, erratic, rapid jerking of the eyes in either the horizontal or the vertical direction. **Myoclonus: Brief, jerklike contractions.**	Breast cancer or neuroblastoma (children).	Anti-Ri.

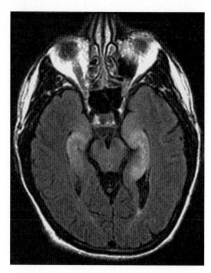

FIGURE 13.14. Limbic encephalitis. MR image from a FLAIR sequence shows symmetric increased signal in the mesial temporal lobes. (Reproduced with permission from Fauci AS et al. *Harrison's Principles of Internal Medicine,* 17th ed. New York: McGraw-Hill, 2008, Fig. 97-2.)

Paraneoplastic Syndromes

A 50-year-old man presents with rapid cognitive decline over the past two months. He has gotten lost in familiar places; has been unable to drive following several minor accidents; and has been neglecting his housework and finances. He has also had numerous episodes of unresponsive staring with lip smacking followed by brief periods of confusion. He has a 60-pack-year history of smoking. On exam, the patient is found to be disheveled and confused, and his MMSE is 23/30 (missing points on orientation and recall). MRI shows symmetric areas of abnormal T2 signal bilaterally in the hippocampus (mesial temporal lobes) with minimal enhancement with gadolinium and no mass effect. What is the most likely diagnosis?

Paraneoplastic limbic encephalitis most commonly associated with small cell lung cancer, and characterized by rapidly progressive cognitive decline in short-term memory and seizures. The anti-Hu antibody is most closely associated.

Neurologic paraneoplastic syndromes may be due to antibodies that cross-react with specific neuronal populations (see Table 13.12).

CHAPTER 14

Oncology

Miten Vasa, MD

Jonathan E. Rosenberg, MD

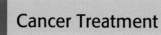

Cancer Treatment

CHEMOTHERAPEUTIC AGENTS

Patterns of Toxicity

Table 14.1 outlines common and serious toxicities of various chemotherapeutic agents. All chemotherapies can cause bone marrow suppression and nausea/vomiting.

TABLE 14.1. Toxicities of Common Chemotherapeutic Agents

DRUG	SIDE EFFECTS	MONITORING REQUIRED
Alkylators (cyclophosphamide, ifosfamide)	**Hemorrhagic cystitis,** neurotoxicity (ifosfamide), severe nausea/vomiting.	UA to monitor for hematuria; **mesna** to bind to toxic metabolite (acrolein).
Anthracyclines (doxorubicin, epirubicin, idarubicin, mitoxantrone)	Dose-dependent **cardiac toxicity** (CHF), nausea/vomiting, bone marrow suppression.	Baseline echocardiogram and echocardiogram after a specified amount of chemotherapy (eg, 300 mg/m² for doxorubicin).
Bleomycin	**Pulmonary fibrosis.**	Baseline PFTs.
Capecitabine	**Hand-foot syndrome** (painful erythema and desquamation of skin on the palms and soles).	No special monitoring.
Cytarabine	Neurotoxicity, rash.	Cerebellar exam prior to each dose; steroids if rash is severe.
5-fluorouracil (5-FU)	**Hand-foot syndrome.**	No special monitoring.
Gemcitabine	**Rare interstitial fibrosis.**	No special monitoring.
Irinotecan	Diarrhea.	Administer with Lomotil.
Methotrexate	Renal failure; hepatic enzyme elevation.	Check for effusions before administration (clearance is slowed if they are present, increasing the risk of renal failure). LFT monitoring is required.
Platinums (carboplatin, cisplatin)	**Neuropathy,** ototoxicity, renal failure, potassium and magnesium wasting, severe nausea/vomiting (cisplatin).	Monitor renal function; conduct a neurologic exam prior to each dose. Conduct an audiologic exam at baseline (cisplatin only) if the patient has any hearing complaints.
Taxanes (docetaxel, paclitaxel)	Allergic reactions, fluid retention, **neuropathy.**	**Premedicate with steroids.**
Vinca alkaloids (vinblastine, vincristine)	**Neuropathy** (including motor neuropathy) with **severe constipation.**	Determine if the patient has had a bowel movement within 48 hours of a dose.

Targeted Therapies

Novel agents or standard treatments that have a specific molecular target and often have fewer and less severe side effects than conventional chemotherapy. Modalities include hormonal therapy, cytokines, monoclonal antibodies, and small molecules that target enzymes. Monoclonal antibodies are often combined with standard chemotherapeutic regimens. Table 14.2 outlines common targeted therapies and their indications.

TABLE 14.2. Common Targeted Therapies and Their Uses

DRUG	APPLICATION	SIDE EFFECTS
HORMONAL AGENTS		
GnRH agonists (goserelin, leuprolide)	Androgen deprivation for prostate cancer.	**Osteoporosis, hot flashes, anemia, weight gain.**
Tamoxifen	Adjuvant therapy for breast cancer.	As above, but **without osteoporosis.**
Aromatase inhibitors (anastrozole, letrozole, exemestane)	Adjuvant therapy for breast cancer.	As above, **with osteoporosis.**
TYROSINE KINASE INHIBITORS		
Erlotinib (EGFR inhibitor)	Non–small cell lung cancer (NSCLC).	**Acneiform rash;** rare pulmonary fibrosis.
Imatinib (BCR-ABL tyrosine kinase inhibitor)	CML, gastrointestinal stromal tumor (GIST).	Edema, transaminitis.
Sorafenib (VEGF inhibitor)	Renal cell carcinoma.	**Diarrhea, rash, hand-foot syndrome, hypertension.**
Sunitinib (VEGF inhibitor)	Renal cell carcinoma, GIST.	**Diarrhea, rash, hypothyroidism.**
Pazopanib (VEGF inhibitor)	Renal cell carcinoma.	**Hypertension, hepatotoxicity.**
CYTOKINES		
Interferon	CML, melanoma, renal cell carcinoma.	**Depression** with suicidal ideation; **bone marrow suppression.**
Interleukin-2	Renal cell carcinoma, melanoma.	**Hypotension, renal failure, edema.**

(continues)

TABLE 14.2. **Common Targeted Therapies and Their Uses** *(continued)*

Drug	Application	Side Effects
Monoclonal Antibodies		
Alemtuzumab (anti-CD52 antibody)	CLL.	Bone marrow suppression.
Bevacizumab (VEGF inhibitor)	Metastatic colorectal cancer, NSCLC.	**Bleeding, hypertension, proteinuria.**
Cetuximab (EGFR inhibitor)	Head and neck cancer, metastatic colorectal cancer.	**Acneiform rash.**
Gemtuzumab (anti-CD33 antibody)	Relapsed AML.	Bone marrow suppression.
Rituximab (anti-CD20 antibody)	B-cell lymphomas.	**Allergic reactions.**
Trastuzumab (HER2/neu antibody)	Breast cancer with HER2/neu overexpression.	**Cardiac toxicity (CHF).**

PRINCIPLES OF ONCOLOGY

Combination Regimens

- Allow for maximum cell kill with less toxicity.
- Prevent cross-resistance (different drugs lead to different mechanisms of resistance).
- Synergistic effects between drugs with nonoverlapping toxicities.

Response to Therapy

- **Complete response:** Disappearance of all evidence of disease for at least four weeks.
- **Partial response: Reduction by at least 30%** of the sum of the largest diameter of all measurable lesions with no new disease appearing, maintained for at least four weeks.
- **Progressive disease:** Growth of existing disease by 20% of the sum of the largest diameter of all measurable lesions, or new lesions during treatment.

Chemotherapy Resistance

- **MDR1:** The multidrug resistance gene; encodes a pump that removes toxins from cancer cells.
- **Drug-specific resistance mechanisms:** Involve upregulation of downstream enzymes, antiapoptotic proteins, and the like.

Adjuvant and Neoadjuvant Chemotherapy

- **Adjuvant chemotherapy:** Chemotherapy given **after surgery** to ↓ the risk of recurrence.
- **Neoadjuvant chemotherapy:** Chemotherapy given **before surgery** to make resection easier and ↓ recurrence by targeting micrometastases.

RADIATION THERAPY

Mechanism of Action

- Radiation induces ionization in biological tissues that damages DNA (cancer cells are less capable of repair than normal cells).
- Side effects include the following:
  - **CNS:** Memory loss, confusion, personality changes, anorexia, lethargy.
  - **GI tract:** Nausea, mucositis, dry mouth.
  - **Hematologic:** Bone marrow suppression, leukemia.
  - **Musculoskeletal:** Osteonecrosis (classically of the jaw; risk ↑ with dental work).
  - **Pulmonary:** Fibrosis.
  - **Skin:** Desquamation, hair loss, scarring.
  - **Spinal cord:** Paralysis (rare).

Methods of Administration

- **External beam radiation therapy:** The most commonly used modality. Toxicities can be minimized through use of the following:
  - **Conformal radiation therapy:** Shaping the radiation beam to precisely fit the tumor outline.
  - **Intensity-modulated radiation therapy:** Shaping the intensity of the radiation beam.
- **Brachytherapy (implants):** The radiation source (in the form of **seeds**) is implanted within the tumor. Most often used in the treatment of **prostate cancer.**
- **Stereotactic radiosurgery:** A three-dimensional technique that delivers the radiation dose in one session, with a high dose of radiation delivered to a very small volume. Used primarily for treating brain tumors to prevent toxicity of whole brain radiation.

SURGICAL ONCOLOGY

- Surgery may be employed to diagnose (through biopsy of lymph node or soft tissue mass) or to treat. Surgical treatment may be curative or palliative.
- Resection is predicated on the ability to achieve ⊖ margins, usually with at least 1 cm of normal tissue if possible (or more in special circumstances).
- **Debulking,** or removal of tumor without obtaining ⊖ margins, plays a role in diseases such as **ovarian cancer.**
- Direct manipulation of tumor is avoided where possible to prevent local recurrence.

Oncologic Emergencies

SUPERIOR VENA CAVA (SVC) SYNDROME

Compression of the SVC by tumor or thrombosis of the SVC.

SYMPTOMS/EXAM

- Presents with facial edema or erythema, shortness of breath, orthopnea, hoarseness, headaches due to increasing ICP, and arm or neck swelling.
- Exam reveals edema of the face, tongue, neck, and arms; dilation of upper body veins; and plethora of the face.

KEY FACT

Cancer and thrombosis cause most cases of SVC syndrome; lung cancer and non-Hodgkin's lymphoma account for most cases of SVC syndrome that are due to cancer.

DIAGNOSIS

CT of the chest and neck, Doppler ultrasound, CXR. **Lack of lower extremity edema distinguishes SVC syndrome from right-sided heart failure.**

TREATMENT

- **Corticosteroids and diuretics** provide symptomatic relief from edema and dyspnea.
- Initiate **radiotherapy or chemotherapy** depending on the malignancy.
- Institute thrombolytic therapy, stent, or anticoagulation if due to thrombosis.

COMPLICATIONS

Laryngeal and cerebral edema are life-threatening complications.

SPINAL CORD COMPRESSION

Affects 1–5% of patients with metastatic cancer. Diagnostic and treatment delays are associated with paralysis and loss of bladder and bowel control.

SYMPTOMS

- **Early:** Presents with pain localized to the spine or radicular pain due to nerve root compression. Pain is exacerbated with movement, coughing, lying down, sneezing, or Valsalva/straining. **Pain generally precedes functional loss by weeks to months.**
- **Late:** Muscle weakness, sensory loss/sensory level, urinary retention, constipation, sphincter dysfunction, paralysis, autonomic dysfunction.

EXAM

- Tenderness to palpation or percussion over the affected area of the spine.
- Focal neurologic findings, UMN signs, abnormal plantar responses, sensory loss, rectal tone.
- **Cauda equina syndrome** refers to compression of the cauda equina (below L1), but the physiology and treatment are the same as those for cord compression.

DIAGNOSIS

- **Plain films are not helpful in ruling out cord compression.**
- **MRI is the gold standard for diagnosis** (see Figure 14.1). Gadolinium enhances the ability to visualize epidural metastases without bony involvement.
- If MRI is unavailable, myelography, CT, or CT myelography can confirm the diagnosis.

TREATMENT

- The outcome depends on rapid assessment and diagnosis.
- If patients can walk at diagnosis, they will likely preserve their function with appropriate treatment.
- Early steroid administration ↓ swelling and pressure on the cord. Administer high-dose bolus dexamethasone 10 mg IV followed by 4–10 mg PO/IV q 6 h.
- Definitive treatment options include immediate surgical decompression, radiation therapy (for radiation-sensitive malignancies), or, rarely, chemotherapy. **Consult neurosurgery, radiation oncology, and oncology early.**

KEY FACT

Spinal cord compression should be considered in any patient with bilateral motor and sensory dysfunction in the extremities in the absence of any signs or symptoms of brain or brainstem dysfunction.

KEY FACT

Vertebral metastases are most frequently found in the thoracic spine (60% of cases), followed by the lumbosacral (30%) and cervical spine (10%).

KEY FACT

Back pain is the cardinal symptom of spinal cord compression. Thus, a patient with a history of cancer who develops new back pain should be suspected of having vertebral metastases until proven otherwise. MRI is the imaging study of choice.

MNEMONIC

Tumors that commonly metastasize to bone–

BLT with Mayo, Mustard, and Kosher Pickle

Breast
Lung
Thyroid
Multiple **M**yeloma
Kidney (renal cell)
Prostate

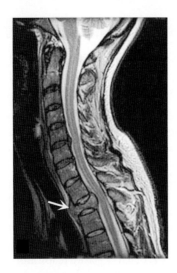

FIGURE 14.1. Spinal cord compression. Sagittal T2-weighted MRI in a patient with breast cancer shows an infiltrated and collapsed T2 vertebral body (arrow), with bony retropulsion compressing the spinal cord at this level. (Reproduced with permission from Fauci AS et al. *Harrison's Principles of Internal Medicine,* 17th ed. New York: McGraw-Hill, 2008, Fig. 372-2B.)

TUMOR LYSIS SYNDROME

Rapid release of intracellular contents due to rapid lysis of cancer cells with life-threatening metabolic consequences. **Most commonly found in rapidly progressing acute leukemias and lymphomas** (particularly Burkitt's lymphoma and ALL), especially after the initial doses of chemotherapy, but can also occur spontaneously. Rarely seen in solid tumors.

SYMPTOMS/EXAM

- **Hyperuricemia, hyperkalemia, hyperphosphatemia, hypocalcemia** (the excess phosphate binds calcium).
- A markedly ↑ LDH points to a risk of tumor lysis.
- May lead to oliguric renal failure.

DIAGNOSIS

Closely monitor serum laboratory values, including potassium, uric acid, calcium, phosphorus, and creatinine (q 4 h initially; then as clinically indicated).

TREATMENT

- Identify patients at risk before starting chemotherapy.
- Urine is often alkalinized with sodium bicarbonate infusion, although supportive evidence for this common practice is lacking.
- Allopurinol should be started before chemotherapy to ↓ the level of hyperuricemia (monitor for changes in creatinine clearance and adjust the dose if necessary).
- Treatment is directed at managing electrolyte abnormalities, maintaining adequate hydration, and instituting dialysis if necessary.
- Consider the use of **uricase,** an expensive enzyme that metabolizes uric acid, in cases of severe tumor lysis (generally considered when uric acid levels are > 10 mg/dL).

KEY FACT

Calcium is **low** in tumor lysis syndrome because excess phosphate binds calcium. Potassium, uric acid, phosphorus, and LDH are ↑.

KEY FACT

IV fluids and allopurinol given prior to the initiation of chemotherapy are critical to preventing tumor lysis syndrome.

NEUTROPENIC FEVER

Generally defined as a fever of $\geq 38.3°C$ with an absolute neutrophil count (ANC) of $\leq 500/\mu L$. An ANC of $< 100/\mu L$ carries the highest risk of rapidly fatal infection. Etiologies are as follows:

- **Bacteria** (gram-$\ominus$ bacilli, gram-$\oplus$ cocci): The most commonly implicated pathogens; increasing in incidence as a result of the growing use of indwelling catheters. **Coagulase-$\ominus$ staphylococci are now the most common cause of bacteremia.**
- **Fungal infections:** More common in patients on broad-spectrum antibacterial therapy, those on corticosteroids, or those with prolonged neutropenia such as that following allogeneic bone marrow transplant. The most common fungal pathogens are *Candida* and *Aspergillus*.
- **Viruses:** Viral infections occurring during neutropenia include the herpesviruses (CMV, HSV, VZV, EBV) and respiratory viruses (RSV, influenza A and B, parainfluenza, rhinovirus, adenovirus).

EXAM

Physical examination is directed at uncovering potential sources of infection and should focus on venous access sites and examination of the oropharynx, lungs, abdomen, and skin.

DIAGNOSIS

- Obtain two sets of blood cultures, a urine culture, a culture of any catheter or catheter drainage, and a CXR.
- Additional evaluation is dictated by signs and symptoms.

TREATMENT

- **Initial empiric antibiotic therapy:** Administer broad-spectrum antibiotics covering gram-$\ominus$ bacilli (including *Pseudomonas*), taking into account local drug resistance patterns.
- **Monotherapy:** Ceftazidime, cefepime, imipenem-cilastatin, meropenem, piperacillin-tazobactam.
- **Combination therapy:** An aminoglycoside plus antipseudomonal penicillin +/– β-lactamase inhibitors.
- **Vancomycin:** Generally not used as part of first-line empiric therapy except under the following conditions:
  - In the presence of a central line that appears infected.
  - If blood culture shows gram-$\oplus$ cocci.
  - In the setting of known colonization with MRSA.
  - In the presence of hypotension or sepsis with no identified pathogen.
  - If the patient was receiving fluoroquinolones or TMP-SMX as prophylaxis prior to the onset of neutropenic fever.
- **G-CSF/GM-CSF:** Not routinely beneficial, but may be considered in the setting of pneumonia, invasive fungal infection, or progressive infection.
- **Duration of treatment:**
  - Generally, broad-spectrum therapy must continue until the ANC recovers to $\geq 500/\mu L$ and the patient is afebrile for 48 hours.
  - If fever resolves and no organism is identified but the patient remains neutropenic, IV broad-spectrum antibiotics should be continued for at least seven days; then consider switching to oral medications.
  - If fever is unresponsive after 3–5 days, consider adding vancomycin and/or antifungals.

Breast Cancer

> A 55-year-old postmenopausal woman was recently diagnosed with lymph node–⊖, ER-⊖, PR-⊕ breast cancer and was treated with wide surgical excision and radiation therapy. She had a hysterectomy 10 years ago for uterine fibroids, but her ovaries remain intact. She also has osteopenia, for which she has been treated with raloxifene for the past two years. Her exam is normal. What is the most appropriate next step in management?
>
> Start adjuvant therapy with an aromatase inhibitor, as this class of drugs is more effective than tamoxifen in preventing breast cancer recurrence in post-menopausal women. This patient's risk of distant recurrence outside the breast over the next 10–15 years is almost 15%. Furthermore, since she was already on a selective estrogen receptor modulator (SERM) when her breast cancer developed, it is unlikely that tamoxifen would be of benefit.

The risk of breast cancer ↑ with age. The lifetime risk for women is roughly 1 in 10. Seventy-five percent of patients with breast cancer have no identifiable risk factors. Known risk factors are as follows:

- **Genetic syndromes:** For most patients, no identified genetic predisposition exists. Those with a genetic predisposition should be screened beginning at least 10 years before the earliest-onset cancer in the family history.
    - **BRCA1:** Associated with a dramatic risk of breast cancer (56–85% lifetime risk), ovarian cancer (15–45% lifetime risk), and prostate cancer (less frequent). Has an autosomal dominant inheritance; Ashkenazi Jews are at highest risk.
    - **BRCA2:** Associated with breast and ovarian cancer as well as with pancreatic cancer and melanoma. **BRCA1 and BRCA2 account for 50% of all inherited breast cancers.**
    - **Li-Fraumeni syndrome:** Breast cancer along with sarcomas, brain tumors, leukemia, lymphoma, and adrenal cancer.
- **Other risk factors:** Include a family history of early-age breast cancer diagnosis in family members, early menarche, late menopause, obesity, nulliparity or late age at first pregnancy, use of estrogen replacement therapy, and OCP use (controversial).

DIFFERENTIAL

Fibrocystic disease, fibroadenoma, atypical hyperplasia, abscess, adenosis, scars, mastitis. Note that no changes in screening intervals are recommended for these findings.

DIAGNOSIS

- Breast cysts can be evaluated with ultrasound and can then be aspirated.
- Breast masses require either fine-needle aspiration (FNA) or core needle biopsy, possibly followed by excisional biopsy.
- **Any mass that is felt on exam must be further evaluated with biopsy even if no abnormality is seen on mammogram** (the sensitivity of mammography is 75–90%, with more false ⊖s found on the denser breast tissue of younger women).

KEY FACT

Genetic syndromes markedly ↑ the risk for breast cancer, although they account for a minority of cases of breast cancer.

KEY FACT

Inflammatory breast cancer is an aggressive form of breast cancer that is characterized by thickened skin (peau d'orange) and is usually accompanied by dermal lymphatic invasion. Breast conservation (lumpectomy) is generally considered inappropriate for local control.

- Algorithm: Palpated mass → mammogram and/or breast ultrasound → biopsy (or aspiration if the lesion is thought to be a cyst) (see also Figure 14.2).
- **Breast MRI:** Has higher sensitivity but much lower specificity than mammography. Currently has two main uses: (1) for screening very high risk women who elect not to have prophylactic surgery; and (2) for evaluating patients with axillary lymph node metastases whose breasts are found to be normal by physical exam and mammography.

TREATMENT

Treatment of **early-stage breast cancer** is as follows:

- **Ductal carcinoma in situ (DCIS):** A premalignant condition that is at high risk of turning into a cancer. Treatment involves excision with ⊖ margins **(lumpectomy) and radiation therapy** to the breast, often with the addition of tamoxifen.
- **Lobular carcinoma in situ (LCIS):** A condition associated with an ↑ risk of breast cancer arising **elsewhere** in **both** breasts. Treatment with tamoxifen may be considered, but close follow-up and observation are indicated.
- **Invasive ductal or lobular carcinoma:**
  - Lumpectomy followed by radiation therapy is equivalent to mastectomy in terms of overall survival, but the risk of local recurrence is lower with mastectomy. Reexcision, often followed by radiation, is indicated in patients with ⊕ tumor margins that are detected after breast-conserving surgery.
  - **Sentinel lymph node biopsy** involves injecting dye or tracer in the tumor and identifying which lymph node takes it up. The node or nodes are then excised and assessed for metastasis. Complete axillary node dissection is warranted only in sentinel node–⊕ or clinically node-⊕ tumors.
  - Mastectomy is appropriate for large or multifocal tumors, for patients with a strong family history, or in accordance with patient preference.

> **KEY FACT**
>
> At the time of surgery for breast cancer, complete axillary node dissection is warranted only in sentinel node–⊕ or clinically node-⊕ tumors.

> **KEY FACT**
>
> DCIS is a premalignant condition that should be treated with lumpectomy and radiation therapy.

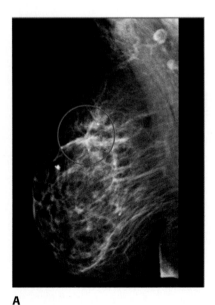
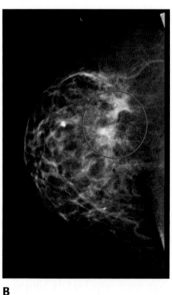
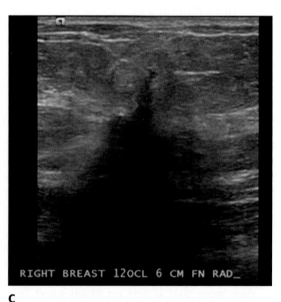

A   B   C

FIGURE 14.2.   Breast cancer. Mediolateral oblique (**A**) and craniocaudal (**B**) views from a mammogram demonstrate a spiculated mass with a satellite mass (circle) in the central and outer upper right breast. A targeted breast ultrasound (**C**) in a different patient demonstrates a hypoechoic mass (arrow) that is taller than it is wide and demonstrates dense posterior acoustic shadowing. (Reproduced with permission from USMLERx. com.)

- **Adjuvant therapy:** Guidelines for the use of adjuvant therapy are as follows:
  - In general, any patient with an **infiltrating** ductal or lobular cancer > **1 cm** or with ⊕ **lymph nodes** should receive adjuvant therapy.
  - Hormone therapy with **tamoxifen** (for **five years**) or an **aromatase inhibitor** is effective **only in patients with ER- or PR-⊕** breast cancers. Aromatase inhibitors should be used only in postmenopausal patients.
  - For ER/PR-⊖ tumors, **chemotherapy** is the recommended adjuvant treatment. For ER- or PR-⊕ tumors, chemotherapy may be needed in addition to hormonal therapy.

Treatment of **advanced (metastatic) breast cancer** is as follows:

- **First-line treatment:** For ER/PR-⊕ postmenopausal women, first-line treatment consists of an aromatase inhibitor.
  - Aromatase inhibitors prevent the conversion of adrenal androgens into estrogens by targeting aromatase enzymes in muscle and fat, resulting in nearly complete elimination of estrogen production.
  - Associated with hot flashes, bone density loss, and sexual dysfunction. These symptoms can be alleviated or ↓ with SSRIs, calcium/vitamin D supplementation, and nonhormonal vaginal lubricants.
- **Second-line hormonal therapy:** For ER/PR-⊕ women, second-line therapy includes tamoxifen, a SERM.
- **Second-line nonhormonal therapy:** If patients progress or are **hormone receptor** ⊖, treat with **chemotherapy.** Active drugs include paclitaxel, docetaxel, doxorubicin, methotrexate, vinorelbine, capecitabine, and 5-FU.
- **Patients with overexpression of HER2:**
  - Comprise 10% of patients with breast cancer.
  - Associated with a poorer prognosis.
  - May respond to trastuzumab (Herceptin), a humanized monoclonal antibody against the HER2 receptor.

PREVENTION

See the discussion of cancer screening in the Ambulatory Medicine chapter.

Lung Cancer

Smoking cessation is the best means of preventing 1° and recurrent lung cancer. Eighty-seven percent of all cases of lung cancer are related to smoking, with the risk significantly higher in patients who have been exposed to asbestos and who also smoke. Lung cancer presents with weight loss, cough, hemoptysis, fatigue, recurrent bronchitis, and chest pain. It is divided into two categories on the basis of pathology: non–small cell lung cancer (NSCLC) and small cell lung cancer (SCLC).

NON–SMALL CELL LUNG CANCER (NSCLC)

The most common type of lung cancer. Has multiple histologies (bronchoalveolar, adenocarcinoma, and squamous), all with the same treatment and natural history. **Accurate staging is key to determining the appropriate therapy.**

DIAGNOSIS

CXR, CT of the chest and abdomen (see Figure 14.3), blood work (including a liver panel); possibly a PET scan.

KEY FACT

For breast cancers that are either ER or PR ⊕, hormonal therapy (with tamoxifen or aromatase inhibitors) is superior to chemotherapy. Tamoxifen and aromatase inhibitors are effective only in patients with ER-⊕ and/or PR-⊕ tumors. Adjuvant therapy for breast cancer should be given to patients with an **infiltrating** ductal or lobular cancer > **1 cm** or with ⊕ **lymph nodes.**

KEY FACT

HER2 is overexpressed in only 10% of breast cancers and confers a poorer prognosis. Treatment should include trastuzumab, a monoclonal antibody against the HER2 receptor.

KEY FACT

Tamoxifen is the only FDA-approved drug for the 1° prevention of breast cancer, resulting in 50% risk reduction in pre- and postmenopausal women who have an ↑ risk for this disease.

KEY FACT

Squamous cell cancers cause hypercalcemia due to the secretion of parathyroid hormone–related protein (PTHrP). Such cancers can also cavitate.

KEY FACT

NSCLC with a malignant pleural effusion is stage IIIB and is unresectable.

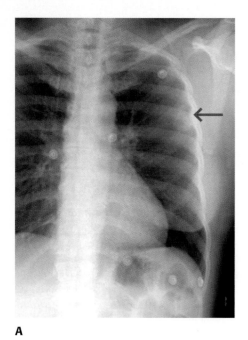

A

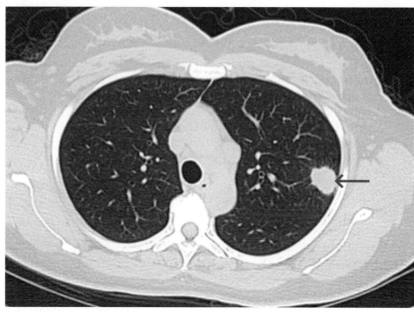

B

FIGURE 14.3. **Non–small cell lung cancer.** Lung adenocarcinoma (arrows) on frontal CXR (**A**) and CT (**B**). (Reproduced with permission from USMLERx.com.)

KEY FACT

Bevacizumab, a VEGF inhibitor, is a new monoclonal antibody sometimes used to treat metastatic NSCLC.

KEY FACT

Bronchioloalveolar cell carcinoma responds uniquely to erlotinib (an epidermal growth factor receptor inhibitor).

TREATMENT

- Treat according to stage:
    - **Stage I or II:** Consider surgical resection.
    - **Stage IIIA (spread to ipsilateral mediastinal lymph nodes):** May warrant resection. Adjuvant chemotherapy may be administered after surgery.
    - **Stage IIIB (spread to contralateral mediastinal lymph nodes or with a malignant pleural effusion):** Consider chemotherapy and radiation.
    - **Stage IV (metastatic disease):** Chemotherapy has been shown to improve quality of life and modestly prolong survival compared with the best supportive care.
- Commonly used drugs for NSCLC include cisplatin, carboplatin, paclitaxel, docetaxel, gemcitabine, pemetrexed, vinorelbine, erlotinib, and, recently, bevacizumab.

SMALL CELL LUNG CANCER (SCLC)

A 70-year-old woman with an extensive smoking history presents with six months of hemoptysis, weakness, and a 50-lb weight loss. She has been bedridden for the past week and was wheelchair bound prior to this from weakness. Her physical exam is normal. Labs show a sodium level of 128 mEq/L, and CT scans of the head, chest, abdomen, and pelvis show a 14-cm left hilar lymph node mass, multiple liver metastases, and three brain metastases; a bone scan shows too many metastases to count. Bronchoscopic biopsy reveals SCLC. What are the most appropriate next steps in management of this patient?

Chemotherapy, whole brain radiation therapy, and monthly bisphosphonate therapy. Most patients with SCLC (even those with widespread metastases) respond dramatically to chemotherapy and whole brain radiation therapy. Although treatment is rarely curative, palliation for 1–2 years is possible in 50% of cases. The bisphosphonates pamidronate and zolendronate help ↓ skeletal pain and fractures. This patient's hyponatremia is most likely caused by SIADH and will resolve following response to chemotherapy.

Characterized by early metastasis; **surgical resection is not part of therapy.** Often associated with neuroendocrine and paraneoplastic features (see Figure 14.4).

DIAGNOSIS

Has two stages (not staged via the TNM system used for most other solid tumors):

- **Limited:** All the visible cancer can be encompassed by a single radiation port in the chest.
- **Extensive:** Anything that is not limited.

TREATMENT

- Chemotherapy and radiation given together improve outcomes in limited-stage disease, but the prognosis remains poor.
- Chemotherapy alone is the treatment of choice for patients with extensive-stage disease, yielding high response rates. However, virtually all patients relapse.
- Inasmuch as **SCLC has high rates of brain metastasis (up to 3–5%),** prophylactic cranial irradiation should be considered in all patients with a complete response to chemotherapy or chemoradiotherapy. Drugs of choice include etoposide and cisplatin.

> **KEY FACT**
>
> The majority of paraneoplastic syndromes are seen with small cell lung cancer. The exception is hypercalcemia due to PTHrP secretion, which is due to squamous cell cancer.

> **KEY FACT**
>
> SCLC metastasizes early and has a unique staging system: "limited" (ie, all the cancer encompassed by a single radiation port in the chest) vs. "extensive" (everything else). Chemotherapy that includes etoposide and cisplatin and prophylactic cranial irradiation should be considered for SCLC.

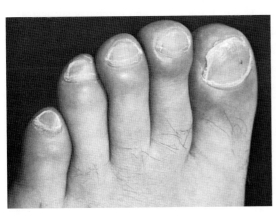

A

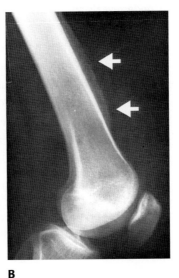

B

FIGURE 14.4. Pulmonary hypertrophic osteoarthropathy associated with small cell lung cancer. (A) Painful clubbing of the toes (close-up). **(B)** The arrows point to new bone formation on the femur. (Reproduced with permission from Brunicardi FC et al. *Schwartz's Principles of Surgery*, 9th ed. New York: McGraw-Hill, 2010, Fig. 19-20B and C.)

Mesothelioma

- A neoplasm arising from the mesothelial surfaces of the peritoneum and pleural cavities, pericardium, and tunica vaginalis. **Asbestos** exposure ↑ the risk. Smoking and asbestos exposure are synergistic.
- **Sx/Exam:** Most commonly presents with dyspnea and a large unilateral pleural effusion; less commonly presents with malignant ascites.
- **Tx:** The prognosis is poor. Debulking of tumor, thoracentesis, and pleurodesis may ↓ the impact of pleural-based disease. Chemotherapy is only modestly effective.

Thymoma

- An anterior mediastinal tumor that is often detected during the workup of **myasthenia gravis.** Most are benign, but some progress to thymic carcinoma. Other paraneoplastic syndromes associated with thymoma include **pure red cell aplasia.**
- **Tx:** Resection is the most effective treatment. If spread occurs outside the mediastinum, chemotherapy and radiation may be used as well but have limited efficacy.

KEY FACT

Ten percent of patients with myasthenia gravis have thymomas. Thirty percent of patient with thymomas have myasthenia gravis.

Squamous Cell Carcinoma (SCC) of the Head and Neck

A 40-year-old man presents with a swelling in his neck of four months' duration. He has a 30-pack-year smoking history. On exam, he is found to have a firm, 3-cm lymph node in the midcervical region. FNA of the lymph node reveals squamous cell carcinoma. What is the most appropriate next diagnostic step?

Upper airway panendoscopy for evaluation and treatment of likely SCC of the head and neck with an unknown 1° site. The location and pathology suggest a head and neck 1° tumor. Treatment with definitive radiation therapy to the pharyngeal axis and bilateral neck, radical neck dissection, or a combination of these local modalities is typically recommended. These result in long-term disease-free survival in about 40–67% of cases.

Many SCCs are curable. Major risk factors include tobacco (cigarettes, chewing tobacco, cigars), alcohol use, and HPV. Lesions progress as follows: leukoplakia → erythroplakia → dysplasia → carcinoma in situ → invasive carcinoma. The highest risk of morbidity and mortality associated with head and neck cancer results from local extension rather than from metastasis.

SYMPTOMS

May present with a hoarse voice, a globus sensation, otalgia, a sore in the mouth or throat, a lump in the throat, numbness in the face or throat, odynophagia, dysphagia, lymphadenopathy, tinnitus, or hearing loss.

EXAM

Evaluate the scalp, cranial nerves, lymph nodes, and oral cavity.

DIAGNOSIS

- Pan–upper endoscopy should be performed under anesthesia to evaluate the entire aerodigestive tract.
- FNA is the standard means of establishing involvement of cervical lymph nodes.
- Core needle biopsy is not done on newly diagnosed lesions owing to concerns over tumor recurrence in the needle tract.
- MRI or CT of the head and neck (see Figure 14.5); CXR.

TREATMENT

Treatment depends on the anatomical site (eg, the oral cavity, base of tongue, oropharynx, pharynx, hypopharynx, or larynx) and on the presence of lymph node involvement.

- **Early-stage tumors in the oral cavity, base of the tongue, or lips:** May be treated with radiation or surgery alone.
- **Early-stage tumors of the oropharynx:** Radiation is the preferred modality.
- **Cervical lymph node involvement:** Treat with surgery, radiation, or chemoradiation. Patients often require a PEG tube, which has significant oral toxicity, to get through radiation. Commonly used chemotherapeutic agents include cisplatin, carboplatin, 5-FU, paclitaxel, docetaxel, methotrexate, and, recently, cetuximab.
- For some patients with laryngeal cancer, voice-sparing treatments (partial laryngectomy, chemoradiotherapy) should be considered; as many as 25% can avoid laryngectomy.

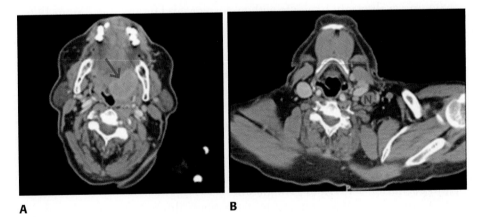

A **B**

FIGURE 14.5. **Squamous cell carcinoma of the tongue base.** (A) Transaxial contrast-enhanced CT image shows a large enhancing mass at the base of the tongue (arrow). (B) Transaxial image lower in the neck shows metastatic left cervical lymph nodes, the largest of which (N) is posterior to the left internal jugular vein. (Reproduced with permission from USMLERx.com.)

Nasopharyngeal Carcinoma

- **Associated with EBV infection,** not tobacco or alcohol. **Endemic to China and parts of Africa.**
- Sx/Exam: Presents with a change in hearing, a sensation of ear stuffiness, tinnitus, nasal obstruction, and/or a mass in the neck.
- **Tx:** Not a surgical disease; requires chemotherapy (**cisplatin**) with concurrent **radiation.** Two-thirds of patients are cured.

Thyroid Cancer

Refer to the Endocrinology chapter for a more detailed discussion of this topic.

Esophageal Cancer

Risk factors include cigarette smoking, alcohol use, obesity, GERD, and **Barrett's esophagus** (associated with a **30-fold ↑ risk**). Other risk factors include HPV infection, achalasia, and vitamin deficiency. SCC is three times more common among African Americans than among Caucasians. Adenocarcinoma is more common in Caucasians.

SYMPTOMS/EXAM

Presents with dysphagia, odynophagia, weight loss, cough, and hoarseness.

DIAGNOSIS

- **Staging evaluation:** Evaluate with endoscopy and biopsy (see Figure 14.6), chest CT, endoscopic ultrasound, and bronchoscopy (to rule out tracheal invasion).
- **Pathology:** The 1° histologies are squamous cell and adenocarcinoma (increasing in incidence; associated with obesity and GERD).

TREATMENT

- **Localized esophageal cancer:** Treat with chemoradiation (5-FU plus cisplatin and external beam radiotherapy) or surgery. Postoperative chemoradiation should be considered for locally advanced cancers.
- **Metastatic disease: Few good options are available;** drugs include cisplatin, paclitaxel, 5-FU, and gemcitabine.
- PEG tubes are often required to get patients through chemoradiation (as in head and neck cancer).

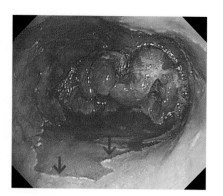

FIGURE 14.6. Esophageal cancer. Esophageal adenocarcinoma (arrowhead) on endoscopy against a background of the pink tongues of Barrett's esophagus (arrows). (Reproduced with permission from Fauci AS et al. *Harrison's Principles of Internal Medicine,* 17th ed. New York: McGraw-Hill, 2008, Fig. 285-3D.)

Gastric Cancer

The most common cancer in Asia; associated with a diet of smoked and pickled foods that is **high in nitrates** and low in vegetables. Working in coal mining and in nickel, rubber, and timber processing are additional risk factors, as is smoking. *H pylori* infection, chronic atrophic gastritis, intestinal metaplasia, and pernicious anemia are associated with gastric cancer.

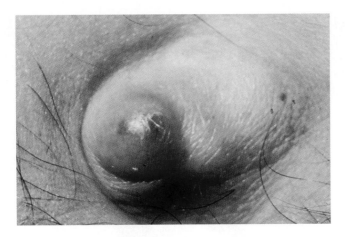

FIGURE 14.7.   Sister Mary Joseph node. A protuberant and firm umbilical nodule, most commonly associated with gastric carcinoma, may also be seen in other abdominal and pelvic malignancies. (Courtesy of the Department of Dermatology, Naval Medical Center, Portsmouth, VA, as published in Knoop KJ et al. *Atlas of Emergency Medicine*, 3rd ed. New York: McGraw-Hill, 2010, Fig. 7-44.)

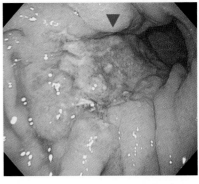

FIGURE 14.8.   Gastric cancer. A malignant gastric ulcer (arrowhead) involving the greater curvature of the stomach is seen on endoscopy. (Reproduced with permission from Fauci AS et al. *Harrison's Principles of Internal Medicine*, 17th ed. New York: McGraw-Hill, 2008, Fig. 285-2B.)

SYMPTOMS/EXAM

Presents with pain, anorexia, weight loss, vomiting, and GI bleeding. Supraclavicular lymphadenopathy (Virchow's node) and periumbilical lymphadenopathy (Sister Mary Joseph node; see Figure 14.7) may also be seen.

DIAGNOSIS

- Endoscopy and biopsy (see Figure 14.8).
- Staging evaluation includes CT of the chest, abdomen, and pelvis as well as endoscopic ultrasound.
- Adenocarcinoma is the predominant histology.

TREATMENT

- Surgery is the preferred therapy for resectable gastric cancer.
- Adjuvant chemoradiotherapy is indicated after surgery for patients with locally advanced gastric cancer.
- Treat metastatic gastric cancer with chemotherapeutic agents such as ECF (epirubicin, cisplatin, 5-FU).

GASTROINTESTINAL STROMAL TUMORS (GISTs)

- Sarcoma of the stomach or small bowel wall (see Figure 14.9). Associated with an activating mutation in the **c-kit** oncogene.
- Tx:
    - Standard treatment is surgery; conventional chemotherapy is ineffective.
    - For patients with metastatic GIST, targeted therapy with **imatinib** (the same agent used for CML), which inhibits c-kit, can lead to dramatic and prolonged responses in patients with previously intractable and incurable disease.

MUCOSA-ASSOCIATED LYMPHOID TISSUE (MALT) LYMPHOMA

Gastric mucosa–associated lymphoma linked to *H pylori* infection; > 80% of cases regress after treatment for *H pylori*.

KEY FACT

Supraclavicular lymphadenopathy (Virchow's node) and periumbilical lymphadenopathy (Sister Mary Joseph node) may represent spread from gastric cancer and other GI malignancies.

KEY FACT

GIST tumors often express c-kit and frequently respond to treatment with imatinib.

KEY FACT

Eradication of *H pylori* is the treatment of choice for MALT lymphomas.

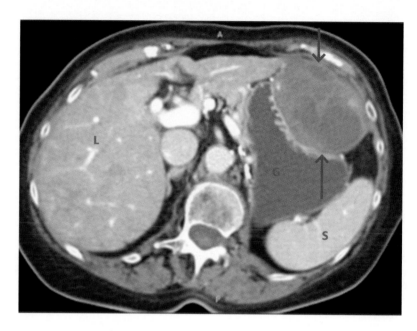

FIGURE 14.9. **Gastrointestinal stromal cell tumor.** Transaxial image from a contrast-enhanced CT demonstrates a large, heterogeneously enhancing mass (arrows) arising from the anterior gastric wall, displacing the gastric lumen posteriorly. L = liver; G = gastric lumen; S = spleen. (Reproduced with permission from USMLERx.com.)

Pancreatic Cancer

A 70-year-old man presents with a one-month history of jaundice, light stools, dark urine, and pruritus. Exam reveals jaundice and fullness in the RUQ. Labs are as follows: AST 99 U/L, ALT 140 U/L, alkaline phosphatase 520 U/L, and total bilirubin 16.2 mg/dL. A CT of the abdomen shows marked intrahepatic bile duct dilatation, a dilated gallbladder, and a mass in the head of the pancreas. What is the most appropriate next step?

ERCP for evaluation of new-onset obstructive jaundice in an elderly patient, which is most often due to pancreatic or biliary tract cancer. ERCP can also be used to obtain biopsy specimens and for therapy with stent deployment. Although long-term survival rates are poor, the best chance for cure is a pancreaticoduodenectomy. Gemcitabine is FDA approved for the treatment of metastatic pancreatic cancer and results in improved clinical benefit and overall survival compared with 5-FU.

A highly lethal cancer with a median survival of 9–12 months and a **five-year survival of 3%**. At diagnosis, > 50% are metastatic or unresectable. Risk factors include tobacco exposure and diabetes mellitus.

SYMPTOMS/EXAM

- Presents with jaundice, pain, glucose intolerance, and a palpable gallbladder (**Courvoisier's sign**).
- **Painless jaundice** is a sign of intrapancreatic bile duct obstruction and may allow for early detection of resectable disease.

KEY FACT

CA 19-9 levels are not specific for pancreatic cancer but may be a useful means of following treatment response in patients with pancreatic cancer.

DIAGNOSIS

- The serum marker **CA 19-9** can be useful in monitoring treatment but is not specific enough to be used for diagnosis.
- CT of the abdomen with fine cuts through the pancreas (pancreatic protocol CT); endoscopic ultrasound; ERCP.

TREATMENT

- **Resectable disease:**
  - Defined as that which does not involve the major vessels or celiac axis, with no distant metastases.
  - The only curative therapy is pancreaticoduodenectomy (the Whipple procedure).
  - **Adjuvant therapy** after the Whipple procedure consists of chemoradiation with 5-FU.
- **Unresectable disease:** Treatment for unresectable cases includes the following:
  - Palliation of symptoms with gemcitabine-based chemotherapy, radiation, a biliary stent, or choledochojejunostomy to ↓ jaundice.
  - A nerve block to the celiac plexus may relieve pain.
- **Advanced pancreatic cancer: Gemcitabine**-based chemotherapy is associated with symptomatic relief and prolonged survival but has a low response rate.

KEY FACT

In pancreatic cancer, invasion into the superior mesenteric artery or vein implies unresectable disease.

Hepatocellular Carcinoma (HCC)

A 55-year-old woman with cirrhosis from HCV presents with fatigue. She has a history of alcohol abuse but has been abstinent for a year. She also has a history of ascites and hepatic encephalopathy, currently controlled with medications. Exam shows mild jaundice, spider angiomata, and mild peripheral edema. Labs are as follows: bilirubin 3.0 mg/dL, INR 1.5, platelet count 80,000/μL, AST 70 U/L, ALT 60 U/L, alkaline phosphatase 120 U/L, normal hematocrit, and serum α-fetoprotein (AFP) 450 ng/mL. Abdominal ultrasonography shows a coarse liver, mild ascites, and a 2.5-cm hyperechoic hepatic mass that was not seen on previous imaging. A CT scan of the liver shows vascular enhancement of the mass, splenomegaly, and evidence of portal hypertension. What is the most likely diagnosis, and what would be the most appropriate next step?

The finding of a new mass with vascular enhancement in a patient with HCV cirrhosis and an ↑ AFP is virtually diagnostic of HCC, and biopsy is unnecessary. Patients with advanced liver disease and HCC should usually be evaluated for liver transplantation. Surgical resection with partial hepatectomy is associated with a very high risk of hepatic decompensation and is not advised for this patient.

Risk factors include HBV (especially vertical transmission), HCV, alcohol abuse (especially in combination with HCV), hemochromatosis, α_1-antitrypsin deficiency, and androgen and estrogen therapy.

DIAGNOSIS

- High-risk patients to be considered for screening are Asian HBV carriers > 40 years of age; cirrhotic HBV carriers; patients with a family history of HCC; those with high HBV DNA concentrations; those with cirrhosis from alcohol, HCV, genetic hemochromatosis, or 1° biliary cirrhosis; and patients on a liver transplant waiting list.
- High-risk patients should be screened with AFP and hepatic ultrasound, although the appropriate interval has not been established (generally 6- to 12-month intervals).
- AFP alone should not be used for screening unless ultrasound is unavailable, as this measure alone does not correlate with the size, stage, or prognosis of HCC. It is ↑ only about 50% of the time in HCC.
- Markedly ↑ AFP in concert with consistent imaging (see Figure 14.10) and high-risk liver disease may obviate the need for a biopsy.

TREATMENT

- Resection is the treatment of choice if liver function is adequate and anatomy permits.
- Patients with cirrhosis may be offered transplantation for single tumors < 5 cm or three tumors < 3 cm each.
- Chemoembolization, intratumoral ethanol injection, cryotherapy, and radiofrequency ablation are all options for unresectable lesions.
- There is no standard chemotherapy with proven efficacy. The multikinase inhibitor sorafenib has been shown to prolong survival in patients with good hepatic function.
- See the Gastroenterology and Hepatology chapter for further details on cirrhosis and liver transplantation.

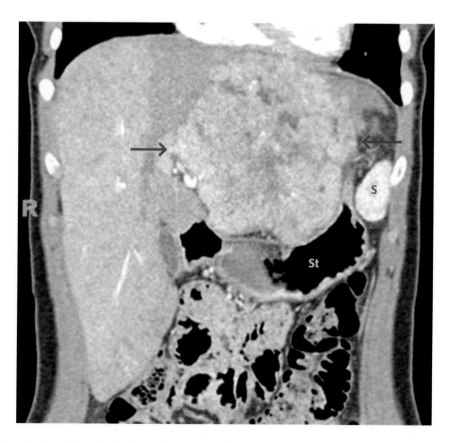

FIGURE 14.10. **Hepatocellular carcinoma.** Coronal reformation from a contrast-enhanced CT shows large left hepatic lobe HCC (arrows). St = stomach; S = spleen. (Reproduced with permission from USMLERx.com.)

Colorectal Cancer

 A 55-year-old man presents for follow-up following surgical resection of stage II colon cancer that was diagnosed three years ago. He received no adjuvant therapy. His exam is normal, and labs show a CEA of 50 ng/mL, which is higher than his previous normal result one year ago. CT scans of the chest and abdomen show multiple pulmonary nodules < 1 cm and five hepatic lesions measuring 3–8 cm. Biopsy of a liver lesion reveals adenocarcinoma consistent with the 1° tumor. What is the most appropriate next step in management?

Patients with colon cancer and unresectable liver metastases require systemic treatment with chemotherapy. This patient likely has pulmonary metastases as well. The response rate of patients who receive chemotherapeutic regimens consisting of oxaliplatin, irinotecan, or bevacizumab is significantly better than that achieved with prior treatments. Hepatic resection of metastatic colon cancer is indicated only for isolated metastatic disease.

Seventy-five percent of cases occur in those with no risk factors (eg, family history, genetic syndrome, IBD, acromegaly). Genetic syndromes include the following:

- **Hereditary nonpolyposis colorectal cancer (HNPCC):** Characterized by few polyps (nonpolyposis); associated with endometrial, gastric, renal, ovarian, and skin cancer and with the mismatch repair genes MLH1/2 and MSH1/2.
- **Familial adenomatous polyposis (FAP):** Characterized by thousands of polyps; the treatment of choice is colectomy. Associated with a mutation in the APC gene.
- **Li-Fraumeni syndrome:** Associated with the p53 mutation.

SYMPTOMS/EXAM

Presentation is highly variable. May be asymptomatic or present with symptoms ranging from abdominal pain to colonic obstruction, lower GI bleeding, or weight loss.

DIAGNOSIS

Diagnosed by a mass detected by DRE or FOBT; confirmed by colonoscopy and biopsy (see Figure 14.11).

TREATMENT

- **Treat according to stage.**
    - **Stage I:** Partial colectomy; no further therapy.
    - **Stage II:** Partial colectomy. Adjuvant therapy is controversial. Consider adjuvant chemotherapy for certain high-risk features (eg, high-grade disease, obstruction, perforation, very large tumors).
    - **Stage III:** Partial colectomy. These cancers with lymph node involvement all merit adjuvant chemotherapy. The standard is 5-FU or 5-FU/leucovorin/oxaliplatin (abbreviated as FOLFOX).
    - **Stage IV:** Palliative colectomy or colon diversion to prevent obstruction. Chemotherapy for metastatic disease is generally palliative. **The exception is stage IV disease due to one or more resectable hepatic metastases, which may still be curable with resection** (the liver is gen-

 KEY FACT

HNPCC has few polyps, but FAP has thousands of polyps; thus, treatment for FAP is colectomy.

KEY FACT

Colon and ovarian cancer are the most frequent causes of malignant large bowel obstruction.

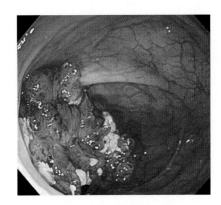

FIGURE 14.11.   Colon cancer. Colonoscopy reveals an adenocarcinoma growing into the lumen of the colon. (Reproduced with permission from Fauci AS et al. *Harrison's Principles of Internal Medicine*, 17th ed. New York: McGraw-Hill, 2008, Fig. 285-6.)

KEY FACT

The liver is the most frequent site of metastasis in colon cancer, whereas rectal cancers may spread through paravertebral venous and lymphatic channels directly to the lungs without liver involvement.

KEY FACT

Colon cancer with one or more resectable liver metastases can still be curable with surgery. This is one of the few metastatic cancers that can be cured.

erally the first site of metastasis). In this case, surgery should be aggressively pursued.

■ **Chemotherapeutic agents:** Two medications are the mainstay of chemotherapy for colon cancer:
  ■ **5-FU:** Converted to F-dUMP; inhibits thymidine production and interferes with DNA synthesis.
  ■ **Leucovorin (folinic acid):** Stabilizes the bond between F-dUMP and thymidylate synthetase, enhancing the efficacy of 5-FU.
  ■ Other drugs include irinotecan, oxiliplatin, cetuximab, and bevacizumab.
■ **Rectal cancer:** Owing to the anatomy of the rectum (and the desire to preserve the rectal sphincter if possible), surgical approaches have less room for adequate margins. Therefore, **radiation therapy is often given either before or after surgery** in addition to or in combination with chemotherapy.

PREVENTION

See the discussion of cancer screening in the Ambulatory Medicine chapter.

Prostate Cancer

A 70-year-old man presents with acute onset of back pain. He was diagnosed with prostate cancer 10 years ago, at which time he underwent external beam radiation therapy; leuprolide therapy was initiated five years later for a rising PSA without evidence of metastases. Labs show a normal hemoglobin, a PSA of < 0.4 ng/mL, and a testosterone level of 16 ng/mL, and x-rays of the thoracic spine reveal a T6 acute fracture. Bone scan reveals intense radioisotope uptake at T6. What is the most likely cause of this patient's back pain?

The fracture causing the back pain is most likely due to osteoporosis rather than to metastases. In patients with prostate cancer, GnRH agonists such as leuprolide can cause bone loss in the lumbar spine by decreasing serum testosterone. Patients with recently diagnosed prostate cancer and a PSA of < 10 ng/mL have a low incidence of bony metastasis. Femoral and tibial fractures are more common than vertebral fractures in metastatic disease.

The most common non–skin cancer diagnosed in men. A ⊕ family history and African American ethnicity are both risk factors.

SYMPTOMS/EXAM

Often associated with urinary obstruction and concurrent prostatitis.

DIAGNOSIS

■ **Screening measures** are as follows:
  ■ All patients with nodules warrant biopsy.
  ■ Those with a PSA of > 4 ng/mL merit biopsy. A PSA that is < 4 ng/mL but rapidly rising should be considered for biopsy.
  ■ A lower **percent free PSA** is associated with a higher risk of prostate cancer being present. In patients with a PSA of < 4 ng/mL, this may aid in determining whether to biopsy.

- The **Gleason score** involves the evaluation of grade under the microscope; tumors are graded from 2 to 10, with 2 being almost benign and 10 being highly aggressive. Has a prognostic impact on outcomes in almost every stage of prostate cancer.

TREATMENT

- **Localized disease:** Four major options are available for the treatment of localized prostate cancer:
  - **Active surveillance:** For those with significant comorbidities, elderly patients, or those with low-risk disease.
  - **External beam radiation therapy:** For patients with a risk of extraprostatic spread or contraindications to surgery.
  - **Brachytherapy:** Implantation of radioactive seeds in the prostate gland.
  - **Radical prostatectomy:** For patients with a long life expectancy and a high likelihood that the cancer is confined to the prostate.
- **Advanced disease: Advanced prostate cancer** (ie, recurrence after local therapies or metastatic disease; see Figure 14.12) is treated in the following manner:
  - **Androgen deprivation:** The most effective medical therapy. Methods are as follows:
    - Bilateral orchiectomy.
    - GnRH agonists (suppress testosterone secretion by inhibiting FSH/LH release from the pituitary).
    - Oral antiandrogens are less proven but have fewer side effects. They are generally used only in combination with GnRH agonists (GnRH agonists + oral antiandrogens = "combined" androgen blockade).

KEY FACT

Most men die with their prostate cancer, not from it.

KEY FACT

The decision to screen for prostate cancer should include a thorough discussion with the patient about risks (false ⊕s, uncertain efficacy in reducing death from prostate cancer, posttreatment complications such as urinary incontinence or proctitis) and benefits (earlier diagnosis and treatment may improve survival). Testing in men over age 75 is not recommended.

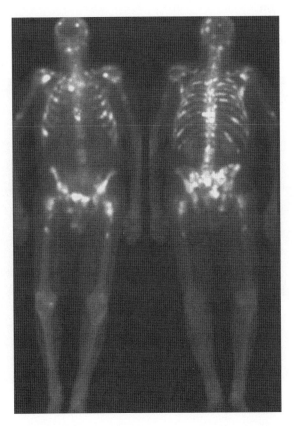

FIGURE 14.12.   Prostate cancer metastases. ^{99m}Tc-MDP bone scan in a patient with a history of prostate cancer shows innumerable areas of abnormal radiotracer uptake throughout the axial skeleton, consistent with bony metastases. (Reproduced with permission from Tanagho EA, McAninch JW. *Smith's General Urology,* 17th ed. New York: McGraw-Hill, 2008, Fig. 22-4.)

- Hormone-refractory metastatic prostate cancer:
  - Treat with chemotherapy; docetaxel with prednisone is currently first-line therapy.
  - Adjunctive therapy with zoledronic acid (a bisphosphonate) to strengthen bones and prevent skeletal complications.

PREVENTION

- **Finasteride** (a 5α-reductase inhibitor that blocks the conversion of testosterone to dihydrotestosterone) ↓ prostate cancer prevalence by 25% in men > 55 years of age. It is associated with higher-grade tumors and more sexual side effects but fewer symptoms of urinary obstruction compared with placebo.
- For further details, see the discussion of cancer screening in the Ambulatory Medicine chapter.

Kidney Cancer

Risk factors include obesity, smoking, and von Hippel–Lindau syndrome (associated with retinal angiomas, CNS hemangioblastomas, and kidney cancer).

EXAM/DIAGNOSIS

- Must be ruled out in patients with hematuria. Pursue IVP or CT (see Figure 14.13).
- Rarely, patients may present with polycythemia due to excess erythropoietin production.
- Diagnosis is based on radiologic appearance. **Biopsy of a renal mass is generally not done given the risk of seeding the tumor.**

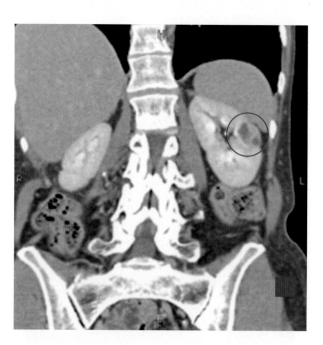

FIGURE 14.13. **Renal cell carcinoma.** (Reproduced with permission from USMLERx.com).

TREATMENT

- **Localized disease:** Nephrectomy.
- **Metastatic disease:**
  - Cytokine-based therapy (**IL-2, interferon**) can induce durable remissions in a small fraction of patients.
  - Other options include **targeted therapy** with sunitinib, pazopanib, bevacizumab, and sorafenib; temsirolimus and everolimus (mTOR inhibitors) are other options.
  - Nephrectomy may be indicated for metastatic disease if the kidney tumor itself represents the bulk of the cancer.

Testicular Cancer

A 25-year-old man presents with an enlarged, painless right testicular mass. Labs reveal a β-hCG of 30 mU/mL, an AFP of 40 ng/mL, and a normal LDH. Chest, abdominal, and pelvic CT scans are unremarkable, but scrotal ultrasound reveals a solid, hypoechoic, 5-cm-diameter right testicular mass. Radical orchiectomy is performed, and the tumor is confirmed as yolk sac carcinoma with chorionic elements. A week after surgery, the patient's β-hCG concentration is 1.8 mU/mL, and his AFP is 16.3 ng/mL. What is the most appropriate next step in management?

Check AFP again 14 days after surgery to evaluate the patient's prognosis, as the half-life of AFP is approximately one week, whereas that of β-hCG is approximately 24 hours. This patient has stage I nonseminomatous testicular cancer confined to the testis and probably has already been cured by the initial surgery. Chemotherapy would be indicated if the patient had metastases or a mixed seminomatous and nonseminomatous tumor. Abdominal radiation is inappropriate in nonseminomatous testicular cancer.

The most common cancer in younger men aged 15–35; a second peak occurs in men > 60 years of age. An **undescended testicle is a major risk factor.** Other risk factors include prior testicular cancer, Klinefelter's syndrome, and a ⊕ family history. The five-year survival rate for all patients with germ cell tumors is roughly 95%.

> **KEY FACT**
>
> An undescended testicle is a major risk factor for testicular cancer.

SYMPTOMS/EXAM

- Presents with a scrotal mass and low back pain (from retroperitoneal lymphadenopathy).
- Testicular pain does **not** indicate a benign etiology.
- Approximately 10% present as extragonadal germ cell tumors with no testis 1°.

DIAGNOSIS

- Evaluate with testicular ultrasound to identify a mass (see Figure 14.14).
- **Never biopsy the testis;** an inguinal orchiectomy is needed to make the diagnosis.
- Serum markers elevated in 80% of germ cell patients are AFP and β-hCG. Monitor serially after surgery to look for recurrence or persistence of tumor.

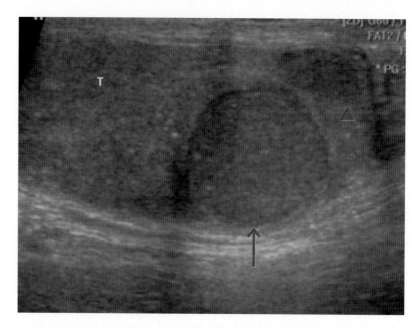

FIGURE 14.14. **Seminoma.** Longitudinal ultrasound image of the testicle (T) showing a homogeneous intratesticular mass (arrow) and an additional, smaller focus of tumor (arrowhead). (Reproduced with permission from USMLERx.com.)

- There are two major pathologic classifications:
    - **Seminoma: Never has an ↑ AFP;** may have ↑ β-hCG.
    - **Nonseminoma:** Includes embryonal carcinoma, yolk sac carcinoma, choriocarcinoma, teratoma, and seminoma (when histology is mixed seminoma and nonseminoma, treat as nonseminoma). Patients may have an ↑ AFP and β-hCG.

TREATMENT

- The treatment of germ cell cancers is determined by prognostic features and stage:
    - **Early-stage seminoma:**
        - If disease is limited to the testis, treat with inguinal orchiectomy alone.
        - Radiotherapy or chemotherapy if there is evidence of retroperitoneal metastasis on imaging.
    - **Early-stage nonseminoma:** Inguinal orchiectomy +/– retroperitoneal lymph node dissection +/– adjuvant chemotherapy.
    - **Advanced seminoma or nonseminoma:** Chemotherapy is standard and results in high cure rates (> 85%). Brain metastases can be treated with whole brain radiation therapy and combination chemotherapy.
- **Prognostic features:** Adverse prognostic factors include high tumor markers, the presence of visceral metastasis outside the lungs (eg, liver, soft tissue, brain), the presence of embryonal carcinoma, and a mediastinal 1° site.
- **Chemotherapeutic regimens for germ cell tumors** include bleomycin, etoposide, and cisplatin (BEP) or etoposide and cisplatin (EP).
- Intensive follow-up is essential, as even relapsed patients have high rates of cure. Follow-up measures to monitor for recurrence include CT scans, markers, and physical examination at frequent intervals.

COMPLICATIONS

- Fertility problems persist in 50% of germ cell tumor patients and are thought to be related as much to underlying pathology as to treatment. Sperm banking should be considered prior to the initiation of chemotherapy.
- Other long-term complications include an ↑ incidence of cardiovascular disease, hypertension, and 2° malignancies (a new testicular 1° tumor and 2° acute leukemia are the most likely).

Bladder Cancer

Risk factors for bladder cancer include cigarette **smoking,** analgesic abuse (phenacetin), chronic urinary tract inflammation, infection with *Schistosoma haematobium*, and aniline dyes.

SYMPTOMS/EXAM

Presents with hematuria, difficulty voiding, renal failure, and bladder irritation/pain.

DIAGNOSIS

- Cystoscopy and biopsy, cytology, CT of the abdomen and pelvis, CXR, and bone scan if alkaline phosphatase is ↑.
- The most common pathology in the United States is transitional cell carcinoma, although SCC is also found, most frequently in parts of the world in which schistosomiasis is common.

TREATMENT

- **Superficial bladder cancer** (not penetrating into the detrusor muscle): Treat with local therapies such as excision, intravesicular BCG, or intravesicular chemotherapy.
- **Muscle-invasive bladder cancer:** Radical cystectomy.
- **Metastatic disease:** The standard of care is **gemcitabine and cisplatin** as first-line chemotherapy.

Cervical Cancer

Almost half of women with cervical cancer are diagnosed before age 35. Risk factors include sexual activity at an early age, **HPV** infection (subtypes 16, 18, 31, 33, and 35), multiple partners, cigarette smoking, and concurrent **HIV** infection.

SYMPTOMS/EXAM

The most common presenting symptom is vaginal bleeding between menses.

DIAGNOSIS

- Colposcopy and biopsy.
- The majority of cancers are squamous cell, although adenocarcinoma accounts for 20% of all cervical cancers.

KEY FACT

Bladder cancer is most often due to transitional cell carcinoma. The exception is bladder cancer due to schistosomiasis, which is SCC.

KEY FACT

Gross hematuria in a patient > 40 years of age should prompt a workup for bladder cancer.

KEY FACT

For metastatic bladder cancer, the standard of care is gemcitabine and cisplatin as first-line chemotherapy.

KEY FACT

For early-stage cervical cancer, treatment options include radiation therapy, cone excisional biopsy, and simple hysterectomy.

KEY FACT

Risk factors for endometrial cancer include unopposed estrogen, tamoxifen, obesity, and a diet high in animal fats.

KEY FACT

Postmenopausal bleeding always requires further evaluation to rule out endometrial cancer.

TREATMENT

- Options for early-stage disease include radiation therapy, cone excisional biopsy, and simple hysterectomy.
- For more advanced disease, combined chemotherapy and radiation therapy is standard; radical hysterectomy/pelvic exenteration is also used.

PREVENTION

See the discussion of cancer screening in the Ambulatory Medicine chapter.

Endometrial Cancer

The most common genital tract malignancy in women, occurring primarily in postmenopausal women. Risks include unopposed estrogen (either endogenous or exogenous), obesity (due to ↑ aromatization of androgens to estrogens), and high levels of animal fat in diet. Childbearing ↓ the risk; tamoxifen is associated with an ↑ risk.

SYMPTOMS/EXAM

Postmenopausal uterine bleeding always requires evaluation.

DIAGNOSIS

- Transvaginal ultrasound, endometrial sampling, or D&C.
- Adenocarcinoma (endometrioid) is the most common histology.

TREATMENT

- Radical hysterectomy, bilateral salpingo-oophorectomy, and lymph node sampling are the treatment of choice, with adjuvant radiation therapy for selected patients.
- Progestins and paclitaxel/doxorubicin/cisplatin play a role in treating metastatic disease.

Ovarian Cancer

 A 55-year-old woman presents with a four-month history of fatigue, shortness of breath, and back pain. Ten years ago she was diagnosed with stage IIB ovarian cancer, for which she was treated with total abdominal hysterectomy and six cycles of adjuvant chemotherapy. Exam reveals dullness to percussion and diminished breath sounds at the posterior lung bases, bulging flanks, abdominal distention, and shifting dullness to percussion on her abdomen. A 3-cm mass is palpated in the right breast. Labs are as follows: alkaline phosphatase 120 U/L, ALT 90 U/L, AST 80 U/L, total bilirubin 3.0 mg/dL, CA-125 200 U/mL, and CA 15-3 350 U/mL. Her mammogram shows a cluster of microcalcifications and a poorly defined mass in her right breast. CT scans of the chest, abdomen, and pelvis show pleural effusions with pleural studding, ascites, several space-occupying hepatic lesions, and mixed lytic/sclerotic lesions in several vertebral bodies. What is the most likely diagnosis?

Despite a history of ovarian cancer with a poor prognosis, this patient's presentation is more consistent with metastatic breast cancer, which more commonly metastasizes to liver and bone. Ovarian cancer rarely metastasizes to bone or liver and rarely metastasizes to the breast. The tumor markers CA-125 (associated with ovarian cancer) and CA 15-3 (associated with breast cancer) may actually be ↑ in both cancers. A breast biopsy should be performed in this patient to determine the status of ER/PR/HER2 expression.

Epithelial ovarian cancer arises from cells that coat the ovary, which are similar to peritoneal epithelial cells. Risk is ↓ by multiparity, OCP use, breastfeeding, and tubal ligation. BRCA1, BRCA2, and HNPCC are genetic risk factors; a ⊕ family history is a risk factor even in the absence of a genetic syndrome. However, screening does not result in ↓ mortality either in general or among high-risk populations.

SYMPTOMS/EXAM

- There are very few symptoms in early-stage disease.
- ↑ abdominal girth, early satiety, rectal pressure, and urinary frequency are found in advanced disease.

DIAGNOSIS

- Close surveillance is warranted for patients with a genetic predisposition. Although an optimal surveillance regimen has not been identified, annual examination, transvaginal ultrasound, and CA-125 are often performed, and prophylactic oophorectomy may be considered.
- Different pathologies are associated with different prognoses:
  - Mucinous and clear cell cancers have a poorer prognosis.
  - Borderline tumors have a good prognosis.

TREATMENT

- **TAH-BSO:** Surgery alone is curative for early-stage ovarian cancer in 90% of cases. Only women who are at high risk for ovarian cancer should consider prophylactic bilateral oophorectomy (associated with osteoporosis, cardiovascular disease, menopausal symptoms, and sexual dysfunction).
- Early-stage tumors can be treated with adjuvant chemotherapy (often paclitaxel/carboplatin) for high-risk features to ↓ the risk of recurrence.
- Advanced tumors require surgical debulking of peritoneal metastasis followed by chemotherapy.
- A survival benefit has been shown for intraperitoneal chemotherapy in advanced (stage III) disease, although it results in added toxicity.
- The treatment of ovarian germ cell tumors is similar to that of testicular cancer.

KEY FACT

CA-125 is ↑ in 50–90% of women with ovarian cancer but is not specific for ovarian cancer. CA-125 screening is not recommended for low-risk women but may play a role in the evaluation of higher-risk women.

KEY FACT

In stage III ovarian cancer, **intraperitoneal** chemotherapy is associated with improved survival.

Sarcoma

- Sarcomas are a heterogeneous group of cancers of mesenchymal tissue that includes osteosarcoma, chondrosarcoma, Ewing's sarcoma, leiomyosarcoma, and other soft tissue sarcomas.
- **Sx/Exam:**
  - Sarcomas typically metastasize hematogenously; the most common site is the lung.
  - Often present with swelling and pain of an extremity.
- **Dx:** MRI is often more effective at imaging sarcomas than CT.
- **Tx:**
  - Limb-salvaging procedures should be attempted when possible.
  - **Ewing's sarcoma** affects children and adolescents, classically arising in the diaphysis. It is highly sensitive to combination chemotherapy; five-year survival rates are high.

KEY FACT

Paget's disease is a risk factor for osteosarcoma.

Anal Cancer

The most common histologies are squamous cell and cloacogenic (transitional cell), which behave similarly. The major risk factor is anal intercourse leading to **HPV** infection; genital warts are a risk factor and are potentiated by **HIV** infection.

KEY FACT

HIV and genital warts due to HPV are independent and additive risk factors for anal cancer.

SYMPTOMS/EXAM

- Patients often present with anal bleeding, pain, or the sensation of a mass in the anal canal.
- Lymph node drainage depends on the anatomic location. If the tumor is located below the dentate line, drainage is to the inguinal lymph nodes, which are the first site of metastasis. If the tumor is located above the dentate line, drainage is to the paravertebral and perirectal nodes.

TREATMENT

- Very small tumors can be surgically removed.
- Larger tumors or those with spread to the lymph nodes require chemoradiotherapy.

PREVENTION

Screen with an anal Pap smear in high-risk patients.

1° Brain Tumors

A 35-year-old woman is evaluated for generalized tonic-clonic seizures that last five minutes. Her exam and labs are unremarkable. CT scan of the head without contrast shows an area of low attenuation with mass effect in the left frontal lobe. MRI of the brain with contrast shows a 4-cm area of ↑ T2 signal in the left frontal lobe. A T1-weighted image with gadolinium shows ring enhancement with some central necrosis. Biopsy reveals that the lesion is a grade 4 astrocytoma (glioblastoma multiforme). What is the most important determinant of prognosis in this patient?

Cell type and tumor grade are the most important determinants of survival in glioma. Grade 4 carries the worst prognosis, with a median survival of only 9–12 months. Oligodendroglial tumors carry a more favorable prognosis than astrocytomas, with a median survival of 10–15 years. Other features indicative of good prognosis are age < 40 years, good performance status, and increasing extent of surgical resection.

Characterized by a bimodal age distribution; affect pediatric patients and those > 20 years of age (the peak is between 75 and 85 years). Subtypes are as follows:

- **Gliomas:** Most common; range from low to high grade (glioblastoma multiforme). Most gliomas in adults are high grade and incurable.
- **Meningiomas:** Benign tumors that cause morbidity by mass effect. Most common in peri- and postmenopausal women.

SYMPTOMS/EXAM

- Present with symptoms referable to ↑ ICP (headache, nausea, vomiting).
- Neurologic deficits, seizures, and strokelike phenomena are also seen.

DIAGNOSIS

- Diagnosis is best made on MRI (see Figure 14.15) followed by biopsy or surgical resection.
- CT scanning in patients with meningioma usually reveals an extra-axial mass with homogeneous enhancement.

TREATMENT

- Radiographic and clinical observation is usually appropriate for small (≤ 3 cm), asymptomatic meningiomas. Surgery is appropriate for symptomatic lesions.
- Surgery is the definitive therapy for brain tumors.
- Radiation may be considered for unresectable, recurrent, atypical, or anaplastic disease.
- Stereotactic or gamma-knife radiotherapy may be used for small tumors in locations where resection is difficult.
- Resection and radiation therapy are indicated for most high-grade gliomas, whereas chemotherapy may benefit younger patients with a good performance status.

KEY FACT

Consider metastases to the leptomeninges (carcinomatous meningitis) as a cause of neurologic deficits or altered mental status in patients with advanced cancer. Leptomeningeal metastases are most common in breast cancer, signify a poor prognosis, and respond poorly to intrathecal chemotherapy.

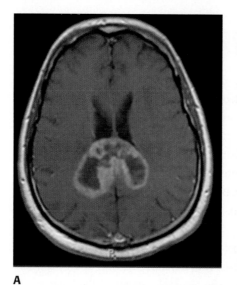 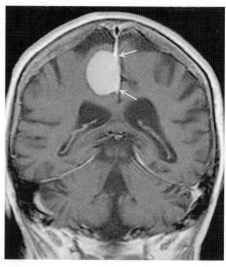

A   B

FIGURE 14.15. **Primary intracranial neoplasms.** (**A**) Transaxial contrast-enhanced MRI showing a centrally necrotic, enhancing intra-axial mass crossing the corpus callosum, in this case a glioblastoma multiforme. (**B**) Coronal contrast-enhanced MRI showing a homogeneously enhancing extra-axial mass with dural tails of enhancement (arrows) arising from the falx cerebrum, representing a meningioma. (Image A reproduced with permission from USMLERx.com. Image B reproduced with permission from Fauci AS et al. *Harrison's Principles of Internal Medicine,* 17th ed. New York: McGraw-Hill, 2008, Fig. 374-5.)

■ Chemotherapy has limited utility in malignant gliomas, although **oligodendrogliomas are highly chemosensitive** (associated with chromosome 1p and 19q loss). Chemotherapy is reserved for unresectable, progressive tumors that fail to respond or recur after radiation therapy.
■ Chemotherapeutic agents for 1° brain tumors include temozolomide, bevacizumab, and combination PCV (procarbazine, CCNU, vincristine).

MNEMONIC

Tumors that commonly metastasize to brain—

"Lots of Bad Stuff Kills Glia"

Lung
Breast
Skin (melanoma)
Kidney (renal cell carcinoma)
Gastrointestinal

KEY FACT

Metastases reach the brain via hematogenous spread, often passing through the lungs first, so check a CXR in any patient with brain metastases.

BRAIN METASTASES

Occur in 15% of patients with solid tumors, most commonly lung and breast cancer. In general, metastases portend a poor prognosis (see Figure 14.16).

■ Leptomeningeal spread may present as a cranial neuropathy or as spinal polyradiculopathy.
■ Occasionally, it presents with encephalopathy due to seizures, diffuse brain infiltration, or communicating hydrocephalus from obstruction of the arachnoid granulations.

TREATMENT

■ Patients with a solitary brain metastasis and no evidence of residual cancer elsewhere may be candidates for surgical resection followed by whole brain radiotherapy to prevent new metastases.
■ For patients with multiple brain metastases, whole brain radiotherapy is the treatment of choice.
■ Stereotactic radiosurgery or gamma-knife radiotherapy may be considered for those with solitary or few metastases.
■ Brain metastases usually respond poorly to systemic chemotherapy due to poor penetration of chemotherapy through the blood-brain barrier.
■ Prophylactic antiepileptic medication is not indicated.

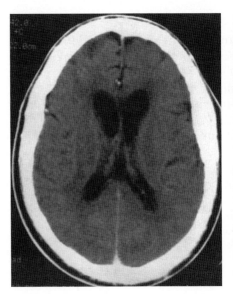 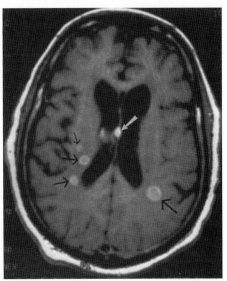

A   **B**

FIGURE 14.16.   Brain metastases. (A) Transaxial unenhanced CT image showing no obvious abnormality. (B) Contrast-enhanced transaxial MRI at the same level, in the same patient, showing multiple enhancing intra-axial masses consistent with metastases (arrows). (Reproduced with permission from Chen MY et al. *Basic Radiology.* New York: McGraw-Hill, 2004, Fig. 12-23.)

Carcinoma of an Unknown 1° Site

A 30-year-old man presents with increasing abdominal girth, intermittent midabdominal pain radiating to the back, and a 15-lb weight loss over the past four months. Exam reveals fullness in the midabdomen without tenderness and normal descended testes. A CT scan of the abdomen shows an 8-cm retroperitoneal mass. Labs reveal a β-hCG of 212 mU/mL and an AFP of 478 ng/mL. Testicular ultrasound is normal. A needle biopsy of the retroperitoneal mass reveals a poorly differentiated carcinoma. What is the most likely diagnosis and the most appropriate next step in management?

Young male patients with poorly differentiated midline carcinomas containing germ cell cancer markers are likely to have extragonadal germ cell cancer and may respond to cisplatin-based chemotherapy.

Comprise 2% of all cancer diagnoses in which a biopsy of a lymph node or other tissue reveals a cancer diagnosis but basic evaluation with history, exam, labs, and imaging fails to point to a 1° site.

DIAGNOSIS

- Pathologic evaluation with immunohistochemical stains or electron microscopy to determine the 1° site of cancer is the key component of workup.
- Evaluation focuses on age- and gender-specific risk factors:
  - Check β-hCG and AFP in all patients (for germ cell tumor). Other tumor markers (eg, CEA, CA-125, CA 19-9, CA 15-3) are useful for monitoring response to treatment but are too nonspecific to aid in diagnosis.
  - CT of the chest, abdomen, and pelvis.
  - PET scan is controversial but may be useful in locating a 1° site.
  - Mammography and breast examination in women; testicular examination, DRE, and PSA testing in men.
  - Colonoscopy in all patients > 50 years of age.

TREATMENT

Some special scenarios are as follows:

- **Women with axillary lymph nodes containing adenocarcinoma:** Should be treated like breast cancer—ie, with mastectomy and axillary lymph node dissection. Consider adjuvant therapy.
- **Patients with cervical lymph nodes and SCC:** Should be treated like SCC of the head and neck following thorough ENT evaluation.
- **Patients with inguinal lymph nodes and SCC:** Carefully evaluate the anal canal, the penis in men, and the vagina, uterus, cervix, and vulva in women.
- **Young men with poorly differentiated carcinoma and a mediastinal or retroperitoneal mass:** Treat as germ cell tumors; evaluate for occult testicular cancer.
- **Men with bone metastasis:** Evaluate with PSA testing for prostate cancer.
- **Women with peritoneal carcinomatosis:** Treat for ovarian cancer.
- **Chemotherapy regimen for patients not falling into the above categories:** Etoposide and a platinum (cisplatin or carboplatin). The addition of paclitaxel may improve response and survival.

Acute Leukemias

Genetic disorders associated with acute leukemia include Down syndrome, Bloom's syndrome, Fanconi's anemia, and ataxia-telangiectasia. Risk factors include chemical exposure (eg, benzene, petroleum products), hair dyes, smoking, and prior chemotherapy or radiation.

SYMPTOMS/EXAM

Present with bone pain and symptoms of pancytopenia (fatigue due to anemia, infection due to leukopenia, and bleeding due to thrombocytopenia). Also look for signs of bony infiltration such as gingival hyperplasia (see Figure 14.17) or sinus headaches from maxillary bone involvement.

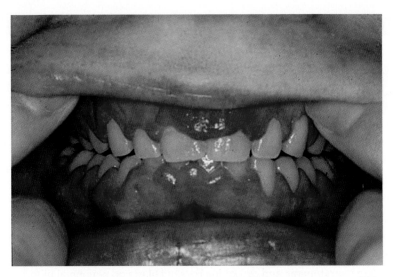

FIGURE 14.17. **Gingival hyperplasia in acute myeloid leukemia.** A 37-year-old female who was recently diagnosed with AML exhibits gingivae that show hyperplasia due to infiltration with leukemic monocytes. (Reproduced with permission from Wolff K, Johnson RA. *Fitzpatrick's Color Atlas & Synopsis of Clinical Dermatology*, 6th ed. New York: McGraw-Hill, 2009, Fig. 34-7.)

DIAGNOSIS

- Evaluate a CBC and a peripheral blood smear for blasts.
- Order a **bone marrow aspirate and biopsy** to assess for blasts, to include immunohistochemistry, cytogenetic evaluation (used to group patients into favorable, intermediate, and unfavorable prognoses), and flow cytometry.
- Check PT, PTT, D-dimer, and fibrinogen to evaluate for DIC.
- Check uric acid, LDH, potassium, creatinine, phosphorus, and calcium to evaluate for tumor lysis.

ACUTE LYMPHOBLASTIC LEUKEMIA (ALL)

May have either B- (75%) or T-cell lineage. For T-cell ALL, test for HTLV-1 (endemic to southern Japan, the Caribbean, the South Pacific, and sub-Saharan Africa). The Philadelphia chromosome, t(9;22), is common and portends a poor prognosis. Adult ALL is more aggressive and less curable than childhood ALL.

TREATMENT

- **Combination chemotherapy:** Vincristine, prednisone, methotrexate, doxorubicin, and asparaginase.
- **Treatment regimen:**
  - Induction chemotherapy.
  - Several cycles of high-dose consolidation chemotherapy.
  - Prolonged maintenance low-dose chemotherapy, often followed by autologous or allogeneic stem-cell transplantation consolidation.
  - **CNS prophylaxis with intrathecal chemotherapy is mandatory for all patients** regardless of CNS involvement (systemic chemotherapy does not sufficiently penetrate the blood-brain barrier).

KEY FACT

In adults, CLL is the most common leukemia, and AML is more common than ALL.

KEY FACT

In patients with ALL, CNS prophylaxis with intrathecal chemotherapy is always mandatory regardless of CNS involvement.

KEY FACT

Poor prognostic factors in ALL include increasing age, t(4;11) (the MLL gene), t9;22 (BCR-ABL genes), or deletion of chromosome 7 or trisomy 8.

ACUTE MYELOID LEUKEMIA (AML)

A 60-year-old woman presents with worsening fatigue, fever, and epistaxis. One year ago she was diagnosed with myelodysplastic syndrome (MDS) and has been receiving intermittent blood transfusions since that time. She had not required platelet transfusions. Her temperature is 38°C (100.5°F), and exam reveals dried blood around the nares as well as numerous ecchymoses and petechiae, particularly on the extremities. There is no abdominal tenderness, splenomegaly, or lymphadenopathy. Labs show a hemoglobin of 6.5 g/dL, a leukocyte count of 2000/μL, and a platelet count of 6000/μL. Her peripheral blood smear shows 50% immature myeloid blasts and a paucity of platelets. In addition to blood transfusion and bone marrow aspiration, what is the most appropriate next step in management, and what is the most likely diagnosis?

Severe pancytopenia and circulating myeloid blasts on peripheral blood smear suggest disease transformation from MDS to AML. Induction chemotherapy for AML should be initiated with cytarabine and anthracycline. Patients with AML arising from MDS have poorer response rates and disease-free survival rates than those with de novo AML.

More common than ALL in adults. Incidence ↑ with age. Idiopathic AML, the most common subtype, carries a better prognosis than treatment-related AML (which results from prior anticancer therapy such as alkylating agents or topoisomerase inhibitors) or 2° AML (which arises following an antecedent MDS).

DIAGNOSIS

Bone marrow biopsy with > 20% marrow blasts. **FAB classification** is as follows:

- **M0:** Undifferentiated.
- **M1:** Myeloid.
- **M2:** Myeloid with differentiation.
- **M3:** Promyelocytic leukemia (APL).
- **M4:** Myelomonocytic leukemia.
- **M5:** Monocytic.
- **M6:** Erythroid.
- **M7:** Megakaryocytic.

TREATMENT

- Before therapy is initiated, patients must be given supportive care to improve their functional status.
- Treat infections.
- Transfusions, electrolyte replacement, allopurinol, and IV hydration to prevent hyperuricemia.
- Give oral hydroxyurea before the start of initial therapy to ↓ leukocyte counts to < 50,000/μL to prevent tumor lysis syndrome.
- Initiate induction chemotherapy with cytarabine (Ara-C) and an anthracycline.
- Consolidation therapy using high-dose cytarabine may result in durable remission or cure.
- Bone marrow transplantation (allogeneic or autologous) may be considered in patients who relapse or who have cytogenetic changes that place them at high risk for recurrence.

KEY FACT

Key steps in the treatment of AML are to induce remission and then to continue consolidation with further chemotherapy.

KEY FACT

Induction chemotherapy for AML is a high-risk time for the development of tumor lysis syndrome.

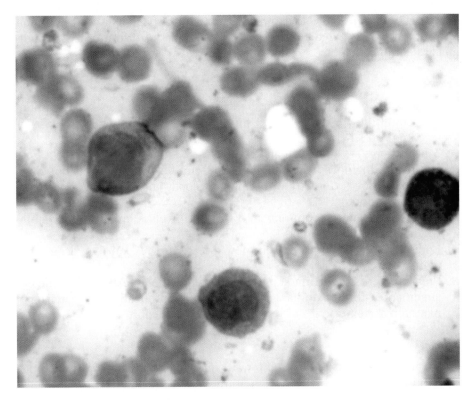

FIGURE 14.18. **Acute promyelocytic leukemia.** Note the **Auer rod** present in the cytoplasm of promyelocytes in bone marrow biopsy specimen. (Reproduced with permission from USMLERx. com.)

ACUTE PROMYELOCYTIC LEUKEMIA (AML-M3, APL)

Characterized by heavily granulated promyelocytic blasts (see Figure 14.18); associated with t(15;17) involving the retinoic acid receptor. DIC is present in the majority of patients at diagnosis.

TREATMENT

- Treatment involves the differentiating agent *all*-trans retinoic acid (ATRA), given during induction chemotherapy and as maintenance therapy. Anthracyclines and arsenic trioxide therapies also work well.
- **Retinoic acid syndrome** is characterized by pulmonary infiltrates, respiratory failure, fever, capillary leak syndrome, and cardiovascular collapse. Treat early with high-dose corticosteroids and temporary cessation of ATRA.

KEY FACT

AML-M3 is unique among AMLs for its propensity to cause DIC and for its high curability when treated with ATRA.

KEY FACT

M4 and M5 AML commonly present with infiltration of the bones of the orbits, sinuses, maxilla (gingival changes), and jaw (numb chin).

Chronic Leukemias

CHRONIC MYELOGENOUS LEUKEMIA (CML)

See the Hematology chapter.

CHRONIC LYMPHOCYTIC LEUKEMIA (CLL)

Abnormal accumulation of morphologically mature-appearing lymphocytes with a characteristic immunophenotype (CD5+, CD20+, and CD23+ B cells) in the blood, bone marrow, or lymphatic tissues. The most common leukemia in adults. Median survival is 10–15 years. **Autoimmune phenomena are common.**

EXAM/DIAGNOSIS

- Patients are often identified in the early stage of disease by an ↑ lymphocyte count, flow cytometry, and **smudge cells** on peripheral blood smear (see Figure 14.19).
- Most patients are asymptomatic.
- Evaluation includes a detailed physical exam for lymphadenopathy, organomegaly, flow cytometry of peripheral blood, and bone marrow biopsy (not always done).
- **Evans' syndrome** is common in CLL and involves autoimmune hemolytic anemia and thrombocytopenia (ITP).
- Long periods of stability or very slow disease progression may occur over many years.
- Progression of CLL is marked by generalized lymphatic and/or splenic enlargement with concomitant pancytopenia. Complications of pancytopenia, such as hemorrhage or infection, are a major cause of death.

TREATMENT

- Treatment should be directed toward relieving disease-related symptoms, rapidly progressive disease, autoimmune hemolytic anemia or thrombocytopenia, and infection.
- Many treatment approaches are available, including alkylating agents (chlorambucil, cyclophosphamide), nucleoside analogs (fludarabine, cladribine, pentostatin), and monoclonal antibodies (alemtuzumab).
- Treatment is highly effective in palliation but is not curative. Patients who are not symptomatic are generally not treated.
- For young patients, allogeneic bone marrow transplantation should be considered.

COMPLICATIONS

Richter's transformation: In 3–10% of patients, CLL may transform into a large cell lymphoma characterized by fever, a rising LDH, and rapid enlargement of nodal disease. Associated with a very poor prognosis.

KEY FACT

Anemia in CLL may be due to warm-antibody autoimmune hemolysis. A direct antiglobulin test (direct Coombs' test) is typically ⊕.

KEY FACT

Treatment for CLL is not curative, and the natural history of CLL is generally indolent, so CLL patients who are not symptomatic are generally not treated.

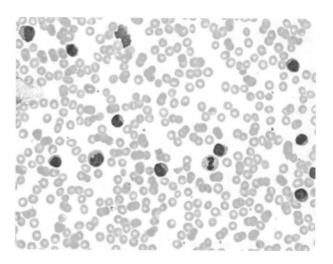

FIGURE 14.19. **Chronic lymphocytic leukemia.** Peripheral blood smear showing mature-appearing lymphocytes. Note the dense chromatin, scant cytoplasm, absence of nucleoli, and smudge cells. (Reproduced with permission from Kantarjian HM et al. *MD Anderson Manual of Medical Oncology.* New York: McGraw-Hill, 2006, Fig. 3-1.)

Hodgkin's Lymphoma

A 35-year-old woman presents for follow-up 15 years after successful treatment for Hodgkin's lymphoma with radiation therapy to the chest and abdominal lymph nodes. She never received combination chemotherapy, has never smoked, lacks any family history of cancer, and has no current medical problems. Her exam is normal. What is she at ↑ risk of developing in the future?

Hodgkin's lymphoma survivors who received extended-field radiation have a 1% risk per year of developing solid tumors. Young women are particularly prone to developing breast cancer, with a lifetime risk of > 50% for a 20-year-old patient treated with mediastinal radiation therapy. CAD is also a risk if the heart was in the radiation field.

The malignant cell is the Reed-Sternberg cell ("owl-eye" cell). Has a bimodal age distribution.

SYMPTOMS/EXAM

- Forty percent of patients present with systemic symptoms (B symptoms), which consist of weight loss, fever, and night sweats.
- Symptoms are also related to the site of involvement.

DIAGNOSIS

- **Excisional** biopsy for architecture (FNA is not sufficient) (see Figure 14.20).
- Staging includes physical examination of lymph nodes, detection of hepatosplenomegaly, CT of the chest/abdomen/pelvis, CXR (see Figure 14.21), and measurement of laboratory values, including CBC, LDH, ESR, and alkaline phosphatase.
- Routine staging laparotomy (splenectomy) has fallen out of favor.

KEY FACT

FNA is often inadequate for diagnosing Hodgkin's disease because it does not allow the pathologist to see the lymph node. Excisional biopsy is preferred.

TREATMENT

- **Early-stage disease (localized lymphadenopathy):**
  - Subtotal nodal irradiation or mantle irradiation.
  - Chemotherapy with ABVD (Adriamycin, bleomycin, vincristine, and dacarbazine) or the Stanford V protocol followed by radiation of the involved field. More than 75% of newly diagnosed disease is cured with combination chemotherapy +/– radiation.
- **Advanced disease:** Combination chemotherapy with ABVD is standard. If the prognosis is unfavorable, the regimen can be escalated to BEACOPP (bleomycin, etoposide, Adriamycin, cyclophosphamide, Oncovin, procarbazine, prednisone).
- **Refractory disease:** Patients with refractory disease should be considered for high-dose chemotherapy followed by autologous stem cell transplantation.

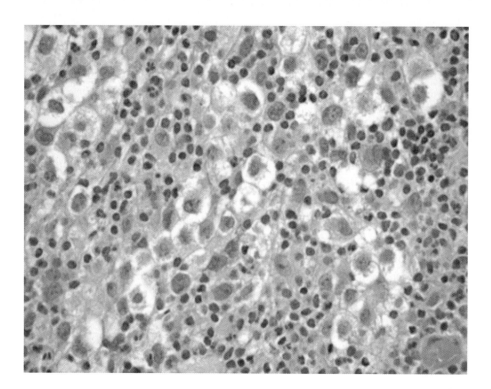

FIGURE 14.20.   Nodular sclerosing Hodgkin's lymphoma. This is the most common form of Hodgkin's lymphoma. The image shows a nodule containing abundant **lacunar cells** that have folded nuclei lying within a prominent clear space caused by retraction of the cytoplasm during processing of the tissue. (Reproduced with permission from USMLERx.com.)

COMPLICATIONS

Long-term complications include myelodysplasia and acute leukemia, 2° cancers (breast cancer in women treated with nodal irradiation), cardiomyopathy (2° to doxorubicin), pulmonary toxicity (2° to bleomycin), infertility, hypothyroidism, and neuropathy.

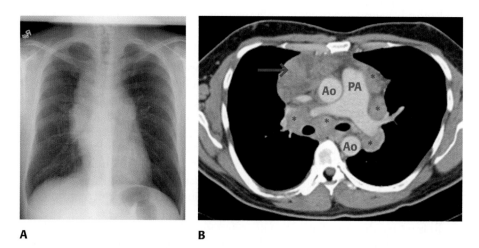

A   **B**

FIGURE 14.21.   Hodgkin's lymphoma. (A) Frontal CXR showing an abnormal mediastinal contour, with widening of the right paratracheal stripe and bilateral hilar enlargement. **(B)** Transaxial image from a follow-up contrast-enhanced CT demonstrates conglomerate lymphadenopathy in the anterior mediastinum (arrow) and multiple other enlarged lymph nodes (*) in the mediastinum and right hilum. Ao = aorta; PA = main pulmonary artery. (Reproduced with permission from USMLERx.com.)

Non-Hodgkin's Lymphoma (NHL)

A 35-year-old man presents with a rapidly enlarging 4-cm lump in the left side of his neck. He has had no fevers, night sweats, weight loss, recent illness, or any other significant history. The remainder of his exam is normal. CBC, chemistry, and LDH are all normal. Examination of the excised lymph nodes reveals CD20+ diffuse large B-cell lymphoma, an aggressive lymphoma. CT scans of the neck, chest, abdomen, and pelvis as well as a PET scan and bone marrow biopsy all confirm the absence of residual disease. What is the most appropriate treatment?

This patient has early-stage (IA) diffuse large B-cell lymphoma, an aggressive but highly curable type of non-Hodgkin's lymphoma. It is considered systemic even when the results of CT and PET scans are ⊖ and requires systemic therapy. The combination of the monoclonal antibody rituximab and CHOP (cyclophosphamide, hydroxydaunorubicin, Oncovin, and prednisone), with or without radiation therapy, is curative for most patients. The disease would most likely recur without any further therapy.

A heterogeneous group of cancers of B and T cells. The incidence of NHL is increasing for unknown reasons.

SYMPTOMS/EXAM

Include B symptoms (weight loss, fever, night sweats) and symptoms referable to lymph node masses or extranodal masses.

DIAGNOSIS/TREATMENT

- Diagnosis is based on histology, immunohistochemistry, and flow cytometry.
- Both FNA and excisional biopsy are acceptable.
- **Lumbar puncture (LP):** To evaluate for CNS involvement (cytology and flow cytometry) in patients with highly aggressive NHL (eg, Burkitt's lymphoma, HTLV-1-associated T-cell leukemia/lymphomas); HIV-⊕ NHL; those with epidural, bone marrow, testicular, or paranasal sinus involvement; or those with at least two extranodal disease sites.
- **CNS prophylaxis:** Can be considered for aggressive lymphomas warranting LP or MRI as outlined above, as CHOP therapy has poor CSF penetration. Prophylactic modalities include intrathecal and/or IV cytarabine or methotrexate, cranial radiation, and/or IV rituximab.
- NHL can be roughly divided into three subtypes based on natural history:
  - **Low grade:** Indolent; demonstrates high response rates to chemotherapy, but **generally not curable.** Treatment is based on reducing symptoms. Median survival is 6–10 years.
  - **Intermediate grade:** Curable. The standard chemotherapy, CHOP, cures approximately half of all patients and is given in 6–8 cycles of therapy. Evidence indicates that adding **rituximab, an anti-CD20 antibody** that targets B-cell lymphoma cells, **improves survival.**
  - **High grade:** Highly aggressive and rapidly growing cancers, but potentially **curable with chemotherapy.** Lymphoblastic lymphomas are treated like ALL. Burkitt's lymphoma is associated with EBV in Africa.

KEY FACT

In lymphomas that express CD20, treatment should include rituximab, a monoclonal antibody against CD20 B cells.

KEY FACT

Poor prognostic features in NHL include age > 60, LDH > 1× normal, poor performance status, late stage of disease, and extranodal disease.

Marginal zone B-cell lymphoma is associated with HCV; treatment of the underlying infection may result in remission of the lymphoma.

There is a risk of tumor lysis syndrome with high-grade lymphomas, so initiate hydration, urinary alkalinization, and administration of a xanthine oxidase inhibitor before chemotherapy by way of prevention.

- **Important subtypes** are as follows:
  - **MALT lymphoma:** See the section under gastric cancer.
  - **Mantle cell lymphoma:** Acts like an intermediate-grade lymphoma in aggressiveness but is not curable with conventional chemotherapy (as with low-grade lymphoma). Median survival is three years.

Important Translocations

- **Burkitt's lymphoma:** t(8;14).
- **Follicular lymphoma:** t(14;18).
- **Philadelphia chromosome:** t(9;22) (CML and a subset of ALL).
- **Good-prognosis AML (M4-Eo):** inv16.
- **Acute promyelocytic leukemia:** t(15;17) retinoic acid receptor and promyelocytic leukemia gene.

HIV and Cancer

- HIV is associated with an ↑ incidence of NHL, anal cancer, cervical cancer, Kaposi's sarcoma, and Hodgkin's disease.
- **Kaposi's sarcoma** is associated with **HHV-8** and is treated with HAART, α-interferon, topical retinoids, localized radiation, or liposomal doxorubicin.
- The optimal treatment of NHL in HIV is not clear, but NHL accounts for 15% of AIDS-related deaths.
- CNS NHL risk is also ↑ in HIV.
- The risk of cervical cancer and anal cancer is ↑ by HPV and impaired cellular immunity.

The 1° side effect of G-CSF is bone pain, most often in the sternum and long bones.

Drug-induced agranulocytosis with severe neutropenia and relatively well-preserved hematocrit and platelet counts can occur after ingestion of TMP-SMX, especially in the setting of sepsis. This usually resolves 10–12 days after stopping the medication, but G-CSF can ↓ the number of days of neutropenia.

Growth Factors

MYELOID GROWTH FACTORS (G-CSF, GM-CSF)

- Used for the prophylaxis of febrile neutropenia, but only in chemotherapy regimens with more than a 40% risk of neutropenic fever or in compromised hosts such as those with diminished bone marrow reserve, open wounds, active infections, or advanced cancer.
- Other uses for myeloid CSFs include mobilization of stem cells for transplant; neutropenia after bone marrow transplantation; congenital, cyclic, or idiopathic neutropenia; neutropenia after leukemia treatment or in MDS; and chemotherapy-induced neutropenic fever with an ANC < 100/μL, uncontrolled cancer, or severe sepsis.
- **Side effects:** The most common G-CSF side effect is bone pain.
- **Administration:** Dosing begins at least 24–48 hours after chemotherapy administration and should always stop at least 24 hours before subsequent chemotherapy.
- **Pegfilgrastim** is a long-acting, pegylated version of G-CSF.

ERYTHROPOIETIN

- ▪ Anemia in cancer and/or chemotherapy impairs quality of life. Erythroid growth factors are approved for use in chemotherapy-associated anemia and has been shown to improve anemia and ↓ transfusion requirements in some patients with transfusion-dependent MDS.
- ▪ **Administration:**
    - ▪ Patients often need supplemental iron to respond to erythropoietin.
    - ▪ Darbepoetin alfa is a new agent with a long half-life; less frequent dosing may be used (q 2–3 weeks).
- ▪ Erythropoietin failure in patients receiving dialysis can be caused by iron deficiency, folate deficiency, ongoing blood loss, or iron overload. Vitamin C can improve the response to erythropoietin in patients receiving dialysis by mobilizing iron stores.

 KEY FACT

Using darbepoetin or erythropoietin to ↑ RBCs above 13 g/dL will ↑ the risk of cardiovascular, thromboembolic events, and stroke.

NOTES

CHAPTER 15

Psychiatry

Anuj Gaggar, MD, PhD
Amin N. Azzam, MD, MA

Psychiatry Pearls

- All psychiatric illnesses can be divided into four major categories (see Figure 15.1). As with other illness, symptoms suggest categories that can then be further clarified. In general, there are no objective laboratory tests for psychiatric diagnostic clarification, so a careful history is essential.
- Some psychiatric syndromes are diagnoses of exclusion; therefore, likely medical etiologies must be ruled out before such diagnoses can be made.
- Pharmacologic treatment follows from the diagnosis or 1° symptoms (see Figure 15.1). Psychotic disorders are treated with antipsychotics; anxiety disorders are treated with anxiolytic agents. Mood disorders are treated with antidepressants or mood stabilizers, depending on unipolarity or bipolarity.
- Some psychiatric syndromes have symptoms from two major disease categories (eg, schizoaffective disorder, which has both psychotic and mood disorder symptoms). For these syndromes, treatment generally involves medication with > 1 category, targeting each symptom separately.
- The choice of medication in each class should be based on several factors:
  - Proven efficacy for the illness being treated.
  - Patient demographics.
  - The likely side effect profile and tolerability to the patient.
  - Patient preference (to maximize patient adherence).
  - Drug-drug interactions with other medications.
  - The choice of benzodiazepine should be based on the nature of the anxiety symptom being treated (see Figure 15.2).
- See Table 15.1 for case presentations of the common psychiatric disorders.

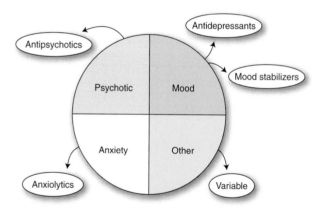

FIGURE 15.1. Pharmacologic management of psychiatric illness.

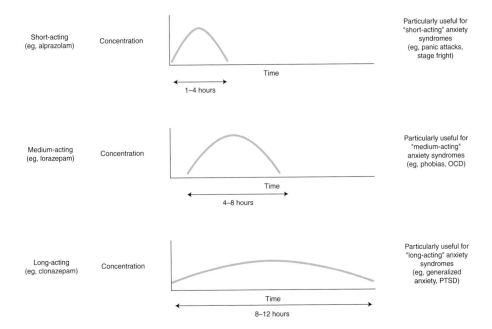

FIGURE 15.2. **Length of action of benzodiazepines.**

TABLE 15.1. **Classic Case Presentations of Common Psychiatric Disorders**

MAJOR DEPRESSIVE EPISODE	GENERALIZED ANXIETY DISORDER	BIPOLAR DISORDER	SCHIZOPHRENIA
▪ A 36-year-old woman with mild psychomotor retardation and dark circles under her eyes complains of excessive fatigue, as well as waking up in the middle of the night and being unable to fall back asleep. ▪ She also has difficulty concentrating on child care, guilt about being a "bad mother," and lack of pleasure in activities she once enjoyed. ▪ Her symptoms began three months ago and have gradually worsened to the point at which she can no longer perform her normal work and child care duties.	▪ A 42-year-old man with mild psychomotor agitation complains that for the past six months "my nerves have been shot." ▪ He mentions that he worries "all the time and over everything" and can't fall asleep, adding that he often "snaps at his wife." ▪ The patient also has chronic neck and shoulder tension as well as mild daily headaches that are relieved by acetaminophen.	▪ A 25-year-old woman you have been treating for depression comes to your office wearing heavy makeup and a revealing red dress "because my husband told me I have to; he says my personality has changed. I think he just can't handle my womanhood." ▪ The woman, previously demure and shy, frequently stands up to admire the artwork in your office, which she describes as "unusually sensual; I might have to test your kissing ability some day." She speaks very quickly and becomes angry whenever interrupted.	▪ A 19-year-old disheveled male is brought to your office by his parents, who state that their son "just got kicked out of college for harassing the dean." They add that they had to fly across the country to come get him because he "couldn't figure out how to get to the airport." ▪ On interview, the man seldom speaks unless asked a question and rarely makes eye contact except to ask you if his eyes look okay, "because I see colors too brightly now." Occasionally he seems to talk to himself, stating, "Yeah, yeah, I know, but I like the doctor."

(continues)

TABLE 15.1. **Classic Case Presentations of Common Psychiatric Disorders** *(continued)*

Major Depressive Episode	Generalized Anxiety Disorder	Bipolar Disorder	Schizophrenia
		▪ The woman's anger dissipates within seconds and is replaced by feelings of exhilaration and joy. She leaves after only a few questions but gives you a $100 "tip," stating that "I'll be rich soon anyway now that I've finally started my consulting business." She sings on her way out of the office.	▪ When asked why he left college, the man states that "no one there can handle the truth—the truth of the elders of the dean and his spies."

Anxiety Disorders

PANIC DISORDER

Consists of at least **two** untriggered panic attacks, with impaired function due to **fear of having another.**

SYMPTOMS

- Panic attacks must develop abruptly and peak within 10 minutes. They must also include at least four of the following: tachycardia, diaphoresis, shortness of breath, chest pain, nausea, dizziness, paresthesias, chills, derealization/depersonalization, and fear of losing control/going crazy/dying.
- A panic attack may be triggered or may occur spontaneously.

DIFFERENTIAL

- **Endocrine:** Hypoglycemia, hypothyroidism, hyperthyroidism, hyperparathyroidism, pheochromocytoma.
- **Neurologic:** Seizure disorders, vestibular dysfunction, neoplasms.
- **Pharmacologic:** Acute intoxication, medication-induced symptoms.
- **Cardiovascular:** Arrhythmias, MI.
- **Pulmonary:** COPD, asthma exacerbation, pulmonary embolus.
- **Psychiatric:**
  - **Generalized anxiety disorder:** Patients typically have more chronic baseline anxiety.
  - **Obsessive-compulsive disorder (OCD):** Patients generally have recurrent repetitive thoughts (obsessions) and mannerisms (compulsions).
  - **Posttraumatic stress disorder (PTSD):** Patients have a history of a traumatic event and no history of panic attacks.

DIAGNOSIS

Rule out all likely medical etiologies (eg, ECG, electrolyte panel, CXR).

TREATMENT

- **Behavioral:** Various forms of behavioral psychotherapies.
- **Medication:** Benzodiazepine anxiolytic agents, β-blockers, antidepressants.

KEY FACT

Panic disorder can occur with or without agoraphobia (fear of open spaces or of being alone in a crowd or leaving the home).

GENERALIZED ANXIETY DISORDER

 A 25-year-old man is seen in the ER for palpitations, dyspnea, and chest heaviness. His symptoms began while he was at home watching television, and he reports having had several similar episodes in the past, two of which required ER visits with ⊖ workups (including a normal TSH). He has recently become concerned about having another episode, and for this reason he has not been attending his classes at the local college. In the ER, he is found to be normotensive with a heart rate of 100 bpm. His ECG is unremarkable, as is his laboratory work, which includes a urine toxicology test. What intervention is most likely to help this patient?

An SSRI and possibly psychotherapy. This patient has generalized anxiety disorder and is now having functional impairment that warrants treatment. Long-acting anxiolytics might prove useful as well, but SSRIs are generally first-line therapy.

Defined as uncontrollable worry about a **broad range of topics** (eg, work/school, relationships, health) over time (ie, more days than not for at least **six months**).

SYMPTOMS

- Patients have poor control over their anxiety and at least **three** of the following: restlessness, poor concentration, irritability, easy fatigue, muscle tension, and sleep disturbances.
- Symptoms **must cause functional impairment** (ie, they must interfere with social or occupational functioning).

DIFFERENTIAL

- **PTSD:** Patients must have a history of a traumatic event.
- **Major depressive disorder:** Patients usually have depressed mood and other physical symptoms.
- **OCD:** Patients typically have recurrent repetitive thoughts (obsessions) and mannerisms (compulsions), and anxiety is only around the obsessions.

DIAGNOSIS

Rule out all likely medical etiologies.

TREATMENT

- **Behavioral:** Various forms of individual and group psychotherapies.
- **Medication: Long-acting** benzodiazepine anxiolytic agents (eg, clonazepam); antidepressants.

COMPLICATIONS

Often leads to **depression** if left untreated.

> **KEY FACT**
>
> Generalized anxiety disorder is characterized by anxiety in many different situations (eg, at work, during mealtimes, in social situations, while falling asleep).

KEY FACT

Specific phobias are the most common anxiety disorder.

SPECIFIC PHOBIAS

Fear of specific items, situations, or activities.

SYMPTOMS

- Presents with excessive or unreasonable fear of a particular trigger; **patients realize that their response is excessive.**
- Must also cause **functional impairment** (ie, must interfere with social or occupational functioning).

DIFFERENTIAL

- **Panic disorder:** Panic attacks can be untriggered.
- **PTSD:** Patients avoid things only after having a traumatic event.
- **Generalized anxiety disorder:** Patients have chronic baseline anxiety about many things, not just when they are exposed to a trigger.

TREATMENT

- **Behavioral:** Exposure-response prevention therapy (exposes the patient to the stressor and prevents their usual fleeing response; desensitizes the patient to the stressor).
- **Medication:** β-blockers; short-acting benzodiazepines (eg, alprazolam).

OBSESSIVE-COMPULSIVE DISORDER (OCD)

Obsessions and compulsions causing significant impairment that are recognized as excessive or unreasonable.

SYMPTOMS

- **Obsessions:** Recurrent or persistent thoughts that **cause** anxiety.
- **Compulsions:** Behaviors or rituals that temporarily **relieve** anxiety.
- **Patients must recognize that their symptoms are unreasonable** and that their obsessions are their own thoughts.

KEY FACT

Obsessions cause ↑ anxiety that is temporarily relieved by compulsions.

DIFFERENTIAL

- **Delusional disorder:** Patients **do not** find the thoughts unreasonable.
- **Schizophrenia:** Patients have psychotic symptoms along with affective flattening, asociality, and avolition.
- **Generalized anxiety disorder:** Patients have anxiety in several different areas of their lives that are generally not relieved by compulsive acts.

TREATMENT

- **Behavioral:** Exposure-response prevention therapy; cognitive-behavioral therapy (teaches patients how to diminish their cognitive distortions of the stressor and how to change their behavioral response).
- **Medication:** Clomipramine, SSRIs (eg, paroxetine, sertraline, fluvoxamine). **Higher doses than those used for depression are usually required.**

COMPLICATIONS

Often leads to depression if left untreated.

POSTTRAUMATIC STRESS DISORDER (PTSD)

A 29-year-old physician returns from an overseas deployment in which he was working in a war zone. He is now spending most of his time at home and has noted poor concentration as well as occasional flashbacks. He wants to return to work but does not feel that he can go back to the hospital because of his experience overseas. What treatments would be best for him?

Cognitive-behavioral therapy, likely combined with an SSRI. Benzodiazepines can be used for short-term symptoms, but SSRIs and cognitive-behavioral therapy will likely achieve the best long-term efficacy.

Reaction to a traumatic event characterized by reexperiencing, avoidance, and ↑ arousal. Prevalence is up to 3%, but up to 30% of veterans are affected.

SYMPTOMS

- Patients must have a perceived life-threatening trauma and all **three** of the following:
  1. Reexperiencing (eg, flashbacks, nightmares).
  2. Avoidance (places, thoughts, feelings, people related to the trauma).
  3. ↑ arousal (insomnia, hyperstartle, poor concentration, anger outbursts).
- Patients must have all symptoms for a minimum of one month.

DIFFERENTIAL

- **Depression:** Patients do not have flashbacks to a traumatic event.
- **Generalized anxiety disorder:** Patients do not have a history of a traumatic event or flashbacks.
- **Adjustment disorder:** Patients have stress, anxiety, depression, or behavioral changes that are related to a specific trigger but do not have all three 1° symptoms of reexperiencing, avoidance, and ↑ arousal.

TREATMENT

- **Behavioral:** Various forms of individual and group psychotherapy.
- **Medication:** SSRIs, sleep agents (eg, trazodone), long-acting benzodiazepines (eg, clonazepam). Prazosin is sometimes given for nightmares.

PREVENTION

Some research suggests that reducing autonomic activation (with β-blockers) shortly after the trauma may ↓ the likelihood of developing PTSD.

COMPLICATIONS

- Long-term use of benzodiazepines can lead to psychological dependence, so prescribe with caution/selectivity.
- Avoidance of stimuli associated with the trauma can generalize to avoidance of wide-ranging things (which become secondarily associated with the trauma in the patient's mind). This leads to a far greater ⊖ impact on the patient's life.

 KEY FACT

In acute stress disorder, symptoms last < 1 month. In PTSD, symptoms last > 1 month.

Mood Disorders

MAJOR DEPRESSIVE DISORDER

The male-to-female ratio is 1:2. Risk is higher if there is a family history. **Untreated episodes usually last ≥ 4 months.**

SYMPTOMS

- Patients must have **depressed mood** or **loss of interest/pleasure (anhedonia)** and **five** of the symptoms outlined in the **SIG E CAPS** mnemonic.
- Symptoms must represent a **change from baseline**; cause **functional impairment** (eg, work, school, or social activities); and **last at least two weeks continuously.**

DIFFERENTIAL

- **Adjustment disorder:** Patients have a known stressor that causes a reaction similar to a depressive episode, but the reaction is less severe and is triggered specifically by that stressor.
- **Dysthymic disorder:** Patients have "low-level depression" (ie, depression involving < 5 **SIG E CAPS** symptoms) that **lasts at least two years.**
- **Anxiety disorders:** Generalized anxiety disorder, PTSD, OCD.
- **Medical "masqueraders":** Hypothyroidism, anemia, pancreatic cancer, Parkinson's disease.
- **Substance-induced mood disorder:** Illicit drugs, thiazide diuretics, digoxin, glucocorticoids, benzodiazepines, cimetidine, ranitidine, cyclosporine, sulfonamides, metoclopramide.

DIAGNOSIS

Eliminate potential medical etiologies (eg, check TSH and CBC).

TREATMENT

- **Behavioral:** Various forms of individual and group psychotherapies.
- **Medication:** SSRIs; other classes of antidepressants. Medication selection should be based on symptom profile and anticipated side effect tolerability as well as on how activating or sedating the medication can be.
    - **Activating:** Bupropion, fluoxetine.
    - **Sedating:** Paroxetine, mirtazapine.
    - **Neutral:** Sertraline, venlafaxine, citalopram.
- **Electroconvulsive therapy (ECT):** Often reserved for medication-resistant depression; **especially useful in the elderly.**

COMPLICATIONS

- Severely depressed patients can develop psychotic symptoms (eg, auditory hallucinations, paranoid ideations, ideas of reference). These symptoms can be treated with a low dose of an antipsychotic agent.
- **Suicidality:** One of the major comorbidities of untreated depression is suicidality (see the mnemonic **SAD PERSONS**).
    - Women generally make more attempts, but attempts made by men are usually more lethal.
    - Clinicians must assess the degree of risk (eg, consider the number of prior attempts, degree of premeditation, lethality of method, and access to the proposed method) and hospitalize if necessary to ensure patient safety.

MNEMONIC

Symptoms of major depressive disorder—

SIG E CAPS

Sleep (hypersomnia or insomnia)
Interest (loss of interest or pleasure in activities)
Guilt (feelings of worthlessness or inappropriate guilt)
Energy (↓)
Concentration (↓)
Appetite (↑ or ↓)
Psychomotor agitation or retardation
Suicidal ideation

KEY FACT

Psychotherapy and antidepressants together are more effective for depression than either treatment alone.

KEY FACT

If a patient has not responded at all after 8–12 weeks of an SSRI given for depression, switch to another medication either of the same class or of a different class.

KEY FACT

Consider augmentation therapy if a patient has achieved only a partial response after maximal treatment with one SSRI for depression. Use a second drug from a different class (eg, bupropion, venlafaxine, mirtazapine).

BIPOLAR AFFECTIVE DISORDER

Extreme mood swings between mania and depression. Risk is higher if there is a family history. There are two types: **type I**, which alternates between mania and depression, and **type II**, which alternates between depression and hypomania (ie, fewer symptoms for a shorter duration).

SYMPTOMS

- The symptoms of manic episodes in bipolar affective disorder are described by the mnemonic **DIG FAST.**
- Manic episodes **must last at least four days or lead to hospitalization** in order to be called mania. Anything less is considered hypomania.
- See the entry on depression for symptoms of the depressive episodes of bipolar disorder; remember the mnemonic **SIG E CAPS.**

DIFFERENTIAL

- **Major depressive disorder:** Patients have no history of a manic episode.
- **Schizoaffective disorder:** Patients have both **psychotic symptoms** and mood symptoms. Psychotic symptoms occur in the **absence** of mood symptoms.
- **Schizophrenia:** Patients do not have mood symptoms.

TREATMENT

- **Acute manic episode:** Hospitalize; consider antipsychotic agents (eg, haloperidol, olanzapine, risperidone). ↑ doses of mood stabilizers (lithium carbonate, valproic acid, carbamazepine).
- **Maintenance treatment:** Give mood stabilizers such as those listed above. Titrate to the lowest effective dose to maintain mood stability.
- **Depressive episodes:** Antidepressants alone may trigger mania, so use carefully; consider individual and group psychotherapies.

PREVENTION

- ↑ the mood stabilizer dose in the presence of imminent symptoms of mania.
- Educate patients to recognize the earliest signs of mania/depression (sleep changes are often the first sign), and encourage them to seek additional help early.

COMPLICATIONS

- In severe phases of mania or depression, patients can have psychotic symptoms.
- **If the condition is left untreated, many patients have progressively more rapid cycling** (more frequent and shorter-duration episodes).

MNEMONIC

Risk factors for suicide—

SAD PERSONS

Sex (male)
Age (elderly or adolescent)
Depression
Previous attempt
Ethanol abuse
Rational thought loss
Sickness
Organized plan
No spouse
Social support lacking

MNEMONIC

Symptoms of manic episodes—

DIG FAST

Distractibility
Insomnia (↓ need for sleep)
Grandiosity (↑ self-esteem)
Flight of ideas (or racing thoughts)
↑ **A**ctivities/psychomotor **A**gitation
Pressured **S**peech
Thoughtlessness (poor judgment—eg, spending sprees, unsafe sex)

KEY FACT

Treating a bipolar patient with antidepressant monotherapy can lead to a manic episode.

Psychotic Disorders

SCHIZOPHRENIA

A 47-year-old man with schizophrenia presents with ↑ "twitching" of his lips and tongue over the past several months. On exam, he is noted to have dyskinetic movements of his tongue and lips but is otherwise doing well. He has no other medical problems and takes haloperidol for his schizophrenia. What would be the most appropriate therapy for his facial movements?

An atypical antipsychotic (eg, olanzapine, quetiapine, risperidone). This patient has likely been on typical antipsychotics (haloperidol) for several years, placing him at risk for tardive dyskinesia. If his symptoms cannot be controlled on atypical antipsychotics, his dose of haloperidol can be ↓. Alternatively, he can be treated with a nonselective β-blocker or a benzodiazepine, but this would not constitute first-line therapy.

A history of **severe** and **persistent** psychotic symptoms (≥ 1 month) in the context of chronic impairment in function (> 6 months). There are several subtypes. **Age of onset is mostly in the late teens or 20s** for men and in the 20s–30s for women; risk is higher if there is a family history.

SYMPTOMS

Patients must have ≥ **2** of the following:

- **Delusions:** Fixed false beliefs.
- **Hallucinations:** Most often auditory, but can be visual, olfactory, gustatory, or tactile.
- **Disorganized speech or thoughts.**
- **Grossly disorganized or catatonic behavior.**
- **Negative symptoms:** Affective flattening, avolition, alogia (poverty of speech), asociality.

DIFFERENTIAL

- **Bipolar affective disorder:** Patients have psychotic symptoms only during extreme manic or depressive episodes.
- **Schizoaffective disorder:** Patients have psychotic symptoms **but also have prominent mood symptoms** (either depression or mania).
- **Delusional disorder:** Patients have **one** fixed false belief that is nonbizarre and that does not necessarily have a broad impact on functioning.
- **Developmental delay:** Patients do not have overtly psychotic symptoms and **have not deteriorated from a higher-functioning baseline.**
- **OCD: Patients are aware** that their obsessions (recurring repetitive thoughts) are their own thoughts.
- **Depression with psychotic features:** Patients have psychotic symptoms that occur only during depressive episodes, and the **depressive symptoms can occur without psychotic symptoms.**
- **Generalized anxiety disorder:** Patients have severe and chronic anxiety but no psychotic symptoms.

KEY FACT

Psychotic = "break with reality."

MNEMONIC

The 4 A's of schizophrenia:

Affective flattening
Asociality
Alogia (paucity of speech)
Auditory hallucinations

- **Substance-induced psychosis:** Especially associated with amphetamine or cocaine, both of which can cause paranoia and hallucinations. Patients have other signs/symptoms of substance use.
- **Medical "masqueraders":** Examples include neurosyphilis, herpes encephalitis, dementia, and delirium.
- **Neurologic "masqueraders":** Include complex partial seizures and Huntington's disease.

DIAGNOSIS

Diagnose by history. **Neuropsychological testing** can be helpful in clarifying the diagnosis but often is not indicated.

TREATMENT

- Choose an antipsychotic agent that minimizes both symptoms and side effect profile.
- **Atypical antipsychotics** (eg, olanzapine, risperidone, quetiapine, ziprasidone, aripiprazole) **are now considered first-line agents** because they have fewer motor side effects than do typical antipsychotics such as haloperidol. However, atypicals are much more expensive and can lead to significant weight gain.
- **Acute psychotic episodes:** Hospitalize; ↑ the dose of antipsychotic agent and consider the use of anxiolytic agents (eg, alprazolam, clonazepam). Group therapy sessions can provide a forum for reality checks if patients can tolerate them.
- **Maintenance treatment: Titrate to the lowest effective dose of antipsychotic agent to maintain stability.** Group therapy and structured day programs provide safety, socialization skills, and reality checks.

COMPLICATIONS

- If left untreated, schizophrenia will lead to a **"downward drift"** in socioeconomic class.
- Long-term use of typical antipsychotics (eg, haloperidol) can lead to **tardive dyskinesia**—ie, involuntary choreoathetoid movements of the face, lips, tongue, and trunk.
  - Tardive dyskinesia should be treated by minimizing doses of neuroleptics or by switching to an atypical neuroleptic (eg, olanzapine, risperidone, quetiapine).
  - Benzodiazepines (eg, alprazolam, clonazepam) or β-blockers (eg, propranolol) can also be given.

DELUSIONAL DISORDER

Patients have a fixed false belief (delusion) that is nonbizarre.

SYMPTOMS

- The delusion is often highly specific and organized into a system (ie, patients can describe wide and varying evidence to support the delusion). This leads to hypervigilance and hypersensitivity.
- There is usually a relative lack of other symptoms, and patients often remain high functioning otherwise.

KEY FACT

There is often a prodromal phase of schizophrenia involving ⊖ symptoms without ⊕ symptoms (delusions or hallucinations).

KEY FACT

Olanzapine and several other atypical antipsychotics can cause significant weight gain and ↑ the risk of type 2 DM.

KEY FACT

Patients newly diagnosed with schizophrenia ("first break") are at high risk for suicide attempts.

DIFFERENTIAL

- **Schizophrenia:** Patients often have a history of auditory hallucinations or other psychotic symptoms, such as prominent ⊖ symptoms (affective flattening, avolition, alogia, asociality). Frequently, there is greater functional impairment.
- **Substance-induced delusions:** Particularly associated with amphetamine and cannabis.
- **Medical conditions:** Hyper-/hypothyroidism, Parkinson's, Huntington's, Alzheimer's, CVAs, metabolic causes (hypercalcemia, uremia, hepatic encephalopathy), other causes of delirium.

TREATMENT

- Patients are often likely to refuse treatment or medications. Low-dose atypical antipsychotics may be helpful.
- Do not pretend that the delusion is true, but do not argue with patients in attempts to prove it false. Instead, gently remind them of your goal of maximizing functionality.

COMPLICATIONS

Many patients do not seek treatment, leading to progressive isolation and to a ↓ in productivity and/or functional status.

Substance Abuse Disorders

CHRONIC ABUSE/DEPENDENCE

Substance abuse is a maladaptive pattern of use that occurs despite adverse consequences. Dependence is abuse and physiologic tolerance.

TREATMENT

All the dependencies are characterized by **relapsing and remitting** patterns. Optimal treatment varies from patient to patient but usually involves **combinations** of the following:

- **Pharmacologic substitutes:** Replace the substance of abuse with a longer-acting and less addictive pharmacologic equivalent. Examples include methadone for heroin, chlordiazepoxide (Librium) for alcohol, and clonazepam for short-acting benzodiazepines. Agents can be used either in a detoxification program (eg, 21 days) or as maintenance therapy (eg, methadone maintenance).
- **Pharmacologic antagonists:** ↓ the pleasurable response associated with the substance of abuse. Examples include the following:
  - **Disulfiram (Antabuse) for alcohol:** Blocks the efficacy of alcohol dehydrogenase, causing buildup of acetaldehyde.
  - **Naltrexone:** Thought to ↓ alcohol craving.
- **Nonpharmacologic treatments:**
  - **Therapeutic communities:** Provide a safe, structured environment in which to boost attempts at maintaining early sobriety. Can be inpatient (residential) or outpatient, brief or long term.
  - **Self-help organizations:** Offer a regular and ongoing community of peers to maintain ongoing sobriety. Examples include Alcoholics Anonymous (AA) and Narcotics Anonymous (NA).

- **Family support/education:** Provide support to family members; offer an environment in which to learn from and commiserate with others. An example is Al-Anon.
- **Individual counseling/therapy:** Various techniques focus on the following:
  - Understanding and eliminating triggers for relapse.
  - **Harm reduction approach:** Minimizing use of the substance, which minimizes its functional impact on patients' lives.
  - **Abstinence model:** Getting patients to accept that they cannot minimize use but must abstain in order to improve their functional quality of life.
  - **Psychoeducation:** Educating patients regarding issues such as the cycle of relapses and remissions; the chronic nature of the illness; and available resources.
- For further information on the treatment of acute intoxication or withdrawal syndromes, see the Hospital Medicine chapter.

COMPLICATIONS

Chronic substance dependence leads to significant loss of productivity, functionality, and quality of life.

Other Disorders

SOMATOFORM DISORDERS

A group of disorders in which patients complain of physical symptoms that have no clear medical etiologies. Certain subtypes are more common in women (eg, conversion disorder, pain disorder); others are more common in men (eg, factitious disorder, malingering). All generally occur more often in those with lower socioeconomic status and education.

SYMPTOMS

- Vary across the specific disorders, but all are insufficiently explained by medical causes alone.
- Demonstrate inconsistent findings and often lead to many unnecessary hospitalizations, procedures, and workups. Specific subtypes include the following:
  - **Somatization disorder:** Complaints are in at least **two** organ systems.
  - **Conversion disorder:** Complaints are in the **neurologic** system.
  - **Pain disorder:** Complaints are predominantly of pain.
  - **Hypochondriasis:** Complaints and fear are of serious diseases.
  - **Body dysmorphic disorder:** Complaints are about a perceived defective body or body part.
  - **Factitious disorder:** Complaints are **consciously simulated by the patient** (vs. somatization disorder).
  - **Malingering:** Complaints are **consciously simulated by the patient with specific 2° goals** as a 1° motivator (vs. factitious disorder).

DIAGNOSIS

- Eliminate likely medical etiologies through standard medical workups. A balance must be struck between sufficient workup to rule out realistic causes and exhaustive workup to rule out extremely rare causes.
- Psychiatric consultation can help clarify specific diagnoses and can therefore elucidate potential treatment options that could be most helpful.

TREATMENT

- **Minimize** the number of providers involved in the care of the patient.
- Establish and maintain a **long-term, trusting doctor-patient relationship;** schedule regular outpatient visits and routinely inquire about psychosocial stressors.
- On each visit, perform at least a partial physical exam directed at the organ system of complaint, and gradually change the agenda to inquire about psychosocial issues in an empathic manner.
- **Refer patients to a mental health professional** to help them express their feelings, thereby minimizing physical symptoms as a proxy for those feelings.
- **Treat any 2° depression** (ie, depression 2° to the sense of hopelessness associated with having the somatoform disorder).
- Some patients may benefit from the use of an anxiolytic agent (eg, alprazolam).
- Be aware that some patients will develop psychological dependence on medications, so prescribe selectively.

> **KEY FACT**
>
> Informal "curbside" consults of colleagues can be quite helpful for somatoform disorders and are preferable to the formal introduction of yet another medical provider.

ATTENTION-DEFICIT HYPERACTIVITY DISORDER (ADHD)

Persistent problems (> 6 months) with **inattention** and/or **hyperactivity and impulsivity.**

SYMPTOMS

Diagnostic criteria are as follows:

- Inattention, including at least **six** of the following:
  1. Poor attention to tasks, play activities, or schoolwork.
  2. Poor listening skills.
  3. Poor follow-through on instructions.
  4. Poor organizational skills.
  5. Avoidance of tasks requiring sustained mental effort.
  6. Frequent loss of things.
  7. Easy distractibility and forgetfulness.
  8. Frequent careless mistakes.
- Hyperactivity-impulsivity, including at least six of the following:
  1. Fidgetiness.
  2. Leaving rooms in which sitting is expected.
  3. Excessive running/climbing.
  4. Subjective thoughts of restlessness.
  5. Difficulties with leisure activities.
  6. Acting as if "driven by a motor."
  7. Talking excessively.
  8. Interrupting others often.

> **KEY FACT**
>
> In order for an adult to be diagnosed with ADHD, symptoms must have been present in childhood and must cause functional impairment.

> **KEY FACT**
>
> Adults tend to have less hyperactivity than do children in ADHD.

DIFFERENTIAL

- **Medication-seeking behavior:** Patients often present with a history of substance abuse (especially amphetamine abuse).
- **Bipolar affective disorder:** Inattention/racing thoughts occur only during manic episodes; are accompanied by a lack of need for sleep and by grandiosity/euphoria; and are cyclical in nature.
- **Substance-induced symptoms:** Especially common with amphetamine intoxication. Look for associated signs and symptoms of substance abuse.

TREATMENT

- **Stimulants** (eg, methylphenidate): ↑ the dose as needed.
- **Nonstimulants** (eg, atomoxetine).
- **Antidepressants:** If there is a risk of abuse/dependence, bupropion (Wellbutrin) is a nonaddictive and reasonable first-line agent.
- **Behavioral therapy:** Focus on changing maladaptive behaviors and on learning more effective ones.

EATING DISORDERS

A 21-year-old woman is brought to the ER following an episode of syncope at home. The patient's mother notes that her daughter is very thin and has not been eating well. She is awake and alert in the ER and has a BMI of 15.5. Her labs show a hematocrit of 28%, a serum potassium level of 2.9 mEq/L, a serum phosphorus level of 2.2 mg/dL, an albumin level of 3.0 g/dL, and an INR of 1.5. The patient wants to go home. What finding puts her at the highest risk for an adverse outcome that would warrant hospitalization?

Hypophosphatemia. This patient has several features that would warrant hospitalization, but having hypophosphatemia puts her at high risk for refeeding syndrome, which could result in cardiovascular collapse. Refeeding syndrome often leads to a further ↓ in intracellular phosphate stores, resulting in lower ATP generation and eventual metabolic collapse.

Marked disturbances in eating behavior. There are **two** major types:

- **Anorexia nervosa:** Patients have misperceptions of body weight, generally weigh < 85% of their ideal body weight, and self-impose severe dietary limitations. The male-to-female ratio is 1:10–20. More common in developed/Western societies and in more affluent socioeconomic strata.
- **Bulimia nervosa:** Episodic uncontrolled binges of food consumption followed by compensatory weight loss strategies (eg, self-imposed vomiting, laxative and diuretic abuse, excessive exercise).

SYMPTOMS

- Both anorexia and bulimia involve a marked misperception of body image and poor self-esteem.
- Distinguished as follows:
  - **Anorexia only:** Actual body weight must be < 85% of ideal body weight (for height and age). Also presents with **lanugo,** dry skin, lethargy, bradycardia, hypotension, cold intolerance, hypothermia, and hypocarotenemia.
  - **Bulimia only:** Patients must have at least **three** months of binge-purging activity that occurs at least **twice a week.** They must also have a sense of **loss of control** during food consumption binges. Patients often have signs of frequent vomiting (eg, low chloride levels, pharyngeal lesions, **tooth enamel decay,** scratches on the dorsal surfaces of the fingers) and **enlarged parotid glands.**

DIFFERENTIAL

Medical causes of weight loss and amenorrhea; failure to thrive.

DIAGNOSIS

Diagnose by history. A collateral history obtained from other family members is often helpful.

TREATMENT

- Correct electrolyte abnormalities.
- Psychotherapy.
- **Antidepressants:** SSRIs.

PERSONALITY DISORDERS

Persistent maladaptive characteristic patterns of behavior **that have been present since childhood** and cause **significant impairment in patients' functioning in society.** All are coded on Axis II.

SYMPTOMS

There are several types, most often subdivided into clusters:

- **Cluster A** (aka the **"weird"** personality disorders):
  - Schizoid
  - Schizotypal
  - Paranoid
- **Cluster B** (aka the **"wild"** personality disorders):
  - Borderline
  - Histrionic
  - Narcissistic
  - Antisocial
- **Cluster C** (aka the **"wimpy"** personality disorders):
  - Dependent
  - Obsessive-compulsive
  - Avoidant

DIFFERENTIAL

Developmental delay (patients have below-normal intelligence).

DIAGNOSIS

Without a significant amount of collateral information, it is difficult to diagnose patients with personality disorders on a single visit. Because there must be a persistent pattern of behavior, patients should ideally be observed over time to ensure accurate diagnosis and referral.

TREATMENT

- Personality disorders are both longstanding and pervasive and are thus **resistant to treatment.**
- **Dialectical behavioral therapy** has been shown to be an effective treatment of **borderline personality disorder.** Brief **cognitive-behavioral therapy** groups may also maximize effective coping strategies and minimize functional impact on patients' lives.
- **Mood stabilizers** (eg, valproic acid, lithium, carbamazepine) may be of use in **antisocial** and **borderline personality disorders.** SSRIs (eg, fluoxetine, sertraline, paroxetine) may be useful in treating **borderline, dependent,** and **avoidant personality disorders.**

KEY FACT

People with cluster B personality disorders will sometimes "split" medical personnel—ie, they will give **incompatible** impressions to different providers about their emotional state and motivation for treatment.

Patient Competence and Decision-Making Capacity

A 30-year-old man on quetiapine for schizophrenia presents to the ER with cough and shortness of breath. He is febrile with an ↑ WBC, and a CXR reveals a necrotizing pneumonia. The patient is told to remain in the hospital to receive IV antibiotics but refuses to do so, noting that he wants to go home. He can understand his medical condition and can repeat the alternative therapy (PO antibiotics) and the potential risks of exercising this option. The admitting physician feels strongly that the patient should remain in hospital and notes that he should not be able to refuse treatment, as he is schizophrenic and thus cannot make appropriate decisions. The physician asks your opinion. What is your response?

If the patient is not actively psychotic, his schizophrenia should be disregarded in any issues regarding decision-making capacity. Since he meets all other criteria for decision-making capacity, he should be evaluated for active psychosis and then discharged with PO antibiotics.

Patient **competence** refers to a patient's ability to regularly make medical decisions on his/her own behalf. It involves a **legal assessment** and is generally a long-term decision made outside the hospital or clinic setting. Patient **capacity** refers to the ability of a person to make an **informed decision** about a particular clinical decision (eg, to operate or not) and always occurs in the context of a specific treatment encounter. Therefore, the fundamental question with regard to **patient decision-making capacity** is, "Does the patient have the ability to make the decision in question on his/her own behalf, or should you (or someone else; see the Ambulatory Medicine chapter) make decisions for him/her?" The answer depends on the **context** of care:

KEY FACT

Competence is a legal assessment made by a judge; patient decision-making capacity can be determined in the health care setting (ie, by clinicians).

- **Patients with acute/emergent medical issues** (eg, massive hemorrhage, delirium): In most states, doctors have the right to perform emergent medical care. Although not explicitly defined, the term *emergent* is generally thought of as "when there is an imminent loss of life or limb." Technically, without explicit patient or representative consent, you must confine your care to the treatment of emergent conditions.
- **Patients with acute psychiatric issues** (eg, those who are actively psychotic, floridly manic, or dangerously suicidal): Again, laws vary from state to state, but most states allow for emergent psychiatric treatment. This may include medications (IM or IV if necessary), locked hospitalization, locked seclusion, or physical restraints.
- **Patients with subacute medical conditions** (eg, nonemergent medical or surgical procedures): Patients have the right to refuse recommended treatment as long as they:
  - **Know and can repeat** the nature of the medical condition.
  - **Know and can repeat** the benefits/risks of and alternatives to the recommended treatment.
  - **Consistently** express their rationale for their decision.
- **Patients with subacute psychiatric conditions** (eg, schizophrenic but not actively psychotic; depressive but not actively suicidal; bipolar but not floridly manic): Recommended medical treatment should be offered just as if there were no psychiatric condition (see above).

- Laws regarding recommended psychiatric care vary significantly across states. Some states allow clinicians significant power in mandating unwanted treatment, while others give patients significant rights to refuse, which can be overturned only in a court of law.
  - Remember that if and when the condition becomes acute or emergent, most states allow psychiatric treatment.
- **Patients with advance directives:** By definition, patients may sign advance directives only when they have the mental capacity to do so.
  - As long as the advance directive explicitly addresses the recommended/anticipated treatment, physicians must adhere to the patient's prestated wishes even if those wishes will lead to a worse outcome (including death).
  - When the directive does not explicitly address an emergent or subacute medical condition (and the patient cannot respond), staff and/or the patient's family/friends must attempt to infer what the patient's wishes would be and treat accordingly.

Confidentiality in Psychiatry

The following are some exceptions to confidentiality in psychiatric practice:

- If the patient is suicidal or homicidal, protective steps may have to be taken that breach confidentiality.
- Child abuse must be reported to protective services.
- If the plaintiff in a lawsuit has made his or her medical or psychiatric condition an issue, the defendant has the right to know about and to obtain the records of the plantiff's evaluation and treatment.
- A court may order a physician to disclose confidential information.
- The results of a court-ordered pretrial evaluation may be available to the defense attorney, the prosecuting attorney, and the judge.
- The results of a disability evaluation will be available to the attorney or agency that requested the evaluation.

Special Populations in Psychiatry

GERIATRIC PATIENTS

See the Geriatrics chapter.

ADOLESCENT PATIENTS

Mid- to late adolescence is the most common time for early signs of schizophrenia or bipolar disorder to begin, with significant impairments in functioning tending to occur in the late teens to early 20s.

- **Depression:** In adolescents (and children), irritability can often be more prominent than sadness or anhedonia when diagnosing depression.
- **Suicidality:** Adolescents are more prone to impulsive acts, so close monitoring when beginning antidepressant medications (which can sometimes cause anxiety or agitation as side effects) is crucial.

KEY FACT

Adolescents on psychiatric medicines should be closely monitored for agitation or anxiety side effects.

PATIENTS WITH HIV/AIDS

Psychomotor slowing and personality change can sometimes be seen in HIV-associated cognitive impairment. Some antiretroviral medications (eg, efavirenz) can have significant psychiatric side effects.

Therapeutic Drugs in Psychiatry

ADVERSE EFFECTS

Table 15.2 outlines both common and potentially serious adverse effects associated with psychiatric drugs.

TABLE 15.2. Adverse Effects of Commonly Administered Psychiatric Drugs

EXAMPLES	COMMON SIDE EFFECTS	MEDICALLY SERIOUS SIDE EFFECTS
SSRIs		
Paroxetine (Paxil), fluoxetine (Prozac), sertraline (Zoloft), citalopram (Celexa), fluvoxamine (Luvox)	Sedation, weight gain, GI discomfort, sexual dysfunction.	Serotonin syndrome (tachycardia, hypertension, fever, hyperthermia, myoclonus, convulsions, coma).
OTHER ANTIDEPRESSANTS		
Bupropion (Wellbutrin)	Insomnia, "jitteriness."	Lowered seizure threshold.
Venlafaxine (Effexor)	Constipation, dizziness.	Lowered seizure threshold, hypertension.
MOOD STABILIZERS		
Lithium	Cognitive dulling, tremor, sedation, nausea, diarrhea, T-wave flattening.	Lithium toxicity, hypothyroidism (with long-term use), nephrogenic diabetes insipidus.
MOOD STABILIZERS/ANTICONVULSANTS		
Valproic acid (Depakote)	Weight gain, sedation, cognitive dulling.	Thrombocytopenia.
Carbamazepine (Tegretol)	Same as above.	SIADH, agranulocytosis, Stevens-Johnson rash.
TYPICAL HIGH-POTENCY ANTIPSYCHOTICS		
Haloperidol (Haldol), fluphenazine (Prolixin)	Sedation.	Acute dystonic reactions, neuroleptic malignant syndrome, tardive dyskinesia (with long-term use); QTc prolongation leading to torsades de pointes with high doses of haloperidol.

(continues)

TABLE 15.2. **Adverse Effects of Commonly Administered Psychiatric Drugs** *(continued)*

Examples	Common Side Effects	Medically Serious Side Effects
Typical Midpotency Antipsychotics		
Thioridazine (Mellaril), chlorpromazine (Thorazine)	Sedation, anticholinergic side effects (dry mouth, constipation, urinary retention, tachycardia).	Acute dystonic reactions, neuroleptic malignant syndrome, tardive dyskinesia (with long-term use).
Typical Low-Potency Antipsychotics		
Perphenazine (Trilafon), trifluoperazine (Stelazine)	Orthostatic hypotension.	Acute dystonic reactions, neuroleptic malignant syndrome, tardive dyskinesia (with long-term use).
Atypical Antipsychotics		
Olanzapine (Zyprexa)	Weight gain, sedation.	Hypercholesterolemia, possible DM.
Risperidone (Risperdal)	Weight gain.	Hyperprolactinemia; side effects of typical antipsychotics (when used in high doses).
Clozapine (Clozaril)	Drooling, weight gain.	Agranulocytosis.
Quetiapine (Seroquel)	Sedation, orthostasis.	Hypotension. QTc prolongation.
Ziprasidone (Geodon)	Sedation.	QTc prolongation.
Aripiprazole (Abilify)	Restlessness.	—

IMPORTANT DRUG-DRUG INTERACTIONS

- Carbamazepine:
    - An autoinducer of cytochrome P-450 isoenzyme, so levels must be re-checked and the dose often ↑ after several weeks of use.
    - ↓ serum level of OCPs.
    - Erythromycin, INH, and H₂ blockers all ↑ carbamazepine levels.
- **Valproic acid:** Levels are ↑ by ASA and anticoagulants.
- **Benzodiazepines:**
    - Levels are ↑ by disulfiram, ketoconazole, valproic acid, erythromycin, and cimetidine.
    - Diazepam (Valium) and alprazolam (Xanax) ↑ levels of digoxin and phenytoin.

NONPSYCHIATRIC MEDICATION CLASSES WITH PSYCHIATRIC SIDE EFFECTS

- **Antiretrovirals** (eg, efavirenz): Delirium, mania, irritability, cognitive impairment.
- **Dopamine agonists** (eg, pergolide, carbidopa-levodopa): Hallucinations, paranoia.
- **Antihistamines** (eg, diphenhydramine, hydroxyzine): Delirium, cognitive impairment.
- **Anticholinergics** (eg, benztropine, oxybutynin): Delirium, cognitive impairment.
- **Steroids** (eg, prednisone): Mania, psychosis, elation, depression.

NOTES

CHAPTER 16

Pulmonary Medicine

Christina A. Lee, MD
Christian A. Merlo, MD, MPH

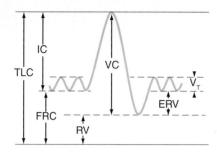

FIGURE 16.1. Lung volumes. Lung volumes, shown by spirogram tracing. VC, vital capacity; IC, inspiratory capacity; V_T, tidal volume.

KEY FACT

Capacities are the sum of two or more volumes.

Physiology Primer

LUNG VOLUMES

Common definitions are as follows (see also Figure 16.1):

- **Residual volume (RV):** Air in the lung at maximal expiration.
- **Expiratory reserve volume (ERV):** Air that can be exhaled after normal expiration.
- **Tidal volume (TV):** Air that enters and exits the lungs during normal respirations; generally 500 cc.
- **Functional reserve capacity (FRC):** RV + ERV.
- **Total lung capacity (TLC):** RV + ERV + TV + IRV.

ALTERATIONS IN LUNG FUNCTION: PULMONARY FUNCTION TESTS (PFTs)

Table 16.1 and the text below outline changes in lung function associated with obstructive and restrictive lung disease. Table 16.2 lists common pulmonary disorders by category.

- **Step 1:** Look at FEV_1/FVC:
  - **Low FEV_1/FVC:** Obstructive lung disease. Look at FEV_1 to determine the severity of disease.
  - **Normal FEV_1/FVC:** Restrictive lung disease.
- **Step 2:** Look at TLC:
  - **Low TLC** (< 80% predicted): Restrictive disease.
  - **High TLC** (> 120% predicted): Hyperinflation.
- **Step 3:** Look at diffusion capacity (DL_{CO}): If DL_{CO} is low (< 80%), DL_{CO} is ↓.

TABLE 16.1. Obstructive vs. Restrictive Lung Disease

	FEV_1/FVC	TLC	RV	VC
Obstructive	↓	Nl to ↑	↑	↓
Restrictive				
Pulmonary parenchymal	Nl to ↑	↓	↓	↓
Extraparenchymal neuromuscular	Nl	↓	↑	↓
Extraparenchymal chest wall	Nl	↓	↑	↓

FEV_1 = forced expiratory volume in one second; FVC = forced vital capacity.

TABLE 16.2.   Diagnostic Categories of Common Pulmonary Disorders by PFTs

OBSTRUCTIVE	RESTRICTIVE—PARENCHYMAL	RESTRICTIVE—EXTRAPARENCHYMAL
Asthma	Idiopathic pulmonary fibrosis	**Neuromuscular:**
COPD	Sarcoidosis	▪ Diaphragmatic weakness/paralysis
Bronchiectasis	Drug- or radiation-related interstitial	▪ Myasthenia gravis
Cystic fibrosis (CF)	lung disease (ILD)	▪ Guillain-Barré syndrome
	Collagen vascular disease–related	▪ Amyotrophic lateral sclerosis (ALS)
	ILD	▪ Cervical spine injury
		Chest wall:
		▪ Kyphoscoliosis
		▪ Obesity
		▪ Postthoracoplasty

Diagnostics in Pulmonary Medicine

ABG INTERPRETATION

ABGs can distinguish respiratory acidosis from respiratory alkalosis.

- **Acute respiratory acidosis:** pH ↓ by 0.08 for each 10-mm Hg rise in P_{CO_2}.
- **Acute respiratory alkalosis:** pH ↑ by 0.08 for each 10-mm Hg fall in Pa_{CO_2}.
- **Chronic respiratory acidosis:** pH ↓ by 0.03 for each 10-mm Hg rise in P_{CO_2}.

THE CHEST X-RAY (CXR)

CXRs can reveal infiltrates, nodules, masses, effusion, and mediastinal/hilar abnormalities (see Tables 16.3 and 16.4).

TABLE 16.3.   Infiltrates Found on CXR

UPPER LOBE ("ASTECS")	LOWER LOBE ("BADASSER")
Ankylosing spondylitis	**B**ronchiectasis
Sarcoidosis	**A**spiration
Tuberculosis	**D**ermatomyositis/polymyositis
Eosinophilic granulomatosis	**A**sbestosis
Cystic fibrosis	**S**cleroderma
Silicosis	**S**LE, **S**jögren's syndrome
	Early Hamman-Rich syndrome
	Rheumatoid arthritis (RA)

TABLE 16.4. Masses Found on CXR

Anterior Mediastinal ("4 T's")	Posterior Mediastinal
Teratoma	Bronchial cysts
Thymoma	Enterogenic cysts
Thyroid	Abscess
"**T**errible" lymphoma	Non-Hodgkin's lymphoma
	Neurogenic tumors
	Pericardial cysts/plasmacytoma
	Hodgkin's lymphoma

KEY FACT

Conventional CT with contrast is used for mediastinal and hilar disease. CT-PA is good for PE.

KEY FACT

HRCT without contrast is used to detect specific lung diagnoses such as bronchiectasis, emphysema, ILD, and nodules. It can also be used to guide lung biopsies.

CT SCAN

- Offers several advantages over routine CXRs:
  - Cross-sectional images allow for the comparison of different lesions that might be superimposed on CXR.
  - Better at characterizing lesions both by density and by size.
  - Particularly valuable in evaluating **mediastinal and hilar** disease; use contrast.
- **CT pulmonary angiography (CT-PA)**, in which contrast is injected and images are rapidly acquired by helical scanning, can be used to detect **pulmonary embolism** (PE) in segmental or larger vessels.
- **High-resolution CT (HRCT)** provides individual cross-sectional images of 1–2 mm and allows for better recognition of lung processes, such as **bronchiectasis, emphysema, ILD,** and **pulmonary nodules.**

PET SCAN

- A useful technique for the evaluation of solitary pulmonary nodules at least 1 cm in size.
- Radiolabeled fluorodeoxyglucose is injected and rapidly transported into neoplastic cells, which then "light up" with PET imaging.

V/Q SCAN

- Often used in the evaluation of PEs.
- Technetium-labeled albumin injected into the vein becomes trapped in the pulmonary capillaries, thereby following the distribution of blood flow.
- Radiolabeled xenon gas is inhaled to demonstrate the distribution of ventilation.
- Defects in perfusion that follow the distribution of a vessel and are not accompanied by defects in ventilation are called **mismatched defects** and may represent PEs.

PULMONARY ANGIOGRAPHY

- Used to visualize the pulmonary arterial system.
- Contrast medium is injected through a catheter placed in the pulmonary artery.
- A **filling defect** or **cutoff** is often seen in cases of PE.
- Can also be used to investigate suspected pulmonary AVMs.

BRONCHOSCOPY

- Allows for the direct visualization of the endobronchial tree.
- **Bronchoalveolar lavage** is a technique used to sample cells and organisms from the alveolar space using aliquots of sterile saline. It is most helpful for diagnosing infectious and neoplastic disease.
- **Transbronchial biopsy** is performed by passing a small forceps through the bronchoscope into the small airways to obtain parenchymal tissue. Transbronchial biopsy may be helpful in differentiating infection, neoplasm, ILD, granulomatous disease, and bronchiolitis obliterans with organizing pneumonia.
- **Transbronchial needle aspiration** involves the passing of a hollow-bore needle through the airway into a mass lesion or an enlarged lymph node. This is particularly useful in cases of mediastinal or hilar adenopathy, allowing for the differentiation of neoplasm, sarcoidosis, fungal disease, and mycobacterial disease.

Cough

Cough is one of the most common conditions for which patients seek medical attention. A systematic approach makes it possible to diagnose the cause in the majority of cases.

SYMPTOMS

- Inquire about postnasal drip syndromes, asthma, GERD, treatment with ACEIs, and smoking.
- A productive cough usually represents an infectious or chronic process such as bronchiectasis. Cough productive of blood may represent malignancy, infection, or the first sign of connective tissue disease (eg, Goodpasture's syndrome, Wegener's granulomatosis).

EXAM

The physical exam should focus on the nasal mucosa, lungs, heart, and extremities (for clubbing). Boggy nasal mucosa may be a sign of postnasal drip. Expiratory wheezing or crackles point to the need for further testing of the lower respiratory tract.

DIAGNOSIS

Estimating the duration of cough is often the first step toward establishing the diagnosis.

- **Acute cough:** Of < 3 weeks' duration.
  - Viral infections are the most common cause.
  - Other causes include allergic rhinitis, acute bacterial sinusitis, COPD exacerbation, and infection with *Bordetella pertussis*.
  - May also be the presenting symptom of left heart failure, asthma, or conditions that predispose patients to aspiration.
- **Subacute cough:** Of 3–8 weeks' duration.
  - Postinfectious cough is the most common etiology.
  - Subacute bacterial sinusitis, asthma, and infection with *B pertussis* may all cause cough lasting 3–8 weeks.

- **Chronic cough:** Of > 8 weeks' duration.
  - Roughly 95% of cases are caused by postnasal drip, GERD, asthma, chronic bronchitis, bronchiectasis, or ACEI use.
  - It is important to remember that cough may have multiple etiologies.

TREATMENT

Treatment depends on symptoms and response to treatment.

Dyspnea

Has five major causes: cardiac (eg, CHF), pulmonary (eg, COPD, asthma, ILD), psychogenic factors, GERD, and deconditioning.

SYMPTOMS/EXAM

Determine the time course (see Table 16.5) and the extent of symptoms. Further distinctions include the following:

- **Orthopnea:** Dyspnea in the supine position; characteristic of CHF.
- **Platypnea:** Dyspnea while sitting upright.
- **Orthodeoxia:** Desaturation while sitting upright that improves when supine.

DIAGNOSIS/TREATMENT

- Review the history and physical (H&P) and obtain a CXR.
- Depending on the findings above, consider the following:
  - PFTs with spirometry and responsiveness to methacholine or a bronchodilator; lung volumes; diffusion capacity; O_2 saturation at rest and with exercise; flow volume loops (see Figure 16.2).
  - **ECG and echocardiography** +/– stress testing.
  - **Chest CT:** Perform CT pulmonary angiography to rule out PE in segmental or larger vessels. High-resolution CT yields smaller and more refined cross-sectional images for bronchiectasis, COPD, and ILD.
  - Twenty-four-hour esophageal pH monitoring to rule out GERD.

KEY FACT

Platypnea-orthodeoxia syndrome is seen in lower lobe pulmonary AVMs or microvascular shunts due to hepatopulmonary syndrome.

TABLE 16.5. Differential Diagnosis of Dyspnea Based on Rapidity of Onset

	ACUTE DYSPNEA (MINUTES TO HOURS)	**CHRONIC DYSPNEA** (DAYS TO YEARS)
Pulmonary disorders	Pneumonia/bronchitis	COPD
	PE	Asthma
	Pneumothorax	ILD
	Bronchospasm (asthma, COPD)	Deconditioning
	Obstruction (anaphylaxis, aspiration)	Pulmonary hypertension
Cardiovascular disorders	Ischemia	Cardiomyopathy
	CHF	
	Cardiac tamponade	

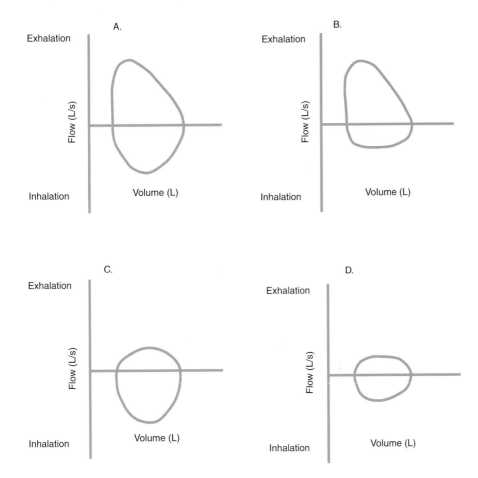

FIGURE 16.2.   Flow volume loops. (A) Normal pattern. (B) Variable extrathoracic obstruction (eg, vocal cord paralysis or dysfunction). (C) Variable intrathoracic obstruction (eg, bronchogenic cysts). (D) Fixed obstruction (eg, prolonged intubation and resultant tracheal stenosis).

Wheezing

SYMPTOMS/EXAM

- Expiratory wheezes suggest asthma, and inspiratory wheezes suggest upper airway obstruction. However, neither type of wheeze is sensitive or specific.
- Think of asthma if the patient has episodic wheezes, especially if they are often expiratory and monophonic (a single musical note) and respond to typical asthma medications (eg, bronchodilators).
- If wheezes do not respond to asthma medications, consider cardiac asthma, vocal cord dysfunction, allergic bronchopulmonary aspergillosis (ABPA), and postnasal drip. Remember that "all that wheezes is not asthma; all that wheezes is obstruction."
- ABPA is suggested by severe asthmatic wheezing and cough with brown mucous plugs, peripheral eosinophilia, ↑ serum IgE levels, immediate wheal-and-flare skin reactivity to *Aspergillus* antigens, and/or serum precipitants. Central bronchiectasis is also present.
- Further distinguished as follows:
  - **Polyphonic wheezes** (consisting of multiple notes): Suggest dynamic compression of the large, more central airways.
  - **Monophonic wheezes:** Suggest disease of the smaller lower airways, most typically asthma (see Figure 16.2 for examples of flow volume loops in patients with upper airway obstruction).

KEY FACT

Remember that "all that wheezes is not asthma." Consider COPD, vocal cord dysfunction, PE, foreign body aspiration, and even GERD.

KEY FACT

In a patient with worsening asthma, always think about concomitant GERD.

DIAGNOSIS/TREATMENT

- The H&P often points to the diagnosis. If it does not, start empiric treatment for common causes such as asthma, especially with symptoms of wheezes combined with chronic cough.
- Lack of improvement following bronchodilator treatment for asthma should suggest the need either to change therapy or to investigate other potential etiologies with PFTs.

Hemoptysis

The expectoration of blood from the lower respiratory tract. Can range from blood-streaked sputum to life-threatening bleeding. **Massive hemoptysis** is defined as the coughing up of > 200 mL of blood in a 24-hour period. The most common causes are bronchitis, bronchogenic carcinoma, and bronchiectasis (see Table 16.6).

SYMPTOMS/EXAM

- A history of TB or sarcoidosis may suggest aspergilloma.
- Frequent, multiple episodes of pneumonia could point to bronchiectasis.
- A diastolic heart murmur may suggest mitral stenosis (a frequently overlooked cause).
- A history of epistaxis, telangiectasias, and a bruit in the posterior aspect of the lungs may represent hereditary hemorrhagic telangiectasia with a ruptured pulmonary AVM.
- Renal insufficiency and hemoptysis may indicate Wegener's granulomatosis or Goodpasture's syndrome.
- Weight loss, tobacco abuse, and cachexia may suggest malignancy.

DIFFERENTIAL

Upper respiratory tract bleeding; upper GI tract bleeding.

TABLE 16.6. Differential Diagnosis of Hemoptysis

MOST COMMON CAUSES	OTHER CAUSES
Bronchitis	Aspergilloma
Bronchogenic carcinoma	CHF
Bronchiectasis	CF
	Goodpasture's syndrome
	Lung abscess
	Mitral stenosis
	Pulmonary AVM
	PE/infarction
	Sarcoidosis
	TB
	Wegener's granulomatosis

DIAGNOSIS

- Routine evaluation should include H&P, CBC, ECG, CXR, UA, and co-agulation studies. Consider **bronchoscopy** if there are risk factors for cancer or chronic bronchitis (especially smoking), or order an **HRCT** if bronchiectasis or AVM is higher on the differential.
- Additional studies, if indicated, include expectorated sputum for acid-fast bacilli and cytology, BUN/creatinine, ANA, ANCA, anti-GBM antibody, ABG, 100% O_2 to evaluate for shunt, and pulmonary arteriography.

TREATMENT

- **Supportive care:** Bed rest with supplemental O_2 and blood products if needed. Avoid antitussives, as an effective cough is needed to clear blood from the airways. If gas exchange becomes compromised, endotracheal intubation may be indicated.
- **Definitive treatment:**
  - **Nonmassive hemoptysis:** Treatment is directed at the specific underlying cause (eg, antibiotics for superinfected aspergilloma).
  - **Massive hemoptysis:** Urgent bronchoscopy or bronchial artery angiography may localize the site of bleeding. Angiography plus embolization stops bleeding in > 90% of cases. Emergency surgery for massive hemoptysis is controversial and reserved for those who have failed embolization.

Hypoxemia

Defined as a ↓ in blood O_2 (in general, a PaO_2 of < 80 mm Hg). An age adjustment given by the formula $80 - [(age - 20)/4]$ is used to define the lower limit of normal PaO_2.

SYMPTOMS/EXAM

Presents with shortness of breath, dyspnea, and tachypnea. Long-standing hypoxia results in fatigue, drowsiness, and delayed reaction time. Severe hypoxia leads to respiratory failure.

DIAGNOSIS

- The alveolar-arterial (A-a) oxygen gradient determines the differential diagnosis (see Table 16.7):

$$\text{A-a gradient} = P_{AO_2} - P_{aO_2}$$

  where $P_{AO_2} = 150 - P_{aCO_2}/0.8$ at sea level and room air.
- A normal A-a gradient = $(age/4) + 4$.

TREATMENT

Supplemental O_2. Long-term O_2 therapy is indicated for a $PaO_2 \leq 55$ mm Hg or an O_2 saturation $\leq 88\%$.

TABLE 16.7. Diagnosis of Hypoxemia by A-a Gradient and Response to Supplemental O_2

ETIOLOGY	A-a GRADIENT	CORRECTS WITH SUPPLEMENTAL O_2?	COMMON CAUSES
↓ inspired Fio_2	Normal	Yes	High altitude.
Hypoventilation	Normal	Yes	Drug overdose, obesity hypoventilation syndrome, muscular weakness, ALS, Guillain-Barré syndrome.
Right-to-left shunt	↑	No	**Physiologic shunt:** Pneumonia, atelectasis. **Anatomic shunt:** Intracardiac shunt, pulmonary AVM.
Impaired diffusion capacity	↑	Yes; characterized by exercise-induced hypoxemia	Emphysema, ILD.
V/Q mismatch	↑	Yes	PE, obstructive lung disease, ARDS.

Chronic Obstructive Pulmonary Disease (COPD)

A 75-year-old man complains of worsening dyspnea on exertion over the past two years. He has a 45-pack-year smoking history and has wheezing on physical exam. His PFTs yield the following results: FEV_1/FVC 55% of predicted; TLC 75%; DL_{CO} 50%. What is your interpretation of his PFTs, and what treatments are indicated assuming that he has COPD?

Mixed obstructive and restrictive ventilatory pattern. Treat with a short-acting bronchodilator for symptomatic relief plus a daily long-acting β_2-agonist and/or anticholinergic bronchodilator (for moderate-severity COPD according to the GOLD criteria).

Progressive chronic airflow limitation that is not fully reversible, resulting from chronic bronchitis and emphysema. Represents the fourth leading cause of death in the United States. Risk factors include cigarette smoking, a ⊕ family history, α_1-antitrypsin deficiency, and occupational dust/chemicals. Distinguished as follows:

- **Chronic bronchitis:** Chronic productive cough for three months over two consecutive years.
- **Emphysema:** Abnormal enlargement of the airspaces distal to the terminal bronchioles with wall destruction.

SYMPTOMS/EXAM

- **Acute exacerbation** is suggested by three features: worsening **dyspnea,** ↑ **cough,** and a **change in sputum volume or purulence.**
- Typically presents with chronic cough in the fourth or fifth decade of life. Dyspnea usually occurs only with moderate exercise.
- Chest wall hyperinflation, prolonged expiration, wheezing, and distant breath and heart sounds are also seen.

- Use of respiratory accessory muscles, cyanosis ("**blue bloater" suggests chronic bronchitis**), and pursed-lip breathing ("**pink puffer" suggests emphysema**) may be seen. Neck vein distention, a tender liver, and lower extremity edema suggest cor pulmonale.

DIFFERENTIAL

Acute bronchitis, asthma, bronchiectasis, CF, CHF.

DIAGNOSIS

- PFTs, particularly FEV_1 (which indicates severity), are important for diagnosis confirmation and for predicting disease progression. Diagnosis is confirmed by postbronchodilator PFTs showing an FEV_1/FVC of < 0.7 and an FEV_1 of $< 80\%$.
- CXR is not required for diagnosis but may show ↓ lung markings, ↑ retrosternal airspace, and hyperinflation with flattened diaphragms (see Figure 16.3).
- If O_2 saturation is abnormal, ABGs will show hypoxemia, hypercarbia, and acute respiratory acidosis during acute exacerbations ($Paco_2$ and Pao_2 are "50/50").
- Obtain an α_1-**antitrypsin level** with early-onset emphysema (fifth decade of life) or in the setting of a suggestive family history. Associated with basilar panlobular emphysema.

TREATMENT

- **Acute COPD:** Treatment of acute COPD differs from that of acute asthma (see also Tables 16.8 through 16.10):
  - **Mild exacerbations:** Give short-acting β_2-**adrenergic** (albuterol) and **anticholinergic** (ipratropium) inhalers or nebulizers.

KEY FACT

The cardinal symptoms of COPD exacerbation are ↑ dyspnea, ↑ cough, and ↑ sputum volume or purulence.

KEY FACT

As long as the patient's GI absorption is not compromised, there is no advantage to IV over oral corticosteroids, and oral corticosteroids are cheaper.

KEY FACT

In acute exacerbations of COPD, **inhaled** corticosteroids are not beneficial.

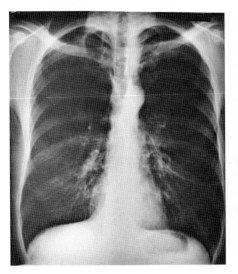
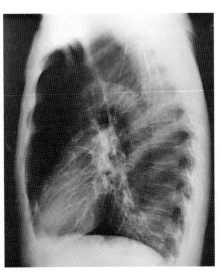

A **B**

FIGURE 16.3. **Chronic obstructive pulmonary disease.** Note the hyperinflated and hyperlucent lungs, flat diaphragms, increased AP diameter, narrow mediastinum, and large upper lobe bullae on PA (**A**) and lateral (**B**) CXR. (Reproduced with permission from Stobo JD et al. *The Principles and Practice of Medicine*, 23rd ed. Stamford, CT: Appleton & Lange, 1996: 135.)

TABLE 16.8. Classification of COPD Severity and Treatment for Stable COPD[a]

Stage	Spirometry	Treatment for Stable COPD
All stages	$FEV_1/FVC < 0.7$	
I (mild)	$FEV_1 \geq 80\%$ of predicted	Short-acting bronchodilator for relief (albuterol, ipratropium).
II (moderate)	FEV_1 50–79% of predicted	Add long-acting β_2-agonists and/or anticholinergic bronchodilators.
III (severe)	FEV_1 30–49% of predicted	Also add an inhaled corticosteroid.
IV (very severe)	$FEV_1 < 30\%$ of predicted or $FEV_1 < 50\%$ of predicted plus chronic respiratory failure	Also add long-term O_2 PRN; consider surgery.

[a]Classification is by the GOLD criteria.

KEY FACT

All patients hospitalized with pneumonia, exacerbations of asthma, or COPD should receive pneumococcal and influenza vaccinations if they are not already up to date.

KEY FACT

General indications for long-term continuous O_2 therapy (24 hours/day):
- $Pao_2 \leq 55$ mm Hg or O_2 saturation $\leq 88\%$

OR
- $Pao_2 \leq 59$ mm Hg or O_2 saturation $\leq 89\%$ with cor pulmonale or erythrocytosis (Hct > 55%)

- **Moderate exacerbations** (may require hospital treatment): In addition to the above, consider the following:
  - O_2 therapy.
  - Short-acting β_2-**agonists and anticholinergics.**
  - Systemic oral or IV corticosteroids help ↓ the length of exacerbations and improve FEV_1.
  - Antibiotics are indicated in the setting of ↑ dyspnea, cough, and sputum production.
- **Stable chronic COPD:** Treatment measures include the following:
  - Smoking cessation.
  - **Immunizations** for influenza and pneumococcus.
  - O_2 if indicated.
  - β_2-**adrenergic and anticholinergic agents** improve pulmonary function and ↓ dyspnea. Long-acting agents should be used as first-line maintenance therapy (β_2-agonists—salmeterol, formoterol; anticholinergics—tiotropium).
  - Inhaled corticosteroids ↓ the frequency of exacerbations but may ↑ the risk of pneumonia and other adverse effects, and their long-term safety is unknown.

TABLE 16.9. Treatment of Acute Exacerbations of Asthma and COPD

Treatment	Asthma	COPD
Peak expiratory flow useful	Yes	No
Systemic corticosteroids	Yes	Yes
Antibiotics	No	Yes
O_2	Yes	Yes
Combination bronchodilator therapy[a]	Yes	Unclear
Noninvasive mechanical ventilation	Unclear	Yes

[a]β_2-agonist and ipratropium bromide.

TABLE 16.10. Treatment of Acute COPD Exacerbations ("ABC-ON")

THERAPY	COMMENTS
Antibiotics	Recommended by the American Thoracic Society for patients with an acute COPD exacerbation with a change in sputum amount, consistency, or color.
Bronchodilators	β_2-**adrenergic agents (eg, albuterol)** and **anticholinergic agents (eg, ipratropium)** are first-line therapy.
Corticosteroids	Oral or IV (but not inhaled) corticosteroids help ↓ the length of exacerbations and improve FEV_1 in hospitalized patients.
Oxygen	Use if the patient is hypoxic. Hypercarbia can result either from a ↓ respiratory drive or from V/Q mismatch, but O_2 therapy must not be withheld for fear of hypercarbia.
Noninvasive mechanical ventilation	Benefits patients with severe acute exacerbations of COPD, as it reduces in-hospital mortality, ↓ the need for intubation, and diminishes hospital length of stay (see the Critical Care chapter).

- Stage IV (very severe) COPD: Home O_2 is the only treatment besides smoking cessation with a proven mortality benefit.
  - **Pulmonary rehabilitation:** Associated with improved exercise tolerance and ↓ pulmonary symptoms.
  - **Lung volume reduction surgery:** ↓ hyperinflation to improve lung mechanics. Best for patients with severe COPD who do not respond to pulmonary rehabilitation and other treatments; have severe emphysema in the upper lobes; and have a low risk of surgery.
  - **Single- or double-lung transplantation** may be indicated for patients with a low FEV_1, hypercarbia, and cor pulmonale.

KEY FACT

O_2 therapy and smoking cessation are the only interventions that ↑ life expectancy in hypoxemic COPD patients.

Bronchiectasis

A 22-year-old woman with CF has experienced frequent cough for the past two years. Her cough is productive of occasionally bloody sputum. She has no fevers, chills, night sweats, or other symptoms suggestive of infection. Her most recent CXR showed peribronchial thickening. What is the most likely etiology of her hemoptysis?

Bronchiectasis. Airway disease is the most common cause of hemoptysis, and patients with CF commonly develop chronic productive cough, chronic bronchitis, and bronchiectasis.

Irreversible dilatation and destruction of bronchi due to cycles of infection and inflammation, with mucopurulent sputum production. Characterized by dilated airways and focal constrictive areas.

Symptoms

- Presents with cough with chronic production of purulent, foul-smelling sputum.
- Dyspnea, wheezing, pleuritic chest pain, and hemoptysis are all possible.
- Patients may have a history of recurrent respiratory tract infections.

- **Most commonly associated with CF.** Other associations include the following:
  - Postinfectious *Pseudomonas, Haemophilus,* TB, pertussis, measles, influenza, RSV, HIV.
  - Immunodeficiency (CVID, IgA deficiency).
  - Congenital conditions (1° ciliary dyskinesia, Kartagener's syndrome).
  - Autoimmune disease (SLE, RA, Sjögren's syndrome, relapsing polychondritis, IBD).
  - Hypersensitivity (ABPA).

EXAM

Exam reveals crackles and wheezing and, rarely, clubbing. Acute exacerbations lead to ↑ sputum production, ↑ dyspnea, ↑ cough and wheezing, and low-grade fever.

DIFFERENTIAL

COPD, interstitial fibrosis, pneumonia, asthma.

DIAGNOSIS

- **CBC, including differential.**
- **Serum immunoglobulins:** Screen for CVID, IgA/IgG deficiency, and ABPA (↑ serum total IgE).
- **HRCT:** The best diagnostic tool for mapping airway abnormalities. Distribution aids in diagnosis (central bronchiectasis suggests ABPA; upper lobe involvement points to CF).
- **Spirometry:** Quantifies the degree of airway obstruction.
- **Sputum sample:** For bacterial, fungal, and mycobacterial cultures.
- **Sweat chloride test for CF.**
- **ANA, RF,** and **anti-Ro/La.**

TREATMENT

- **Antibiotics:** Use a fluoroquinolone +/− an inhaled tobramycin solution for acute exacerbations.
- **Bronchodilators:** For probable airway inflammation.
- **Inhaled corticosteroids:** Can ↓ inflammation and improve dyspnea, cough, and pulmonary function in severe cases.
- **Airway clearance:** Chest physiotherapy, flutter devices, percussive vests.
- **Mucolytic agents: DNAse** is helpful in stable CF but potentially harmful in patients with non-CF bronchiectasis.
- **Surgical resection.**

Cystic Fibrosis (CF)

Caused by mutations in the CF transmembrane conductance regulator (CFTR), leading to chloride channel dysfunction. Consider especially in young adults with a history of bronchiectasis, infertility, or recurrent pancreatitis.

SYMPTOMS/EXAM

- Look for a history of failure to thrive as a child, persistent respiratory infections (*Pseudomonas*), nasal polyposis, sinusitis, intestinal obstruction, malabsorption (steatorrhea, diarrhea), recurrent pancreatitis, hepatobiliary disease, and male infertility.

- Bronchiectasis and *S aureus* and *Pseudomonas aeruginosa* (mucoid variant) pneumonias are common.
- Exam reveals an ↑ AP chest diameter, upper lung field crackles, nasal polyps, hepatomegaly, and clubbing. Additional findings are as follows:
  - **Acute exacerbations:** ↑ sputum production, dyspnea, fatigue, weight loss, and a decline in FEV_1.
  - **Chronic exacerbations:** Hypoxemia and compensated respiratory acidosis.

DIFFERENTIAL

Immunodeficiency, asthma, ABPA.

DIAGNOSIS

- A **sweat chloride test** shows ↑ sodium and chloride concentration. Considered the screening test of choice, but a normal test does not rule out CF.
- If the sweat chloride test is normal but there is high clinical suspicion for CF, do **genotyping** for CFTR mutations and a **nasal potential difference test** (measures ion transport in the nose).
- On CXR, early CF may present as hyperinflation. More advanced disease can manifest with peribronchial cuffing, interstitial markings, and bronchiectasis (see Figure 16.4).

TREATMENT

- **Acute pulmonary exacerbations:** Chest physical therapy to clear lower airway secretions. Also give bronchodilators and two antipseudomonal antibiotics. Inhaled recombinant DNAse, given to cleave extracellular DNA in viscous sputum, will improve FEV_1 and ↓ exacerbations.

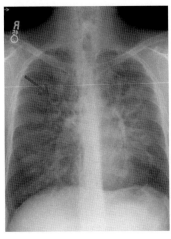

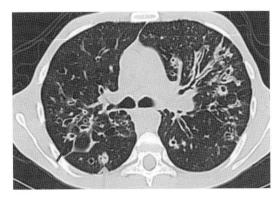

A   **B**

FIGURE 16.4. **Cystic fibrosis.** (A) Frontal CXR showing central cystic bronchiectasis (arrow) in a patient with CF. (B) Transaxial CT image showing cystic bronchiectasis (red arrow), with some bronchi containing impacted mucus (yellow arrow). (Reproduced with permission from USMLERx.com.)

- Chronic stable CF:
    - Inhaled tobramycin, nebulized DNAse, azithromycin.
    - **Airway clearance:** Aerobic exercise, flutter devices, external percussive vests.
    - Pancreatic enzymes and vitamins A, D, E, and K.
    - Nutritional counseling.
    - Pneumococcal and influenza vaccines.
- **Lung transplantation** for severe progressive pulmonary disease.
- Genetic counseling and screening of family members.

Interstitial Lung Disease (ILD)

A 65-year-old woman with well-controlled hypertension presents to her primary care physician with gradual onset of dyspnea and nonproductive cough for the past year. Her physical exam is normal except for bibasilar crackles. What is the most likely diagnosis?

Idiopathic pulmonary fibrosis.

Represents > 100 disorders; also known as diffuse parenchymal lung disease. The most common known causes are **occupational/exposure, connective tissue disease, and drugs** (see Table 16.11). Idiopathic interstitial pneumonia is a broad category of ILDs of unknown etiology, classified by histopathologic characteristics on lung biopsy (see Table 16.12). Consider in patients with dyspnea on exertion, nonproductive cough, and an abnormal CXR.

TABLE 16.11. Categories of Interstitial Lung Disease

CATEGORY	EXAMPLES	PRESENTATION
		OCCUPATIONAL/EXPOSURE
Hypersensitivity pneumonitis		Caused by an allergic reaction to inhaled organic agents.
		Acute symptoms: Fever, chills, cough, dyspnea 4–8 hours after exposure; inspiratory crackles; ground-glass opacities on CT (see Figure 16.5A).
		Chronic symptoms: Gradual cough and dyspnea, malaise, weight loss; diffuse fibrosis on biopsy.
		Treatment: Avoid common inciting agents such as mold, dust, bird droppings, aerosolized/humidified water, and pesticides. Give corticosteroids if severe.
Pneumoconioses	Asbestosis, silicosis, coal workers' pneumoconiosis, berylliosis	Fibrotic lung diseases from inhalation of agents.
		Asbestosis: Construction and shipyard workers are at risk. Presents decades after exposure with dyspnea and inspiratory crackles. CXR shows pleural calcifications and plaques. Mesothelioma and pleural cancer are most often due to asbestos.
		Silicosis: Usually asymptomatic, but may see "eggshell calcification" (calcified periphery of hilar lymph nodes). Associated with an ↑ incidence of TB, so check PPD and CXR.

TABLE 16.11. Categories of Interstitial Lung Disease *(continued)*

CATEGORY	EXAMPLES	PRESENTATION
DRUG AND RADIATION INDUCED		
Drug reactions	Amiodarone, nitrofurantoin, chemotherapeutic agents (bleomycin, cyclophosphamide), amphotericin, cocaine	Symptoms improve 24–48 hours after the drug is stopped. Crack cocaine inhalation presents with edema, pulmonary hemorrhage, and talc depositions.
Radiation exposure	Radiation pneumonitis	Occurs several months after radiotherapy for cancer (eg, breast, lung, lymphoma). Acute pneumonitis presents with fever, chest pain, cough, and dyspnea and is responsive to steroids. May progress to pulmonary fibrosis after 6–12 months of radiation (steroids do not help).
CONNECTIVE TISSUE DISEASES		
SLE		Pleural effusion or pleural thickening is common, but ILD is rare.
RA		Pleural effusion is common; rheumatoid nodules may be seen. Some treatments for RA (eg, methotrexate) can lead to ILD.
Dermatomyositis/ polymyositis		Presents with symmetric and proximal muscle weakness, elevated muscle enzymes, and ANA/anti-Jo-1 antibody. ILD occurs in > 10% of patients; diaphragmatic and chest wall weakness may also be seen.
Scleroderma		ILD is often seen (especially with diffuse cutaneous disease), as is pulmonary hypertension.
GRANULOMATOUS DISEASE		
Sarcoidosis		Stage I hilar adenopathy (spontaneous remission is common). Progresses to stage IV: fibrosis and architectural distortion with no spontaneous remission.
Langerhans cell histiocytosis		Also known as eosinophilic granuloma or histiocytosis X. Young smokers are at risk.
VASCULITIS		
Wegener's granulomatosis		Presents with cough, hemoptysis, sinus symptoms, and glomerulonephritis. ⊕ c-ANCA; necrotizing granulomas.
Churg-Strauss syndrome		Asthma with eosinophilia.

(continues)

TABLE 16.11. **Categories of Interstitial Lung Disease** *(continued)*

CATEGORY	EXAMPLES	PRESENTATION
	OTHER	
Eosinophilic pneumonias		**PIE** syndrome: "**P**ulmonary **I**nfiltrates with peripheral blood **E**osinophilia." Present with eosinophilic lung infiltrates, dyspnea, and cough, often with constitutional symptoms.
Lymphangio-leiomyomatosis		Affects premenopausal women; associated with tuberous sclerosis. Presents in childbearing years with dyspnea, cough, and chylous effusions. Pneumothorax is common.
Idiopathic interstitial pneumonias		See Table 6.12.

TABLE 16.12. **Categories of Idiopathic Interstitial Pneumonia**

	EPIDEMIOLOGY	SYMPTOMS/EXAM	DIAGNOSIS	TREATMENT
Idiopathic pulmonary fibrosis (IPF)	The **most common ILD.**	Affects middle-age or older patients (> 50 years); presents with chronic, nonproductive cough and gradually worsening dyspnea over many months. Exam reveals bibasilar inspiratory crackles (Velcro-like), restrictive lung disease (↓ FVC, TLC, FRC), and ↓ gas exchange (DL$_{CO}$).	Lung biopsy reveals **usual interstitial pneumonia (UIP).** HRCT shows bibasilar, reticular patchiness with honeycombing and bronchiectasis in subpleural areas (see Figure 16.5B).	Has a poor prognosis despite immunosuppressive therapy; lung transplantation can improve survival and quality of life.
Nonspecific interstitial pneumonitis		Similar to IPF, but patients are younger, and inspiratory crackles are less common.	See Figure 16.5C.	More responsive to treatment than IPF with less fibrosis; consider corticosteroids or other immunosuppressive agents (eg, azathioprine, cyclophosphamide).
Cryptogenic organizing pneumonia		Mimics community-acquired pneumonia symptoms and may have initial flulike symptoms (eg, fever, fatigue, nonproductive cough). Dyspnea on exertion and weight loss are also common.	CXR and CT show bilateral patchy opacities with normal lung volumes. Lung biopsy reveals organizing pneumonia but is not diagnostic.	Responsive to corticosteroids.
Acute interstitial pneumonia	Also known as Hamman-Rich syndrome or idiopathic diffuse alveolar damage.	Presents with abrupt fever, cough, and dyspnea in previously healthy patients; progresses to acute **hypoxemic** respiratory failure over days to weeks. Clinically appears to be ARDS, including diffuse alveolar damage.		Treatment is supportive; has a poor prognosis.

SYMPTOMS/EXAM

- The most common symptom is dyspnea.
- Ask about symptom onset, family history, and exposures (drugs, occupational/environmental, tobacco, radiation).
- Exam reveals **dry bibasilar crackles.**

DIAGNOSIS

- **Labs:** Obtain **serologies for exposure-related ILD and connective tissue disease.**
- **CXR:** Shows a bibasilar interstitial pattern +/– a nodular pattern or honeycombing.
- **HRCT:** Characterizes and quantifies the extent of disease; directs further diagnostic workup, including biopsy. Patterns include honeycombing, reticulations, nodules, consolidation, ground-glass opacification, mosaic perfusion, air trapping, and inflammatory or traction bronchiectasis (see Figure 16.5).
- **PFTs:** A restrictive pattern is commonly seen consisting of a normal or ↑ FEV$_1$/FVC, a ↓ TLC, and a ↓ DL$_{CO}$.
- **Lung biopsy:** For diagnosis/confirmation and activity. Can be either transbronchial/bronchoscopic lung biopsy or open surgical lung biopsy. **Open lung biopsy is preferred if IPF is suspected.**

TREATMENT

- Eliminate potential occupational/environmental exposures.
- O$_2$ for hypoxemia (PaO$_2$ < 55 mm Hg) at rest or with exercise.
- **Glucocorticoids** are usually recommended, but they confer no survival benefit, and the prognosis may still be poor.
- **Immunosuppressive therapy** with cyclophosphamide or azathioprine +/– steroids has been used with varying success.
- Lung transplantation is reserved for patients < 65 years of age with severe, refractory disease.

KEY FACT

Nonspecific interstitial pneumonia (NSIP) has a clinical presentation similar to that of IPF; however, NSIP responds to corticosteroids and has a better prognosis.

KEY FACT

When ILD is suspected, HRCT is the starting point (after CXR, of course). Lung biopsy also has an important role in diagnosis.

KEY FACT

IPF has a characteristic pattern of UIP on HRCT and biopsy. Although HRCT is sufficient to diagnose IPF, an open lung biopsy can help make a definitive diagnosis.

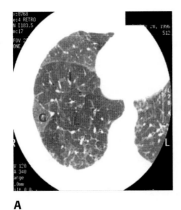

A

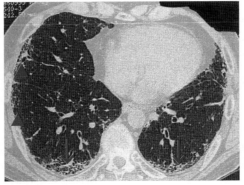

B

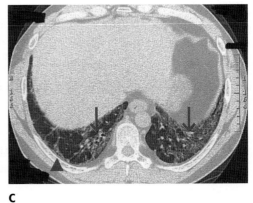

C

FIGURE 16.5.   Diffuse lung diseases on high-resolution CT. (A) Hypersensitivity pneumonitis, subacute. The "headcheese sign" consists of lung parenchyma of three different densities. Geographic areas of lucency (L) are due to bronchiolar inflammation–induced air trapping and resultant decreased perfusion of these areas. Intermediate-density (I) lung is normally perfused. Ground-glass opacities (G) are a result of alveolitis. **(B)** Idiopathic pulmonary fibrosis. Early honeycombing (arrows), reticulation (arrowheads), and traction bronchiectasis with a basilar, subpleural predominance. **(C)** Nonspecific interstitial pneumonitis showing ground-glass opacities (arrows) and reticulation (arrowhead) in the absence of honeycombing with a basilar predominance, sparing the immediate subpleural lung. (Image A reproduced with permission from Hanley ME, Welsh CH. *Current Diagnosis & Treatment in Pulmonary Medicine.* New York: McGraw-Hill, 2003, Fig. 32-1A. Images B and C reproduced with permission from Fauci AS et al. *Harrison's Principles of Internal Medicine,* 17th ed. New York: McGraw-Hill, 2008, Figs. 255-3 and 255-4.)

Pleural Effusion

Abnormal accumulation of fluid in the pleural space. In the United States, the most common causes are CHF, pneumonia, and cancer. Distinguished as follows (see also Table 6.13):

- **Transudative effusion:** Due to an imbalance between hydrostatic and oncotic pressures.
- **Exudative effusion:** Due to altered vascular permeability or impaired lymphatic drainage of fluid from pleural space.

Symptoms/Exam

- Presents with dyspnea and pleuritic chest pain.
- Exam reveals dullness to percussion, ↓ or absent fremitus, and ↓ breath sounds on the affected side.

Diagnosis

- **CXR:** May demonstrate blunting of the costophrenic angle (see Figure 16.6). Decubitus films help determine if fluid is free flowing or loculated. A finding of > 1 cm of fluid on decubitus CXR suggests a significant amount of fluid.
- **Diagnostic thoracentesis:**
    - Performed on clinically significant effusions; can distinguish transudate from exudate using Light's criteria (see below).
    - Also send for Gram stain, bacterial/fungal/mycobacterial cultures, and cytology. Pleural fluid amylase, triglycerides, cholesterol, and hematocrit may be analyzed if appropriate (see Table 16.14).
- **Light's criteria:** Pleural effusion is exudative if any of these criteria are met:
    - Pleural fluid/serum protein ratio > 0.5.
    - Pleural fluid/serum LDH ratio > 0.6.
    - Pleural fluid LDH > 2/3 the upper limit of normal for serum LDH.

> **KEY FACT**
>
> Consider pleural effusion if the etiology remains unknown. Pleural effusion usually presents as exudates but can be transudative.

TABLE 16.13. Transudative vs. Exudative Effusion

	TRANSUDATES ("-OSIS")	EXUDATES
1° mechanisms	↑ hydrostatic or ↓ oncotic pressures.	↑ fluid production due to abnormal capillary permeability; impaired lymphatic drainage of fluid from the pleural space.
Pleural effusion clues	If fluid is transudative by Light's criteria (0 of 3 criteria met), no further pleural labs are needed.	↑ WBC count (> 1000): Indicates exudate (>100,000 points to empyema). ↓ glucose (< 60 mg/dL) or ↑↑ LDH (> 1000 IU/L): Cancer, empyema, RA. ↓ pH (< 7.4): Exudate; < 7.3 suggests cancer, infection, or inflammation.
Examples	**Cardiosis (CHF):** The most common cause. Bilateral. **Cirrhosis:** Generally bilateral but can be unilateral (hepatic hydrothorax, often on the right side). **Nephrosis** (nephrotic syndrome). **Thrombosis** (pleural effusion; most often exudative, but occasionally transudative).	Parapneumonic (viral, bacteria), cancer, TB, pancreatitis. **Chylothorax:** Due to thoracic duct trauma or lymphoma. **Other:** Collagen vascular disease, esophageal rupture, hemothorax.

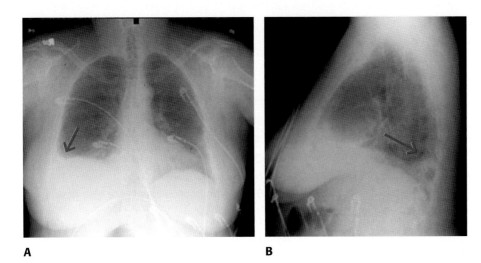

A   **B**

FIGURE 16.6. **Pleural effusion.** PA (**A**) and lateral (**B**) CXRs show blunting of the right costophrenic sulcus (arrows). (Reproduced with permission from USMLERx.com.)

■ **If the etiology remains unclear,** consider (1) **pleural biopsy,** which may aid in the diagnosis of cancer or TB effusion, and (2) **evaluation for PE.**

TREATMENT

■ **Transudative pleural effusion:** Treatment is aimed at the underlying cause; therapeutic thoracentesis if the patient is symptomatic.
■ **Malignant:** Pleurodesis (in which an irritant is placed into the drained pleural space to obliterate the space) may be considered in symptomatic patients who are unresponsive to chemotherapy or radiation.
■ **Parapneumonic:** Drainage of the pleural space is indicated with evidence of empyema (pH < 7.2, pus, glucose < 40 mg/dL, gram ⊕). If otherwise free flowing with a ⊖ Gram stain, it is acceptable to observe for resolution with antibiotics for pneumonia.
■ **Hemothorax:** Requires drainage or fibrothorax will likely develop.

> **KEY FACT**
>
> Drain a pleural effusion if pH is < 7.2, glucose is < 40 mg/dL, or Gram stain is ⊕.

TABLE 16.14. **Pleural Fluid Analysis and Interpretation**

PLEURAL FLUID TEST	INTERPRETATION
pH	If pleural pH is < 7.2 with parapneumonic effusion, drainage is required.
Hematocrit	> 50% of peripheral hematocrit suggests hemothorax.
Glucose	< 60 mg/dL suggests a complicated parapneumonic effusion or malignancy. If especially low (< 30), think rheumatoid.
Triglycerides	> 110 mg/dL points to chylothorax (thoracic duct lymph disruption); milky white. Due to lymphoma, cancer, trauma, or lymphangioleiomyomatosis.
Lymphocytes	> 50% lymphocytes is likely TB or malignancy.
Eosinophils	> 10% eosinophils is seen if **air or blood** is present, but most commonly due to pneumothorax. Also consider drug reaction, asbestos, paragonimiasis, Churg-Strauss syndrome, and pleural effusion.

Pneumothorax

A 34-year-old woman presents to the ER with chest pain and shortness of breath. A review of systems reveals dyspnea and cough of several months' duration. CXR shows a right-sided pneumothorax. For what underlying disorder should she be evaluated?

Lymphangioleiomyomatosis (LAM). This is a progressive cystic disease in child-bearing women, often presenting with pneumothorax. Patients can also develop chylous pleural effusions.

Air in the pleural space. Can be spontaneous, iatrogenic, or traumatic.

- **Spontaneous:** Can be 1° (no known lung disease and no obvious precipitating factor) or 2° (occurring with underlying lung disease, usually COPD). Associated diseases include ILD, PCP, CF, and LAM.
- **Iatrogenic:** A result of diagnostic (thoracentesis) or therapeutic intervention (central venous catheter placement).
- **Traumatic:** Occurs with penetrating or blunt trauma that causes air to enter the pleural space or with acute compression of the chest that results in alveolar rupture.

Symptoms/Exam

- Presents with unilateral chest pain (sharp or steady pressure) and acute shortness of breath. Consider 1° spontaneous pneumothorax in young, thin, tall men who smoke.
- Exam may be normal if the pneumothorax is small. Large pneumothoraces present with ↓ chest movement, hyperresonance, ↓ fremitus, and ↓ breath sounds. In the setting of tachycardia, hypotension, and tracheal deviation, consider tension pneumothorax.

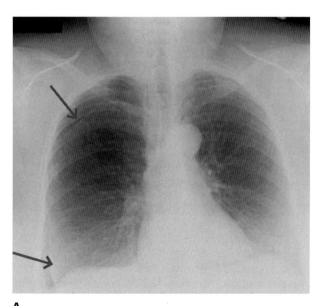

A

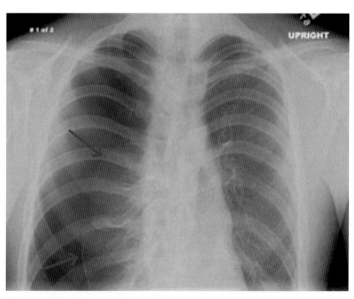

B

FIGURE 16.7. **Pneumothorax.** (A) Small right pneumothorax. (B) Right tension pneumothorax with collapse of the right lung and shifting of mediastinal structures to the left. Arrows denote pleural reflections. (Reproduced with permission from USMLERx.com.)

DIFFERENTIAL

Acute PE, MI, pleural effusion, pneumonia, pericardial tamponade.

DIAGNOSIS

Confirmed through the identification of a thin visceral pleural line away from the chest wall on upright PA CXR. A CT scan of the thorax may help when the CXR is difficult to interpret because of severe underlying lung disease (eg, CF) (see Figure 16.7).

TREATMENT

- **Small 1° pneumothoraces:** Observation and O_2 therapy. Supplemental O_2 accelerates the reabsorption of gas from the pleural space by ~ 8–9% per day.
- **Larger, more symptomatic 1° spontaneous pneumothoraces:** Drain with simple aspiration or a small-bore chest tube.
- **2° spontaneous pneumothorax:** Aspiration initially; if persistent, then use a chest tube.
- Persistent air leaks and recurrences are more common with 2° than with 1° spontaneous pneumothorax.
- Smoking ↑ the risk of recurrence; counsel for smoking cessation.

> **KEY FACT**
>
> Tension pneumothorax is a medical emergency requiring immediate decompression of the pleural space with a 14-gauge needle in the second intercostal space at the midclavicular line.

Pulmonary Complications of HIV

 A 45-year-old man with a history of IV drug abuse presents with 3–4 weeks of severe progressive dyspnea and dry cough. On physical exam, he is cachectic and hypoxic with ambulation (82% on room air) and has bilateral crackles on auscultation. His CXR shows bilateral interstitial infiltrates, and a rapid HIV test is ⊕. What is the most likely diagnosis?

Pneumocystis jiroveci pneumonia (PCP) in a patient with newly diagnosed HIV. The standard treatment is TMP-SMX (with steroids if Pao_2 is < 70 mm Hg).

Table 16.15 outlines both infectious and noninfectious pulmonary disorders associated with HIV. See the Infectious Disease chapter for further details.

TABLE 16.15. Infectious and Noninfectious Pulmonary Manifestations of HIV

INFECTIOUS	NONINFECTIOUS
Bacterial pneumonia	Emphysema
PCP	Lung carcinoma
TB	Non-Hodgkin's lymphoma
Fungal pneumonia	Lymphocytic interstitial pneumonia
CMV, VZV	Kaposi's sarcoma
Nocardia	Pulmonary hypertension

SYMPTOMS

Evaluate for the following:

- TB risk factors.
- Adherence to TMP-SMX prophylaxis.
- Timing of the initiation of highly active antiretroviral therapy (HAART) to evaluate for immune reconstitution inflammatory syndrome (IRIS).

EXAM

Focus on extrapulmonary manifestations of a systemic disease. Skin, lymph node, and funduscopic exams can narrow the differential to fungal, mycobacterial, or neoplastic etiologies. The CD4 count and viral load are also helpful in narrowing the differential.

DIAGNOSIS

- Obtain a CXR and an expectorated sputum sample. The pattern of infiltrate can suggest a diagnosis. CXR may show diffuse ground-glass opacities +/– pneumatoceles, but CXR can be normal in PCP.
- A chest CT is helpful if CXR is normal but suspicion for PCP remains high. ABGs and DL_{CO} may also be useful adjuncts in some situations.
- In patients who are critically ill and those not responding to empiric therapy, fiberoptic bronchoscopy should be performed.

TREATMENT

Unless a patient is critically ill, it is preferable to establish a diagnosis before empiric treatment is started.

Pulmonary Embolism (PE)

A 56-year-old woman with metastatic breast cancer presents with mild dyspnea, pleuritic chest pain, and left leg edema for three days. Her exam is normal except for an HR of 110 bpm and RR of 20. Contrast-enhanced helical CT of the chest shows several segmental pulmonary emboli. Her creatinine level is 0.7 mg/dL. What is the most appropriate treatment?

SQ injections of low-molecular-weight heparin (LMWH). Patients with PE are typically treated acutely with LMWH in the short term and started on long-term warfarin. In patients with underlying malignancy, long-term use of LMWH instead of warfarin has been associated with improved mortality.

Obstruction of blood flow through the pulmonary vasculature due to deep venous thrombosis (DVT), air, tumor, fat, or other material. Risk factors are **Virchow's triad:**

- **Hypercoagulable state:** May be inherited (protein C or S deficiency, factor V Leiden, prothrombin gene mutation, antithrombin III deficiency) or acquired (drugs [estrogen/OCPs]).
- **Endothelial damage:** Previous DVTs, leg trauma, hip/knee replacement.
- **Venous stasis:** Immobilization, recent surgery, CHF, morbid obesity, venous obstruction.

SYMPTOMS/EXAM

- Classically presents with acute-onset shortness of breath and pleuritic chest pain +/– cough or hemoptysis.
- Exam may reveal low-grade fever, tachypnea, tachycardia, a loud P2, and JVD. Homans' sign and palpable cords on the calf may be present with DVT.

DIFFERENTIAL

MI, aortic dissection, pneumonia, pneumothorax, pericarditis, anxiety.

DIAGNOSIS

Workup may include the following:

- **ABGs:** May demonstrate **respiratory alkalosis,** hypoxemia, and an ↑ A-a gradient.
- **CXR:** Often normal, but may show **Hampton's hump** (a wedge-shaped infarct), **Westermark's sign** (relative oligemia in the region of the embolus), pleural effusion, or atelectasis.
- **ECG:** The most common finding is sinus tachycardia. Less commonly seen is an S1Q3T3 pattern (S in lead I, Q in lead III, and an inverted T in lead III), which suggests right heart strain.
- **D-dimer:** A nonspecific breakdown product of fibrin. Helpful only to rule out embolism if the patient has a low pretest clinical probability for embolism.
- **CT pulmonary angiography:** First line for PE detection. Detects PEs in larger proximal pulmonary arteries (see Figure 16.8), but can miss subsegmental PEs.
- **V/Q scan:** Comparable to helical CT scan. Segmental regions of ventilation without perfusion suggest PE. "Low-probability" results do not rule out PE in the setting of high clinical probability. Perform a V/Q scan if a patient has a contraindication to CT pulmonary angiography.

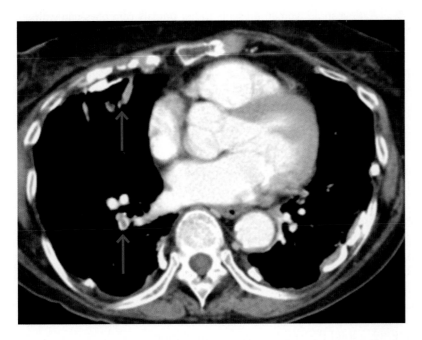

FIGURE 16.8.   Pulmonary emboli. Transaxial image from a contrast-enhanced CT shows multiple filling defects (arrows) in the pulmonary arteries of a patient with a history of pancreatic cancer. (Reproduced with permission from USMLERx.com.)

- **Lower extremity ultrasound:** May be used in conjunction with low or indeterminate V/Q scans to aid in the diagnosis of venous thromboembolism.
- **Pulmonary arteriography:** The gold standard for diagnosis, but requires an invasive procedure, IV contrast, and skilled personnel. Consider if the diagnosis is in doubt, despite initial workup, in the setting of a high pretest probability for PE.
- **Echocardiography:** May demonstrate right heart strain in massive or submassive PE, but its effect on management is controversial.

TREATENT

- **Unfractionated heparin (UFH) and LMWH:** Equally efficacious in the acute treatment of DVT and PE. LMWH is preferred initially because of its more predictable properties and ease of administration.
    - **UFH:** Bolus intravenously and continue using a weight-based nomogram.
    - **LMWH:** Given subcutaneously. Requires less monitoring than UFH. Avoid in the setting of severe renal impairment.
- **Warfarin:** Used for long-term maintenance, not acute anticoagulation. Can be introduced at the same time as UFH or LMWH. The duration of treatment is 3–6 months if the DVT/PE was provoked and there are no risk factors for future PEs. For unprovoked or thrombophilia-related DVT/PE, consider indefinite administration.
- **Thrombolytics:** Consider in hemodynamically unstable patients (persistent shock requiring pressors). Confers no mortality benefit for submassive PE (right ventricular strain without hemodynamic compromise).

Pulmonary Hypertension

A 46-year-old woman presents to her primary care physician with complaints of increasing dyspnea for the past six months. Her exercise tolerance has ↓ from running several miles to walking four city blocks with associated shortness of breath. She also acknowledges dysphagia, heartburn symptoms, and Raynaud's phenomenon. Her physical exam is notable for mild skin thickening and tightness. What is the most likely etiology of her dyspnea? Pulmonary artery hypertension from scleroderma or CREST.

Defined as a mean pulmonary artery pressure of > 25 mm Hg at rest (see Table 16.16).

SYMPTOMS/EXAM

- Presents with progressive dyspnea on exertion. In more advanced stages, patients may have exertional dizziness or syncope.
- Raynaud's phenomenon is common and may suggest an underlying collagen vascular disease.
- Elevated pulmonary arterial pressure and right ventricular strain on exam are associated with JVD, right ventricular heave, a right-sided S4, a fixed/split S2, a loud P2, and tricuspid regurgitation.
- Hepatomegaly, a pulsatile liver, and ascites from progressive right ventricular overload are seen in advanced disease.

TABLE 16.16. **World Health Organization Classification of Pulmonary Hypertension**

Group 1: Pulmonary Arterial Hypertension	Group 2: Pulmonary Venous Hypertension	Group 3: Lung Disease or Chronic Hypoxia	Group 4: Thrombotic or Embolic Disease	Group 5: Directly Affecting Vessels
Idiopathic	Left heart disease (mitral	COPD	Chronic	Sarcoidosis
Collagen vascular	valve, atrial myxoma)	ILD	thromboemboli	Vasculitis
disease		Sleep apnea		Tumor, lymphadenopathy
HIV				
Drugs/toxins				
(amphetamines,				
chemotherapy,				
cocaine)				

DIFFERENTIAL

Left ventricular systolic failure; left ventricular diastolic dysfunction.

DIAGNOSIS

- **Echocardiogram:** Estimates pulmonary arterial pressure and identifies left heart disease and congenital heart disease.
- **CXR:** Enlargement of pulmonary arteries with "pruning" of the peripheral vessels; ↑ right ventricular and right atrial pressure.
- **PFTs: Characterize underlying lung disease.**
- **V/Q scan:** To evaluate for chronic thromboembolic disease. If ⊕, a pulmonary angiogram (CT) is needed.
- **Sleep study:** Obstructive sleep apnea is a potentially reversible cause of pulmonary hypertension.
- **Serologic testing:** For SLE, RA, scleroderma, and HIV. LFTs should also be performed as part of the workup.
- **Right heart catheterization:** To confirm the diagnosis, determine the severity of the disease, and evaluate for pulmonary venous hypertension (left heart failure). Can also assess the response to a vasodilator challenge trial (eg, inhaled nitric oxide, prostacyclin), which usually predicts response to long-term therapy with oral calcium channel blockers (CCBs).

TREATMENT

- Treat the underlying disease if possible.
- **Vasodilator therapy:**
    - **Prostacyclin analogs:** Epoprostenol, treprostinil.
    - **Endothelin-1 antagonists:** Bosentan (survival advantage).
    - **Phosphodiesterase inhibitors:** Sildenafil.
- Diuretics for right heart failure.
- **O_2:** Critical if O_2 saturation is < 90% (hypoxemia worsens pulmonary vessel vasoconstriction).
- **Anticoagulation** (↑ risk for thrombus formation).
- **Oral CCBs:** Use only if pulmonary arterial pressure ↓ during a vasodilator challenge.
- Consider lung transplantation if the disease worsens despite treatment.

Solitary Pulmonary Nodule

A 60-year-old nonsmoking man presents for follow-up of an incidental solitary lung nodule detected on noncontrast CT scan. The nodule is 7 mm in diameter with smooth borders. What is the most appropriate follow-up?

Serial CT scans. The characteristics of this nodule are consistent with a benign etiology (< 1 cm diameter, smooth borders), and he has no risk factors for lung cancer. High-risk patients or nodules with concerning features (spiculated borders, > 2 cm diameter) should prompt biopsy or further imaging with contrast CT or PET scan.

An isolated lesion < 3 cm in diameter surrounded by pulmonary parenchyma. Abnormalities > 3 cm are lung masses and are usually malignant. Most benign lesions are infectious granulomas.

SYMPTOMS/EXAM

Often asymptomatic, but cough, hemoptysis, or dyspnea may be seen. Older age and a history of cigarette smoking raise the suspicion of cancer. Exam is often normal; lymphadenopathy may be seen.

DIFFERENTIAL

Granuloma (old TB, histoplasmosis, foreign body reaction), bronchogenic carcinoma, metastatic disease (usually > 1), bronchial adenoma, round pneumonia.

DIAGNOSIS

- **Comparison of serial CXRs:** If nodule size has been stable for two years, the nodule is considered benign.
- **Chest CT:** Characterizes nodules more effectively than CXR (see Table 16.17). IV contrast will detect lymphadenopathy.
- **PET scan:** May help determine if a lesion is malignant and provide staging information for lung cancer.

> **KEY FACT**
>
> Lesions that ↑ in size or change in character are likely malignant and should be resected, assuming a low surgical risk and no evidence of metastatic disease.

TABLE 16.17. Chest CT Patterns and Other Risks for Malignancy

MALIGNANT FEATURES	BENIGN FEATURES
Spiculated border or corona radiata sign (linear strands radiating from lesion); scalloped is intermediate risk.	Smooth border.
No or minimal calcification, or eccentric or stippled.	Laminated ("eggshell"), diffuse, central, or "popcorn" calcification (see Figure 16.9).
Doubling time one month to one year.	No growth over two years.
Size > 2 cm.	
Smoking history.	

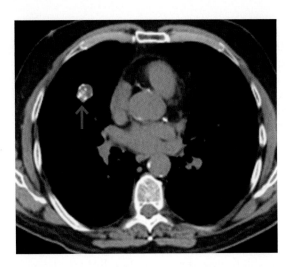

FIGURE 16.9.   Solitary pulmonary nodule, hamartoma. Transaxial image from an unenhanced CT shows the characteristic "popcorn" calcification of a pulmonary hamartoma (arrow). (Reproduced with permission from USMLERx.com.)

TREATMENT

- Most nodules > 2 cm are malignant.
- **Low risk for cancer and nonconcerning radiographic pattern:** Serial CT scans.
- **High risk for cancer or concerning radiographic features:** Biopsy/excision.
- **Intermediate risk for cancer:** Consider PET scan prior to biopsy. Uptake of glucose on PET scan is higher in malignant than in benign lesions (false ⊕s are also seen in infection and sarcoid).

Sarcoidosis

A 27-year-old woman presents with two weeks of fevers and painful nodules on her shins. Her exam is notable for painful, erythematous nodules on her lower extremities and bilateral ankle effusions. What is the most appropriate next step in diagnosis?

CXR. This patient's presentation is suspicious for sarcoidosis. Löfgren's syndrome is a form of sarcoidosis involving fever, erythema nodosum, polyarthralgia, and hilar lymphadenopathy. Staging the disease requires documentation of the extent of hilar lymphadenopathy and parenchymal involvement.

A systemic disease of unknown etiology that primarily affects the lungs and lymphatics and is characterized by **noncaseating granulomas.** Commonly affects young and middle-age adults, often presenting with **bilateral hilar adenopathy, pulmonary infiltrates, and skin lesions.** The liver, lymphatics, salivary glands, heart, CNS, and bones may be involved as well.

   KEY FACT

Do not biopsy erythema nodosum, because it will show only panniculitis, not granulomas.

SYMPTOMS/EXAM

- Presents with nonspecific constitutional symptoms such as fever, fatigue, anorexia, weight loss, and arthralgias.
- Löfgren's syndrome presents with fever, erythema nodosum, polyarthralgias, and hilar lymphadenopathy.
- Exam reveals dry crackles, lymphadenopathy, parotid enlargement, splenomegaly, uveitis, or skin changes (erythema nodosum).

DIFFERENTIAL

Mycobacterial, fungal, bacterial (tularemia and brucellosis), and parasitic (toxoplasmosis) infection. Also includes berylliosis, lymphoma, hypersensitivity pneumonitis, Wegener's granulomatosis, and Churg-Strauss syndrome.

DIAGNOSIS

- There is no one definitive diagnostic test, but transbronchial biopsy is the preferred procedure if an accessible lesion (eg, palpable lymph nodes or nodules) is not present for biopsy.
- Diagnosis requires (1) **noncaseating** granulomas on histopathology, (2) compatible clinical and radiographic findings, and (3) exclusion of other diseases that have a similar clinical picture.
- **Baseline studies** include the following:
  - **History:** Emphasis on occupational and environmental exposure.
  - **Physical exam:** Emphasis on the lung, skin, eye, liver, spleen, and heart.
  - Biopsy to obtain histologic confirmation of noncaseating granulomas.
  - CXR allows for staging of sarcoidosis. Stages according to CXR findings are as follows:
    - **Stage 0:** Normal CXR.
    - **Stage 1:** Hilar lymphadenopathy.
    - **Stage 2:** Hilar lymphadenopathy and interstitial infiltrates.
    - **Stage 3:** Interstitial infiltrates.
    - **Stage 4:** Fibrocystic changes.
  - HRCT is often performed after CXR to review for suggestive findings, although chest CT is not a component of official staging (see Figure 16.10).
  - LFTs, calcium, BUN/creatinine.
  - ACE level is not sensitive, and its value for disease monitoring is unclear.

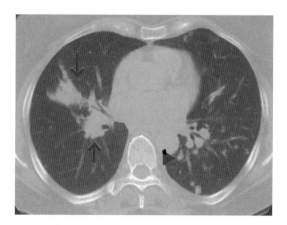

FIGURE 16.10. Pulmonary sarcoidosis. Transaxial CT image demonstrating nodules in the left lung (arrowhead) and consolidations in the right lung (arrows) centered around bronchovascular bundles. (Reproduced with permission from Fauci AS et al. *Harrison's Principles of Internal Medicine,* 17th ed. New York: McGraw-Hill, 2008, Fig. 322-3.)

TREATMENT

■ Treatment remains controversial for many reasons, including spontaneous remission, which is common; difficulty in assessing disease activity and severity; and variability in clinical course.

■ The goal is to ↓ inflammatory response and prevent fibrosis. Systemic (oral) glucocorticoids are the mainstay of treatment.

■ Indications for treatment of pulmonary sarcoidosis include worsening pulmonary symptoms, declining PFTs, and worsening radiographic findings.

■ Indications for treatment of extrapulmonary sarcoidosis include disabling symptoms. Treat earlier if the patient has hypercalcemia or has ocular, neurologic, cardiac, or renal involvement in view of the potential for end-organ damage.

KEY FACT

Do not treat if patients are asymptomatic with stage 1 disease (bilateral hilar lymphadenopathy with or without erythema nodosum). There is also no need to treat stage 2 or 3 disease if patients are without symptoms and still have relatively preserved lung function.

Sleep-Disordered Breathing

Patients with **obstructive sleep apnea** (OSA) have episodic closure of the upper airway during sleep with continued respiratory efforts. Patients with **central sleep apnea** (CSA) have cessation of both airflow and respiratory efforts. CSA is often associated with CNS disorders, respiratory muscle weakness, cardiovascular disease, or pulmonary congestion, but it may also be idiopathic.

SYMPTOMS/EXAM

■ Presents with daytime hypersomnolence, morning headache, impaired cognition, snoring, witnessed gasping or choking at night, and witnessed apneic episodes while sleeping.

■ Patients with severe disease may have significant hypoxemia during sleep, pulmonary hypertension, systemic hypertension, heart failure, arrhythmias, and 2° erythrocytosis.

DIAGNOSIS

Polysomnography. The sum of apneas and hypopneas per hour of sleep (the apnea-hypopnea index) is used to determine severity.

TREATMENT

See Table 16.18.

KEY FACT

In CSA, apneic episodes are not accompanied by respiratory effort; patients breathe faster after apneic episodes (periodic breathing = Cheyne-Stokes respiration). Polysomnography can distinguish between CSA and OSA.

TABLE 16.18.   Obstructive vs. Central Sleep Apnea

	OBSTRUCTIVE SLEEP APNEA	**CENTRAL SLEEP APNEA**
Definition	Apnea due to transient obstruction of the upper airway, but ventilatory effort is present.	Apnea occurs, but there is no compensatory ventilatory effort during apneic episode. Tachypnea occurs after the apneic episode.
Risk factors	Obesity (large neck circumference), large tonsils, upper airway soft tissue abnormalities, hypothyroidism, craniofacial abnormalities.	Systolic-dysfunction CHF is most common. CNS disorders, respiratory muscle weakness, opioids, and renal/liver failure also ↑ risk.
Treatment	Weight loss (10–20% of weight), nasal CPAP, avoidance of EtOH and sedatives, oral devices or upper airway surgery (uvulopalatopharyngoplasty).	Treat underlying disease; O₂ if hypoxemic; consider BiPAP or CPAP.

NOTES

CHAPTER 17

Rheumatology

Miten Vasa, MD
Jonathan Graf, MD

Approach to Arthritis

Tables 17.1 through 17.3 outline general approaches toward the differential diagnosis of arthritis and other rheumatic diseases. **Contraindications to arthrocentesis** include the following:

- Overlying soft tissue infection or cellulitis.
- Severe coagulopathy or bleeding disorder (INR > 3.0).

TABLE 17.1. Differential Diagnosis of Arthritis

DISEASE	INFLAMMATION	JOINT PATTERN	PERIPHERAL JOINT INVOLVEMENT	SPINAL DISEASE	KEY DISTINGUISHING FEATURES
Rheumatoid arthritis (RA)	+	Symmetric/ polyarticular	Wrist/MCPs, PIPs/ MTPs, ankles, knees; DIPs are spared	No (except C-spine)	Polyarticular, symmetric, small joints, ulnar deviation, boutonnière deformity.
SLE	+	Symmetric/ polyarticular	Wrist/MCPs/PIPs	No	Extra-articular manifestations of SLE.
Ankylosing spondylitis	+	Usually oligoarticular	Hips, shoulders, knees	Yes	Low back pain.
Psoriatic arthritis	+	Asymmetric/ oligoarticular	Dactylitis, DIPs	Yes	History of cutaneous psoriasis.
Reactive arthritis	+	Asymmetric/ oligoarticular	Larger, weight-bearing joints; knees/ankles	Yes	History of URI, diarrheal illness, or STD.
IBD-associated arthritis	+	Oligoarticular	Larger joints	Yes	GI manifestations (eg, diarrhea, bloody stools).
Gout	+	Monoarticular, polyarticular	First MTP, ankle, knee, MCPs/PIPs	No	Acute, exquisitely painful to touch.
Osteoarthritis (see Figures 17.1 and 17.2)	–	Monoarticular/ oligoarticular, polyarticular	DIPs, first carpal-metacarpal, knees, hips	Yes	Noninflammatory, ie, worse at the end of the day and with activity; improves with rest; Bouchard's nodes, Heberden's nodes.

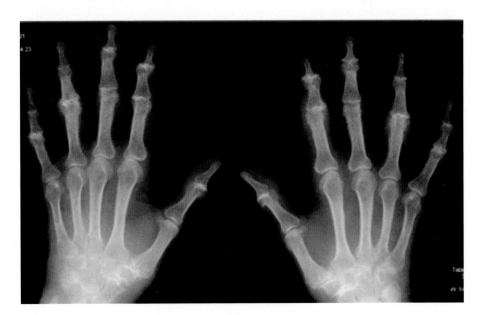

FIGURE 17.1. **Osteoarthritis of the hands.** Plain radiographs show joint space narrowing, osteophytes, and subchondral degenerative cysts involving the interphalangeal joints in a 68-year-old female with chronic hand pain; note sparing of the MCP and carpal joints. (Reproduced with permission from USMLERx.com.)

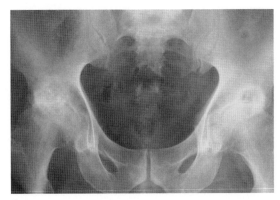

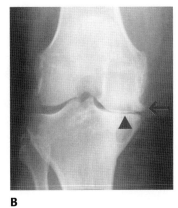

A   **B**

FIGURE 17.2. **Osteoarthritis of the hips and knee.** (A) Frontal radiograph of both hips shows articular space narrowing, sclerosis, and subchondral cyst formation bilaterally. (B) AP knee radiograph shows a narrowed joint space on the medial side of the joint only, subchondral sclerosis (arrowhead) and cyst (lucency below arrowhead), and osteophytes (arrow). (Reproduced with permission from Chen MY et al. *Basic Radiology*. New York: McGraw-Hill, 2004, Figs. 7-34 and 7-40.)

TABLE 17.2.   Characteristics of Synovial Fluid

Sign	Normal	Group 1: Noninflammatory (Osteoarthritis, Hypothyroidism)	Group 2: Inflammatory (RA, Gout, CPPD, Spondyloarthropathy)	Group 3: Septic
Clarity	Transparent	Transparent	Slightly opaque	Opaque
Color	Clear	Yellow	Yellow-opalescent	Yellow-green
Viscosity	High	High	Low	Usually low
Culture	⊖	⊖	⊖	Often ⊕
WBCs/mm³	< 200	200–2000	2000–50,000	> 50,000
PMNs (%)	< 25	< 25	> 50	> 75

TABLE 17.3.   Laboratory Serologies in SLE and Other Rheumatic Diseases

Test	RA	SLE	SS	DS	LS	P/DM	Wegener's	Comments
						% Disease Association		
				ANA Tests				
ANA	30–60	95–100	95	80–95	80–95	80–95	0–15	Often used as a screening test; a ⊖ test virtually excludes SLE.
Anti-dsDNA	0–5	60						Titer generally correlates with disease activity. Also seen in drug-induced lupus from anti-TNF agents and interferon-α.
Anti-Smith		10–25						Specific for SLE.
Anti-RNP	0–10	30		20–30	20–30			Antibody must be present to make the diagnosis of mixed connective tissue disease.
Anti-SSA (Ro)	0–5	15–20	60–70					Associated with neonatal lupus and subacute cutaneous lupus erythematosus.
Anti-SSB (La)	0–2	5–20	60–70					Associated with neonatal lupus.
Anticentromere					50			
Antitopoisomerase I (anti-SCL-70)				33	20			

TABLE 17.3.   Laboratory Serologies in SLE and Other Rheumatic Diseases *(continued)*

| | % DISEASE ASSOCIATION | | | | | | | |
TEST	RA	SLE	SS	DS	LS	P/DM	WEGENER'S	COMMENTS
	NON-ANA TESTS							
RF	70–80	20	75	25	25	33	50	
Anti-CCP	47–76							Appears earlier than RF in RA; specificity for RA is 95%; associated with the development of erosive RA.
ANCA		1–5					93–96	Also in drug-induced lupus from minocycline, hydralazine.
Anti-Jo-1						20–30		

SS = Sjögren's syndrome; DS = diffuse scleroderma; LS = limited scleroderma; P/DM = polymyositis/dermatomyositis.

Rheumatoid Arthritis (RA)

 A 35-year-old house cleaner presents with a three-month history of proximal interphalangeal and wrist swelling and pain. These joints are stiff in the morning, interfering with her work. On exam, the patient has symmetric synovitis of the MCP and wrist joints. Her labs show ⊖ ANA, ⊖ RF, and ⊕ anti–cyclic citrullinated peptide (anti-CCP) antibodies. Radiographs of the hand show juxta-articular osteoporosis and marginal erosions in the MCP joints. What is the most likely diagnosis?

RA, a symmetric, inflammatory arthritis that has been present for > 6 weeks and involves the MCP and wrist joints. RF is ⊕ in 85% of cases, but only 33% of cases are ⊕ in the first six months of disease. Anti-CCP has 90–95% specificity for RA, is often present early in disease, and has significant predictive value when combined with RF.

Has a female-to-male predominance of 3:1. Prevalence ↑ with age, with a typical age at onset of 20–40.

SYMPTOMS/EXAM

- Symptoms and signs include the following:
  - **Morning pain and/or stiffness for > 30 minutes.**
  - Gelling phenomenon, or worsening of symptoms with prolonged joint inactivity.
  - Improvement in symptoms with use of the joint.
  - The presence of erythema, warmth, and/or swelling in the joint (see Figure 17.3).
  - A symmetric pattern of joint involvement.

> **KEY FACT**
>
> In a young woman with bilateral symmetric arthritis of the hands and wrists, the differential is RA, SLE, and viral infection. If the symptoms abate within six weeks, RA is less likely. Plain x-rays may not distinguish early RA from SLE, as radiographic erosions take time to develop.

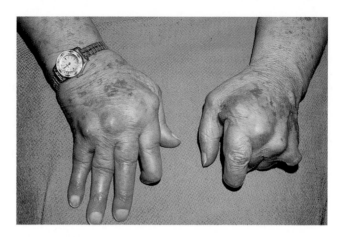

FIGURE 17.3. Rheumatoid arthritis involving the hands. Typical ulnar deviation of the MCP joints and swelling of the PIP joints in a patient with RA. Multiple subcutaneous rheumatoid nodules are also seen. (Reproduced with permission from Wolff K et al. *Fitzpatrick's Dermatology in General Medicine,* 7th ed. New York: McGraw-Hill, 2008, Fig. 161-1A.)

KEY FACT

Most extra-articular manifestations of RA are observed in patients who are RF ⊕ and have long-standing erosive articular disease.

- Rheumatoid nodules over bony prominences, on extensor surfaces, or in juxta-articular regions but also in the lungs or on heart valves. Nodules occur in 25% of cases (see Figure 17.4).
- A prodrome of low-grade fever and malaise.
- The most common joints affected are the hands, wrists, toes, ankles, and knees, although all joints with movable articulations can be involved.

DIAGNOSIS

- **Classification criteria** were revised in 2010 and are outlined in Table 17.4.

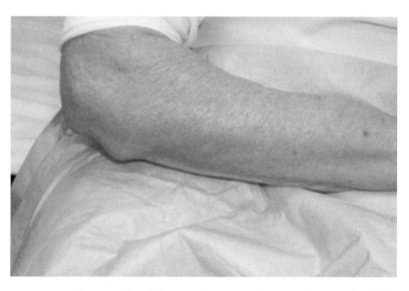

FIGURE 17.4. Rheumatoid nodule over a bony prominence. A rheumatoid nodule in a typical location on the extensor surface of the forearm is apparent in this patient with seropositive, erosive RA. (Reproduced with permission from Imboden JB et al. *Current Rheumatology Diagnosis & Treatment,* 2nd ed. New York: McGraw-Hill, 2007, Fig. 15-5.)

TABLE 17.4.   **Criteria for the Classification of RA[a]**

CRITERION	DESCRIPTION	POINTS
Joint involvement (swollen, tender, or erosions seen on x-ray)	1 large joint	0
	2–10 large joints	1
	1–3 small joints	2
	4–10 small joints	3
	> 10 joints	5
Serology[b]	⊕ RF or anti-CCP at low level	2
	⊕ RF or anti-CCP at high level	3
Acute-phase reactants	Elevated CRP or ESR	1
Duration	≥ 6 weeks	1

[a]The diagnosis of RA requires a score of 6 or higher and no other disease to explain the symptoms.

[b]A ⊕ serology is now required for diagnosis.

- **Classic radiographic findings:** Periarticular osteopenia, joint space narrowing, juxta-articular erosions, erosions of the ulnar styloids (see Figures 17.5 and 17.6).
- **Aggressive RA** is probable with high titers of RF, ⊕ anti-CCP, ⊕ HLA-DR4 antigen, insidious onset, constitutional symptoms, early erosive disease on x-ray, and early appearance of rheumatoid nodules.
- **Common laboratory findings:**
  - **RF:**
    - Usually an IgM antibody directed against an Fc fragment of IgG.
    - Extremely high titers correlate with severe RA and nodular disease.
    - Not specific for RA; can be seen in other collagen vascular diseases and in chronic infections (eg, HCV).

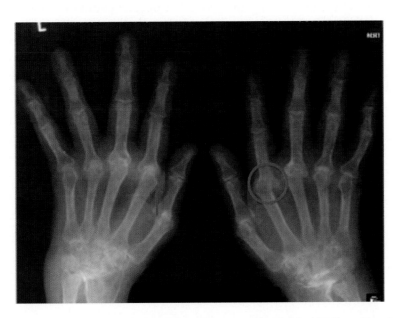

FIGURE 17.5.   **Radiographic appearance of rheumatoid arthritis.** AP bilateral hand radiograph in a patient with advanced RA shows joint space narrowing involving the carpal, MCP, and PIP joints as well as subluxation at multiple MCP joints (circle) and periarticular erosions (arrow). (Reproduced with permission from USMLERx.com.)

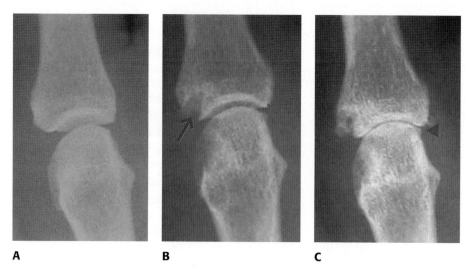

FIGURE 17.6. Progression of radiographic findings of rheumatoid arthritis. (A) Normal MCP joint one year before the onset of RA. **(B)** Six months following the onset of RA, there is a bony erosion (arrow) adjacent to the joint and joint space narrowing. **(C)** After three years of disease, diffuse loss of articular cartilage has led to marked joint space narrowing (arrowhead). (Reproduced with permission from Imboden JB et al. *Current Rheumatology Diagnosis & Treatment,* 2nd ed. New York: McGraw-Hill, 2007, Fig. 15-3.)

KEY FACT

In an RA patient being treated with methotrexate who develops new-onset dyspnea and interstitial infiltrates on CXR, consider opportunistic infections and hypersensitivity pneumonitis from methotrexate and stop the drug.

KEY FACT

Infliximab is associated with higher rates of infusion reactions and of neutralizing antibodies than other TNF inhibitors.

- Anti-CCP:
  - More specific (90–95%) than RF antibody.
  - Testing for both RF and anti-CCP is more effective for diagnosing RA than testing for either antibody alone and is likely better for excluding the diagnosis of RA if both are ⊖, especially in patients with polyarthritis. Early RA may be seronegative.
  - Anti-CCP-⊕ patients are at ↑ risk for radiographic progression of RA.
- **Other findings** are as follows:
  - ESR and CRP are frequently ↑ but are neither sensitive nor specific.
  - Anemia of chronic disease is common.
  - Platelet count is normal or ↑ (vs. a low platelet count in SLE).
  - C1–C2 subluxation is seen in patients with chronic severe disease and can cause posterior headaches starting at the base of the skull and cervical myelopathy. The lumbar spine and sacroiliac joints are spared.
  - Neutropenia and splenomegaly can be seen with Felty's syndrome.
- **Extra-articular manifestations:**
  - Rheumatoid nodules, vasculitis, interstitial lung disease (ILD).
  - Serositis (pleuritis, pericarditis, myocarditis, effusions with ↓ glucose, ↑ LDH).
  - Ocular disease (episcleritis, uveitis, scleritis, keratitis).
  - Sjögren's syndrome.
  - Caplan's syndrome (large nodulosis of the lungs associated with anthracite coal exposure; dust-mining pneumoconiosis).
  - Amyloidosis.
  - Accelerated atherosclerosis (associated with a threefold ↑ risk of CAD).
  - Carpal tunnel syndrome.

TREATMENT

- **Early use of disease-modifying antirheumatic drugs (DMARDs) is key.** NSAIDs are important for symptom flares but do not alter the disease course. The American College of Rheumatology recommends starting DMARD therapy within three months of diagnosis, either with single agents or with combination therapy, particularly for those predicted to have active, erosive disease, sparing those with milder disease from the potential side effects of DMARDs.
- Table 17.5 outlines indications for the various antirheumatic drugs as well as their appropriate dosages, contraindications, and potential side effects. The recommended protocol is as follows:
  - **First-line DMARDs:** Methotrexate (or sulfasalazine/leflunomide).
  - **Second-line DMARDs:** Combination therapy with two first-line DMARDs or a TNF-α inhibitor.
  - **Third-line DMARDs:** If no response is achieved after 3–6 months of a TNF-α inhibitor, consider changing to a different class of biologic medication or adding azathioprine.
- As patients improve with early, aggressive use of DMARDs, the more toxic drugs are usually withdrawn, and therapy is continued with the least toxic drugs.

KEY FACT

For patients with RA or SLE, prednisone and hydroxychloroquine are the preferred anti-inflammatory agents during pregnancy.

TABLE 17.5. **Comparison of the Most Commonly Used Antirheumatic Drugs**

DRUG	INDICATION	DOSAGE	INITIAL MONITORING	ROUTINE MONITORING	CONTRA-INDICATIONS	SIDE EFFECTS
Methotrexate	First-line DMARD.	Weekly.	CXR, hepatitis serologies, CBC, LFTs, creatinine.	CBC, LFTs every 4–8 weeks.	Renal disease, hepatic disease, EtOH abuse.	Myelosuppression, hypersensitivity pneumonitis, pulmonary fibrosis, hepatotoxicity, cirrhosis, GI intolerance, stomatitis, alopecia.
Sulfasalazine	First- or second-line DMARD.	Daily.	CBC, G6PD (if suspected).	CBC, LFTs.	G6PD deficiency (can cause hemolysis), sulfa allergy.	GI intolerance, transaminitis, neutropenia, thrombocytopenia.
Leflunomide	First- or second-line DMARD.	Daily, but $t_{1/2}$ is > 2 weeks.	Hepatitis serologies, CBC, LFTs, creatinine.	CBC, LFTs, creatinine.		Myelosuppression, hepatotoxicity, rash, diarrhea, alopecia.

(continues)

TABLE 17.5.   Comparison of the Most Commonly Used Antirheumatic Drugs *(continued)*

Drug	Indication	Dosage	Initial Monitoring	Routine Monitoring	Contra-indications	Side Effects
TNF-α inhibitors	Second-line DMARDs/ biologics; usually added after 3–6 months if there is little or no response to other DMARDs.	**Infliximab:** Infusion q 6–8 weeks. **Adalimumab:** SQ injection q 2 weeks. **Etanercept:** SQ injection 1–2 times per week. **Certolizumab:** SQ injection 1–2 times/mo. **Golimumab:** SQ injection 1 time/mo.	PPD, CXR, CBC, LFTs.	CBC, LFTs.	Malignancy; active or untreated latent TB.	Immuno-suppression with an ↑ incidence of opportunistic infections and malignancy. All can cause drug-induced lupus (⊕ anti-ds-DNA). Infliximab is hepatotoxic.
Anakinra	Second-line DMARD/ biologic IL-1 receptor antagonist; can be used instead of anti-TNF agents.	SQ injection daily.	PPD, CXR, CBC, creatinine.	CBC.		Neutropenia, infection, thrombocytopenia, hypersensitivity, malignancy, GI intolerance.
Antimalarials (hydroxy-chloroquine)	Weak DMARD used in mild RA.	Daily.		Yearly eye exam.		Retinopathy, especially with renal dysfunction.
Corticosteroids	First-line DMARD, but use lowest dose possible and wean off to prevent long-term complications.	Daily oral. Injections are very helpful for symptoms.	BP, glucose, metabolic panel, lipids.	Bone densitometry (DEXA), glucose, lipids.		Glucose intolerance, hypertension, cataracts, osteoporosis, avascular necrosis.
Azathioprine	Used for severe/ refractory RA.	Daily.	CBC, LFTs, creatinine.	CBC with change in dose, LFTs.	Not to be used concomitantly with allopurinol.	Myelosuppression, immuno-suppression, hepatotoxicity, lymphoproliferative disorders.
Minocycline	Weak DMARD.	Daily.				Dizziness, hyperpigmentation, deposition into bone.

Systemic Lupus Erythematosus (SLE) and Drug-Induced Lupus

SYSTEMIC LUPUS ERYTHEMATOSUS (SLE)

 A 25-year-old African American woman presents with three weeks of diffuse joint pain, fatigue, and easy bruisability about six weeks after she had a severe sunburn on her face and chest. On exam, she is found to have an erythematous rash extending from the bridge of her nose to both cheeks but sparing the nasolabial folds, together with ecchymoses on her lower extremities, a few painless oral ulcers, cervical lymphadenopathy, bibasilar crackles, and splenomegaly. Her PIP and MCP joints are tender to palpation. Labs reveal a hemoglobin level of 8 g/dL, a leukocyte count of 3000/µL, and a platelet count of 55,000/µL. What is the most likely diagnosis?

SLE is characterized by arthralgias, a photosensitive rash, a malar rash, oral ulcers, pancytopenia, and serositis. Lymphadenopathy and splenomegaly may also be seen.

Has a female-to-male predominance of 9:1. Three times more common among African Americans than among Caucasians. Both genetic and environmental factors are involved. Nearly 90% of patients have joint symptoms.

DIFFERENTIAL

The differential diagnosis of SLE is outlined in Table 17.6.

DIAGNOSIS

- Four of the 11 clinical and laboratory criteria listed in Table 17.7 can classify patients as having SLE.
- ANA testing is nearly 100% sensitive but is not specific for SLE (see Table 17.3).
- Antibodies to dsDNA and Smith are specific (> 90% and > 95%, respectively) but not sensitive (50–60% and 30%, respectively).
- Antibody titers to dsDNA can correlate with disease activity, particularly renal disease.

 KEY FACT

In active SLE, antibodies to dsDNA may ↑ and serum complement level may ↓.

TABLE 17.6. **Differential Diagnosis of SLE**

DIFFERENTIAL	DISTINGUISHING FACTORS
Drug-induced lupus (must be excluded)	See text.
RA	Erosive arthritis is seen in RA.
Mixed connective tissue disease (MCTD)	MCTD has features of systemic sclerosis and/or inflammatory myopathy and less severe renal disease.
Acute drug reaction	Identification of offending agent.
Systemic sclerosis	Predominance of skin changes.

TABLE 17.7. Diagnostic Criteria for SLE[a]

Variable	Criteria
Skin/**S**unlight	1. Malar rash
	2. Discoid rash
	3. Photosensitivity
Serosa/mucous membranes	4. Oral ulcers
	5. Serositis (pleuritis/pericarditis)
Synovitis	6. Arthritis
Seizures, "**S**"ychosis	7. Neurologic disease
"**S**"ellular casts, proteinuria	8. Renal disease (any one of the following):
	a. > 0.5 g/day proteinuria
	b. ≥ 3+ dipstick protein
	c. Cellular casts
"**S**"ytopenias	9. Hematologic disorders (any one of the following):
	a. Hemolytic anemia
	b. Leukopenia (< 4000/mL)
	c. Lymphopenia (< 1500/mL)
	d. Thrombocytopenia (< 100,000/mL)
Serologies	10. ⊕ ANA
	11. Immunologic abnormalities (any one of the following):
	a. Antibodies to native DNA
	b. Anti-Smith antibodies
	c. Antiphospholipid antibodies:
	(1) False-⊕ serologic test for syphilis
	(2) Evidence of anticardiolipin antibodies
	(3) Evidence of lupus anticoagulant

[a]Four out of 11 yield high specificity in classifying a patient as having SLE.

KEY FACT

An ↑ PTT in a patient with SLE suggests the presence of antiphospholipid antibodies.

- Antibody titers to Smith and ANA do not correlate with disease activity.
- Depressed serum complement levels (CH50, C3, C4) are frequently seen in SLE but can normalize in remission.

Treatment

Nonpharmacologic treatment includes sun avoidance, sun protection, rest, and avoidance of stress. Pharmacologic treatment can be broken down according to disease severity:

- **Mild disease** (skin/joint involvement, oral ulcers, serositis) (see Figures 17.7 and 17.8):
  - NSAIDs.
  - Topical corticosteroids for skin disease.
  - Low-dose oral corticosteroids (< 10 mg/day).
  - Antimalarial medications (ie, hydroxychloroquine; good for mild symptoms and skin disease).

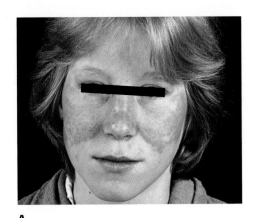

A

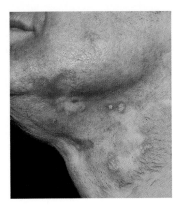

B

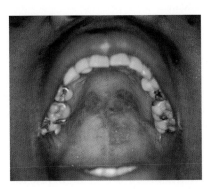

C

FIGURE 17.7. **Mucocutaneous manifestations of SLE.** (A) Malar rash. This type of rash is typically photosensitive. (B) Discoid rash. (C) Oral ulcer. (Image A reproduced with permission from Wolff K, Johnson RA. *Fitzpatrick's Color Atlas & Synopsis of Clinical Dermatology,* 6th ed. New York: McGraw-Hill, 2009, Fig. 14-20. Image B reproduced with permission from Wolff K et al. *Fitzpatrick's Dermatology in General Medicine,* 7th ed. New York: McGraw-Hill, 2008, Fig. 156-7. Image C reproduced with permission from Wolff K et al. *Fitzpatrick's Dermatology in General Medicine,* 7th ed. New York: McGraw-Hill, 2008, Fig. 156-8C.)

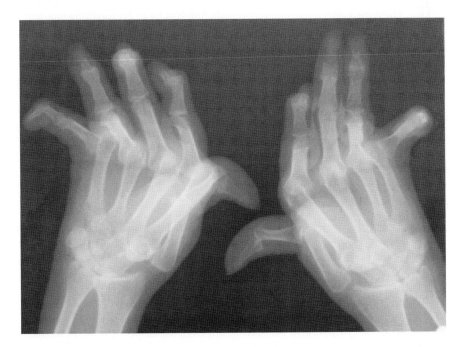

FIGURE 17.8. **Lupus arthritis.** Characteristic ulnar deviation at the MCP joints with subluxation at multiple joints. Note the absence of bony erosions. (Reproduced with permission from Chen MY et al. *Basic Radiology.* New York: McGraw-Hill, 2004, Fig. 7-43.)

- **Moderate disease** (cytopenias/hemolytic anemia, serositis, mild pneumonitis, mild myocarditis):
  - Moderately dosed systemic corticosteroids (~ 0.5 mg/kg/day).
  - Steroid-sparing agents such as azathioprine, methotrexate (good for skin and arthritis), and mycophenolate mofetil.
- **Severe disease** (nephritis, severe CNS disease, vasculitis, pulmonary hemorrhage):
  - High-dose corticosteroids (≥ 1 mg/kg/day).
  - IV cyclophosphamide (proven efficacy for nephritis; less established for other indications).
  - Azathioprine.
  - Rituximab.
  - IVIG (for antibody-mediated cytopenias).
  - Plasmapheresis (in extreme circumstances).

COMPLICATIONS

In addition to disease-related organ-specific damage, complications are as follows:

- Accelerated atherosclerosis; CAD.
- An ↑ risk of venous thromboembolism, especially in SLE patients who also have antiphospholipid antibodies.
- Transitional cell carcinoma and hematologic malignancies if the patient received cyclophosphamide.
- Opportunistic infections (SLE patients on rituximab are at high risk for **progressive multifocal leukoencephalopathy**).

> **KEY FACT**
>
> The leading causes of death in patients with SLE are active organ disease and infection early on; later in the disease, accelerated atherosclerosis, end-stage organ disease (especially renal), and infections predominate.

DRUG-INDUCED LUPUS

A 40-year-old woman with a 10-year history of RA presents with worsening symmetrical joint pain in her hands and feet together with pleuritic chest pain and a macular malar rash. She has been on methotrexate and infliximab for one year, which greatly improved her severe erosive RA. On exam, she is found to have synovitis of her hands and feet and a pericardial friction rub. Which of the following is the most likely cause of the patient's symptoms?

Drug-induced SLE, most likely induced by the anti-TNF agent infliximab, which should be discontinued. About 20% of RA patients treated with anti-TNF agents can develop ⊕ ANA, and some develop drug-induced lupus. Corticosteroid therapy may be needed to treat the arthritis, pericarditis, and rash.

DIFFERENTIAL

Hallmarks that distinguish drug-induced lupus from SLE include the following:

- Equal prevalence in both sexes.
- Lack of severe renal and neurologic involvement.
- Lack of antibodies to DNA.
- Frequently normal levels of serum complement.
- Abatement of clinical and laboratory features on discontinuation of the inciting agent.

> **KEY FACT**
>
> The medications most commonly associated with drug-induced lupus are hydralazine, procainamide, INH, quinidine, methyldopa, anti-TNF agents, and chlorpromazine.

- The presence of **antihistone antibodies** (sensitive but not specific for drug-induced lupus):
  - Seen in 95% of drug-induced lupus cases and 50% of SLE cases.
  - Most helpful in ruling out drug-induced lupus caused by procainamide, hydralazine, chlorpromazine, and quinidine. Anti-TNF drugs and interferon-α can cause drug-induced lupus with a ⊕ anti-dsDNA; minocycline and hydralazine can cause a lupuslike syndrome with a ⊕ ANCA.

KEY FACT

In a patient taking hydralazine who develops a pericardial effusion, arthralgias, and ⊕ ANA and antihistone antibodies, suspect drug-induced lupus and stop the hydralazine.

NEONATAL LUPUS

Clinical features of neonatal lupus are as follows:

- A photosensitive rash, **complete heart block,** hepatitis, thrombocytopenia, and hemolytic anemia.
- Passive transfer of maternal **anti-Ro/SSA and anti-La/SSB antibodies** in utero associated with disease.
- Most features remit when titers of antibodies wane in the neonate.
- Complete heart block is permanent.

KEY FACT

Neonatal lupus is classically associated with anti-SSa (anti-Ro) and anti-SSb (anti-La) antibodies and may cause complete heart block.

Sjögren's Syndrome

A 50-year-old woman presents with a 20-pound weight loss over two months together with fatigue and night sweats. She has a history of dental caries and tooth loss. In addition, her mouth is often very dry, and her eyes feel as though there is sand in them. On exam, she is found to be cachectic with dry mucous membranes, symmetric parotid gland enlargement, dry eyes, and splenomegaly. Labs show an ANA titer of 1:320, ⊕ anti-Ro/SSA antibodies, and an ↑ gamma globulin level on serum protein electrophoresis. What diagnostic study should be done next to evaluate for a complication of this woman's disease?

CT of the chest and abdomen. This patient has Sjögren's syndrome, which carries a 44-fold ↑ risk for non-Hodgkin's lymphoma and other lymphoproliferative conditions. 1° Sjögren's syndrome occurs in women 40–60 years of age. Patients often have ⊕ antibodies, including ANA and RF, along with hypergammaglobulinemia.

Characterized by lymphocytic and plasma cell infiltration of affected exocrine glands throughout the body. Can be 1° in etiology or 2° to another autoimmune disorder. Sjögren's exhibits a significant female-to-male predominance (9:1) and most commonly affects middle-aged individuals.

SYMPTOMS/EXAM

The clinical characteristics of Sjögren's syndrome are as follows (common boards associations are in boldface):

- **Dry mouth (xerostomia), dental caries,** impaired taste and/or smell, dysphagia.
- **Keratoconjunctivitis sicca: Burning, itching eyes;** diminished lacrimation; thickened/sticky tears; photophobia.
- Parotid enlargement.
- Dryness of the skin and vaginal mucosa.

- Pancreatitis.
- ILD, **lymphocytic interstitial pneumonitis,** tracheobronchitis sicca.
- **Type 1 RTA;** interstitial nephritis (the leading cause of interstitial nephritis among Caucasian patients in the United States).
- Neuropsychiatric diseases of various etiologies.
- Vasculitis.

DIFFERENTIAL

Drugs (eg, anticholinergic medications), HCV, HIV, and sarcoidosis may present with dry eyes and dry mouth. HIV and sarcoidosis may also present with glandular infiltration.

DIAGNOSIS

- **Biopsy** of minor lip/salivary gland reveals lymphocytic foci in glands.
- **Labs:** ANA, RF, and anti-SSA/anti-SSB antibodies are frequently ⊕ (see Table 17.3); hypergammaglobulinemia.
- **Other:** Ancillary testing can demonstrate ↓ tear production and low salivary flow.

TREATMENT

Seek symptom relief with the following:

- Artificial tears and saliva.
- Sugar-free candies and frequent sipping of water.
- Aggressive oral hygiene.
- Avoidance of anticholinergic and decongestant medications.
- Cholinergic agonist medications such as pilocarpine to stimulate saliva production.

COMPLICATIONS

Lymphoproliferative disorders, including lymphomas; Waldenström's macroglobulinemia.

Seronegative Spondyloarthropathies

Include four disorders: ankylosing spondylitis, psoriatic arthritis, IBD-associated arthritis, and reactive arthritis (see Table 17.8).

TABLE 17.8. Features of Seronegative Spondyloarthropathies

DISEASE	SACROILIITIS	% WITH ⊕ HLA-B27	OTHER MANIFESTATIONS
Ankylosing spondylitis	Symmetric	90%	Uveitis, aortitis.
Psoriatic arthritis	Asymmetric	75%	Skin disease in 80% of cases; DIP arthritis is common.
Reactive arthritis	Asymmetric	80% of Caucasians, 50–60% of African Americans	The classic triad is conjunctivitis, urethritis, and arthritis (more commonly of larger peripheral joints than of the spine); keratoderma blennorrhagicum (a pustular rash on the soles of the feet).
IBD-associated arthritis	Symmetric	50% (when sacroiliitis is present)	GI disease is usually present; more commonly Crohn's disease than ulcerative colitis.

ANKYLOSING SPONDYLITIS

A 30-year-old man presents with a two-year history of worsening lower back stiffness that is present for a few hours after he awakens in the morning, accompanied by buttock pain throughout the day when he is seated. He is currently on corticosteroid eye drops for left eye uveitis that has improved over the past week. His exam is notable for bending forward of the spine during walking and tenderness over the sacroiliac joints and lumbar spine. He also has a 2/6 diastolic blowing murmur at the left base and a BP of 160/50 mm Hg. Labs show an ESR of 100 mm/hr, and a pelvic x-ray reveals narrowing and erosions of the sacroiliac joints and syndesmophytes (bony growth attached to ligaments). What is the most likely diagnosis?

Ankylosing spondylitis, a systemic inflammatory disorder in which sacroiliac damage can occur 6–12 months after disease onset. Extra-articular manifestations include aortitis with aortic insufficiency, upper lobe pulmonary fibrocystic disease, amyloidosis, cardiac conduction disease, and recurrent uveitis.

Shows a predominance of **males over females**; characterized by an early age of onset (generally < 35 years). Prevalence is 0.2–0.5% among Caucasians in the United States (has a higher prevalence among Scandinavians).

SYMPTOMS

- Presents with inflammatory low back pain that worsens in the morning and with inactivity but improves with exercise.
- Also characterized by progressive pain and stiffening of the spine and transient acute arthritis (pain and swelling) of the larger peripheral joints.

EXAM

- Tenderness of the sacroiliac joints to palpation.
- ↓ lumbar lordosis; ↓ chest expansion diameter.
- Limited range of motion of the neck.
- Enthesitis—ie, pain of the Achilles tendon on palpation (see Figure 17.9).

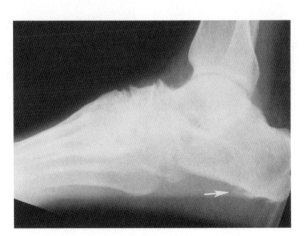

FIGURE 17.9. **Enthesitis.** Lateral foot radiograph in a patient with sacroiliitis and heel pain, most commonly due to ankylosing spondylitis or reactive arthritis. Note the prominent calcaneal spur representing enthesopathic change (abnormalities at bony insertion points of tendons, in this case the plantar fascia tendon) (arrow). (Reproduced with permission from Chen MY et al. *Basic Radiology.* New York: McGraw-Hill, 2004, Fig. 7-44.)

DIFFERENTIAL

- RA (affects numerous symmetric, small peripheral joints).
- Noninflammatory, mechanical low back pain.
- Diffuse idiopathic skeletal hyperostosis.
- Osteitis condensans ilii (sclerosis of the iliac bone in childbearing women).
- Infectious sacroiliitis (eg, TB, brucellosis).

DIAGNOSIS

- Diagnosed in the setting of a consistent history.
- **Imaging:** Look for radiographic evidence of sacroiliitis and/or spinal involvement (see Figure 17.10):
  - Bilateral sclerosis of the sacroiliac joints.
  - Squared-off vertebral bodies.
  - "Shiny" corners of vertebral bodies.
  - Symmetric, bamboo-like syndesmophytes between vertebral bodies.
- **Labs:**
  - HLA-B27 is ⊕ in the majority of cases but is **not diagnostic** (seen in 8% of the normal Caucasian population).
  - ↑ ESR and ⊖ RF.

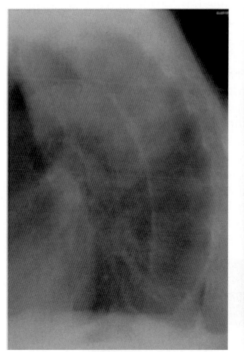 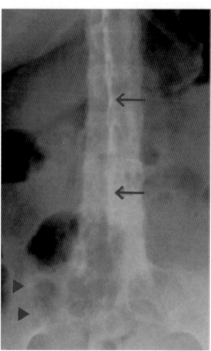

A   B

FIGURE 17.10. **Ankylosing spondylitis.** (**A**) Cropped image from a lateral CXR shows the characteristic "bamboo spine," with squared vertebral bodies and thin syndesmophytes bridging the entire thoracic spine. (**B**) AP radiograph of the lumbar spine in a different patient also demonstrates thin symmetric syndesmophytes bridging the lumbar spine, as well as ossification of the interspinous/supraspinous ligaments ("dagger sign," arrows) and sclerosis and near-fusion of the right sacroiliac joint (arrowhead). The left sacroiliac joint is not well visualized here but typically is symmetrically involved in ankylosing spondylitis. (Image A reproduced with permission from USMLERx.com. Image B reproduced with permission from Chen MY et al. *Basic Radiology.* New York: McGraw-Hill, 2004, Fig. 7-45.)

TREATMENT

- NSAIDs.
- Sulfasalazine or methotrexate for peripheral arthritis.
- TNF-α antagonists.
- Aggressive **physical therapy** to enable spinal fusion in an advantageous position.

COMPLICATIONS

All of the following are classic associations:

- Anterior uveitis.
- Aortitis and aortic regurgitation (more rarely, cardiac conduction system involvement).
- Apical pulmonary fibrosis (mimics TB—be careful!).
- Pseudoarthroses can occur when a fused spine is severed in a traumatic accident, which can cause spinal cord compromise.

KEY FACT

Before initiating TNF inhibitor medication, always place a PPD to screen for active or latent TB.

KEY FACT

Apical pulmonary fibrosis in ankylosing spondylitis can look like TB.

PSORIATIC ARTHRITIS

A 55-year-old man with a three-year history of psoriatic arthritis presents with worsening symptoms. He has been on oral methotrexate 20 mg weekly with some improvement after an unsuccessful trial of naproxen, but over the past year he has had worsening functional capacity with new areas of joint inflammation and stiffness together with cutaneous psoriasis on the back, arms, legs, and buttocks. Exam reveals swelling, erythema, and tenderness over the PIPs and DIPs of both hands as well as the wrists; dactylitis of the toes; and bilateral knee effusions. The patient also has lower lumbar and sacroiliac tenderness and limited range of motion of the torso, and he finds it difficult to turn his head without turning his body. What is the next best treatment for this patient?

Add an anti-TNF agent. This patient has severe, active, destructive psoriatic arthritis that is unresponsive to full-dose methotrexate and NSAIDs. Anti-TNF therapy produces excellent clinical responses for the spinal inflammation of psoriatic arthritis and ankylosing spondylitis.

Peripheral arthritis, dactylitis, and enthesitis (inflammation of the tendinous insertions of the joints; seen with other HLA-B27-related diseases as well). Found in 15–20% of patients with psoriatic skin disease. Skin disease precedes arthritis in 80% of cases.

SYMPTOMS/EXAM

The clinical presentation of psoriatic arthritis is further outlined in Table 17.9.

TABLE 17.9. Five Major Patterns in Psoriatic Arthritis

Pattern	Joint Involvement
DIP involvement	Can be monoarticular or asymmetric; nail pitting and onycholysis (see Figure 17.11).
Pseudorheumatoid	Symmetric, smaller-joint polyarthritis.
Oligoarticular	Erosive arthritis, dactylitis ("sausage digit").
Arthritis mutilans	Severe, osteolytic, deforming (telescoping digits).
Spondylitis	Sacroiliitis and/or ankylosing spondylitis.

DIAGNOSIS

- Characteristic presentation.
- Radiographic findings include the following:
    - Marginal erosions of bone.
    - "Sausage digits" (diffuse soft tissue swelling of the entire digit).
    - Characteristic "pencil-in-cup" deformities of distal digits (see Figure 17.12).
    - Periosteal bone formations and calcifications of entheses.
    - Sacroiliitis and spondylitic changes of the spine (frequently asymmetric).

TREATMENT

- NSAIDs; methotrexate, sulfasalazine, and other DMARDs for peripheral arthritis; TNF-α inhibitors.
- **Avoid corticosteroids if possible** (tapering can cause skin disease to flare).

KEY FACT

Psoriasis precedes most cases of psoriatic arthritis.

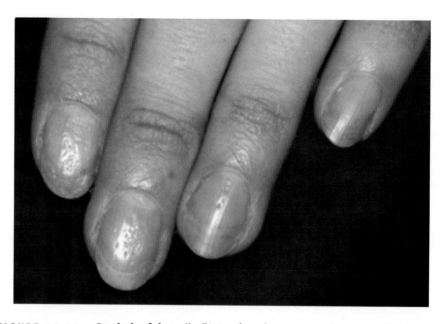

FIGURE 17.11. Psoriasis of the nails. Pitting describes punctate depressions. The brownish to salmon discolorations of the nails of the fourth and fifth digits represent "oil stains." (Reproduced with permission from Wolff K, Johnson RA. *Fitzpatrick's Color Atlas & Synopsis of Clinical Dermatology,* 6th ed. New York: McGraw-Hill, 2009, Fig. 3e-PS-50.)

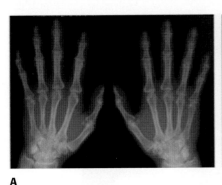 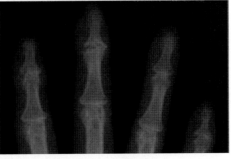

A   **B**

FIGURE 17.12. **Psoriatic arthritis, DIP predominant.** (A) AP radiograph of the hands shows periarticular erosions involving the PIP and DIP joints with sparing of the carpal and carpometacarpal joints and absence of periarticular osteopenia. (B) Magnified, cropped view of the interphalangeal joints of the right hand better demonstrates the joint space narrowing and marginal erosions that predominate in the DIP joints but also affect the PIP joints. (Reproduced with permission from USMLERx.com.)

REACTIVE ARTHRITIS

An 18-year-old boy presents with three months of fatigue together with swelling and pain in the ankles and knees. He had an episode of gastro-enteritis about one month ago and has had two episodes of anterior uveitis in the past year. On exam, his right knee is warm and tender with an effusion, and both ankles are swollen and warm with pain on ankle motion, particularly with stretching of the Achilles tendon or palpation of the posterior heel. Hepatitis serologies and RF are ⊖, but ESR is 70 mm/hr. What is the most likely diagnosis?

Reactive arthritis, which is characterized by large joint oligoarthritis (≤ 4 joints), enthesitis involving tendon insertion sites, and extra-articular manifestations, including uveitis. It is triggered by infections in the intestines, the urogenital tract, and, less commonly, the throat or respiratory tract.

Males (particularly young men) are affected more often than females. Eighty percent of Caucasian and 50–60% of African American patients are HLA-B27 ⊕. May be idiopathic or may develop within days to weeks of antecedent infection:

- **GI disease:** *Salmonella, Shigella, Campylobacter, Yersinia.*
- **GU disease (urethritis):** *Chlamydia.*

SYMPTOMS/EXAM

- Presents with frequently asymmetric involvement of larger, weight-bearing joints.
- Spinal involvement is seen in 20% of patients.
- Conjunctivitis, urethritis, cervicitis, and mucocutaneous ulcerations are seen, as is keratoderma blennorrhagicum (pustular eruptions on the palms and soles; see Figure 17.13).
- Systemic signs (fever, weight loss) are not unusual.

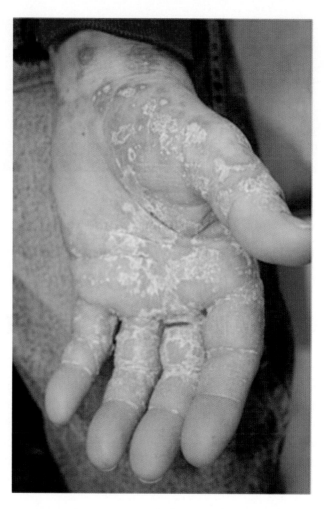

FIGURE 17.13. Keratoderma blennorrhagicum in reactive arthritis. Hyperkeratotic scaled erythematous plaques of the hand of a 33-year-old man with eye irritation, joint pain, and a recent history of diarrhea. (Reproduced with permission from USMLERx.com.)

DIFFERENTIAL

Septic and gonococcal arthritis, crystal-induced arthritis, seronegative RA, other seronegative spondyloarthropathies.

DIAGNOSIS

- An inflammatory pattern is seen on arthrocentesis.
- Culture of affected joints is sterile.
- Test for chlamydia if the history or exam is suggestive.

TREATMENT

- NSAIDs; antibiotics for chlamydia-related reactive arthritis.
- Sulfasalazine, methotrexate, and other DMARDs can be given for recalcitrant peripheral arthritis.

COMPLICATIONS

Aortitis and aortic regurgitation (rare).

INFLAMMATORY BOWEL DISEASE (IBD)–ASSOCIATED ARTHRITIS

Twenty percent of patients with IBD have associated arthritis. Associated more often with Crohn's disease than with ulcerative colitis. Arthritis usually appears after the onset of GI disease.

SYMPTOMS/EXAM

- **Peripheral arthritis, enthesitis, and dactylitis:**
  - Asymmetric, oligoarticular.
  - Large joint involvement.
  - Frequently nonerosive.
  - Flares in concert with intestinal disease.
- **Spinal arthritis:**
  - Symmetric inflammatory sacroiliitis and spondylitis.
  - Mimics ankylosing spondylitis.
  - The course of the disease is independent of intestinal disease.

DIFFERENTIAL

Ankylosing spondylitis, enteropathic reactive arthritis, Whipple's disease, sero-negative RA.

TREATMENT

NSAIDs; treatment of intestinal disease (controls peripheral arthritis).

Crystalline-Induced Arthropathies

Include gout, pseudogout, and calcium pyrophosphate dihydrate deposition disease.

KEY FACT

Asymptomatic hyperuricemia does not need to be treated. The majority of patients with hyperuricemia do not develop gout.

HYPERURICEMIA

The causes of hyperuricemia and its relation to gout are delineated in Table 17.10.

TABLE 17.10. Causes of Hyperuricemia

OVERPRODUCTION OF URIC ACID (< 10%)	UNDEREXCRETION OF URIC ACID (> 90%)
Genetic metabolic defects:	Idiopathic
Lesch-Nyhan syndrome	CKD
Glycogen storage diseases	Medication induced:
Psoriasis	Thiazide diuretics
Myeloproliferative disorders/large tumor	Loop diuretics
burden malignancies	Cyclosporine
Idiopathic	Metabolic:
	Lactic acidosis
	Alcoholism
	Ketoacidosis
	Lead nephropathy (saturnine gout)

GOUT

> A 60-year-old man with hypertension and gout presents with his third episode of disabling left knee pain in the past year. He is on HCTZ and lisinopril for hypertension and does not drink alcohol. His labs show a normal CBC and a uric acid level of 10.4 mg/dL, and arthrocentesis of the left knee reveals urate crystals. His gout is treated successfully with intra-articular corticosteroids, and low-dose colchicine therapy is started to prevent future attacks. What is the most appropriate next step in the management of his gout?
>
> Given this patient's frequent and severe attacks of gout and hyperuricemia, it would be reasonable to start allopurinol with a target uric acid level of ≤ 6 mg/dL, checking levels every 3–4 weeks after a change in dose. He will be at risk for more frequent gouty attacks during the first few months of treatment as uric acid levels change, so low-dose colchicine prophylaxis is indicated unless the patient has severe kidney disease. Colchicine may be discontinued if tophi resolve, uric acid levels stabilize, and the patient has no gout attacks for six months. Allopurinol is equally effective in the setting of inefficient excretion or overproduction of urate.

Usually associated with abnormal uric acid metabolism and hyperuricemia; can be associated with uric acid stones and urate nephropathy (renal toxicity). Males are affected more often than females (9:1). Onset is generally after age 30; almost always **postmenopausal** in women.

Symptoms

- Presents with sudden-onset, self-limited, recurrent, acute mono- or oligoarticular arthritis.
- Can progress to chronic deforming polyarthritis after multiple attacks.
- Additional features are as follows:
  - **Tophi:** Deposits of uric acid crystals in joints, bone, tendon, cartilage, and subcutaneous tissues.
  - **Podagra:** Refers to gout of the first MTP, the most commonly affected joint (see Figure 17.14).
  - Other affected joints include the knees, ankles, feet, elbows, and hands.
- Asymptomatic periods (**intercritical periods**) can last months or years.

Exam

- Exam reveals erythema, swelling, warmth, and tenderness to palpation of affected joints.
- Cellulitis-like erythema of overlying skin and soft tissue is also seen.
- Classically exhibits a monoarticular presentation, but can be oligoarticular or polyarticular in long-standing disease.
- Look for the presence of **tophi** on the external ears, elbows, hands, and feet (see Figure 17.15).
- Fever is common but rarely exceeds 39°C (102.2°F).

Differential

Cellulitis, septic arthritis, pseudogout, reactive arthritis, RA, lead poisoning.

KEY FACT

Gout and hyperuricemia are strongly associated with metabolic syndrome, hypertension, thiazide diuretic use, alcohol abuse, CAD, and CKD.

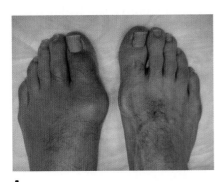

A

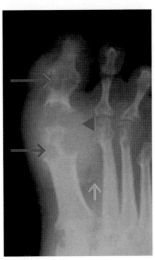

B

FIGURE 17.14. **Gout.** (A) Swollen left first MTP joint with overlying erythema and warmth, characteristic of an acute gout attack of the first MTP (podagra). (B) AP radiograph showing the severe consequences of long-standing gout, including large, nonmarginal erosions with overhanging edges of bone (red arrows), soft tissue swelling, and destruction of the first MTP joint (arrowhead). Note the subtle calcification of a gouty tophus (orange arrow). (Image A reproduced with permission from LeBlond RF et al. *DeGowin's Diagnostic Examination,* 9th ed. New York: McGraw-Hill, 2009, Plate 30. Image B reproduced with permission from USMLERx.com.)

Diagnosis

- Uric acid is abnormally ↑ at some point in 95% of cases, but **this is not diagnostic, does not correlate with disease activity, and is not needed to make a diagnosis.**

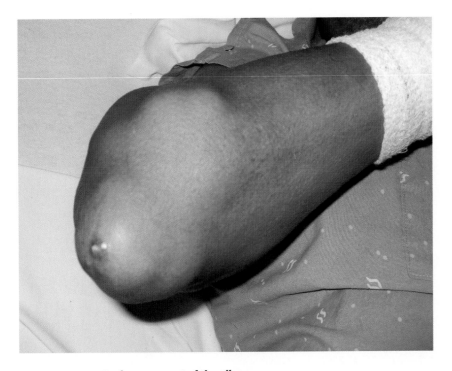

FIGURE 17.15. **Tophaceous gout of the elbow.**

- Synovial fluid aspiration reveals the following:
  - An inflammatory pattern.
  - Sterile cultures.
  - Negatively birefringent, needle-like crystals (the crystals are yellow under polarized light, when the red compensator is pointed in parallel to the crystals (think **yeLLow = paraLLel;** see Figure 17.16). Radiographs of chronic tophi show "rat-bite" erosions adjacent to affected joints (see Figure 17.17).
- Measure urinary uric acid excretion to distinguish underexcreters from overproducers of uric acid (< 600–800 mg/day = underexcretion).

TREATMENT

Guidelines for the treatment of gout are outlined in Table 17.11.

COMPLICATIONS

Complications associated with treatment are as follows:

- **Allopurinol:**
  - An acute gouty attack may occur if allopurinol is used without a concomitant NSAID, colchicine, or corticosteroid.
  - Hypersensitivity syndrome may also be seen (↑ in renal disease and ↑ serum metabolite levels).
  - Fever, desquamating rash, hepatitis, vasculitis.
  - Allopurinol ↑ the effect and toxicity of azathioprine by blocking its metabolism.
- **Probenecid:**
  - Hypersensitivity.
  - Loss of efficacy in patients with advanced renal disease.
  - Precipitates urate nephropathy and nephrolithiasis if used in tophaceous gout or in patients with a history of urate calculi.

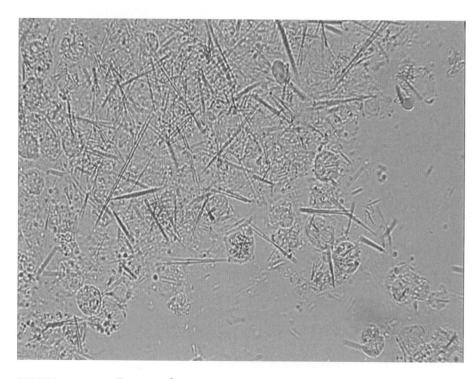

FIGURE 17.16.   Gout crystals.

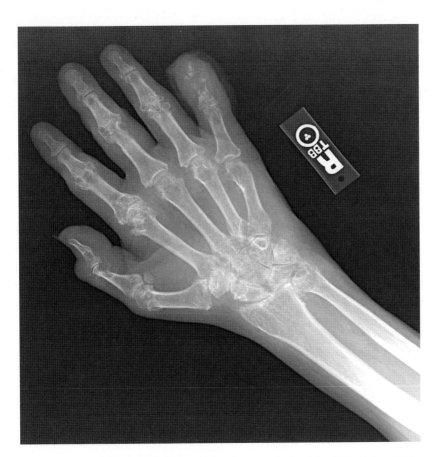

FIGURE 17.17. Radiograph of the hand showing osteolysis of the fifth digit and PIP, MCP, and carpal erosions 2° to tophaceous gout.

TABLE 17.11. Treatment of Gout

DRUG	USAGE
Acute attack:	
NSAIDs (indomethacin)	Use until symptoms resolve (1–2 weeks, 50–75 mg TID).
Colchicine	Use within 48 hours of onset of attack (0.6 mg/hr until resolution of toxicity).
Corticosteroids	Oral steroids in NSAID-intolerant patients; intra-articular injections for monoarticular disease.
After attack:	
Nothing	Many patients experience few if any future attacks and choose to discontinue uric acid therapy.
Diet	Low purine (at best, can lower uric acid 1 mg/dL); alcohol avoidance.
Medication management	Discontinue precipitating medications (eg, thiazides, low-dose salicylates, niacin).
Colchicine	Give 0.6 mg QD BID to prevent future attacks; give 0.6 mg/day × 1–2 weeks while initiating uric acid–lowering therapies.
Allopurinol (xanthine oxidase inhibitor)	Best for uric acid overproducers, tophaceous gout, and urate nephropathy. The usual dose is 300 mg/day; ↓ the initial starting dose if the patient has ↓ creatinine clearance.
Febuxostat	Uric acid–lowering agent; use if the patient cannot tolerate allopurinol.
Probenecid	Best for uric acid underexcreters (promotes uricosuria). Give 500 mg/day (starting) to 2 g/day.

CALCIUM PYROPHOSPHATE DIHYDRATE DEPOSITION DISEASE (CPPD)

 A 68-year-old man with hyperparathyroidism presents with worsening left knee pain and swelling of one week's duration; these episodes have been occurring intermittently for the past four years and usually last several days. Between attacks, he experiences knee stiffness and discomfort. On exam, he is found to have synovitis of the left knee and a suprapatellar joint effusion, and his knee is tender. An x-ray of the knee shows linear deposits of calcium in the articular space and marked joint space narrowing. What is the most likely diagnosis?

CPPD as demonstrated by chondrocalcinosis of the fibrocartilage of the knee, joint space narrowing, and the episodic nature of the attacks. Arthrocentesis would show calcium pyrophosphate crystals. CPPD can be mono- or oligoarticular and can affect the fibrocartilage of the knee, symphysis pubis, glenoid and acetabular labra, and wrist as well as the elbow and MCP (ie, atypical distribution of osteoarthritis).

Arthritis associated with CPPD crystal deposition may be hereditary or associated with metabolic disease, or it may be 2° to aging. Four percent of the adult population are found to have articular CPPD deposits at the time of death, and by the ninth decade nearly half of the population have been found to have chondrocalcinosis.

SYMPTOMS/EXAM

There are three patterns of CPPD disease:

- **Pseudo-osteoarthritis (pseudo-OA) pattern:**
  - Accounts for 50% of symptomatic CPPD patients.
  - The knee is most commonly affected.
- **Pseudogout pattern:**
  - Accounts for roughly 25% of CPPD cases.
  - Acute pseudogout is marked by inflammation in one or more joints that lasts for several days to two weeks.
  - Fifty percent of attacks affect the knee.
  - Differentiation from gout or infection may be difficult and requires arthrocentesis.

> **KEY FACT**
>
> Accelerated or unusual distribution of degenerative joint disease should raise suspicion for CPPD.

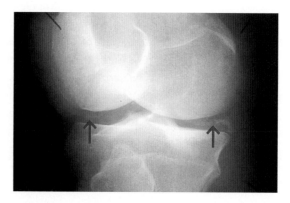

FIGURE 17.18. **Chondrocalcinosis.** Deposition of calcium pyrophosphate (chondrocalcinosis) in the medial and lateral menisci (arrows). (Reproduced with permission from Imboden JB et al. *Current Rheumatology Diagnosis & Treatment,* 2nd ed. New York: McGraw-Hill, 2007, Fig. 46-2.)

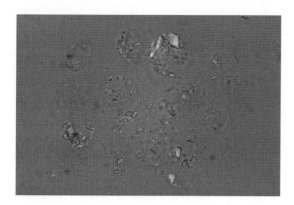

FIGURE 17.19. **Pseudogout.** Positively birefringent calcium pyrophosphate dihydrate crystals from a joint aspirate. (Reproduced with permission from Imboden JB et al. *Current Rheumatology Diagnosis & Treatment,* 2nd ed. New York: McGraw-Hill, 2007, Fig. 46-1.)

- **Pseudo-RA pattern:**
  - Five percent of patients with CPPD have multiple joint involvement resembling RA.
  - The presence of RF or anti-CCP antibodies favors the diagnosis of true RA over CPPD.

DIAGNOSIS

- Serum urate level is normal.
- **Chondrocalcinosis** is visualized on radiographs of the knees and wrists (see Figure 17.18).
- Synovial fluid aspiration reveals the following:
  - An inflammatory fluid profile in acute attacks.
  - Weakly positively birefringent **rhomboid-shaped crystals** (the opposite of urate; see Figure 17.19).

TREATMENT

- There are no drugs that ↓ CPPD crystal formation except treatment of the underlying etiology.
- NSAIDs and intra-articular injection of corticosteroids are used to treat inflammation; colchicine is used for chronic chemoprevention.

Inflammatory Myopathies

Presumed autoimmune diseases of skeletal muscles. Major types are **polymyositis, dermatomyositis, and inclusion body myositis,** each of which has distinctive patterns of muscle weakness, associated symptoms, and muscle pathology. May be confused with polymyalgia rheumatica. Table 17.12 outlines the clinical characteristics of various inflammatory myopathies.

KEY FACT

CPPD as part of underlying metabolic disorders:
- Hemochromatosis
- Hypophosphatemia
- Hypomagnesemia
- Hyperparathyroidism
- Hypothyroidism
- Diabetes

KEY FACT

Colchicine toxicity can cause GI intolerance, bone marrow suppression, alopecia, and severe myopathy, all of which are potentially reversible by stopping the drug. The risk is ↑ in renal insufficiency and with concomitant use of macrolides and statins.

TABLE 17.12.   **Characteristics of Inflammatory Myopathies and Polymyalgia Rheumatica**

	POLYMYOSITIS	**DERMATOMYOSITIS**	**INCLUSION BODY MYOSITIS**	**POLYMYALGIA RHEUMATICA**
Age at onset	30–50.	40–60.	> 60.	> 50.
Gender	Women >> men.	Women >> men.	**Men** >> women.	Women > men.
Key features	Proximal muscle weakness **without skin findings.**	Proximal muscle weakness and skin findings: Gottron's papules, heliotrope rash, "mechanic hands."	Insidious onset with prominent wasting of the **finger and forearm flexors and quadriceps.**	Proximal shoulder and pelvic muscle **pain without weakness.**
CK	Elevated.	Elevated.	**Normal.**	**Normal.**
Response to steroids	Good.	Good.	**Poor.**	**Excellent.**
Comments	Biopsy distinguishes polymyositis from dermatomyositis.	Strongest association with **underlying malignancy.**	Most patients lose the ability to walk within 10 years of diagnosis.	Look for signs of giant cell arteritis.

POLYMYOSITIS

A 55-year-old woman presents with four months of generalized weakness, especially when she climbs stairs, reaches for things overhead, and combs her hair. She also has myalgias and dyspnea on exertion. She is on prednisone and methotrexate for RA. Exam reveals proximal muscle weakness and neck flexor weakness. Her CK level is 5000 U/L, and a needle EMG shows diffuse spontaneous fibrillations associated with myopathic motor unit potentials, repetitive discharges, and positive sharp waves. What is the most likely diagnosis?

Polymyositis with characteristic findings; respiratory symptoms may be related to an associated ILD. This inflammatory myopathy is autoimmune and can coexist with other autoimmune disorders. Steroid myopathy would have normal CK levels and a normal EMG but similar weakness.

Targets the proximal musculature, typically in women 40–60 years of age. May have a mild association with malignancy.

SYMPTOMS/EXAM

- Presents with progressive muscle weakness of the neck and upper and lower extremities.
- **Weakness** is more common than **pain.**
- **Proximal muscles are affected more than distal muscles.**
- Patients may have difficulty swallowing.

DIFFERENTIAL

- Inclusion body myositis (**distal muscles are affected more than proximal muscles**).
- Polymyalgia rheumatica (**pain** is more common than weakness).
- Myositis 2° to other autoimmune diseases.
- Myositis 2° to malignancy.
- Medication-related myopathies (steroid, statin, colchicine).
- Toxin- or endocrine/metabolic-related myopathy.
- Myasthenia gravis.
- Genetic myopathies.

DIAGNOSIS

- Requires supportive clinical features, ↑ muscle enzymes, and consistent muscle biopsy.
- Look for elevated markers of muscle enzymes (CK and/or aldolase) for both diagnosis and disease follow-up.
- MRI is the best imaging modality for identifying muscle edema and localizing a site for muscle biopsy. It does not establish a diagnosis of polymyositis by itself.
- EMG is nonspecific and shows abnormal polyphasic potentials, fibrillations, and high-frequency action potentials.
- Biopsy of affected muscle shows endomysial lymphocytic inflammatory infiltrate.

TREATMENT

- Corticosteroids (0.5–1.0 mg/kg/day).
- DMARDs (methotrexate, azathioprine) for steroid sparing or recalcitrant disease.

COMPLICATIONS

- **Antisynthetase syndrome:** ILD, Raynaud's phenomenon, arthritis (associated with **anti-Jo-1 antibodies**).
- **Other:** Myocarditis, respiratory muscle failure, swallowing difficulties and aspiration.

DERMATOMYOSITIS

Often associated with occult malignancy. Amyopathic dermatomyositis is a variant with a characteristic skin disease but no clinically apparent muscle involvement.

SYMPTOMS/EXAM

- Symptoms are similar to those of polymyositis.
- Additional features are as follows:
  - **Gottron's papules:** A scaly rash over the extensor surfaces (see Figure 17.20).
  - **Shawl sign:** Erythema in a sun-exposed V-neck or shoulder distribution (see Figure 17.21).
  - **Heliotrope rash:** A violaceous rash over the eyelids, sometimes with periorbital edema.
  - **Facial erythema:** A diffuse, dusky rash.
  - **Mechanic hands:** Dystrophic cuticles of the hands.
  - **Other:** Periungual erythema and dilated periungual capillaries.

KEY FACT

The risk of malignancy is ↑ in dermatomyositis, polymyositis, and inclusion body myositis, but of these the highest risk is associated with dermatomyositis. The malignancy may occur several years before or after myositis. Patients require aggressive screening for malignancy, including the consideration of abdominal and pelvic imaging in females.

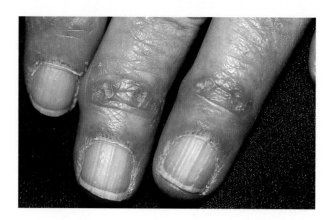

FIGURE 17.20. **Gottron's papules, nail fold telangiectasias, and dystrophic cuticles in dermatomyositis.** (Reproduced with permission from Wolff K et al. *Fitzpatrick's Dermatology in General Medicine,* 7th ed. New York: McGraw-Hill, 2008, Fig. 157-5.)

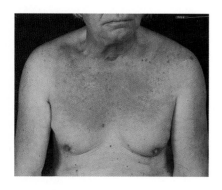

FIGURE 17.21. **Dermatomyositis.** The confluent, macular, violaceous erythema of the "V" area of the upper chest and neck ("V sign"), when persistent over time, can evolve into poikilodermatous skin changes. (Reproduced with permission from Wolff K et al. *Fitzpatrick's Dermatology in General Medicine,* 7th ed. New York: McGraw-Hill, 2008, Fig. 157-6.)

DIAGNOSIS

- Similar to polymyositis.
- Muscle biopsy shows perivascular and perifascicular lymphocytic inflammatory infiltrate with destruction of microvasculature.

TREATMENT

- Similar to that of polymyositis.
- IVIG for refractory cases.
- Age-appropriate and symptom-directed cancer screening. Consider screening women for ovarian cancer with pelvic ultrasound and/or CA-125 level.
- Treat underlying malignancy (if present).

INCLUSION BODY MYOSITIS

- Characterized by distal more than proximal muscle weakness; weakness is more often asymmetric than symmetric. Older Caucasian males are more frequently affected.
- More insidious in onset than polymyositis or dermatomyositis.
- **Dx:** CK levels may be normal or ↑. Characteristic inclusion bodies (intranuclear and cytoplasmic) are seen on muscle biopsy.
- **Tx:** "Treatment resistant" compared to other inflammatory myopathies.

KEY FACT

Inclusion body myositis involves asymmetric weakness of distal more than proximal muscles and is seen more often in men than in women.

Other Myopathies

METABOLIC MYOPATHIES

A 25-year-old Asian man is brought by friends to the ER because of sudden profound weakness and inability to get out of bed. The patient felt normal earlier in the day, has no medical conditions, and takes no medications or illicit substances. He had eaten a large bowl of pasta several hours before symptom onset. On further questioning, he describes a 10-pound weight loss over three weeks along with palpitations. His heart rate is 120 bpm, and he is unable to lift his limbs. Labs reveal a serum potassium level of 1.8 mEq/L. What diagnosis do you suspect, and what other lab test would you order?

Periodic paralysis is suggested by the patient's low potassium and sudden weakness following the ingestion of a high-carbohydrate meal. It is associated with hyperthyroidism, so a TSH level would be indicated. The prognosis is generally benign. Multiple endocrine abnormalities are associated with myopathies; CK is often normal, and EMG shows nonspecific myopathic changes.

Hyperthyroidism, hypothyroidism, and glucocorticoid excess, whether endogenous (eg, Cushing's) or exogenous (eg, steroid treatment), may all produce myopathy.

DRUG-INDUCED AND TOXIC MYOPATHIES

 A 30-year-old woman with dermatomyositis diagnosed two years ago presents with six months of progressive lower extremity muscle weakness. The patient had initially been treated with high-dose prednisone, which had improved her rash, strength, and CK levels, and had continued on prednisone 20 mg/day. On exam, she is found to have proximal thigh and hip muscle weakness but no rashes. Her CK level is 150 U/L. What is the most likely cause of her recurrent weakness?

Corticosteroid-induced myopathy, which is characterized by continued or worsening proximal muscle weakness, particularly in the lower extremities, after a ↓ in or normalization of muscle enzyme levels. Muscle wasting and upper extremity involvement may be seen, but there is usually no tenderness.

Many medications are associated with toxic myopathies, and the condition is usually reversible upon withdrawal of the offending toxin. Common offending medications include **statins,** cimetidine, penicillamine, chloroquine, niacin, corticosteroids, and zidovudine (AZT). Other toxins associated with myopathy include alcohol and heroin.

Systemic Sclerosis (Scleroderma)

The clinical characteristics of systemic sclerosis are outlined below and in Table 17.13.

TABLE 17.13. **Characteristics of Systemic Sclerosis**

DISEASE TYPE	FREQUENCY OF CASES	ORGANS INVOLVED	ANTIBODIES
Limited scleroderma	80%	CREST, pulmonary hypertension	ANA, anticentromere
Progressive systemic sclerosis	20%	Proximal skin, kidney, heart, lung, GI tract	ANA, anti-SCL-70

> **KEY FACT**
>
> Hypothyroid myopathy is characterized by muscle pain, cramps, stiffness, fatigue, paresthesias, and a delay in the relaxation phase of the muscle stretch reflex. CK levels may be 10–100 times normal. Check TSH before EMG or muscle biopsy.

> **KEY FACT**
>
> Many patients taking statins develop nonspecific myalgias and muscle weakness. Rhabdomyolysis occurs in < 1% of patients taking these meds. Concomitant use of fibrates or cyclosporine, or kidney disease, ↑ the risk of statin myopathy.

> **KEY FACT**
>
> There is no disease-modifying treatment for scleroderma. Therapy for scleroderma involves systematic management of end-organ involvement.

LIMITED SCLERODERMA

A 60-year-old woman with a 15-year history of limited cutaneous systemic sclerosis presents with abdominal pain, bloating, large-volume watery diarrhea for a week preceded by a week of constipation, and episodes of fecal incontinence. She is on nifedipine for Raynaud's phenomenon and omeprazole for GERD. She has not taken any antibiotics recently, nor has she traveled or had contact with anyone having similar symptoms. On exam, she is found to be mildly orthostatic and has sclerodactyly with digital pitting. She also has hyperactive bowel sounds, distention, and diffuse abdominal tenderness but no rebound or guarding. CBC, chemistry, and upright AXRs are all normal. What is the most appropriate next step in this patient's management?

A course of oral ciprofloxacin (for 7–10 days) for small bowel bacterial growth from GI dysmotility. In scleroderma, smooth muscle disease may lead to chronic intestinal pseudo-obstruction of the small bowel. Coverage for gram-$\ominus$ rods and anaerobes is indicated. Opioid antidiarrheal therapy such as loperamide is not indicated for patients with scleroderma because it may worsen intestinal motility disorders.

SYMPTOMS/EXAM

- Characterized primarily by **CREST** syndrome: **C**alcinosis, **R**aynaud's phenomenon, **E**sophageal dysmotility, **S**clerodactyly (sclerodermatous skin changes confined to the upper extremity distal to the wrist), and **T**elangiectasias.
- Lung disease tends to be pulmonary hypertension.
- Also presents with arthralgia and arthritis, fever and malaise, abnormal periungual capillary dropout or dilatation, digital ulcerations, and tapering of the distal digits.

TREATMENT

Treatment is outlined in Table 17.14.

COMPLICATIONS

The prognosis is generally more favorable than that of diffuse scleroderma, but later-onset pulmonary hypertension and other vasculopathic processes affect mortality.

TABLE 17.14. Symptomatic Treatment of Limited Scleroderma

DISORDER	TREATMENT
Raynaud's phenomenon	Body-warming techniques, calcium channel blockers (CCBs).
Digital ulcerations	Raynaud's therapies as above; ASA, sildenafil, topical nitrates, prostacyclin analogs.
Esophageal dysmotility	Elevate the head of the bed and avoid late-night meals; H_2 blockers or PPIs.
Pulmonary hypertension	O_2, CCBs, sildenafil, prostacyclin analogs, endothelin receptor antagonists.

PROGRESSIVE (DIFFUSE) SYSTEMIC SCLEROSIS

A 40-year-old woman presents with two weeks of worsening headaches. Over the past year she was diagnosed with scleroderma after having developed Raynaud's phenomenon, GERD, and skin thickening. Her BP is 170/95 mm Hg, whereas at a prior visit it was normal. She also has digital pitting and skin thickening of the face, trunk, and extremities; flexion contractures of the PIPs and elbows; and 2+ lower extremity edema. Labs are as follows: hemoglobin 9 g/dL, platelets 100,000/μL, and creatinine 2 mg/dL. What is the most appropriate next step in this patient's management?

Admit her to the hospital and start a short-acting ACEI such as captopril for scleroderma renal crisis. This condition requires aggressive BP control starting with an ACEI even if creatinine is increasing, or the patient will require hemodialysis. In scleroderma patients, moderate- or high-dose corticosteroids may be associated with a normotensive renal crisis, microangiopathic hemolytic anemia, and thrombocytopenia. Low doses can be used as second-line treatment for associated inflammatory arthritis.

SYMPTOMS/EXAM

- Presents with skin involvement **proximal to the wrists,** including the arms, chest, and face (see Figures 17.22 and 17.23).

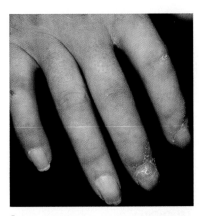

A

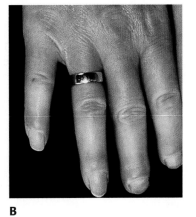

B

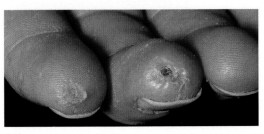

C

FIGURE 17.22. **Scleroderma of the hand.** (**A**) Sclerodactyly. The hands and fingers are edematous (nonpitting); the skin is without skin folds and taut. The distal fingers are tapered ("madonna fingers"). (**B**) **Raynaud's phenomenon.** The fingers show both bluish erythema and vasoconstriction (blue and white). The distal phalanges (index and third finger) are shortened, a characteristic that is associated with bony resorption. (**C**) **Acrosclerosis.** Typical "rat bite" necroses and ulcerations of the fingertips are seen. (Reproduced with permission from Wolff K, Johnson RA. *Fitzpatrick's Color Atlas & Synopsis of Clinical Dermatology,* 6th ed. New York: McGraw-Hill, 2009, Figs. 14-28 and 14-29A.)

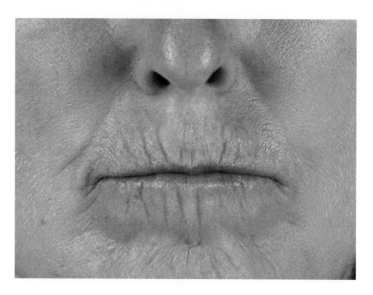

FIGURE 17.23. Facial features in scleroderma. Note the thinning of the lips, or microstomia (which is more evident when patients attempt to open the mouth), along with radial perioral furrowing. Also note the sharp, beaklike nose. (Reproduced with permission from Wolff K, Johnson RA. *Fitzpatrick's Color Atlas & Synopsis of Clinical Dermatology,* 6th ed. New York: McGraw-Hill, 2009, Fig.14-29B.)

- Also characterized by the following:
  - Tendon friction rubs.
  - Early **scleredema** (soft tissue swelling of affected joints).
  - Lung disease tends to be interstitial lung disease.
  - Features of CREST.

DIFFERENTIAL

Morphea and linear scleroderma (characteristic localized skin disease), limited scleroderma, scleromyxedema, eosinophilic fasciitis, eosinophilia-myalgia syndrome.

TREATMENT

Treatment is outlined in Table 17.15.

KEY FACT

Lung disease is the most common cause of morbidity and mortality in systemic sclerosis. Pulmonary hypertension and ILD can occur independently or together.

TABLE 17.15. Symptomatic Treatment of Diffuse Scleroderma

ORGAN	COMPLICATIONS	TREATMENT
Kidney	Renal crisis (malignant hypertension, renal failure, and microangiopathic hemolytic anemia).	ACEIs.
Lung	Interstitial pneumonitis, interstitial fibrosis.	Corticosteroids,[a] cytotoxic (eg, cyclophosphamide) and immunosuppressant therapies.
Heart	Myocarditis, myocardial fibrosis, heart failure, pericardial effusions, conduction system disease.	Corticosteroids,[a] immunosuppressants, CHF therapy, pacemakers.
GI	Delayed gastric emptying, intestinal malabsorption, bacterial overgrowth.	Frequent small meals, promotility agents, antibiotics.

[a]Corticosteroids are usually avoided in scleroderma (unless severe organ-related disease leaves little other choice) because they may precipitate a renal crisis.

Vasculitis

APPROACH TO VASCULITIS

Vasculitis can be classified as either 1° or 2°. Figure 17.24 categorizes 1° vasculitis according to vessel size. 2° causes of vasculitis are as follows:

- **Infections:** Particularly indolent, chronic infections such as subacute bacterial endocarditis and HCV.
- **Medications:** Hypersensitivity vasculitis, leukocytoclastic vasculitis, ANCA-associated vasculitis.
- **Other:** Collagen vascular disease, malignancy.

1° VASCULITIS SYNDROMES

Wegener's Granulomatosis

A 30-year-old man presents with two months of epistaxis, intermittent night sweats, cough, and a 10-pound weight loss without any recent travel. Exam reveals a large perforation of the nasal septum. UA reveals 3+ protein, erythrocytes, and erythrocyte casts, and a CT of the chest shows bilateral cavitary nodules. What is the most likely diagnosis?

Wegener's granulomatosis, which is characterized by a necrotizing granulomatous vasculitis that particularly affects the upper and lower respiratory tract (lower lobe cavitary nodules) and kidneys (glomerulonephritis). Ground-glass opacities may be seen on chest imaging. Nasal and sinus mucosal inflammation may cause cartilaginous ischemia with perforation of the nasal septum and/or saddle-nose deformity. A ⊕ c-ANCA (anti–proteinase 3) is highly associated with Wegener's.

A necrotizing **granulomatous** arteritis of small- to medium-sized arteries, arterioles, and capillaries. Characterized by cavitating **nodules of the upper and lower respiratory tract (lungs and sinuses)** and by **glomerulonephritis.** Organs and systems affected include the upper and lower respiratory tract, kidney, eye, ear, nerve, skin, gingiva, and joints.

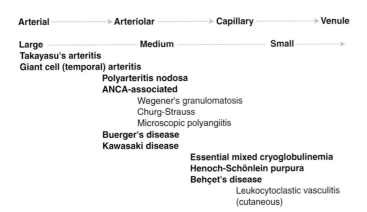

FIGURE 17.24.   **Classification of 1° vasculitis according to size of vessel involved.**

Symptoms/Exam

- Fever, malaise, weight loss.
- Sinusitis, epistaxis, otitis media, gingivitis, stridor, mastoiditis.
- Cough, hemoptysis, dyspnea.
- Arthritis, scleritis, neuropathy, skin rashes, hematuria.

Diagnosis

- **Labs:**
  - ↑ ESR; normal serum complement levels.
  - ⊕ **c-ANCA** (anti–proteinase 3) more than p-ANCA (antimyeloperoxidase).
- **Imaging:** CXR and chest CT show pulmonary nodules or cavities (see Figure 17.25).
- UA with active sediment.
- Characteristic biopsy.

Treatment

- **Induction:** Cyclophosphamide, corticosteroids, and/or rituximab.
- **Remission:** Methotrexate, azathioprine.

Churg-Strauss Angiitis

A 40-year-old man with a long history of severe asthma presents with fever, skin rash, and worsening respiratory symptoms with frequent daily use of albuterol during the day and night. The patient is also on high-dose inhaled corticosteroids, a long-acting β-agonist, and 15–20 mg/day of prednisone for the past six months. About one month ago he started a leukotriene receptor antagonist in an attempt to taper off prednisone. His CXR shows bilateral patchy infiltrates, and his leukocyte count is 20,000/μL with 30% eosinophils. What is the most appropriate next step in management?

Stop the leukotriene receptor antagonist and restart or ↑ the prednisone to treat Churg-Strauss syndrome. Neuropathic, cardiac, renal, and GI symptoms can also occur. ↑ inflammatory markers and a ⊕ p-ANCA (antimyeloperoxidase ANCA) support the diagnosis.

A small- and medium-vessel necrotizing vasculitis that presents as eosinophilic pneumonia and corticosteroid-dependent asthma. Males are affected more often than females. Organs and systems affected include the lung, heart, nerve, and kidney.

Symptoms/Exam

- **Asthma,** nasal polyps, allergic rhinitis.
- Mono- and peripheral neuropathy (mononeuritis multiplex).
- Fever, rash, myalgias, arthralgias, weight loss.
- Cough, dyspnea, angina pectoris (due to myocarditis or coronary artery involvement).
- Glomerulonephritis is less common than in other ANCA-associated diseases.

KEY FACT

Hemorrhagic cystitis is a possible complication of cyclophosphamide therapy, presenting with hematuria without erythrocyte casts or protein on UA. Patients also have an ↑ risk of transitional cell carcinoma of the bladder even years after treatment has been discontinued. For this reason, lifelong screening for bladder cancer with cystoscopy is indicated.

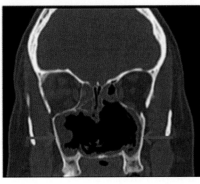
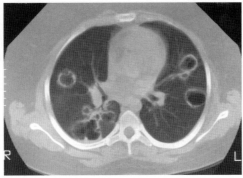

A   **B**

FIGURE 17.25.   Wegener's granulomatosis. (A) Coronal reformation from CT of the paranasal sinuses shows destruction of the nasal septum and turbinates and mucoperiosteal thickening of the maxillary sinuses (arrows) due to upper respiratory tract involvement of Wegener's granulomatosus. **(B)** Transaxial CT image through the lungs demonstrates multiple cavitary pulmonary nodules due to lower respiratory tract involvement with Wegener's granulomatosus. (Image A reproduced with permission from USMLERx.com. Image B reproduced with permission from Fauci AS et al. *Harrison's Principles of Internal Medicine,* 17th ed. New York: McGraw-Hill, 2008, Fig. 319-3.)

DIAGNOSIS

- Labs:
    - Peripheral eosinophilia.
    - Normal serum complement levels (antimyeloperoxidase).
    - ⊕ p-ANCA (antimyeloperoxidase), **although not specific for the disease.**
- **Imaging:** CXR shows fleeting pulmonary infiltrates.
- Biopsy of affected tissue demonstrates extravascular eosinophils.

TREATMENT

- High-dose corticosteroids.
- Immunosuppressants for renal or nerve/CNS involvement or for steroid-unresponsive disease.

Microscopic Polyangiitis

A 60-year-old woman presents with two weeks of progressive dyspnea and a productive cough with blood-streaked sputum. She has no history of asthma and was born in the United States. On exam, she is hypertensive and has bilateral crackles at the lung bases, 1+ edema of the extremities, and a palpable petechial rash. Labs are as follows: CBC with no eosinophils, creatinine 4 mg/dL, C3 100 mg/dL, and C4 30 mg/dL; numerous dysmorphic erythrocytes and erythrocyte casts are found on UA. Her CXR shows bilateral pulmonary infiltrates. What is the most likely diagnosis?

Microscopic polyangiitis causing a pulmonary-renal syndrome, with alveolar bleeding from capillaritis. Seventy-five percent of patients have a ⊕ ANCA. Complement levels would be abnormal in cryoglobulinemia or lupus. Classic polyarteritis nodosa typically spares the lungs.

KEY FACT

The triad of asthma, eosinophilia, and a ⊕ **p-ANCA** strongly suggests Churg-Strauss syndrome.

A medium- or, more commonly, small-vessel nongranulomatous vasculitis and capillaritis characterized by pulmonary hemorrhage and by glomerulonephritis and renal failure. Organs and systems affected include the lung, kidney, nerve, and skin. Often confused with polyarteritis nodosa (see Table 17.16).

SYMPTOMS/EXAM

- Fever, malaise, myalgias, arthralgias, weight loss.
- Hemoptysis, dyspnea.
- Hematuria/active sediment.
- Mono-/polyneuropathy; skin rashes (palpable purpura).

DIAGNOSIS

- Labs:
  - ↑ ESR; normal serum complement levels.
  - ⊕ p-ANCA (antimyeloperoxidase).
- Tissue biopsy demonstrates alveolar hemorrhage/necrotizing capillaritis/glomerulonephritis.

TREATMENT

Corticosteroids; cytotoxic agents.

Polyarteritis Nodosa (PAN)

> A 60-year-old woman presents with six months of inability to fully raise her left foot along with painful paresthesias on the dorsum of that foot and in her right hand. She has also had fevers, night sweats, arthralgias without joint swelling or stiffness, myalgias, and a 20-pound weight loss. On exam, she is found to have a fever of 38.8°C (102°F) and a BP of 175/96 mm Hg. She has livedo reticularis on her lower extremities, is unable to dorsiflex her left foot, and has weakness in her right hand. Labs are as follows: ESR 110 mm/hr, hemoglobin 11g/dL, creatinine 1.9 mg/dL, AST 90 U/L, ALT 80 U/L, ⊕ hepatitis B surface antigen and core antibody but ⊖ surface antibody, ⊖ cryogobulins, ⊖ hepatitis C antibody, and normal UA. What is the most likely diagnosis?
>
> PAN presents with mononeuritis multiplex in up to 60% of affected patients and frequently affects the renal arteries, GI tract, and skin as well. Patients with PAN often have a ⊕ hepatitis B surface antigen.

TABLE 17.16. **Polyarteritis Nodosa vs. Microscopic Polyangiitis**

	POLYARTERITIS NODOSA	**MICROSCOPIC POLYANGIITIS**
Vessel size	Medium	Medium and small
Skin	Ulcer/nodule/livedo reticularis	Palpable purpura
Lung	Rare	Capillaritis/alveolar hemorrhage
Renal	Renal artery aneurysms/renal infarction	Glomerulonephritis

A necrotizing arteritis of small and medium-sized vessels. Active infection with **HBV** predisposes to the development of disease (prevalent in 5–10% of these patients). Organs affected include the kidney, nerves, GI/mesentery, brain, skin, heart, testes, and joints. Often confused with microscopic polyangiitis (see Table 17.16).

SYMPTOMS/EXAM

- Fever, malaise, weight loss, hypertension, testicular pain, **abdominal pain.**
- Arthritis or arthralgias; myalgias.
- **Neuropathies** (mono- or polyneuritis).
- **Skin rash** (livedo reticularis, nodules, ulcerations).

DIAGNOSIS

- **Labs:**
  - ↑ ESR.
  - The majority of cases are **ANCA** ⊖.
  - Normal serum complement levels.
  - HBV serologies.
- **Imaging:** Angiography shows aneurysmal dilations of affected arteries.
- Site-directed biopsy.

KEY FACT

In a patient with newly diagnosed PAN, check for evidence of hepatitis B infection, which is associated with PAN.

TREATMENT

- High-dose corticosteroids.
- Cytotoxic immunosuppressive agents (eg, cyclophosphamide).

Polymyalgia Rheumatica (PMR)

A 62-year-old woman presents with six months of fatigue, malaise, and significant shoulder and hip pain, especially in the morning. She cannot do her usual daily exercise and is unable to sleep at night because of the pain. On exam, she is found to have full range of motion of the shoulders and hips, albeit with discomfort, along with tenderness at the deltoid and trochanteric areas. Her ESR is 70 mm/hr and CK 100 U/L, and her CBC and LFTs are normal. What is the most likely diagnosis?

PMR, which is characterized by pain and morning stiffness in the axial joints and proximal muscles, an absence of restricted motion, and no swelling, pain, or warmth of the proximal joints. Patients usually have an ↑ ESR and a normal CK and are typically > 50 years of age.

Associated with proximal/axial skeletal pain and stiffness; fever, malaise, and weight loss; and an ↑ ESR. Rare before age 50; usually affects **older females.** Associated with giant cell (temporal) arteritis.

KEY FACT

CK is normal in PMR, and there is no weakness. Remember that poly**myalgia** is not poly**myositis**.

SYMPTOMS/EXAM

- Joints affected include the shoulders, hip girdles, and low back and, less commonly, the peripheral joints.
- **No muscular weakness is seen** (vs. polymyositis).
- Fever, malaise, and weight loss can be profound.

DIAGNOSIS

Presents as follows (see also Table 17.12):

- Characteristic joint involvement (shoulders, hips).
- ↑ ESR (> 40 mm/hr).
- Constitutional features.
- Prompt response to corticosteroids.

TREATMENT

Small to moderate doses of corticosteroids (prednisone 5–20 mg day). The mean duration of therapy is 2–3 years with an average dose of 9–10 mg/day.

Giant Cell Arteritis (GCA)

A 70-year-old man presents with fever, fatigue, a severe bitemporal headache, jaw discomfort when chewing, and episodes of transient diplopia for the past two days. He has scalp tenderness on exam, and his ESR is 85 mm/hr. A temporal artery biopsy is scheduled in three days. What is the most appropriate course of management before the biopsy?

Whenever GCA is suspected, prednisone should be started immediately to ↓ the risk of visual loss. Symptoms of GCA also include neck pain (carotidynia), jaw and tongue claudication, and ptosis. Biopsy of the temporal artery will show panmural mononuclear cell infiltration with occasional giant cells. Prednisone use for about two weeks will not affect biopsy results, but a biopsy should be done as soon as possible.

Granulomatous arteritis of large and medium-sized vessels of the extracranial branches of the carotid artery. The most common vasculitis in North America and Europe; affects patients > 50 years of age. Blindness results from involvement of posterior ciliary arteries/ischemic optic neuritis. Has a strong association with PMR.

SYMPTOMS/EXAM

- Severe headache.
- Scalp/temporal artery tenderness.
- Jaw claudication, sore throat, amaurosis fugax.
- Fever, malaise, and weight loss.

DIAGNOSIS

- Age > 50.
- ↑ ESR (> 50 mm/hr).
- New-onset headache.
- A tender, nodular, or pulseless temporal artery.
- Characteristic angiographic findings.
- A characteristic temporal artery biopsy showing mononuclear cell infiltration with occasional giant cells.

TREATMENT

High-dose corticosteroids (prednisone 40–60 mg/day) usually for 1–2 years, titrated on the basis of symptoms and ESR.

Takayasu's Arteritis

> A 24-year-old woman presents with one year of worsening fatigue and malaise and has started to feel feverish. She has had worsening upper extremity pain with exertion that resolves with rest in about five minutes, along with lightheadedness. On exam, her BPs in the left and right arm are 155/85 and 165/95 mm Hg, respectively, with 1+ pulses in the right carotid and left brachial and radial arteries as well as the right dorsalis pedis, and an abdominal bruit is present. Her musculoskeletal exam is normal, and her CBC shows a normal WBC count, a hemoglobin of 11 g/dL, a platelet count of 400,000/μL, and an ESR of 40 mm/hr. What is the most likely diagnosis?
>
> Takayasu's arteritis, which primarily affects the aorta and its main branches and occurs mostly in reproductive-age women. This disorder can commonly cause "subclavian steal" syndrome, compromising posterior cerebral blood flow. BP measurements are often inaccurate and asymmetric due to vascular stenoses. CT, MRA, or arteriography can confirm the diagnosis.

A pulseless aortitis and vasculitis of the large vessels/branches of the aorta. Most prevalent in East Asia; **women < 40 years of age** are most commonly affected.

SYMPTOMS/EXAM

- Fever, malaise, myalgias, arthralgias, weight loss, progressive claudication.
- Evidence of limb and/or organ ischemia.
- Hypertension, bruits, and abnormal pulses; **systolic BP discrepancies measured between limbs;** aortic valvular regurgitation murmur.

DIAGNOSIS

- ↑ ESR is common but not universal.
- CXR may suggest aortic abnormalities.
- Angiography of the aorta/branches shows stenoses and occasional aneurysms (see Figure 17.26).
- Biopsy reveals granulomatous arteritis +/– variable numbers of giant cells.

TREATMENT

- Corticosteroids, methotrexate.
- Aggressive BP control.
- Surgical bypass of ischemic vessels once systemic disease is controlled.

KEY FACT

Takayasu's arteritis is also known as "pulseless disease" because the arteries it involves—the aorta and its branches—can narrow, resulting in ↓ radial and femoral pulses and BP.

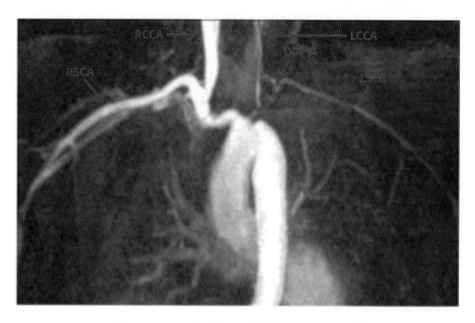

FIGURE 17.26. Takayasu's arteritis. Coronal MIP image from an MRA shows normal appearance of the right subclavian and common carotid arteries (RSCA, RCCA) but severe diffuse narrowing of the left common carotid artery (LCCA) and occlusion of the origin of the left subclavian artery (LSCA), which is diffusely narrowed distally but fills via retrograde flow from the left vertebral artery (LVA) ("subclavian steal"). (Reproduced with permission from USMLERx.com.)

OTHER VASCULITIDES

Cryoglobulinemia

A 40-year-old woman who is a former IV drug user presents with a lower extremity rash of four months' duration along with a year of Raynaud's cold-induced acral cyanosis. On exam, she is hypertensive and has hepatomegaly, 1+ lower extremity edema, and a purpuric rash. Her labs are as follows: hemoglobin 10 g/dL, creatinine 1.5 mg/dL, C3 80 mg/dL, C4 10 mg/dL, AST 50 U/L, and ALT 80 U/L. Her UA shows 3+ hematuria, 1+ protein, and dysmorphic erythrocytes. What is the most likely cause of her renal disease?

Cryoglobulinemic glomerulonephritis. Cryoglobulinemia and associated small vessel vasculitis are characterized by Raynaud's phenomenon, a palpable purpuric rash, abnormal LFTs, arthritis, neuropathy, membranous glomerulonephritis, cryoglobulins, and a C4 level that is ↓ to a greater extent than the C3 level. It is highly associated with hepatitis C, which should be strongly suspected in this former IV drug user with an abnormal ALT. ESR may be ↑ and RF can be ⊕.

- All cryoglobulins are immune complexes that precipitate at ≤ 4°C. Cryoglobulinemias are divided into three types:
    - **Type 1:** Monoclonal (seen in multiple myeloma and Waldenström's macroglobulinemia). Acrocyanosis (blue digits) and hyperviscosity complications are more common than vasculitis.
    - **Type 2:** Monoclonal antibodies (RF) against polyclonal immune targets.
    - **Type 3:** Polyclonal antibodies (RF) against polyclonal immune targets.
- Types 2 and 3 can both be **idiopathic** or caused by **HCV** or other chronic infections, malignancies, or collagen vascular diseases (especially Sjögren's syndrome).
- **Sx/Exam:** Clinically, signs of vasculitis are seen—eg, glomerulonephritis, palpable purpura, and neuropathy.

Buerger's Disease (Thromboangiitis Obliterans)

- Thromboses of medium-sized arteries and veins, usually of the hands or feet. Most commonly affects **males who smoke** heavily.
- **Tx:** Treat by discontinuing smoking.

Behçet's Disease

A 30-year-old woman presents with a week of headache and left eye pain along with a vaginal ulcer; she has also had intermittent oral ulcers for the past two years. She is monogamous, takes no medications, and has no fevers, neck stiffness, or joint pain. Exam shows oral ulcers, an inflamed left eye with a ciliary flush and hypopyon, and a vaginal ulcer. Her leukocyte count is 16,000/μL, her head CT is normal, and an LP shows a leukocyte count of 15/μL (100% lymphocytes) with a ⊖ Gram stain. What is the most ikely diagnosis?

Behçet's disease, a multisystem inflammatory disease characterized by recurrent aphthous oral ulcers and at least two or more of the following: recurrent painful genital ulceration, eye or cutaneous lesions, or ⊕ findings on pathergy testing. Features associated with the greatest morbidity or mortality include CNS disease, ocular disease, vascular thrombosis, arterial aneurysms, and GI disease (ulcers in the terminal ileum, cecum, and ascending colon). This patient has aseptic meningitis and anterior uveitis with hypopyon.

- **Sx/Exam:** Recurrent **oral and genital ulcerations**, skin ulcerations, **pathergy** (worsening of ulcerations with provocation), and erythema nodosum. Other characteristics are as follows:
    - **Ocular disease:** Keratitis, hypopyon, uveitis, retinal vasculitis, blindness.
    - **CNS abnormalities:** Cerebral vasculitis, meningoencephalitis, myelitis, cranial neuropathies.
    - Seronegative arthritis, pulmonary artery aneurysms, thrombophlebitis.
- **Tx:** Treat with corticosteroids, colchicine, dapsone, or thalidomide for aphthous and mucocutaneous disease, and/or immunosuppressants such as azathioprine in severe ocular or CNS disease.

KEY FACT

HCV infection is the most common cause of cryoglobulinemia in the United States.

KEY FACT

Three rheumatic diseases associated with oral ulcers are Behçet's, SLE, and reactive arthritis.

Relapsing Polychondritis

A 40-year-old woman presents with acute-onset shortness of breath and nasal pain. She has been treated for left ear cellulitis in the past year. On exam, she is found to be in respiratory distress, has stridor localized to the trachea, and has a collapsed nasal bridge with an early saddle-nose deformity. Her CBC, chemistry, and UA are normal. Her CXR is normal as well, and laryngoscopy shows dynamic laryngeal collapse with inspiration but a normal mucosa. What is the most likely diagnosis?

Relapsing polychondritis with a history of auricular inflammation, saddle-nose deformity, and collapse of the tracheal cartilage. The most common presenting feature is auricular chondritis. Relapsing polychondritis is a systemic inflammatory connective tissue disease characterized by inflammation and destruction of cartilaginous structures.

- Episodic inflammatory attacks involving the **cartilage of the ears, nose, larynx, and trachea.**
  - May be idiopathic or 2° to another autoimmune, collagen vascular, or malignant disease.
  - Noncartilaginous involvement includes fever, polyarthritis, scleritis, uveitis, middle/inner ear inflammation, hearing loss, and vasculitis.
- **Tx:** Treat with corticosteroids, dapsone, colchicine, and immunosuppressants (for refractory disease).
- **Cx:** Complications include chronic deformities of the ear (cauliflower ear), nasal septum collapse (**saddle nose**), laryngotracheal chondritis and stenoses, hearing loss, vertigo, tinnitus, and valvular heart disease.

Infectious Arthritis

NONGONOCOCCAL ARTHRITIS

A 70-year-old woman presents with severe right hip pain of one week's duration that is causing difficulty with walking. Two weeks ago she had extensive dental surgery. She denies any fevers or chills, and hip x-rays show mild joint space narrowing. On exam her temperature is 38.1°C (100.6°F), and range of motion testing elicits right groin pain that limits her mobility. Blood cultures are drawn. What is the next best step in establishing a diagnosis?

Imaging-guided hip joint aspiration with ultrasound or fluoroscopy to rule out septic arthritis. About 50% of patients with nongonococcal arthritis have ⊕ blood cultures, and 70–90% have ⊕ synovial fluid cultures. Up to 65% of cases are caused by *S aureus*. Bacteremia usually precedes this (dental surgery), and patients often have extra-articular sites of infection. Radiographic evidence is usually delayed 7–10 days.

Acute-onset, **monoarticular** joint pain, swelling, warmth, and erythema. The knee is the most commonly involved joint (affecting 50% of cases). Gram-⊕ species (**S aureus, Streptococcus**) are common causative organisms. Gram-⊖ species (*E coli, Pseudomonas*) are less commonly involved. Risk factors include the following:

- Age > 80
- Diabetes mellitus
- IV drug use
- Endocarditis
- Recent joint surgery
- Skin infection
- RA
- Joint prostheses

SYMPTOMS/EXAM

Fevers, chills, inability to bear weight or pain with joint motion, large joint effusions, a very hot and tender joint.

DIAGNOSIS

- Blood cultures are ⊕ in < 50% of cases.
- Arthrocentesis reveals leukocytosis (usually > 50,000 with > 90% PMN predominance) and a ⊕ culture; Gram stain is ⊕ in only 75% of cases (*S aureus*).
- X-rays are nonspecific but may reveal demineralization, bony erosions, joint narrowing, and periosteal reactions.

TREATMENT

- IV antibiotics are often needed for up to six weeks.
- Serial arthrocentesis if effusion reaccumulates; surgical drainage if the patient fails medical therapy or the disease involves inaccessible sites (eg, the hip).

COMPLICATIONS

Articular destruction; septicemia. The mortality rate for in-hospital septic arthritis is 7–15% despite antibiotic therapy.

GONOCOCCAL ARTHRITIS (DISSEMINATED INFECTION)

A 20-year-old sexually active woman presents with an acutely painful and swollen right wrist and left knee. Six days ago she had flulike symptoms and migratory joint pains, and now she is having difficulty holding things. On exam, the affected joints are found to be warm, swollen, and tender, and there is scant mucoid cervical discharge. Blood, pharyngeal, cervical, rectal, and left knee cultures are obtained, with arthrocentesis showing a leukocyte count of 15,000/ μL with 90% neutrophils and a ⊖ Gram stain. IV ceftriaxone is started, but two days later she is only minimally improved and cultures are ⊖. What is the most appropriate next step in management?

Continue ceftriaxone, as a complete response to appropriate antibiotic therapy for disseminated gonorrhea may take up to 72 hours. This is based on a high suspicion with asymmetric migratory arthralgias in a sexually active woman, oligoarthritis, and tenosynovitis in the wrist, but the rash is not always present. Screening for chlamydia, HIV, and other STDs should be performed once gonorrheal infection is established. Gonorrheal infection must be excluded by ⊖ culture results and a lack of response to antibiotic therapy before a diagnosis of reactive arthritis is established.

> ### KEY FACT
>
> Septic arthritis should be suspected and empirically treated in all patients with otherwise unexplained acute inflammatory mono- or oligoarthritis if crystals are not seen on synovial fluid analysis. Oral antibiotics are not appropriate in a closed-space infection because these conditions may rapidly lead to joint destruction.

> ### KEY FACT
>
> A synovial WBC count of > 100,000 is 99% specific for nongonococcal septic arthritis.

Most common in patients < 40 years of age; women are more frequently affected than men.

SYMPTOMS/EXAM

- **Migratory** polyarthralgias and **tenosynovitis** (see Figure 17.27).
- A papulopustular skin rash that may involve the palms and soles.
- Fever.

DIAGNOSIS

- Arthrocentesis reveals leukocytosis (commonly > 50,000); 10% Gram stain $\oplus$, and < 50% culture $\oplus$.
- Blood cultures, rectal and throat swab cultures, urethral cultures (70–86% sensitive).

TREATMENT

- Give IV antibiotics (third-generation cephalosporin) until clinical improvement is seen, followed by the oral equivalent or a quinolone antibiotic for a 7- to 10-day total course.
- Empiric therapy or testing for chlamydia is recommended.

TUBERCULOUS ARTHRITIS

Most common in children, immunosuppressed patients, and the elderly. Can occur shortly after 1° infection or as a reactivation phenomenon. Fewer than 50% of patients with tuberculous arthritis will have an abnormal CXR. Patients with spinal disease (Pott's) rarely have extraspinal involvement.

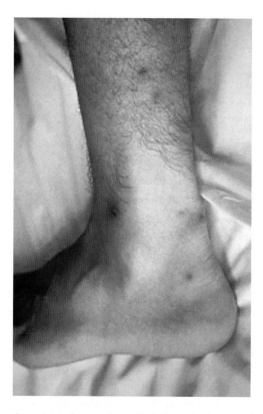

FIGURE 17.27. **Disseminated gonorrhea skin lesions.** Lesions may be a clue to the etiology of migratory arthritis and tenosynovitis. (Reproduced with permission from USMLERx.com.)

Symptoms/Exam

- Insidious-onset, subacute or chronic monoarticular joint swelling, pain, and warmth followed by destructive arthritis, contractures, and abscess/sinus drainage.
- **Pott's disease** presents as insidious onset of back pain with involvement of the thoracic and lumbar spine.

Diagnosis

Isolation of acid-fast bacilli from joint fluid or synovial biopsy.

Treatment

As for pulmonary TB, but a longer treatment course may be necessary.

Complications

Joint destruction, invasion of adjacent soft tissues and bone, paraplegia (Pott's disease).

LYME ARTHRITIS

Early Lyme disease (stages 1 and 2) may have migratory arthralgias and myalgias along with flulike symptoms and an erythema migrans rash. **Advanced Lyme disease** (stage 3) presents as an **acute monoarthritis of the knee;** oligo- or polyarthritis is less common.

Diagnosis

- **Arthrocentesis:** PMN-predominant leukocytosis (average ~ 25,000); cultures for *Borrelia burgdorferi* are typically ⊖.
- **American College of Physicians recommendations for diagnosis:** Objective arthritis with both ELISA and Western blot confirmatory tests to *B burgdorferi*.

Treatment

Treat advanced Lyme arthritis (stage 3) with doxycycline (4 weeks) or ceftriaxone (2–4 weeks).

> **KEY FACT**
>
> The joint most commonly involved in Lyme arthritis (stage 3) is the knee; this stage occurs several months after the initial infection if the condition is left untreated.

Fibromyalgia

A 30-year-old woman presents with diffuse muscle and joint pains of two years' duration along with insomnia, difficulty getting out of bed in the morning due to fatigue and pain, difficulty concentrating, and chronic headaches that are not relieved by ibuprofen, acetaminophen, or naproxen. On exam, she is found to have diffuse soft-tissue tenderness to palpation at multiple sites (trapezius, coracoid processes, bicipital tendons, lateral epicondyles, trochanteric bursa, and gluteal muscles) but no weakness or synovitis. Her CBC, ESR, LFTs, chemistries, serum B_{12} level, and TSH are normal, and a head CT is normal as well. What is the most appropriate next step in this patient's management?

This patient has fibromyalgia. Graded exercise therapy and cognitive-behavioral therapy are the nonpharmacologic therapies of choice. Medications that may benefit patients with fibromyalgia include TCAs, SSRIs, and pregabalin. Narcotic analgesics are contraindicated as first-line treatment for this disorder.

Criteria for the diagnosis of fibromyalgia include the following:

- A history of widespread pain involving all four quadrants of the body (and axial spine) for ≥ 3 months.
- Pain in ≥ 11 of 18 tender points (occiput, low cervical trapezius, supraspinatus, second rib, lateral epicondyle, gluteal, greater trochanter, knee) on digital palpation by 4 kg of pressure—the approximate amount of pressure required to blanch the examiner's nail (see Figure 17.28).

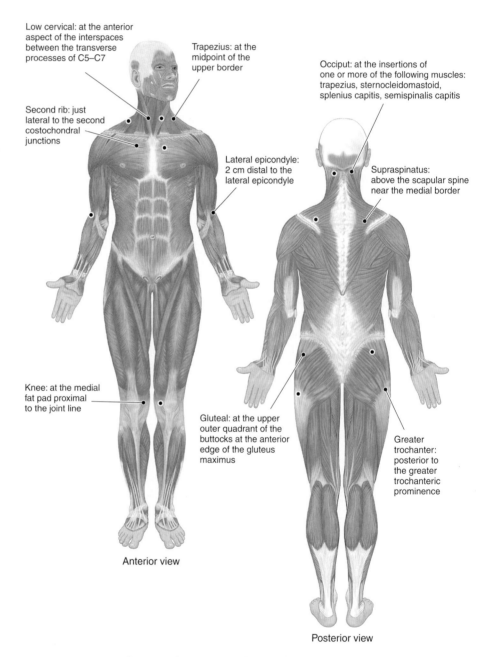

Low cervical: at the anterior aspect of the interspaces between the transverse processes of C5–C7

Trapezius: at the midpoint of the upper border

Occiput: at the insertions of one or more of the following muscles: trapezius, sternocleidomastoid, splenius capitis, semispinalis capitis

Second rib: just lateral to the second costochondral junctions

Lateral epicondyle: 2 cm distal to the lateral epicondyle

Supraspinatus: above the scapular spine near the medial border

Knee: at the medial fat pad proximal to the joint line

Gluteal: at the upper outer quadrant of the buttocks at the anterior edge of the gluteus maximus

Greater trochanter: posterior to the greater trochanteric prominence

Anterior view

Posterior view

FIGURE 17.28. The 18 tender points used in the diagnosis of fibromyalgia. Classification criteria are those of the American College of Rheumatology. (Reproduced with permission from Imboden JB et al. *Current Rheumatology Diagnosis & Treatment,* 2nd ed. New York: McGraw-Hill, 2007, Fig. 13-1.)

DIFFERENTIAL

The differential diagnosis of fibromyalgia is outlined in Table 17.17.

TREATMENT

- **Nonpharmacologic treatment** is as follows:
  - Education; cognitive-behavioral therapy.
  - Treat sleep disturbances and depression if present.
  - **Aerobic exercise:** "Start low and go slow" with a focus on adherence to a lifelong program.
  - **Complementary therapies:**
    - Almost all patients with fibromyalgia use complementary and alternative medicine, at least in part because of distrust of physicians and frustration with the limited efficacy of much traditional care.
    - Acupuncture, hypnotherapy, relaxation techniques (yoga, Tai Chi, and meditation), and osteopathic manipulation appear to have some efficacy.
- **Pharmacologic treatment** options include low-dose TCAs (eg, **amitriptyline**), SSRIs (eg, fluoxetine), and pregabalin.

COMPLICATIONS

The adverse impact of fibromyalgia on the patient, family, and society is high. More than 25% of patients receive some type of disability or other compensation payment.

TABLE 17.17. **Differential Diagnosis of Fibromyalgia**

DISEASE CATEGORY	EXAMPLES
Endocrine disorders	Hypothyroidism,[a] Addison's disease, Cushing's disease, hyperparathyroidism.
Autoimmune disorders	PMR,[a] RA, SLE, polymyositis.
Medications	Lipid-lowering drugs, antiviral agents, tapering of corticosteroids.
Infection	HCV,[a] HIV, parvovirus, Lyme disease, subacute bacterial endocarditis.
Malignancy	Myeloma; breast, lung, or prostate cancer.
Neurologic disorders	Carpal tunnel syndrome,[a] MS,[a] sleep apnea,[a] cervical stenosis.[a]
Psychiatric disorders	
Vitamin D deficiency	

[a]Commonly encountered diagnoses.

Miscellaneous Diseases

ADULT STILL'S DISEASE

A 30-year-old man presents with one month of arthralgias, daily fevers, a sore throat, and a rash that is present during febrile episodes. His temperature is 38.3°C (101°F), and he appears ill. On exam, he is found to have a pink macular rash on his extremities, cervical and axillary lymphadenopathy, splenomegaly, and synovitis of the wrists and knees. Labs are as follows: hemoglobin 10 mg/dL, leukocyte count 15,000/μL, AST 110 U/L, LDH 300 U/L, ferritin 4000 ng/mL, iron 90 μg/dL, and TIBC 350 μg/dL. What is the most likely diagnosis?

Adult-onset Still's disease, an inflammatory disease characterized by daily high spikes of fever; arthritis; a salmon-colored evanescent rash on the trunk, extremities, palms, soles, or face, particularly in the evening; the absence of infection or other disease (SLE, PAN, other rheumatic disease); and **ferritin levels of > 3000 ng/mL.** Patients can also have serositis, lymphadenopathy, sore throat, splenomegaly, leukocytosis, and an ↑ LDH.

- **Sx/Exam:** Presents with high-spiking **fevers,** diaphoresis, chills, sore throat, an evanescent salmon-colored **rash** coincident with fevers, erosive arthritis, serositis, and lymphadenopathy.
- **Dx:** Laboratory findings include **leukocytosis,** anemia, seronegativity, transaminitis, and **hyperferritinemia.**
- **Tx:** Treat with NSAIDs and corticosteroids.

SARCOIDOSIS

A 25-year-old man presents with one week of right ankle pain and multiple painful, nonpruritic "bug bites" on his legs that appeared after he mowed the lawn, causing him to walk with a limp. On exam his temperature is 38.3°C (101°F), his right ankle is swollen and tender, and he has tender erythema nodosum of the lower extremities. His CBC, chemistries, UA, and arthrocentesis are normal. What is the most appropriate next step in the patient's management?

Order a CXR to evaluate for hilar lymphadenopathy of Löfgren's syndrome, a variant of sarcoidosis characterized by acute erythema nodosum, hilar adenopathy, arthritis or periarthritis, and fever. Löfgren's carries a good prognosis and can be treated with NSAIDs and/or low-dose corticosteroids.

- Arthritis associated with sarcoidosis is either acute or chronic. See the Pulmonary Medicine chapter for nonarticular manifestations of sarcoidosis.
- Acute sarcoid arthritis = Löfgren's syndrome, which presents with **periarthritis** (most commonly of the ankle/knee), **erythema nodosum,** and **hilar adenopathy** on CXR.
- Resolution of acute disease occurs in 2–16 weeks with minimal therapy, NSAIDs, and colchicine.
- **Chronic sarcoid arthritis** usually involves minimally inflamed joints with synovial swelling/granulomata. Treat with NSAIDs, corticosteroids, and immunosuppressants.

CHOLESTEROL EMBOLI SYNDROME

Precipitated by invasive arterial procedures in patients with atherosclerotic disease. Features include fever, livedo reticularis, cyanosis/gangrene of the digits, vasculitic/ischemic ulcerations, **eosinophilia, renal failure,** and other end-organ damage (see Figures 17.29 and 17.30).

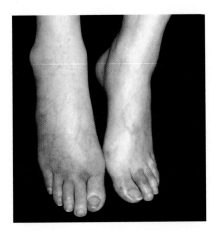

FIGURE 17.29. Cholesterol emboli. Typical appearance of blue toes due to multiple atheromatous emboli to the lower limbs in a patient with extensive atheromatous disease of the aorta. (Reproduced with permission from Wolff K et al. *Fitzpatrick's Dermatology in General Medicine,* 7th ed. New York: McGraw-Hill, 2008, Fig. 174-5A.)

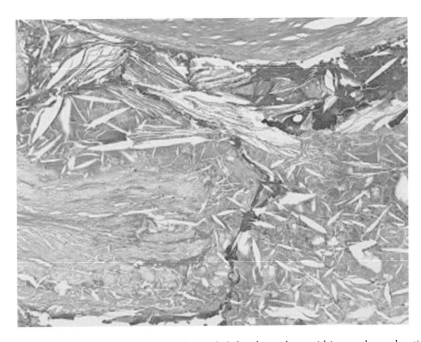

FIGURE 17.30. Needle-shaped cholesterol clefts, shown here within an atherosclerotic plaque, may also be seen in skin or kidney biopsy specimens in patients with cholesterol emboli syndrome. (Reproduced with permission from USMLERx.com.)

NOTES

CHAPTER 18

Women's Health

Christina A. Lee, MD
Linda Shiue, MD

Breast Masses

SYMPTOMS/EXAM

- May be found on clinical exam or by the patient.
- Ask about associations with menstrual cycle, pain, and risk factors for breast cancer.

DIAGNOSIS/TREATMENT

- The clinical breast exam should include palpation of the axillae and nipples, inspection for skin changes, and examination of the asymptomatic breast.
- If a dominant mass is present, proceed to mammography +/– ultrasound and surgical evaluation for biopsy (see Figure 18.1).
- Women with benign findings on imaging and biopsy require close follow-up. Consider excision in the setting of continued growth or patient preference.
- The management of breast malignancies is discussed in detail in the Oncology chapter.

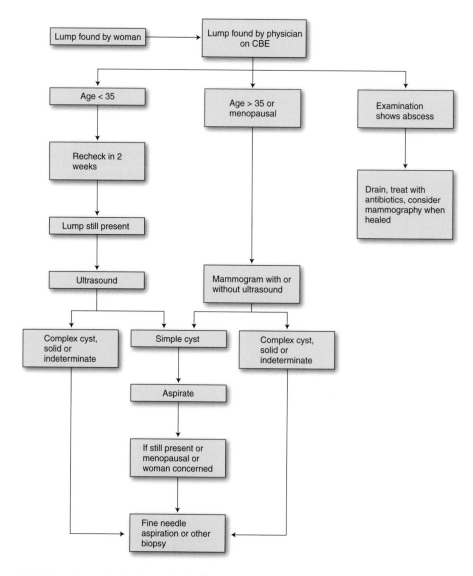

FIGURE 18.1. Evaluation of palpable breast masses. (Reproduced with permission from South-Paul JE et al. *Current Diagnosis & Treatment in Family Medicine,* 2nd ed. New York: McGraw-Hill, 2008: 272.)

Contraception

A 36-year-old woman seeks advice on her options for contraception. Her past medical history is significant for migraines with aura. She is a non-smoker. What type of hormonal birth control is most appropriate?

According to the World Health Organization (WHO), the best method for this patient is a copper IUD. It may be acceptable to initiate progestin-only pills, long-acting depot medroxyprogesterone or norethisterone implants, and levonorgestrel-releasing IUDs as well, but the risks of continuing these methods may outweigh the advantages of doing so. The WHO recommends **against** initiating combined oral or injectable contraceptives, transdermal patch, or vaginal rings in women with migraines with aura at any age.

Table 18.1 describes common contraceptive methods and outlines their contraindications and side effects.

KEY FACT

Women > 35 years of age who are heavy smokers should not be prescribed combination OCPs because of the ↑ risk of MI and DVT.

KEY FACT

Emergency contraception in the form of progestin (+/– estrogen) should be taken within five days (ideally < 24 hours) of intercourse to suppress ovulation or discourage implantation. Levonorgestrel alone (Plan B) is more effective and has fewer side effects than combined estrogen/progestin.

TABLE 18.1.   Contraceptive Methods

METHOD	DESCRIPTION	PROS/CONS
BARRIER METHODS		
Diaphragm, cervical cap	A domed sheet of latex filled with spermicide and placed over the cervix.	Allergy to latex or spermicide; ↑ **risk of UTI.**
Male or female condoms	A latex or polyurethane sheath placed over the penis during intercourse.	Allergy to latex or spermicide. **The only contraceptive method that also prevents STD transmission.**
INTRAUTERINE DEVICES (IUDs)		
Copper IUD (ParaGard)	A copper device placed into the endometrial cavity. Produces a local inflammatory reaction that has a spermicidal effect and also impairs implantation.	↑ vaginal bleeding/cramping; lasts a long time (up to 12 years). IUDs do **not** ↑ the risk of infertility in patients who are at low risk of STDs. **IUDs are the most commonly used reversible method of contraception worldwide.**
Progesterone-releasing IUD (levonorgestrel [Mirena])	Releases progestin, which thins the endometrium and thickens cervical mucus. Local effects are the same as those of the copper IUD.	Amenorrhea may occur. Lasts a shorter time (up to five years). ↓ menstrual blood loss may be beneficial for women with menorrhagia or dysmenorrhea.

(continues)

TABLE 18.1. Contraceptive Methods *(continued)*

METHOD	DESCRIPTION	PROS/CONS
HORMONAL METHODS		
Combined estrogen/progestin contraceptives (OCPs, transdermal ["the patch"], vaginal ring ["the ring"])	Suppress ovulation; thicken cervical mucus; thin endometrium.	Nausea, breast tenderness, acne, mood changes, hypertension, hepatic adenoma, weight gain. **↑ risk of venous thromboembolism (VTE) and arterial thrombosis** (MI, CVA), particularly among women with other cardiovascular risk factors. Commonly used.
Progestin-only oral contraceptive ("mini-pill")		No apparent ↑ in the risk of VTE. A good option for women who are intolerant of estrogen or who are breast-feeding.
Depot medroxyprogesterone acetate (Depo-Provera)	IM injection lasts three months.	Irregular vaginal bleeding, depression, weight gain, breast tenderness, delayed restoration of ovulation after discontinuation (6–18 months). Easy for patients, although some may be bothered by the irregular bleeds.
Etonogestrel implant (Implanon)	A single-rod subdermal implant that is effective for three years.	Irregular vaginal bleeding; small possibility of device migration and difficult removal.
SURGICAL STERILIZATION		
Vasectomy	The vas deferens is cut.	Very low risk of local complications. More than 50% of men with reversed vasectomies are fertile.
Tubal ligation	The fallopian tubes are ligated, cauterized, or mechanically occluded.	Tubal ligation may result in bleeding, infection, failure, or ectopic pregnancy; the procedure is essentially irreversible.

Medical Conditions in Pregnancy

TERATOGENIC DRUGS

Table 18.2 lists common teratogens.

HYPERTENSION IN PREGNANCY

Table 18.3 lists hypertensive disorders during pregnancy.

Preeclampsia

Currently known as pregnancy-induced hypertension. Develops in the third trimester and resolves after delivery. Patients present with new hypertension (BP > 140/90 mm Hg), generalized weight gain, and rapid swelling and are found to have proteinuria. Risk factors include the following:

> **KEY FACT**
>
> Drugs that are safe to use in pregnancy include heparin (thrombosis), β-lactam antibiotics, prednisone (SLE or RA), and insulin.

TABLE 18.2.   Teratogenic/Fetotoxic Drugs

Drug Class	Examples
Antibiotics	Doxycycline and other tetracyclines, sulfonamides, **quinolones, streptomycin.**
Anticonvulsants	Carbamazepine, valproic acid, phenytoin.
Psychotropics	Lithium, benzodiazepines.
Immunomodulatory/ antiangiogenic drugs	Methotrexate, thalidomide.
Miscellaneous	**NSAIDs, ACEIs, warfarin, isotretinoin,** iodide.

- First pregnancy.
- Multiple gestation.
- Certain medical conditions (eg, DM, obesity, autoimmune/renal disease).
- Advanced maternal age.
- Gestational trophoblastic disease.
- Factor V Leiden mutations; antiphospholipid antibody syndrome.

TABLE 18.3.   Hypertensive Disorders of Pregnancy

	Chronic Hypertension	Preeclampsia/Eclampsia	Gestational Hypertension
Timing	Present before pregnancy or persisting > 6 weeks postpartum.	Onset after 20 weeks' gestation (can occur up to six weeks postpartum).	Onset after 20 weeks' gestation. Resolves after delivery.
Clinical features	Hypertension prior to pregnancy.	**Preeclampsia: Hypertension (> 140/90 mm Hg) and proteinuria with onset after 20 weeks.** Often associated with edema. **Uric acid level is often ↑.** Eclampsia = preeclampsia + seizures.	Hypertension without proteinuria during pregnancy.
Complications	↑ risk of preeclampsia. Intrauterine growth restriction (IUGR), placental abruption, fetal demise.	**Fetal:** IUGR, oligohydramnios, demise. **Maternal:** Edema, **HELLP syndrome** (hemolysis, elevated liver enzymes, low platelets), seizures, death.	May develop into preeclampsia. ↑ risk of subsequent essential hypertension.
Treatment	Treat BP if > 145–150/95–100 mm Hg. Target a diastolic BP of 80–100 mm Hg. **Methyldopa, β-blockers, hydralazine, and calcium channel blockers** (CCBs) are often used **(ACEIs and ARBs are contraindicated).**	**After 36 weeks' gestation:** Immediate delivery. **Before 36 weeks' gestation:** Bed rest, close monitoring of mother and fetus, BP management (goal diastolic BP 90–100 mm Hg). Hospitalization and delivery at any stage of gestation for severe preeclampsia, HELLP, or eclampsia. Magnesium sulfate is given after delivery to prevent seizures.	Same as that for chronic hypertension.

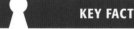
Treatment

- See Table 18.3 for an overview of preeclampsia management. The treatment of choice is delivery.
- For women with chronic hypertension, evaluate the BP regimen prior to conception.
    - **Eliminate teratogenic agents** (eg, **ACEIs and ARBs**).
    - Diuretics are usually avoided unless they are needed for volume overload.
    - β-blockers and CCBs are generally acceptable for use during pregnancy.
    - Methyldopa has the longest record of safety during pregnancy but has many side effects.

HELLP Syndrome

- **H**emolysis, **E**levated **L**iver enzymes, and **L**ow **P**latelets. Considered a variant of preeclampsia. May be associated with renal dysfunction.
- **Dx:**
    - Microangiopathic hemolytic anemia.
    - AST > 70 IU/L.
    - Platelets < 100K.
- **Tx:** Prompt delivery; supportive measures.
- **Cx:** Although most patients recover fully within weeks, there is a 3–5% maternal mortality rate.

DIABETES IN PREGNANCY

Preexisting type 2 DM or impaired glucose tolerance may be unmasked in pregnancy. Guidelines for testing are as follows:

- **High risk:** Administer an oral glucose tolerance test (OGTT) to pregnant women at high risk for gestational diabetes mellitus (GDM). Risk factors include the following:
    - Marked obesity.
    - A personal history of GDM.
    - Previous delivery of a large-for-gestational-age infant.
    - Glycosuria.
    - Polycystic ovarian syndrome (PCOS).
    - A strong family history of DM.
- **Average risk:** Test between 24 and 28 weeks' gestation.
- **Low risk:** Women at low risk do not need testing if they:
    - Are < 25 years of age.
    - Are of normal weight prior to pregnancy.
    - Are not members of high-risk ethnic groups (ie, not African American, Asian, Hispanic, or Native American).
    - Have no first-degree relatives with DM.
    - Have no history of abnormal glucose tolerance.
    - Have had no prior poor obstetric outcome.

Diagnosis

- Conduct initial screening with a 50-g glucose load. Then perform a 100-g diagnostic **OGTT** in patients with a one-hour glucose level ≥ 130–140 mg/dL (see Table 18.4).
- Women with preexisting type 1 or type 2 DM should have baseline chemistries, HbA_{1c}, 24-hour urine protein and creatinine clearance, a funduscopic exam, and an ECG.

TABLE 18.4. **Diagnostic Criteria for GDM: 100-g Oral Glucose Tolerance Test**

TIME	GLUCOSE LEVEL (mg/dL)
Baseline (fasting)	≥ 95
One hour	180
Two hours	155
Three hours	140

TREATMENT

- Maternal and fetal outcomes are improved with tight glycemic control. **Tight control should be established before conception (HbA$_{1c}$ < 6%)** in women with preexisting DM.
    - Obese women should be placed on a calorie-restricted diet.
    - Insulin may be indicated to achieve target glycemic control.
    - Oral agents are generally not preferred to insulin, although sulfonylureas and metformin are likely safe and effective. **Insulin is standard in pregnancy; sulfonylureas are commonly used, and metformin is sometimes used.**
- Fetal size should be monitored, and patients may be referred for cesarean section if macrosomia is present.

COMPLICATIONS

- **Maternal:** DKA, preeclampsia, preterm labor, polyhydramnios; the need for C-section due to fetal macrosomia.
- **Fetal/neonatal:** Macrosomia; cardiac, renal, and neural tube defects; birth injury (shoulder dystocia); neonatal hypoglycemia; perinatal mortality.

KEY FACT

The goal in a mother with preexisting diabetes is good control (HbA$_{1c}$ < 6%) before conception.

THYROID DISEASE IN PREGNANCY

Normal Changes in Thyroid Function During Pregnancy

- ↑ thyroid-binding globulin.
- This will ↑ total serum levels of T$_4$ and T$_3$, but free hormone levels should remain normal.
- The normal range for TSH in pregnancy is lower (< 2.5 mIU/L).

Hyperthyroidism

- Affects 0.05–0.20% of pregnant women.
- In general, Graves' disease improves during pregnancy but may **flare in the early postpartum period.**
- **Dx:** Similar to the approach in nonpregnant patients except that **radioactive iodine is contraindicated during pregnancy.**
- **Tx:**
    - **Antithyroid medications:** All antithyroid medications cross the placenta and have the potential to cause fetal hypothyroidism in the newborn. **Propylthiouracil (PTU) is preferred** over methimazole because of concerns about embryogenesis ("**P** for **PTU** in **P**regnancy")
    - **Other medications: Avoid iodine** therapy, as it can lead to fetal goiter. **Propranolol** may be used to control cardiovascular symptoms.

- **Surgery:** In the setting of uncontrolled hyperthyroidism, thyroidectomy should be considered and performed during the second trimester if necessary.
- **Cx:** Complications of untreated hyperthyroidism may include spontaneous abortion, premature delivery, and an ↑ risk of a small-for-gestational-age newborn.

Hypothyroidism

- New-onset hypothyroidism is rare during pregnancy.
- **Tx:**
  - **Thyroid hormone replacement:** Women with preexisting hypothyroidism may require up to 50% higher levothyroxine dosages.
  - Monitor thyroid function closely. Consider an empiric ↑ of levothyroxine by 30% after pregnancy is confirmed. Consider treating subclinical hypothyroidism.
- **Cx:**
  - **Fetal complications:** Congenital anomalies, perinatal mortality, impaired mental and somatic development.
  - **Maternal complications:** Anemia, preterm labor, preeclampsia, placental abruption, postpartum hemorrhage.

Postpartum Thyroiditis

A 35-year-old woman who delivered a healthy baby three months ago presents with restlessness, weight loss, and heat intolerance. Her BP is normal and HR is 130 bpm, and her thyroid is enlarged but not tender. Her ECG shows sinus tachycardia. Her TSH is < 0.01 mIU/L. She has no history of Graves' disease and is diagnosed with painless postpartum thyroiditis. What would be expected on radioactive iodine uptake (RAIU), and what is the treatment of choice?

RAIU should be ↓, distinguishing this condition from Graves' disease. Treat hyperthyroid symptoms with a β-blocker; antithyroid medications have no role in postpartum thyroiditis.

- **Sx/Exam:**
  - Presents with painless goiter 1–6 months postpartum.
  - Patients first develop transient hyperthyroidism and then develop hypothyroidism, which evolves over the postpartum year.
- **Tx:**
  - Hyperthyroid symptoms should be treated with β-blockers; antithyroid drugs are not used.
  - Although hypothyroidism is usually self-limited, temporary treatment with levothyroxine may be necessary.
  - Patients need annual follow-up because they are at risk of developing permanent hypothyroidism.

VALVULAR DISEASE IN PREGNANCY

- Cardiac conditions that are major risk factors for maternal or fetal complications include pulmonary hypertension (particularly Eisenmenger's syndrome), cyanotic congenital heart disease, dilated cardiomyopathy with severe CHF, and severe valvular disease. Patients with these conditions should be strongly advised against pregnancy.
- The safest and most effective contraceptive device for cardiac patients is a levonorgestrel-releasing IUD. Low-estrogen OCPs are another possibility. Depo-Provera can lead to fluid retention in CHF patients.

> **KEY FACT**
>
> Think of a new diagnosis of mitral stenosis if a pregnant woman presents with atrial fibrillation and edema. Digoxin can be used in pregnancy. Electrocardioversion is also allowed.

Infertility

Inability to conceive after **one year** of unprotected intercourse, or six months in women ≥ 35 years of age. Etiologies include the following:

- **Male infertility:** Disorders of sperm transport (posttesticular defects), seminiferous tubule dysfunction, 1° hypogonadism, hypothalamic pituitary disease.
- **Ovulatory disorders:** Hypogonadism, PCOS, ovarian failure.
- **Oocyte aging.**
- **Luteal phase defects:** Implantation defects.
- **Uterine abnormalities:** Congenital, DES exposure, fibroids, polyps, synechiae from prior manipulation.
- **Tubal and peritoneal abnormalities:** Scarring from prior PID, severe endometriosis, adhesions.
- **Cervical abnormalities.**

EXAM

Often unremarkable. Look for hirsutism, goiter, galactorrhea, an abnormal pelvic exam in the female partner, and testicular size/masses in the male partner.

DIAGNOSIS

- Semen analysis.
- Obtain serum FSH, LH, TSH, and prolactin.
- Assess ovulation with a basal body temperature chart or a urine LH kit for the female partner.
- Consider hysterosalpingography, pelvic ultrasound, endometrial biopsy, and/or laparoscopy.

> **KEY FACT**
>
> Rule out male infertility first, as it is the source of the problem in 40% of cases and is easy to evaluate with a semen analysis.

TREATMENT

Treat the underlying cause:

- Urologic treatment for male factor infertility.
- Ovulation induction (clomiphene, gonadotropins, GnRH).
- Laparoscopy (eg, to remove endometriosis implants).
- Assisted reproductive technologies (intrauterine insemination, IVF).
- Sperm or egg donation.

Menstrual Disorders

ABNORMAL UTERINE BLEEDING

A 30-year-old African American woman presents to your clinic with one year of menorrhagia and dysmenorrhea. Her menses typically last 8–9 days and require that she change her tampons as often as every hour. What is the most likely diagnosis?

Uterine fibroids. Fibroids are extremely common, with a higher incidence, earlier clinical presentation, and more severe symptoms in African American women than in Caucasian women. Abnormal uterine bleeding (heavy and/or prolonged menses) is the most common symptom. The diagnosis is usually made on the basis of physical exam findings of an enlarged, mobile uterus with irregular contours on bimanual exam. Ultrasound may be used to confirm the diagnosis and to rule out the presence of an adnexal mass.

> **KEY FACT**
>
> **Dysfunctional uterine bleeding** refers to heavy and irregular bleeding due to anovulation and not to anatomic problems, leading to estrogen-induced stimulation of endometrium without progesterone to stabilize growth. It is a diagnosis of exclusion and should be considered in a woman with irregular bleeding in the absence of pelvic exam abnormalities or medical illness.

Defined as abnormalities in the frequency, duration, volume, and/or timing of menses. Etiologies are listed in Table 18.5. Subtypes include the following:

- **Intermittent/postcoital bleeding:** Think cervical lesions, endometrial polyps, cervicitis, and endometritis.
- **Menorrhagia:** Prolonged and/or excessive uterine bleeding. Think fibroids, adenomyosis, and coagulopathy.
- **Menometrorrhagia:** Heavy bleeding at irregular intervals. Think anovulation, some myomas, adenomyosis, **hyperplasia**, and **cancer.**
- **Amenorrhea:** Absence of menses for ≥ **3 usual cycle lengths** (see below).

TABLE 18.5. Causes of Abnormal Uterine Bleeding

CAUSE	UNDERLYING DISORDERS	CLINICAL FEATURES
Anovulation	PCOS, hypothalamic-pituitary-ovarian axis dysfunction, hypothyroidism, prolactinoma, ovarian or adrenal tumor.	Irregular cycles. Check for other endocrinologic signs, physical or mental stress, eating disorders, or high-intensity exercise.
Cervical lesions	Cervical polyps, cervicitis, dysplasia/malignancy.	Spotting, often postcoital; vaginal discharge (infection).
Bleeding disorder	von Willebrand's disease; acquired or other congenital coagulopathies.	Menorrhagia, intermenstrual heavy bleeding; other sites of bleeding.
Fibroids, endometrial cancer or hyperplasia		Dysmenorrhea +/– pelvic mass on exam; menorrhagia or intermenstrual bleeding.
Hormonal medications	OCPs, HRT.	Intermenstrual spotting, amenorrhea, postmenopausal bleeding.
Dysfunctional uterine bleeding (DUB)	Idiopathic. Often anovulatory.	Irregular menstrual pattern without an identifiable underlying cause.

Symptoms/Exam

- **History:** Determine whether bleeding is anatomic or anovulatory (irregular cycles with no premenstrual symptoms). Check for signs of PCOS (hirsutism, acne, obesity).
- **Exam:** Pelvic exam; Pap smear and urine pregnancy test.

Diagnosis

- **Labs:** May include TSH, prolactin, and CBC/coagulation studies.
- If you suspect chronic anovulation, confirm the presence of estrogen with a ⊕ **progesterone withdrawal test.** Give a medroxyprogesterone pill daily for five days; if withdrawal bleed is present, estrogen is present.
- **Additional testing:** Ultrasound (fibroids), hysteroscopy (endometrial polyps, some fibroids), and endometrial biopsy (endometrial polyps, hyperplasia, cancer). **Women > 35 years of age should routinely undergo endometrial biopsy for irregular bleeding to rule out cancer.**

Treatment

Treat the underlying cause:

- **Ovulatory, heavy bleeding:** NSAIDs and OCPs ↓ the amount of bleeding.
- **Anovulatory bleeding:** Hormonal treatment. OCPs, levonorgestrel IUDs, and cyclic progestins regularize cycles.
- **Profuse bleeding:** High-dose estrogen, D&C, endometrial ablation, hysterectomy.

AMENORRHEA

 An 18-year-old woman presents to her primary care physician for irregular menstrual periods. The onset of menarche was at age 13, and she had monthly menses until two years ago. Her last menstrual period was six months ago. She is an active marathon runner and will be on the cross-country team when she enters college in the fall. On physical exam, her BMI is found to be 18, and her urine pregnancy test is ⊖. TSH, prolactin, and FSH are all within normal limits. What is the next most appropriate step, and what is the most likely diagnosis?

When basic lab tests are normal, the next best step is to administer a progestin challenge test (medroxyprogesterone acetate daily × 10 days). If there is no withdrawal bleeding, the cause is either low estrogen (hypothalamic-pituitary axis dysfunction) or anatomic obstruction—most likely the former in this patient given her history of exercise and low BMI. If withdrawal bleeding occurs and if estrogen production and the uterine outflow tract are normal, the most likely diagnosis is PCOS (the presence of withdrawal bleeding indicates lack of progesterone or anovulation).

May be 1° or 2°.

- **1°:** Absence of menses by age 16, or by age 14 in the absence of 2° sexual characteristics.
- **2°:** Previously normal menses; absence for **three consecutive months.** **The most common cause (with the exception of pregnancy) is PCOS,** followed by **hypothalamic hypoestrogenism, hyperprolactinemia,** and **premature ovarian syndrome.**

Symptoms/Exam

- Ask about pregnancy symptoms, galactorrhea, headaches, visual changes, hirsutism, acne, stress or illness, medications, and menopausal symptoms. There may also be weight loss (eg, in eating disorders or exercise).
- Look for 2° sexual characteristics, virilization (male-pattern hair loss/growth, acne, clitoromegaly), galactorrhea, and pelvic exam abnormalities.

Differential

- **Hypothalamus-pituitary axis dysfunction** (↓ pulsatile GnRH activity of the hypothalamus leads to **low estrogen levels**): Physical or emotional stress, anorexia, heavy exercise; hyperprolactinemia and hypothyroidism.
- **Hyperandrogenism (normal estrogen levels):** PCOS, Cushing's syndrome, prolactinoma, 21-hydroxylase deficiency.
- **Uterine structural disorders:** Endometrial scarring after a procedure or infection (Asherman's syndrome).
- **Premature ovarian failure:** Autoimmune disease, Turner's syndrome, postchemotherapy.
- **Other:** Pregnancy, menopause.

Diagnosis

To diagnose 2° amenorrhea:

- Always rule out pregnancy.
- Check **TSH, FSH, LH, and prolactin. High FSH** points to **premature ovarian failure.**
  - **Abnormal TSH:** Thyroid dysfunction.
  - **High prolactin:** Hyperprolactinemia.
  - **High FSH and LH:** Premature ovarian failure.
  - **Low FSH and LH:** Low GnRH due to hypothalamus-pituitary axis dysfunction ("hypothalamic hypoestrogenism"), often due to stress, anorexia, or exercise.
  - **LH/FSH > 3:** PCOS.
- If all tests are normal (particularly FSH), **administer a progestin challenge.**
  - **"Positive test" (withdrawal bleed in response to progestin challenge):** This indicates normal estrogen production and a normal outflow tract, but progesterone is lacking. It suggests anovulation, with the most common cause PCOS.
  - **"Negative test" (no withdrawal bleed after progestin challenge):** Indicates one of the following:
    - **Hypothalamus-pituitary axis dysfunction (low GnRH):** Most commonly due to stress, weight loss, anorexia, or heavy exercise.
    - **Abnormal outflow tract:** Asherman's syndrome (endometrial adhesions) or cervical stenosis. Proceed to pelvic ultrasound to rule out an anatomic defect.
- To distinguish between hypoestrogenism and outflow obstruction, give combined estrogen/progesterone oral contraceptives for 1–2 cycles.
  - **If no bleeding occurs:** Outflow obstruction.
  - **If bleeding occurs:** Amenorrhea is due to hypothalamus-pituitary axis dysfunction or premature ovarian failure.

Treatment

Treat the underlying cause.

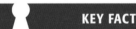

KEY FACT

A ⊕ progestin challenge test (the presence of a withdrawal bleed after progestin is given) suggests anovulation as a cause for amenorrhea. PCOS is the most common cause.

KEY FACT

Amenorrhea and high FSH in young women indicate premature ovarian failure and put women at risk for osteoporosis from estrogen deficiency. Consider starting hormone replacement.

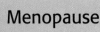

Menopause

One year of amenorrhea after the final menstrual period.

SYMPTOMS/EXAM

- Irregularity of cycle length may begin during the perimenopause state (lasts ~ 4 years).
- The most common complaints are vasomotor symptoms (hot flashes, night sweats, vaginal atrophy/dryness).

DIFFERENTIAL

If indicated by the history and exam, consider thyroid disease, prolactinoma, and chronic medical conditions that cause night sweats (eg, TB, lymphoma).

DIAGNOSIS

Clinical diagnosis is generally adequate. A high FSH level is diagnostic but usually unnecessary.

TREATMENT

- **Hormone replacement therapy (HRT):** The most effective treatment for vasomotor and urogenital symptoms, but associated with an ↑ risk of VTE, breast cancer, stroke, and CAD. Current recommendations for HRT use are as follows:
    - Use the lowest dose for the shortest duration needed to treat symptoms (attempt to taper or discontinue every six months).
    - Do not use HRT to prevent a chronic health condition.
    - A history of breast/endometrial cancer, CAD, or VTE are **absolute contraindications.**
    - Women with a uterus need to take **estrogen plus a progestin** to protect against endometrial cancer. Women who have undergone hysterectomy may take estrogen alone.
- **Non-HRT treatment** of menopausal symptoms includes the following:
    - **Vaginal symptoms:** Intravaginal estrogen (low dose), moisturizers, lubricants.
    - **Vasomotor instability:** Some evidence supports the efficacy of clonidine, venlafaxine and paroxetine, and gabapentin. Complementary/alternative medications such as black cohosh and soy are probably of no benefit.

KEY FACT

Estrogen works best for the symptoms of menopause, but the associated risks of ↑ breast cancer, CAD, and VTE must be weighed against its benefits. Consider short-term replacement only for refractory menopausal symptoms; do not use as first-line therapy.

KEY FACT

HRT has no role in the prevention of CAD.

Postmenopausal Bleeding

 A 70-year-old woman presents to your clinic with a six-month history of intermittent vaginal spotting. What is the most appropriate diagnostic test?
Endometrial biopsy to rule out endometrial cancer.

All women with postmenopausal bleeding should be evaluated for endometrial carcinoma. Other etiologies include endometrial atrophy (most common), exogenous hormones, nongynecologic sources, endometrial hyperplasia or polyps, and cervical cancer.

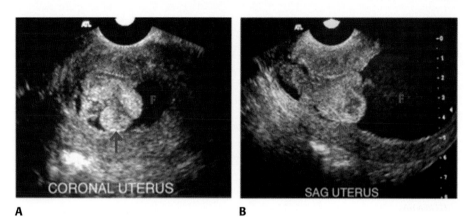

A   B

FIGURE 18.2. **Endometrial cancer.** Transvaginal coronal (**A**) and sagittal (**B**) ultrasound images of the uterus demonstrate a large echogenic mass in the uterine cavity (arrow) with adjacent fluid or blood (F). (Reproduced with permission from USMLERx.com).

SYMPTOMS

Patients may complain of "spotting" or of heavier, menses-like bleeding.

EXAM

- Pelvic exam reveals vaginal atrophy, vaginal lesions, cervical polyps, or uterine masses.
- Pap smear.

DIAGNOSIS

- Endometrial biopsy is the gold standard for diagnosis.
- Ultrasound is an alternative first test (see Figure 18.2); if the endometrial lining is < 5 mm thick, endometrial biopsy may be deferred unless unexplained bleeding continues.

TREATMENT

Bleeding is usually light and self-limited. Once malignancy has been ruled out, there is generally no need for treatment.

Osteoporosis

A 68-year-old woman with a history of tobacco use presents for a routine physical exam. Her medications include ASA and a combined calcium/vitamin D pill (500 mg/200 IU twice daily). As part of routine screening, she undergoes a DEXA scan (T-score = –2.0) and 25-OH vitamin D level (9 ng/mL; normal range > 30). What is the best treatment plan at this time?

This patient has osteopenia and vitamin D deficiency. Her vitamin D deficiency should be treated with 50,000 IU of ergocalciferol weekly for 6–8 weeks; her 25-OH vitamin D level should then be rechecked to ensure repletion before she is switched to vitamin D 800 IU daily for osteopenia. She should also take oral calcium supplementation at a dosage of 1500 mg daily, participate in weight-bearing exercises, and stop smoking.

Low bone mass and ↑ skeletal fragility leading to ↑ risk of fractures, particularly of the vertebrae, hip, and long bones (proximal femur and distal radius). Genetic and environmental risk factors include the following:

- Female sex, although men are also at risk (due to androgen deficiency).
- Advanced age.
- Caucasian or Asian ethnicity.
- Previous fracture.
- **Long-term glucocorticoid use** (prednisone ≥ 5 mg/day for at least three months).
- Low body weight.
- A family history of osteoporosis or hip fracture.
- **Tobacco or alcohol** use.

See the Endocrinology chapter for details on the 2° causes of osteoporosis.

SYMPTOMS/EXAM

- May be asymptomatic or present with back pain, loss of height, or nonspinal fractures.
- Exam may be normal. Patients may be thin and have a "dowager's hump" (kyphosis).

DIAGNOSIS

- Dual-energy x-ray absorptiometry (**DEXA**) **imaging** measures bone mineral density (BMD) at the spine and hip.
  - **Osteoporosis is diagnosed if the BMD T-score is ≥ 2.5 standard deviations below that of young, healthy women.**
  - Osteopenia is diagnosed if the T-score is between –1.0 and –2.5.
- Z-scores compare a patient's BMD with age- and gender-matched norms. A low Z-score (< –2) should raise suspicion for 2° causes of osteoporosis. Think **Z**-score for "**Z**ebra" (unusual causes of osteoporosis).
- Osteoporosis can be diagnosed clinically in the presence of vertebral or other fragility fractures—eg, hip fractures, compression fractures (see Figure 18.3), and Colles' fracture of the wrist.
- Details on the workup for 2° causes of osteoporosis can be found in the Endocrinology chapter.

KEY FACT

Caucasians and Asians are at higher risk for osteoporosis than African Americans.

KEY FACT

Screen for osteoporosis with DEXA in all women > 65 years of age and all men ≥ 70 years of age. Consider screening all postmenopausal women and men ≥ 50 years of age if risk factors are present.

KEY FACT

Osteopenia is defined as a T-score of –1.0 to –2.5. Osteoporosis is diagnosed when the T-score is < –2.5.

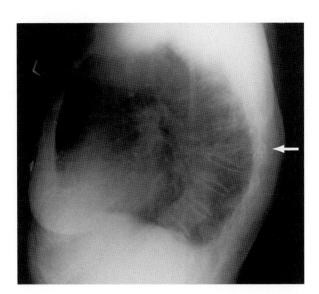

FIGURE 18.3. Osteoporotic compression fracture. Lateral chest radiograph shows a severe anterior wedge compression deformity of a midthoracic vertebral body (arrow). The bones are diffusely osteopenic. (Reproduced with permission from Fauci AS et al. *Harrison's Principles of Internal Medicine*, 17th ed. New York: McGraw-Hill, 2008, Fig. 348-2.)

TREATMENT

Treatment measures include the following (see also Table 18.6):

- Calcium 1500 mg QD; vitamin D 800 IU QD; weight-bearing exercises for all women unless contraindications exist. For severe vitamin D deficiency, replete with ergocalciferol 50,000 IU weekly × 6–8 weeks.
- Smoking cessation.
- Fall prevention measures for frail patients (handrails, assistive devices for ambulation, balance exercises).

TABLE 18.6. First- and Second-Line Therapy for Osteoporosis

TREATMENT	NOTES	TREATMENT CONSIDERATIONS
FIRST-LINE THERAPY		
Oral bisphosphonates		
Alendronate/ risedronate	Pill taken daily or, more commonly, given weekly at a higher dose. ↓ all types of fractures; improve BMD. Side effects include esophagitis.	Most patients should start with these oral bisphosphonates. Also first-line therapy to prevent and treat osteoporosis from glucocorticoids. Must be taken on an empty stomach to ↓ the risk of esophagitis.
Ibandronate	Pill taken monthly; ↓ vertebral fractures only.	Beware of osteonecrosis of the jaw, which is seen primarily in cancer patients treated with high-dose IV formulation.
IV bisphosphonates (zolendronate)	IV annually; ↓ all types of fractures.	See above. Give to patients who cannot tolerate oral bisphosphonates.
SECOND-LINE THERAPY		
Selective estrogen receptor modulators (SERMs) (raloxifene)	Improve BMD. ↓ the risk of vertebral fractures but not nonvertebral (eg, hip) fractures.	Hot flashes are common. ↑ the risk of VTE but ↓ that of breast cancer. Use in patients who are at high risk of breast cancer or are unable to tolerate a bisphosphonate.
Intranasal calcitonin	Not as effective as other medications for long-term therapy.	Use only for acute pain after a recent fracture.
Teriparatide (recombinant PTH) injections	↑ bone formation (all other drugs are antiresorptive). ↓ risk of fracture, but may ↑ the risk of stroke in older women.	Use in postmenopausal patients with severe osteoporosis who are at high risk for fracture, have failed other treatments, or have contraindications to other treatments.
Estrogen or HRT	↓ the risk of all fractures, but ↑ the risk of breast cancer, stroke, VTE, and CAD.	No longer widely used for osteoporosis.

Hirsutism

Symptoms

- ↑ hair growth in androgen-dependent areas such as the lip, chin, chest, abdomen, and back.
- May present with associated amenorrhea and signs of virilization (eg, deepening voice, male-pattern baldness, clitoromegaly, male body habitus).

Exam

- Note body habitus (obesity).
- Look for male-pattern hair growth and/or androgenic alopecia, acne, signs of Cushing's syndrome, and virilization.
- Conduct an abdominal and pelvic exam for mass lesions.

Differential

- Many cases are idiopathic or familial. **PCOS** is the most common medical condition associated with hirsutism (see below). Other etiologies include the following:
    - **Congenital adrenal hyperplasia** (late-onset 21-hydroxylase deficiency): Rare.
    - **Medications:** Androgenic progestins in OCPs, danazol, minoxidil, cyclosporine.
    - **Cushing's syndrome:** Excess cortisol production; characterized by rapid weight gain, fat pads ("buffalo hump," "moon facies"), hypertension, and hyperglycemia.
    - **Androgen-secreting ovarian tumors** (eg, Sertoli-Leydig tumor: very high testosterone but normal DHEAS).
    - **Androgen-secreting adrenal neoplasm** (50% are malignant): ↑↑ DHEAS.
- Features associated with neoplastic causes of hirsutism are as follows:
    - Abrupt onset, short duration (< 1 year), or sudden progressive worsening.
    - Onset in the third decade of life or later (not peripubertal).
    - Virilization (acne, deepened voice, male-pattern baldness, clitoral hypertrophy, rare menses).

Diagnosis

- No labs are indicated for patients with long-standing hirsutism who have regular menses and familial factors.
- Consider checking testosterone, androstenedione, and DHEAS (a precursor of adrenal androgens) to rule out ovarian or adrenal neoplasm.
- Image the adrenals (CT) and ovaries (ultrasound or MRI) if androgen levels are significantly ↑. Mild elevations of testosterone levels are common in PCOS.

Treatment

- Treat the underlying cause.
- **Nonpharmacologic treatment:** Shaving, depilatories, electrolysis, laser treatment, eflornithine hydrochloride cream.
- **Antiandrogen therapy:** Try OCPs and/or spironolactone first. Finasteride, which ↓ 5α-reductase and thus testosterone, is also an option.

KEY FACT

PCOS is the most common cause of hirsutism but is not associated with virilization. Virilization and/or abrupt onset of hirsutism in an older woman may point to an androgen-secreting cancer in the ovaries or adrenal glands; check testosterone and DHEAS.

Polycystic Ovarian Syndrome (PCOS)

A 26-year-old Caucasian woman with an ↑ HbA$_{1c}$ (7.3%) presents with six months of absent periods. Previously, she had had normal periods since menarche at age 14. On exam, her BP is found to be 150/76 mm Hg, and she is noted to have facial acne, hair in the chin area, and balding in a male pattern. Her BMI is 29. What is the most likely diagnosis, and what would you expect to find on labs and imaging?

PCOS. Expect an LH/FSH ratio of > 3 and mildly ↑ testosterone. Ultrasound may show large ovaries with cysts.

A syndrome characterized by menstrual irregularity (chronic anovulation) and hyperandrogenism (acne, hirsutism, balding). Diabetes and obesity are often present. Can present as 1° or 2° amenorrhea; onset is typically **peripubertal** and slowly progressive.

Symptoms/Exam

- Patients seek treatment for **hirsutism, acne, oligomenorrhea/amenorrhea, or infertility.**
- Obesity, acne, hypertension, and acanthosis nigricans may be present. Enlarged, cystic ovaries may be found on bimanual exam.

Differential

- **Irregular menses:** See the section on menstrual disorders.
- **Androgen excess:** Adrenal or ovarian tumor, congenital adrenal hyperplasia, Cushing's syndrome.

Diagnosis

- **Rotterdam criteria:** Requires two of the following: (1) anovulation or oligo-ovulation (leading to irregular menses); (2) hyperandrogenism by clinical or laboratory evidence; and (3) polycystic ovaries on ultrasound. Other characteristics may include infertility and insulin resistance.
- **Labs:** A serum LH-to-FSH ratio of > 3:1 is suggestive but not diagnostic of PCOS, and serum testosterone is **often mildly** ↑. Labs are most helpful for excluding other causes of amenorrhea or hirsutism (see the sections on those topics above).
- **Imaging:** Ultrasound may reveal enlarged ovaries with numerous large cysts. However, such polycystic ovaries are seen in up to 25% of normal women, so their presence is not specific for PCOS.
- Many patients with PCOS have insulin resistance and are **at risk for type 2 DM and metabolic syndrome.** Fasting lipids and glucose should be measured periodically.

Treatment

- Treatment depends on the target symptom, but **weight loss (in obese patients) and OCPs are best overall.** OCPs ↓ ovarian androgen secretion.

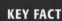

KEY FACT

The presence of polycystic ovaries is neither necessary nor sufficient to make the diagnosis of PCOS. The LH/FSH ratio is often > 3:1. Serum testosterone is only mildly ↑ in PCOS, whereas stromal ovarian cancers have very high testosterone.

- Symptom-specific treatment is as follows:
    - **Insulin resistance:** Weight reduction and metformin. It is unclear whether metformin improves ovulation, but it does improve insulin action.
    - **Infertility:** Clomiphene induces ovulation.
    - **Hirsutism, acne:** OCPs, spironolactone, other acne treatment, hair removal methods.
    - **Endometrial hyperplasia:** OCPs or intermittent progestin therapy.

Chronic Pelvic Pain

Pain below the umbilicus lasting at least six months and severe enough to cause functional disability or require treatment. Often multifactorial and challenging to diagnose and treat. The most common underlying conditions leading to a chronic pelvic pain syndrome are as follows:

- **Gynecologic:** Endometriosis, chronic PID, adenomyosis, uterine fibroids, pelvic adhesions.
- **GI/renal:** IBS, interstitial cystitis.
- **Musculoskeletal:** Fibromyalgia.
- **Other:** Depression, somatization, domestic violence, narcotic and other substance abuse.

DIAGNOSIS

- Conduct a careful history and physical exam focusing on features of the common etiologic conditions above.
- Evaluate psychosocial status, including mood and abuse history.
- **Labs:** CBC, vaginal cultures/STD testing, UA, pregnancy testing.
- **Imaging:** Pelvic ultrasound, laparoscopy.

TREATMENT

- Treat the underlying cause when one is apparent.
- Effective treatment of idiopathic chronic pelvic pain requires a multidisciplinary approach, including psychological counseling.

Domestic Violence

The leading cause of injury in women. Abuse may be physical, mental (including denial of financial or health care access), or sexual. Affects all socioeconomic groups; may also occur in same-sex relationships. Pregnancy may initiate or exacerbate abuse.

SYMPTOMS

- All patients should be screened. See the mnemonic **SAFE** for screening and follow-up questions.
- Patients may present with no symptoms or with a variety of clinical scenarios, including the following:
    - Multiple somatic complaints.
    - Chronic pain syndromes.
    - Depression.
    - Injuries unexplained by the history (especially multiple injuries in various stages of healing).
    - A possible delay in seeking care.

EXAM

Conduct a mental status exam, and look for signs of new, old, or chronic trauma. Ask the partner to leave the room so that the patient can be interviewed alone.

DIFFERENTIAL

Psychological illness, physical illness, somatization.

TREATMENT

- Conduct a risk assessment (frequency, weapons, substance abuse, threats of suicide, homicide).
- Determine if the patient has a safety plan.
- Refer to appropriate support services, and report the abuse to law enforcement. Accurate documentation of any injuries is important for potential future legal proceedings.

STD Screening

See the Ambulatory Medicine chapter for a detailed discussion of HSV, chancroid, and 1° syphilis. HIV and HBV are discussed in the Infectious Diseases chapter.

CHLAMYDIA SCREENING

- The most commonly diagnosed sexually transmitted bacterial infection in the United States. Can lead to PID, ectopic pregnancy, and infertility. Patients are frequently asymptomatic.
- Risk factors include age < 25, new or multiple sexual partners, inconsistent use of barrier methods, and a prior history of any STD.
- Annual screening is recommended for all sexually active women ≤ 25 years of age. Women > 25 years of age may be screened if STD risk factors are present.
- Tx: See below.

CERVICITIS

SYMPTOMS

Presents with vaginal discharge, dysuria, pelvic pain, or spotting. Chlamydia infection is frequently asymptomatic (see above).

EXAM/DIAGNOSIS

- Look for evidence of systemic illness.
    - **Gonorrhea and chlamydia:** A mucopurulent discharge and cervical friability are common. In the setting of cervical motion tenderness (a sign of coexisting PID), obtain cervical or vaginal specimens for gonorrhea and chlamydia culture or DNA amplification assays.
    - **HSV:** Consider HSV cultures in the presence of diffuse vesicular lesions or ulcerations.
    - ***Trichomonas vaginalis* infection:** Look for punctate hemorrhages ("strawberry cervix").

KEY FACT

All women ≤ 25 years of age should be screened for chlamydia. Asymptomatic chlamydia infection can lead to PID, ectopic pregnancy, and tubal infertility.

■ Most STDs are reportable to the local public health department.
■ Anyone who presents for testing should be offered the **HBV vaccine.**
■ Women with chlamydia should be rescreened at 3–4 months and no later than 12 months to check for reinfection.

TREATMENT

Treat cervicitis or urethritis as follows (the partner should also be treated):

■ **Gonorrhea:** Cefixime PO × 1 or ceftriaxone IM × 1; fluoroquinolones are no longer recommended owing to high resistance rates.
■ **Chlamydia:** Azithromycin 1 g PO × 1 or doxycycline × 7 days.

PELVIC INFLAMMATORY DISEASE (PID)

Infection of the upper genital tract in women. May be acute, subacute, or chronic. Risk factors include multiple sexual partners, unprotected intercourse, young age at first intercourse, mucopurulent cervicitis, IUD use, and prior PID.

SYMPTOMS/EXAM

■ Presents with lower abdominal pain, possibly accompanied by fever, nausea, and vomiting. May occur after recent menses, and may present with abnormal uterine bleeding or discharge.
■ Pelvic exam reveals cervical motion tenderness, discharge, and adnexal tenderness.

DIFFERENTIAL

Ectopic pregnancy, endometriosis, ovarian tumors or cysts, adnexal torsion, UTI/pyelonephritis, appendicitis, diverticulitis, IBD.

DIAGNOSIS

Diagnostic criteria are as follows:

■ **Minimal criteria:** Lower abdominal or pelvic pain plus cervical motion or adnexal tenderness on exam.
■ **Helpful for establishing the diagnosis:**
  ■ Fever > 38.3°C (100.9° F).
  ■ A mucopurulent cervical or vaginal discharge.
  ■ ↑ ESR or CRP.
  ■ Numerous WBCs on saline wet mount microscopy.
■ ⊕ gonococcal/*Chlamydia trachomatis* (GC/CT) cultures or inflammation/abscess seen on imaging or in the OR can confirm the diagnosis if a patient has pelvic pain but does not meet the other criteria.

TREATMENT

■ Treat for gonorrhea, chlamydia, and anaerobes.
■ **Outpatient regimens:** Cefoxitin IM plus probenecid PO or ceftriaxone IM × 1 plus doxycycline × 14 days. May also give metronidazole × 14 days in addition to either regimen.
■ **Inpatient regimens (indications for hospitalization below):**
  ■ Cefoxitin IV; cefotetan IV plus doxycycline.
  ■ Clindamycin IV plus gentamicin.
  ■ Once patients improve, continue PO regimens for 14 days.

KEY FACT

When treating gonorrhea, also treat for chlamydia, as coinfection frequently exists and diagnostic tests may be ⊖. Partners should also be treated.

MNEMONIC

Complications of PID—

I FACE PID

Infertility
Fitz-Hugh–Curtis syndrome (perihepatitis or inflammation of the liver capsule and adjacent peritoneal surfaces)
Abscess
Chronic pelvic pain
Ectopic pregnancy
Peritonitis
Intestinal obstruction
Disseminates (sepsis, endocarditis, arthritis, meningitis)

- Indications for hospitalization include the following:
  - Severe symptoms such as a high fever, nausea, vomiting, severe abdominal pain, and a high WBC count.
  - Pelvic abscess or peritonitis.
  - Noncompliance or inability to tolerate PO medications.
  - Pregnancy.
  - Lack of response to oral therapy.
  - Possible need for percutaneous abscess drainage or surgical intervention.

Urinary Tract Infection (UTI)

Infection of the bladder and/or kidneys. May be complicated or uncomplicated.

- **Uncomplicated:** UTI in a premenopausal, healthy, nonpregnant woman. Species most commonly involved are *E coli* and *Staphylococcus saprophyticus.* Less common are *Proteus mirabilis, Klebsiella* spp., *Enterococcus,* and *Chlamydia.*
- **Complicated:** UTI in anyone else (male, elderly, hospital acquired, pregnant, indwelling catheter, recent catheterization, anatomic abnormalities, neurogenic bladder, obstruction, recent antibiotics, symptoms of > 1 week at presentation, fever, immunosuppression, diabetes, recurrent UTI, history of resistant UTI).

SYMPTOMS

- Presents with dysuria, frequency, and urgency.
- Gross hematuria, fever, flank pain, and suprapubic pain are also common.

EXAM

- Fever, abdominal exam, flank tenderness.
- Conduct a pelvic exam if gynecologic etiologies are suspected.

DIFFERENTIAL

STDs (gonorrheal or chlamydial urethritis, HSV, trichomoniasis); infectious, atrophic, or irritant vaginitis; interstitial cystitis (recurrent UTI-like symptoms without objective evidence of infection).

DIAGNOSIS

- Order a UA and urine culture if complicated infection or pyelonephritis is suspected.
- Consider urine testing for gonorrhea and chlamydia if urethritis is suspected.

TREATMENT

- **Uncomplicated infections:** Give a **three-day** course of an oral fluoroquinolone or a **seven-day course of nitrofurantoin.** A three-day course of TMP-SMX can be used in areas with low resistance to this antibiotic.
- **Complicated infections:** Give a 7- to 14-day course of a typically used fluoroquinolone.
- **Recurrent UTIs:** Self-treatment is appropriate in women who can recognize recurrent symptoms; consider antibiotic prophylaxis after sexual intercourse.

Vaginitis

A change in normal vaginal flora that leads to bacterial overgrowth. Can be due to medications, illness, or frequent intercourse.

SYMPTOMS

- May present with normal discharge (fishy odor; thin, grayish-white discharge) and with symptoms such as itching, burning, soreness, dysuria, and dyspareunia.
- Most women are asymptomatic.

EXAM

Conduct a pelvic exam and note:

- Vulvar edema/erythema.
- **Discharge:** Quantity, color, adherence, odor.
- **Cervicitis:** Friability, purulent discharge, **"strawberry cervix"** (petechiae in trichomonal infection).

DIFFERENTIAL

UTI, normal (physiologic) discharge, noninfectious/irritants (spermicide, douching), atrophy.

DIAGNOSIS

- Wet mount (pH and microscopy in saline and KOH) (see Table 18.7 and Figure 18.4).
- Consider UA and/or STD testing.

TREATMENT

Treat the underlying cause:

- **Bacterial vaginosis:** Metronidazole (500 mg PO BID × 7 days or 2 g × 1, or topical × 5 days) or clindamycin (PO or topical × 7 days). May resolve spontaneously; recurrence is common.
- **Candidiasis:** Fluconazole 150 mg PO × 1 or various topical azoles (several are available OTC).
- **Trichomoniasis:** Oral metronidazole at the same doses as for bacterial vaginosis.

TABLE 18.7.   Wet Mount Criteria in Diagnosing Vaginitis

DIAGNOSIS	DISCHARGE	CELLS	pH	"WHIFF TEST"
Bacterial vaginosis	Grayish-white, thin, fishy odor.	Clue cells.	> 4.5	⊕ with KOH
Yeast	Thick, white, clumpy, adherent ("cottage cheese").	Pseudohyphae with KOH.	3.5–4.5	⊖
Trichomoniasis	Profuse, yellow-green, frothy, malodorous.	Motile trichomonads.	> 4.5	⊕

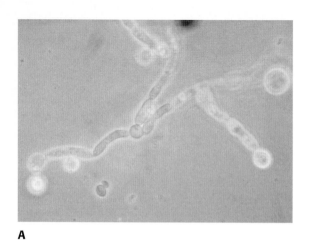

A

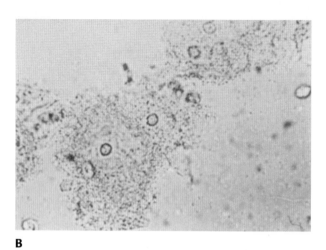

B

FIGURE 18.4. **Causes of vaginitis.** (A) Candidal vaginitis. *Candida albicans* organisms are evident on KOH wet mount. (B) *Gardnerella vaginalis.* Note the granular epithelial cells ("clue cells") and indistinct cell margins. (Image A reproduced with permission from Wolff K et al. *Fitzpatrick's Color Atlas & Synopsis of Clinical Dermatology,* 5th ed. New York: McGraw-Hill, 2005: 717. Image B reproduced with permission from Kasper DL et al. *Harrison's Principles of Internal Medicine,* 16th ed. New York: McGraw-Hill, 2005: 767.)

Abbreviations and Symbols

Abbreviation	Meaning
AA	Alcoholics Anonymous
A-a	alveolar-arterial (oxygen gradient)
AAA	abdominal aortic aneurysm
ABG	arterial blood gas
ABI	ankle-brachial index
ABPA	allergic bronchopulmonary aspergillosis
ABPA-CB	allergic bronchopulmonary aspergillosis with central bronchiectasis
ABPA-S	allergic bronchopulmonary aspergillosis—seropositive
ACA	anterior cerebral artery
ACC	American College of Cardiology
ACD	anemia of chronic disease
ACEI	angiotensin-converting enzyme inhibitor
ACh	acetylcholine
AChE	acetylcholinesterase
ACL	anterior cruciate ligament
ACLS	advanced cardiac life support (protocol)
ACTH	adrenocorticotropic hormone
AD	autosomal dominant
ADA	American Diabetes Association
ADH	antidiuretic hormone
ADHD	attention-deficit hyperactivity disorder
ADL	activities of daily living
ADPKD	autosomal dominant polycystic kidney disease
AED	automated external defibrillator
AF	atrial fibrillation
AFB	acid-fast bacillus
AFP	α-fetoprotein
AGMA	anion-gap metabolic acidosis
AHA	American Heart Association
AI	adrenal insufficiency
AIDS	acquired immunodeficiency syndrome
AIN	acute interstitial nephritis
ALI	acute lung injury
ALL	acute lymphoblastic leukemia
ALS	amyotrophic lateral sclerosis
ALT	alanine aminotransferase
AMA	antimitochondrial antibody
AMD	age-related macular degeneration
AML	acute myeloid leukemia
ANA	antineutrophil antibody
ANC	absolute neutrophil count

Abbreviation	Meaning
ANCA	antineutrophil cytoplasmic antibody
AP	anteroposterior
APL	acute promyelocytic leukemia
APLA	antiphospholipid antibody (syndrome)
APO	apolipoprotein
AR	autosomal recessive
ARB	angiotensin receptor blocker
ARDS	acute respiratory distress syndrome
ARF	acute renal failure
5-ASA	5-aminosalicylic acid
ASA	acetylsalicylic acid
ASCA	anti–*Saccharomyces cerevisiae* antibody
ASD	atrial septal defect
ASMA	anti–smooth muscle antibody
ASO	antistreptolysin O
AST	aspartate aminotransferase
AT	angiotensin, atrial tachycardia
ATN	acute tubular necrosis
ATP	adenosine triphosphate
ATP III	National Cholesterol Education Program Adult Treatment Panel III
ATRA	*all*-trans retinoic acid
AV	arteriovenous, atrioventricular
AVF	arteriovenous fistula
AVM	arteriovenous malformation
AVN	avascular necrosis
AVNRT	atrioventricular nodal reentrant tachycardia
AVP	arginine vasopressor
AVRT	atrioventricular reentrant tachycardia
AXR	abdominal x-ray
AZT	azidothymidine (zidovudine)
BAL	bronchoalveolar lavage
BCC	basal cell carcinoma
BCG	bacille Calmette-Guérin
BG	blood glucose
BID	twice daily
BiPAP	bilevel positive airway pressure
BIW	biweekly
BMD	bone mineral density
BMI	body mass index
BP	blood pressure
BPH	benign prostatic hyperplasia
BPPV	benign paroxysmal positional vertigo
BRAT	bran, rice, applesauce, toast (diet)

Abbreviation	Meaning
BSE	breast self-examination
BUN	blood urea nitrogen
BV	bleomycin and vincristine
CABG	coronary artery bypass graft
CaCO$_3$	calcium carbonate
CAD	coronary artery disease
c-ANCA	cytoplasmic antineutrophil cytoplasmic antibody
CAP	community-acquired pneumonia
CBC	complete blood count
CBE	clinical breast examination
CCB	calcium channel blocker
CCK	cholecystokinin
CCP	cyclic citrullinated peptide
CD	cluster of differentiation
CDC	Centers for Disease Control and Prevention
CEA	carcinoembryonic antigen
CF	cystic fibrosis
CFS	chronic fatigue syndrome
CFTR	cystic fibrosis transmembrane regulator
CHF	congestive heart failure
CI	confidence interval
CIDP	chronic inflammatory demyelinating polyneuropathy
CIWA	Clinical Institute Withdrawal Assessment
CK	creatine kinase
CKD	chronic kidney disease
CK-MB	creatine kinase, MB fraction
CLL	chronic lymphocytic leukemia
CML	chronic myelogenous leukemia
CMML	chronic myelomonocytic leukemia
CMV	cytomegalovirus
CN	cranial nerve
CNS	central nervous system
COMT	catechol-O-methyltransferase
COPD	chronic obstructive pulmonary disease
COX	cyclooxygenase
CP	ceruloplasmin
CPAP	continuous positive airway pressure
CPPD	calcium pyrophosphate dihydrate deposition
CPR	cardiopulmonary resuscitation
Cr	creatinine
CrAg	cryptococcal antigen
CRBSI	catheter-related bloodstream infection
CrCl	creatinine clearance
CREST	calcinosis, Raynaud's phenomenon, esophageal involvement, sclerodactyly, telangiectasia (syndrome)
CRF	corticotropin-releasing factor
CRP	C-reactive protein
CRPS	complex regional pain syndrome
CSA	central sleep apnea

Abbreviation	Meaning
CSF	cerebrospinal fluid
CT	computed tomography
CTCL	cutaneous T-cell lymphoma
CTP	Child-Turcotte-Pugh (scoring)
CT-PA	CT pulmonary angiography
CVA	cerebrovascular accident, costovertebral angle
CVID	common variable immunodeficiency
CXR	chest x-ray
D$_2$	ergocalciferol
D$_3$	cholecalciferol
d4T	didehydrodeoxythymidine (stavudine)
DASH	Dietary Approaches to Stop Hypertension
DBP	diastolic blood pressure
DCIS	ductal carcinoma in situ
DDAVP	1-deamino (8-D-arginine) vasopressin
ddI	dideoxyinosine
DEET	N,N-diethyl-meta-toluamide
DES	diethylstilbestrol
DEXA	dual-energy x-ray absorptiometry
DF	discriminant function
DFA	direct fluorescent antibody
1,25-DHD	1,25-dihydroxyvitamin D
DHEAS	dehydroepiandrosterone sulfate
DI	diabetes insipidus
DIC	disseminated intravascular coagulation
DIP	distal interphalangeal (joint)
DKA	diabetic ketoacidosis
DL$_{CO}$	diffusing capacity for carbon monoxide
DM	diabetes mellitus
DMARD	disease-modifying antirheumatic drug
DNA	deoxyribonucleic acid
DNase	deoxyribonuclease
DNR	do not resuscitate
2,3-DPG	2,3-diphosphoglycerate
DPOA-HC	durable power of attorney for health care
DRE	digital rectal examination
dsDNA	double-stranded DNA
DTRs	deep tendon reflexes
DTs	delirium tremens
DVT	deep venous thrombosis
DWI	diffusion-weighted imaging
EBNA	Epstein-Barr nuclear antigen
EBV	Epstein-Barr virus
ECG	electrocardiography
ECT	electroconvulsive therapy
ED	erectile dysfunction
EEG	electroencephalography
EF	ejection fraction
EGD	esophagogastroduodenoscopy
EGFR	epidermal growth factor receptor
EHEC	enterohemorrhagic *E coli*
EIA	enzyme immunoassay
EIEC	enteroinvasive *E coli*
ELISA	enzyme-linked immunosorbent assay

Abbreviation	Meaning
EM	electron microscopy, erythema multiforme
EMG	electromyography
ENT	ears, nose, and throat
EP	evoked potential
ER	emergency room, estrogen receptor
ERCP	endoscopic retrograde cholangiopancreatography
ERV	expiratory reserve volume
ES	elastic stockings
ESR	erythrocyte sedimentation rate
ESRD	end-stage renal disease
ETEC	enterotoxigenic *E coli*
EtOH	ethanol
EUS	endoscopic ultrasound
EVH	esophageal variceal hemorrhage
FAP	familial adenomatous polyposis
FCH	familial combined hyperlipidemia
FDA	Food and Drug Administration
F-dUMP	5-fluorodeoxyuridine monophosphate
Fe_{Na}	fractional excretion of sodium
FEV_1	forced expiratory volume in one second
FFP	fresh frozen plasma
FH	familial hypercholesterolemia
Fio_2	fraction of inspired oxygen
FLAIR	fluid-attenuated inversion recovery (imaging)
FNA	fine-needle aspiration
FOBT	fecal occult blood test
FRC	functional reserve capacity
FSBG	fingerstick blood glucose
FSH	follicle-stimulating hormone
FT_3	free triiodothyronine
FT_4	free thyroxine
5-FU	5-fluorouracil
FUO	fever of unknown origin
FVC	forced vital capacity
G6PD	glucose-6-phosphate dehydrogenase
GABA	gamma-aminobutyric acid
GABHS	group A β-hemolytic streptococcus
GAD	glutamic acid decarboxylase
GBM	glomerular basement membrane
GBS	Guillain-Barré syndrome
GCA	giant cell arteritis
G-CSF	granulocyte colony-stimulating factor
GDM	gestational diabetes mellitus
GERD	gastroesophageal reflux disease
GFR	glomerular filtration rate
GGT	γ-glutamyltransferase
GH	growth hormone
GHRH	growth hormone–releasing hormone
GI	gastrointestinal
GIST	gastrointestinal stromal tumor
GLP	glucagon-like peptide
GM-CSF	granulocyte-macrophage colony-stimulating factor

Abbreviation	Meaning
GnRH	gonadotropin-releasing hormone
GOLD	Global Initiative for [Chronic Obstructive] Lung Disease
GU	genitourinary
HAART	highly active antiretroviral therapy
HACEK	*Haemophilus, Actinobacillus, Cardiobacterium, Eikenella, Kingella*
HAEM	herpes simplex–associated erythema multiforme
HAV	hepatitis A virus
Hb	hemoglobin
HbA_{1c}	hemoglobin A_{1c}
HBeAg	hepatitis B early antigen
HBIG	hepatitis B immune globulin
HBsAg	hepatitis B surface antigen
HBV	hepatitis B virus
HCAP	health care–associated pneumonia
HCC	hepatocellular carcinoma
hCG	human chorionic gonadotropin
HCM	hypertrophic cardiomyopathy
HCO_3	bicarbonate
HCTZ	hydrochlorothiazide
HCV	hepatitis C virus
25-HD	25-hydroxyvitamin D
HDL	high-density lipoprotein
HDV	hepatitis D virus
HELLP	hemolysis, elevated LFTs, low platelets (syndrome)
HEV	hepatitis E virus
HGA	human granulocytic anaplasmosis
HHV	human herpesvirus
5-HIAA	5-hydroxyindole acetic acid
HIDA	hepato-iminodiacetic acid (scan)
HIPAA	Health Insurance Portability and Accountability Act
HIT	heparin-induced thrombocytopenia
HIV	human immunodeficiency virus
HL	hearing loss
HLA	human leukocyte antigen
HME	human monocytic ehrlichiosis
HNPCC	hereditary nonpolyposis colorectal cancer
HOCM	hypertrophic obstructive cardiomyopathy
HPV	human papillomavirus
HR	heart rate
HRCT	high-resolution computed tomography
HRS	hepatorenal syndrome
HRT	hormone replacement therapy
HSV	herpes simplex virus
5-HT	5-hydroxytryptamine
HTLV	human T-cell leukemia virus
HUS	hemolytic-uremic syndrome
IABP	intraaortic balloon pump
IAHG	International Autoimmune Hepatitis Group

Abbreviation	Meaning
IBD	inflammatory bowel disease
IBS	irritable bowel syndrome
ICA	internal carotid artery
ICD	implantable cardioverter-defibrillator
ICH	intracranial hemorrhage
ICP	intracranial pressure
ICS	inhaled corticosteroid
ICU	intensive care unit
IF	intrinsic factor
IFE	immunofixation electrophoresis
Ig	immunoglobulin
IGF	insulin-like growth factor
IL	interleukin
ILD	interstitial lung disease
IM	intramuscular
INH	isoniazid
INR	International Normalized Ratio
IPC	intermittent pneumatic compression
IPF	idiopathic pulmonary fibrosis
IPSS	inferior petrosal sinus sampling
IRIS	immune reconstitution inflammatory syndrome
ITP	idiopathic thrombocytopenic purpura
IUD	intrauterine device
IUGR	intrauterine growth retardation
IV	intravenous
IVC	inferior vena cava
IVF	in vitro fertilization
IVIG	intravenous immunoglobulin
IVP	intravenous pyelography
JNC 7	Joint National Committee on Prevention, Detection, Evaluation, and Treatment of High Blood Pressure
JVD	jugular venous distention
JVP	jugular venous pressure
KOH	potassium hydroxide
KS	Kaposi's sarcoma
LAD	left anterior descending (artery)
LAM	lymphangioleiomyomatosis
LBBB	left bundle branch block
LBP	lower back pain
LCIS	lobular carcinoma in situ
LDH	lactate dehydrogenase
LDL	low-density lipoprotein
LDUH	low-dose unfractionated heparin
LES	lower esophageal sphincter
LFT	liver function test
LGIB	lower GI bleeding
LH	luteinizing hormone
LKM	liver/kidney microsomal (antibody)
LLQ	left lower quadrant
LMN	lower motor neuron
LMWH	low-molecular-weight heparin
LP	lumbar puncture
LR	likelihood ratio

Abbreviation	Meaning
LT_4	levothyroxine
LTBI	latent tuberculosis infection
LTOT	long-term oxygen therapy
LUQ	left upper quadrant
LVH	left ventricular hypertrophy
MAC	*Mycobacterium avium* complex
MAHA	microangiopathic hemolytic anemia
MALT	mucosa-associated lymphoid tissue
MAOI	monoamine oxidase inhibitor
MCA	middle cerebral artery
MCL	midclavicular line
MCP	metacarpophalangeal (joint)
MCTD	mixed connective tissue disease
MCV	mean corpuscular volume
MDI	metered-dose inhaler
MDMA	3,4-methylene-dioxymethamphetamine ("Ecstasy")
MDR	multidrug-resistant
MDS	myelodysplastic syndrome
MELD	Model for End-stage Liver Disease
MEN	multiple endocrine neoplasia
MG	myasthenia gravis
MGUS	monoclonal gammopathy of undetermined significance
MI	myocardial infarction
MIBG	metaiodobenzylguanidine (scan)
MMA	methylmalonic acid
MMI	methimazole
MMR	measles, mumps, rubella (vaccine)
MMSE	mini-mental status exam
6-MP	6-mercaptopurine
MPA	microscopic polyangiitis
MPGN	membranoproliferative glomerulonephritis
MPO	myeloperoxidase
MR	magnetic resonance
MRA	magnetic resonance angiography
MRCP	magnetic resonance cholangiopancreatography
MRI	magnetic resonance imaging
MRSA	methicillin-resistant *S aureus*
MS	multiple sclerosis
MSM	men who have sex with men
mTOR	mammalian target of rapamycin
MTP	metatarsophalangeal (joint)
MUGA	multigated acquisition (scan)
MV	minute ventilation
MVP	mitral valve prolapse
NA	Narcotics Anonymous
NAAT	nucleic acid amplification test
nAChR	nicotinic acetylcholine receptor
NAEPP	National Asthma Education and Prevention Program
NAGMA	non-anion-gap metabolic acidosis
$NaHCO_3$	sodium bicarbonate

Abbreviation	Meaning
NCS	nerve conduction study
NF	neurofibromatosis
NG	nasogastric
NHL	non-Hodgkin's lymphoma
NNT	number needed to treat
NPO	nil per os (nothing by mouth)
NPPV	noninvasive positive pressure ventilation
NPV	negative predictive value
NREM	non–rapid eye movement
NS	normal saline
NSAID	nonsteroidal anti-inflammatory drug
NSCLC	non–small cell lung cancer
NSIP	nonspecific interstitial pneumonia
NSTEMI	non-ST-elevation myocardial infarction
NVE	native valve endocarditis
NYHA	New York Heart Association
O&P	ova and parasites
OA	osteoarthritis
OCD	obsessive-compulsive disorder
OCP	oral contraceptive pill
OGTT	oral glucose tolerance test
OSA	obstructive sleep apnea
OTC	over the counter
PA	pernicious anemia, posteroanterior
PAC	plasma aldosterone concentration
Pa_{CO_2}	partial pressure of carbon dioxide in arterial blood
PAN	polyarteritis nodosa
p-ANCA	perinuclear antineutrophil cytoplasmic antibody
Pa_{O_2}	partial pressure of oxygen in arterial blood
PCI	percutaneous coronary intervention
P_{CO_2}	partial pressure of carbon dioxide
PCOP	pulmonary capillary occlusion pressure
PCOS	polycystic ovarian syndrome
PCP	phencyclidine, *Pneumocystis carinii* (now *jiroveci*) pneumonia
P_{Cr}	plasma creatinine
PCR	polymerase chain reaction
PCT	porphyria cutanea tarda
PCWP	pulmonary capillary wedge pressure
PDA	patent ductus arteriosus
PDE	phosphodiesterase
PE	pulmonary embolism
PEEP	positive end-expiratory pressure
PEF	peak expiratory flow
PEG	polyethylene glycol
PET	positron emission tomography
PFO	patent foramen ovale
PFT	pulmonary function test
PHN	postherpetic neuralgia
PICA	posterior inferior cerebellar artery
PID	pelvic inflammatory disease
PIP	posterior interphalangeal (joint)
P_{K+}	plasma potassium

Abbreviation	Meaning
PLED	periodic lateralizing epileptiform discharge
PLMD	period limb-movement disorder
PLMS	periodic limb movements of sleep
PMI	point of maximal insertion
PMN	polymorphonuclear (leukocyte)
PMR	polymyalgia rheumatica
P_{Na}	plasma sodium
PNH	paroxysmal nocturnal hemoglobinuria
PO	per os (by mouth)
P_{O_2}	partial pressure of oxygen
P_{osm}	plasma osmolality
PPD	purified protein derivative (of tuberculin)
PPI	proton pump inhibitor
PPN	peripheral parenteral nutrition
PPV	positive predictive value
PR	progesterone receptor
PRA	plasma renin activity
PRCA	pure red cell aplasia
PRN	pro re nata (as needed)
PSA	prostate-specific antigen
PSVT	paroxysmal supraventricular tachycardia
PT	prothrombin time
PTA	percutaneous transluminal angioplasty
PTH	parathyroid hormone
PTHC	percutaneous transhepatic cholangiography
PTHrP	parathyroid hormone–related protein
PTSD	posttraumatic stress disorder
PTT	partial thromboplastin time
PTU	propylthiouracil
PUD	peptic ulcer disease
PUVA	psoralen and ultraviolet A
PVC	premature ventricular contraction
PVD	peripheral vascular disease
PVE	prosthetic valve endocarditis
PVT	portal vein thrombosis
QD	once daily
QHS	at bedtime
QID	four times daily
QOD	every other day
RA	refractory anemia, rheumatoid arthritis
RADS	reactive airway dysfunction syndrome
RAEB	refractory anemia with excess blasts
RAI	radioactive iodine
RAIU	radioactive iodine uptake
RARS	refractory anemia with ringed sideroblasts
RAST	radioallergosorbent test
RBBB	right bundle branch block
RBC	red blood cell
RCT	randomized clinical trial
RDW	red cell distribution width
REM	rapid eye movement
RF	rheumatoid factor

Abbreviation	Meaning
RIBA	recombinant immunoblot assay
RICE	rest, ice, compression, and elevation
RLQ	right lower quadrant
RLS	restless leg syndrome
RNA	ribonucleic acid
RNV	radionuclide ventriculogram
ROM	range of motion
RPGN	rapidly progressive glomerulonephritis
RPR	rapid plasma reagin
RR	respiratory rate
RSV	respiratory syncytial virus
RTA	renal tubular acidosis
RUQ	right upper quadrant
RV	residual volume
RVH	right ventricular hypertrophy
SAAG	serum-ascites albumin gradient
SADNI	selective antibody deficiency with normal immunoglobulins
SAH	subarachnoid hemorrhage
SAMe	S-adenosyl-methionine
SARS	severe acute respiratory syndrome
SBP	spontaneous bacterial peritonitis, systolic blood pressure
SCA	superior cerebellar artery
SCC	squamous cell carcinoma
SCD	sequential compression device
SCLC	small cell lung cancer
SERM	selective estrogen receptor modulator
SIADH	syndrome of inappropriate secretion of antidiuretic hormone
SIRS	systemic inflammatory response syndrome
SJS	Stevens-Johnson syndrome
SLE	systemic lupus erythematosus
SMA	smooth muscle antibody
SNRI	serotonin-norepinephrine reuptake inhibitor
SOD	superoxide dismutase
SPEP	serum protein electrophoresis
SQ	subcutaneous
SSPE	subacute sclerosing panencephalitis
SSRI	selective serotonin reuptake inhibitor
STARI	southern tick–associated rash illness
STD	sexually transmitted disease
STEMI	ST-elevation myocardial infarction
SVC	superior vena cava
SVR	systemic vascular resistance
SVT	supraventricular tachycardia
T_3	triiodothyronine
T_4	thyroxine
TB	tuberculosis
TBG	thyroid-binding globulin
3TC	dideoxycytidine (lamivudine)
TC	total cholesterol
TCA	tricyclic antidepressant

Abbreviation	Meaning
Td	tetanus and diphtheria (vaccine)
Tdap	tetanus, diphtheria, acellular pertussis (vaccine)
TEDS	thromboembolic disease stockings
TEE	transesophageal echocardiography
TEN	toxic epidermal necrolysis
TFT	thyroid function test
TG	triglyceride
TIA	transient ischemic attack
TIBC	total iron-binding capacity
TID	three times daily
TIPS	transjugular intrahepatic portosystemic shunt
TLC	therapeutic lifestyle changes, total lung capacity
TMP-SMX	trimethoprim-sulfamethoxazole
TNF	tumor necrosis factor
tPA	tissue plasminogen activator
TPN	total parenteral nutrition
TPO	thyroperoxidase
TRALI	transfusion-related acute lung injury
TRH	thyrotropin-releasing hormone
T_{sat}	transferrin saturation
TSH	thyroid-stimulating hormone
TSI	thyroid-stimulating immunoglobulin
TSS	toxic shock syndrome
TSST	toxic shock syndrome toxin
TTE	transthoracic echocardiography
TTG	tissue transglutaminase
TTKG	transtubular K^+ gradient
TTP	thrombotic thrombocytopenic purpura
TURP	transurethral resection of the prostate
TV	tidal volume
TZD	thiazolidinedione
UA	urinalysis
UAG	urine anion gap
U_{Cr}	urine creatinine
UFH	unfractionated heparin
UGIB	upper GI bleeding
U_{K+}	urine potassium
UKPDS	United Kingdom Prospective Diabetes Study
ULN	upper limit of normal
UMN	upper motor neuron
U_{Na}	urine sodium
U_{osm}	urine osmolality
UPEP	urinary protein electrophoresis
URI	upper respiratory infection
USPSTF	United States Preventive Services Task Force
UTI	urinary tract infection
UV	ultraviolet
VAP	ventilator-associated pneumonia
VATS	video-assisted thoracoscopy
VBI	vertebrobasilar insufficiency

Abbreviation	Meaning
VC	vital capacity
VDRL	Venereal Disease Research Laboratory
VEGF	vascular endothelial growth factor
VF	ventricular fibrillation
VIP	vasoactive intestinal peptide
VMA	vanillylmandelic acid
V/Q	ventilation-perfusion (ratio)
VSD	ventricular septal defect

Abbreviation	Meaning
VT	ventricular tachycardia
VTE	venous thromboembolism
vWD	von Willebrand disease
vWF	von Willebrand factor
VZV	varicella-zoster virus
WBC	white blood cell
WHO	World Health Organization
WPW	Wolff-Parkinson-White (syndrome)

NOTES

Index

About the Authors

Tao Le, MD, MHS

Tao is a well-recognized figure in medical education. As senior editor, he has led the expansion of *First Aid* into a global educational series. In addition, he is the founder of the *USMLERx* online test bank series as well as a cofounder of the *Underground Clinical Vignettes* series. As a medical student, he was editor-in-chief of the University of California, San Francisco (UCSF) *Synapse*, a university newspaper with a weekly circulation of 9000. Tao earned his medical degree from UCSF in 1996 and completed his residency training in internal medicine at Yale University and fellowship training at Johns Hopkins University. At Yale, he was a regular guest lecturer on the USMLE review courses and an adviser to the Yale University School of Medicine curriculum committee. Dr. Le subsequently went on to cofound Medsn and served as its chief medical officer. He is currently conducting research in asthma education at the University of Louisville.

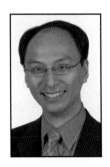

Peter Chin-Hong, MD, MAS

Peter is Associate Professor of Medicine in the Division of Infectious Diseases at UCSF; is Director of the Transplant Infectious Diseases program; and is co-leader of the clinical and translational research programs for predoctoral students. He is course director of the second-year microbiology block for medical students and is a member of the Academy of Medical Educators at UCSF. He was born and raised in Trinidad, West Indies, and received his undergraduate and medical degrees at Brown University in Providence, Rhode Island. Seeking a balmier clime, he completed internal medicine residency training and a fellowship in infectious diseases at UCSF. He is board certified in internal medicine and infectious diseases. He is a frequent speaker for UCSF continuing medical education courses, including the annual Internal Medicine Board Certification and Recertification Review. He has authored chapters in various medical texts (including *Current Medical Diagnosis & Treatment*) and actively publishes in scientific journals based on an active research program in infectious diseases of immunocompromised hosts.

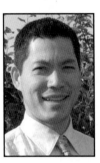

Tom Baudendistel, MD, FACP

Tom is the Internal Medicine Residency Program Director at Kaiser Permanente in Oakland, California. He is the Deputy Editor and CME Editor of the *Journal of Hospital Medicine* and is past Chair of the Society of Hospital Medicine's national ethics committee. Prior to joining Kaiser Oakland, he was the Dean's Award recipient at the University of Missouri–Columbia School of Medicine, where he received his MD in 1995. He completed his internal medicine residency and chief residency at UCSF and was a member of UCSF's Hospitalist faculty. He is board certified in internal medicine and has lectured nationally on numerous clinical and bioethical topics. He has been a contributor on *Current Consult Medicine*, *The Patient History: Evidence-Based Approach*, *Hospital Medicine for the PDA*, *The Saint-Frances Guide to Inpatient Medicine*, and the *UCSF Housestaff Handbook*, and edited the companion Web page for *Current Medical Diagnosis & Treatment*.

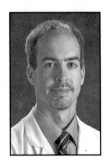

Cindy Lai, MD

Cindy is Associate Professor of Medicine at UCSF, where she serves as the Site Director for the Internal Medicine Clerkships. Cindy completed medical school at the University of Southern California; a primary care internal medicine residency at Massachusetts General Hospital; and a clinician-educator fellowship at UCSF. Board certified in internal medicine, she attends on the medicine wards and has a primary care practice. In addition to teaching and advising students and residents, Cindy directs Intersessions, an interdisciplinary course where third-year medical students learn about clinical decision making, health policy, advances in medical sciences, medical ethics, and professional development. Cindy is a member of UCSF's Academy of Medical Educators and has authored chapters in medical education texts and journals. She currently serves as a deputy editor for the *Journal of General Internal Medicine*.

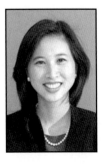